Evidence-based Hematology

Evidence-based Hematology

EDITED BY

MARK A. CROWTHER MD, MSC, FRCPC
Professor and Division Director
Division of Hematology
McMaster University
Hamilton, Canada

JEFF GINSBERG MD, FRCPC
Professor, Department of Medicine
McMaster University
Hamilton, Canada

HOLGER J. SCHÜNEMANN MD, PHD, MSC, FACP, FCCP
Professor
Italian National Cancer Institute "Regina Elena"
Rome, Italy, and
McMaster University
Hamilton, Canada

RALPH M. MEYER MD, FRCPC
Edith Eisenhauer Chair in Clinical Cancer Research
Professor, Departments of Oncology and Medicine
Queen's University
Kingston, Canada

RICHARD LOTTENBERG MD, FACP
Professor of Medicine
University of Florida
Gainesville, USA

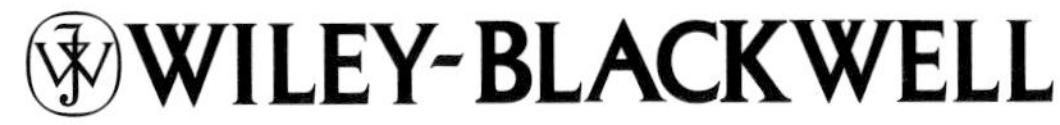
A John Wiley and Sons, Ltd., Publication

BMJ | Books

This edition first published 2008, © 2008 by Blackwell Publishing Ltd

BMJ Books is an imprint of BMJ Publishing Group Limited, used under licence
by Blackwell Publishing which was acquired by John Wiley & Sons in February 2007.
Blackwell's publishing programme has been merged with Wiley's
global Scientific, Technical and Medical business to form Wiley-Blackwell.

Registered office: John Wiley & Sons Ltd, The Atrium, Southern Gate, Chichester, West Sussex, PO19 8SQ, UK

Editorial offices: 9600 Garsington Road, Oxford, OX4 2DQ, UK
The Atrium, Southern Gate, Chichester, West Sussex, PO19 8SQ, UK
111 River Street, Hoboken, NJ 07030-5774, USA

For details of our global editorial offices, for customer services and for information about how to apply for permission to reuse the copyright material in this book please see our website at www.wiley.com/wiley-blackwell

Library of Congress Cataloging-in-Publication Data

Evidence-based hematology/edited by Mark A. Crowther . . . [et al.].
p. ; cm.
Includes bibliographical references and index.
ISBN 978-1-4051-5747-6 (alk. paper)
1. Blood—Diseases. 2. Hematology. 3. Evidence-based medicine. I. Crowther, Mark, 1966-
[DNLM: 1. Hematologic Diseases–therapy. 2. Evidence-Based Medicine. 3. Hematologic Diseases–diagnosis. WH 120 E93 2008]
RC636.E94 2008
616.1′5—dc22

2007047284

ISBN: 978-1-4051-5747-6

A catalogue record for this book is available from the British Library.

Set in 9.25/12 by Aptara, Inc.
Printed in Singapore by Fabulous Printers Pte Ltd

1 2008

Contents

Companion website: www.blackwellpublishing.com/medicine/bmj/hematology

List of contributors

Syed A. Abutalib MD
Northwestern University Feinberg School of Medicine
Robert H. Lurie Comprehensive Cancer Center
Chicago
Illinois, USA

Walter Ageno MD
Department of Clinical Medicine
University of Insubria
Varese, Italy

Julia A. M. Anderson MBChB, BSc(Hons), MD FRCP(Edin), FRCPath, FACP
Department of Medicine
McMaster University
Hamilton
Ontario, Canada

Karl E. Anderson MD
Departments of Preventive Medicine and Community Health
Internal Medicine and Pharmacology and Toxicology
University of Texas Medical Branch
Galveston
Texas, USA

Lucas M. Bachmann MD, PhD
Reader in Clinical Epidemiology
Deputy Director, Horten Centre for Patient Oriented Research
University of Zürich
Zürich, Switzerland

Tiziano Barbui MD
Department of Hematology-Oncology
Ospedali Riuniti di Bergamo
Bergamo (Bg), Italy

Giovanni Barosi MD
Director, Unit of Epidemiology Center for the Study of Myelofibrosis
IRCCS Policlinico S. Matteo Foundation
Pavia, Italy

Charles Bennett MD PhD
Division of Hematology/Oncology
Department of Medicine
Feinberg School of Medicine
Mid-West Center for Health Services Policy Research
Chicago VA/Lakeside Division
Northwestern University Medical School
Chicago
Illinois, USA

Ernest Beutler MD
Department of Molecular and Experimental Medicine
The Scripps Research Institute
La Jolla
California, USA

Patrick M. M. Bossuyt PhD
Department of Clinical Epidemiology and Biostatistics
Academic Medical Center
University of Amsterdam
Amsterdam
The Netherlands

Brian Boulmay MD
Department of Medicine
Health Science Center
University of Florida
Gainesville
Florida, USA

Jan L. Brozek MD, PhD
Italian National Cancer Institute "Regina Elena"
Rome, Italy
Polish Institute for EBM
Krakow, Poland

George R. Buchanan MD
Division of Hematology-Oncology
Department of Pediatrics
University of Texas
Southwestern Medical Center at Dallas
Dallas
Texas, USA

Harry R. Büller MD
Department of Vascular Medicine
Academic Medical Center
University of Amsterdam
Amsterdam, The Netherlands

Arina ten Cate-Hoek MD
Department of Epidemiology
Care and Public Health Research Institute
University of Maastricht
Maastricht, The Netherlands

Anthony K. C. Chan MBBS, FRCPC
Department of Pediatrics
McMaster University
Hamilton
Ontario, Canada

Wee-Shian Chan MD, FRCPC, MSc
Department of Medicine
Women's College Hospital
Department of Obstetrics and Gynecology
Sunnybrook Health Sciences Centre
Toronto
Ontario, Canada

Christine I. Chen MD, MMED, FRCP
Department of Medical Oncology and Hematology
Princess Margaret Hospital
University of Toronto
Toronto
Ontario, Canada

Bruce D. Cheson MD
Division of Hematology/Oncology
Georgetown University Hospital
Washington, DC, USA

Matthew Cheung MD, SM, FRCP(C)
Division of Hematology/Oncology
Department of Medicine
University of Toronto Sunnybrook Health Sciences Centre
Toronto, Ontario
Canada

Richard W. Childs MD
Hematology Branch
National Heart, Lung, and Blood Institute
National Institutes of Health
Bethesda
Maryland, USA

Elie Cogan MD, PhD
Department of Internal Medicine
Erasme Hospital, Brussels
Université Libre de Bruxelles (ULB)
Belgium

Stephen Couban MD, FRCPC
Queen Elizabeth II Health Sciences Centre
Halifax
Nova Scotia, Canada

Mark A. Crowther MD, MSc, FRCPC
Professor and Division Director
Division of Hematology
McMaster University, and
St. Joseph's Hospital
Hamilton
Ontario, Canada

Michael Crump MD, FRCPC
Princess Margaret Hospital
Division of Medical Oncology and Hematology
Department of Medicine
University of Toronto
Toronto
Ontario, Canada

David C. Dale MD, FACP
Department of Medicine
University of Washington
Seattle
Washington, USA

Sally C. Davies MB, FRCP, FRCPath
Faculty of Medicine
Imperial College at Central Middlesex Hospital
London, UK

Marcello Di Nisio MD, PhD
Department of Medicine and Aging
School of Medicine, and Aging Research Center, Ce.S.I.
"Gabriele D'Annunzio"
University Foundation
Chieti-Pescara, Italy

Benjamin Djulbegovic MD, PhD
Department of Interdisciplinary Oncology
H. Lee Moffitt Cancer Center and Research Institute
University of South Florida
Tampa
Florida, USA

James D. Douketis MD, FRCP(C)
Department of Medicine
McMaster University and St Joseph's Healthcare
Hamilton
Ontario, Canada

John W. Eikelboom MBBS, MSc, FRACP, FRCPA
Department of Medicine
McMaster University
Hamilton
Ontario, Canada

Miguel A. Escobar MD
Department of Pediatrics and Internal Medicine
Division of Hematology
University of Texas Health Science Center at Houston
Houston
Texas, USA

Guido Finazzi MD
Director, Transfusion Medicine and Haemostasis and Thrombosis Services
Ospedali Riuniti
Bergamo, Italy

Jonathan W. Friedberg MD
James P. Wilmot Cancer Center
University of Rochester
Rochester
New York, USA

Patrick G. Gallagher MD, FAAP
Department of Pediatrics
Yale School of Medicine
New Haven
Connecticut, USA

James N. George MD
Hematology–Oncology Section
University of Oklahoma Health Sciences Center
Oklahoma City
Oklahoma, USA

John Gerecitano MD, PhD
Department of Medicine
Lymphoma Service
Memorial Sloan-Kettering Cancer Center
New York, USA

Michel Goldman MD, PhD
Institute for Medical Immunology
Université Libre de Bruxelles
Charleroi-Gosselies, Belgium

Andreas Greinacher
Department of Immunology and Transfusion Medicine and Transfusion Medicine
Thrombosis and Hemostasis Service
Universitätsklinikum Greifswald
Ernst-Moritz-Arndt University Greifswald
Greifswald, Germany

Gordon G. Guyatt MD, MSc
CLARITY Research Group
Department of Clinical Epidemiology and Biostatistics
McMaster University
Hamilton
Ontario, Canada

Christine L. Hann MD, PhD
Department of Oncology
Johns Hopkins University School of Medicine
Baltimore
Maryland, USA

R. Brian Haynes MD, PhD
Health Information Research Unit
Department of Clinical Epidemiology and Biostatistics
McMaster University Faculty of Health Sciences
Hamilton
Ontario, Canada

Davide Imberti MD
Head of Thrombosis Center
Emergency Department
Hospital of Piacenza
Piacenza, Italy

Kevin Imrie MD, FRCPC
Chair, Cancer Care Ontario Hematology Disease Site Group, and
Toronto-Sunnybrook Regional Cancer Centre
Toronto
Ontario, Canada

Scott Kaatz DO, MSc, FACP
Henry Ford Health System
Detroit
Michigan, USA

Marc J. Kahn MD
School of Medicine
Tulane University School of Medicine
New Orleans
Louisiana, USA

Tyler Y. Kang MD
Hematology/Oncology Fellow
Taussig Cancer Center
Cleveland Clinic
Cleveland
Ohio, USA

Clive Kearon MB, MRCPI, FRCPC, PhD
McMaster University
Hamilton
Ontario, Canada

Andrea Kew MD, FRCPC
Queen Elizabeth II Health Sciences Centre
Halifax
Nova Scotia, Canada

Nigel S. Key MB, ChB, FRCP(UK)
Department of Medicine
University of North Carolina at Chapel Hill
Chapel Hill
North Carolina, USA

Craig S. Kitchens MD, MACP
Veterans Affairs Medical Center
University of Florida
Gainesville
Florida, USA

C. Tom Kouroukis MD, MSc, FRCPC
Hematology-Oncology
Juravinski Cancer Centre
Department of Oncology
McMaster University
Hamilton
Ontario, Canada

Ambuj Kumar MD, MPH
Department of Health Outcomes and Behavior and Oncologic Sciences
H. Lee Moffitt Cancer Center and Research Institute
University of South Florida
Tampa
Florida, USA

Richard A. Larson MD
Section of Hematology/Oncology
Department of Medicine and Cancer Research Center
University of Chicago
Chicago
Illinois, USA

Pieter Leffers
Department of Epidemiology
Care and Public Health Research Institute
Maastricht University
Maastricht, The Netherlands

Wendy Lim MD, MSc
St. Joseph's Hospital
Department of Medicine
McMaster University
Hamilton
Ontario, Canada

Lori-Ann Linkins MD, MSc, FRCPC
Henderson Research Centre
Hamilton Health Sciences Corporation
Hamilton
Ontario, Canada

Richard Lottenberg MD, FACP
Division of Hematology/Oncology
Department of Medicine
University of Florida College of Medicine
Gainesville
Florida, USA

Alice D. Ma MD
University of North Carolina School of Medicine
Division of Hematology/Oncology
Harold R. Roberts Comprehensive Hemophilia Center CB
Chapel Hill
North Carolina, USA

Nicola Magrini MD
CeVEAS NHS Centre for the Evaluation of the Effectiveness of Health Care
Modena Local Health Authority
Modena, Italy

Roberto Marchioli MD
Laboratory of Clinical Epidemiology of Cardiovascular Disease
Department of Clinical Pharmacology and Epidemiology
Consorzio Mario Negri Sud
Santa Maria Imbaro, Italy

K. Ann McKibbon MLS, PhD
Health Information Research Unit
Department of Clinical Epidemiology and Biostatistics
McMaster University Faculty of Health Sciences
Hamilton
Ontario, Canada

Brandon McMahon MD
Northwestern University
Feinberg School of Medicine
Robert H. Lurie Comprehensive Cancer Center
Chicago
Illinois, USA

Simon J. McRae MBBS, FRACP, FRCPA
The Queen Elizabeth Hospital
Woodville
South Australia
Australia

Ralph M. Meyer MD, FRCP(C)
Director, National Cancer Institute of Canada Clinical Trials Group
Edith Eisenhauer Chair in Clinical Cancer Research
Professor, Departments of Oncology and Medicine
Queen's University
Kingston, Ontario
Canada

Paul Monagle MBBS, MSc, MD, FRACP, FRCPA, FCCP
Department of Haematology
Royal Children's Hospital
Department of Pathology
University of Melbourne
Melbourne
Victoria, Australia

Isaac Odame MB, ChB, FRCPCH, FRCPath, FRCPC
Division of Hematology/Oncology
The Hospital for Sick Children
Toronto
Ontario, Canada

Antonello Pietrangelo MD. PhD
Department of Medicine
Center for Hemochromatosis
University of Modena and Reggio Emilia
Modena, Italy

Martin Prins MD, PhD
Department of Epidemiology
Care and Public Health Reseach Institute
University of Maastricht and Department of Epidemiology and Medical Technology Assessment
Academic Hospital Maastricht
Maastricht, The Netherlands

Cara A. Rosenbaum MD
Section of Hematology/Oncology
Department of Medicine and Cancer Research Center
University of Chicago
Chicago
Illinois, USA

Florence Roufosse MD, PhD
Department of Internal Medicine
Hôpital Erasme
Université Libre de Bruxelles (ULB)
Institute for Medical Immunology
Université Libre de Bruxelles (ULB)
Gosselies
Brussels, Belgium

Deborah Rund MD
Hematology Department
Hebrew University
Hadassah University Hospital
Ein Kerem
Jerusalem, Israel

Kerry Savage BSc, MD, MSc, FRCPC
University of British Columbia
Division of Medical Oncology
British Columbia Cancer Agency
Vancouver, British Columbia
Canada

Sam Schulman MD, PhD, FRCPS
Clinical Thromboembolism Program
McMaster University
Hamilton
Ontario, Canada

Holger J. Schünemann MD, PhD, MSc, FACP, FCCP
CLARITY Research Group
Department of Epidemiology Italian National Cancer Institute Regina Elena
Rome, Italy

Michael Sebag MD, PhD, FRCPC
Mayo Clinic Arizona
Scottsdale
Arizona, USA

Tamara Shenkier MDCM, FRCPC
Department of Medical Oncology
University of British Columbia
British Columbia Cancer Agency
Vancouver
British Columbia, Canada

Heloisa P. Soares MD
Department of Internal Medicine
Mount Sinai Medical Center
Miami Beach
Florida, USA

Gagan Sood MD
Division of Gastroenterology and Hepatology
Department of Internal Medicine
The University of Texas Medical Branch
Galveston
Texas, USA

Alessandro Squizzato MD
Department of Clinical Medicine
University of Insubria
Varese, Italy

Shivani Srivastava MD
Bone Marrow and Stem Cell Transplantation
IU Simon Cancer Center
Indiana University
Indianapolis
Indiana, USA

Martin Stanulla MD, MSc
Department of Pediatric Hematology and Oncology
Children's Hospital
Hannover Medical School
Hannover, Germany

A. Keith Stewart MBCHB, FRCPC, FACP
College of Medicine, Mayo Clinic
Scottsdale
Arizona, USA

John M. Storring MD
McGill University Health Centre
Montreal
Quebec, Canada

David J. Straus MD
Lymphoma Service
Department of Medicine
Memorial Sloan–Kettering Cancer Center
New York
New York, USA

Michael B. Streiff MD
Department of Medicine
Johns Hopkins Medical Institutions
Baltimore
Maryland, USA

John W. Sweetenham MD, FRCP
Taussig Cancer Center
Cleveland Clinic
Cleveland
Ohio, USA

Martin S. Tallman MD
Northwestern University Feinberg School of Medicine
Robert H. Lurie Comprehensive Cancer Center
Chicago
Illinois, USA

Victor F. Tapson MD
Division of Pulmonary and Critical Care Medicine
Duke University Medical Center
Durham
North Carolina, USA

Sara K. Vesely PhD
Department of Biostatistics and Epidemiology
University of Oklahoma Health Sciences Center
Oklahoma City
Oklahoma, USA

Cynthia J. Walker-Dilks MLS
Health Information Research Unit
Department of Clinical Epidemiology and Biostatistics
McMaster University Faculty of Health Sciences
Hamilton
Ontario, Canada

Irwin Walker MBBS, FRACP, FRCPC
Hematology and Bone Marrow Transplantation
McMaster University Medical Centre
Hamilton
Ontario, Canada

Theodore E. Warkentin MD, BSc(Med), FRCP(C), FACP
Department of Pathology and Molecular Medicine, and Department of Medicine McMaster University
Transfusion Medicine
Hamilton Regional Laboratory Medicine Program
Service of Clinical Hematology
Hamilton, Ontario
Canada

Karen W. L. Yee MD
Department of Medical Oncology and Hematology
University Health Network—Princess Margaret Hospital
Toronto
Ontario, Canada

Marc S. Zumberg MD
Department of Medicine
Division of Hematology/Oncology
University of Florida
Gainesville
Florida, USA

Preface

Evidence-based medicine is defined variably, however fundamental to its practice, it is the systematic appraisal of available evidence and the formulation of therapeutic plans, which take into account this evidence. Evidence-based medicine is flexible and uses "best practice" evidence as broadly as possible to answer clinically relevant questions.

Evidence-based Hematology focuses on clinical questions within all domains of hematology. The questions are designed to address clinical problems seen in day-to-day practice. We have systematically reviewed the literature available as it applies to each of these questions and have made recommendations that reflect this evidence. We hope that this text will assist readers in understanding how to formulate and answer their own clinical questions using the best available evidence.

Although most texts such as this are inevitably delayed in their production and, as a result, the evidence presented may be already out of date, we have made every effort to update the material, making *Evidence-based Hematology* a timely addition to the literature. We hope that readers will use the techniques employed in this text (formulation of a clinically relevant question, systematic literature review, and grading of evidence) to update their knowledge in specific content areas using their own personal continuous learning techniques. Our hope is that you will find this text useful in your day-to-day clinical practice. Additionally, we hope that it spurs your interest in evidence-based hematology, thus assisting you in providing the best possible care to your patients.

Mark A. Crowther
Hamilton, Ontario, April 1, 2008

Companion Website

A companion site for this book is available at the following URL:
www.blackwellpublishing.com/medicine/bmj/hematology

The site includes the following:

- web-only tables (Tables 22.5 and 22.6, Appendix 22.1)
- updates section
- more about the Wiley–Blackwell evidence-based products.

1 A Guide to the Evidence

Holger J. Schünemann

1 Rating the Quality of Evidence and Making Recommendations

A Guide to the Spectrum of Clinical Research

Holger J. Schünemann, Martin Stanulla, Jan L. Brozek, Gordon G. Guyatt

Introduction

Clinicians require clinical expertise to integrate a patient's circumstances and values with the best-available evidence to initiate decision making in health care (1). Using "best evidence" implies that a hierarchy of evidence exists and that clinicians are more confident about decisions based on evidence that offers greater protection against bias and random error.

Protection against bias and greater confidence in decisions result from high-quality research evidence. We can consider quality of evidence a continuum that reflects the confidence in estimates of the magnitude of effect of alternative patient management interventions on the outcomes of interest. However, gradations of this continuum are useful for communication with practicing clinicians, providing useful summaries of what is known because specific clinical questions aid interpretation of clinical research (see chapter 4).

Aiding interpretation becomes increasingly important considering that much of clinicians' practice is guided by recommendations from experts summarized in clinical practice guidelines and textbooks such as this new book *Evidence-based Hematology*. To integrate recommendations with their own clinical judgment, clinicians need to understand the basis for the clinical recommendations that experts offer them. A systematic approach to grading the quality of evidence and the resulting recommendations for clinicians represent an important step in providing evidence-based recommendations.

In this chapter, we will describe the key features of the "quality of evidence" and how we asked the authors of individual chapters to evaluate the available evidence and formulate their recommendations using a pragmatic approach that falls short of the full development of evidence-based guidelines. Most authors used an approach based on the work of the Grading of Recommendations Assessment, Development, and Evaluation Working Group (GRADE) (2–5). Over 20 international organizations, including the World Health Organization, the American College of Physicians, the American College of Chest Physicians, the American Thoracic Society, the European Respiratory Society, UpToDate®, and the Cochrane Collaboration, are now using the GRADE system.

Evidence-based Hematology. Edited by Mark A. Crowther, Jeff Ginsberg, Holger J. Schünemann, Ralph M. Meyer, and Richard Lottenberg.

Question formulation and recommendations in this book

We asked chapter authors to ask clinical questions that are particularly relevant to hematology practice using the framework of identifying the patient population(s), the interventions examined (or exposure), alternative interventions (comparison), and the outcomes of interest (see chapter 4). We then asked them to identify relevant studies related to these questions or sets of questions.

For instance, McRae and Eikelboom asked whether thrombolytic therapy compared with anticoagulant therapy has favorable effects on death, recurrent venous thrombosis, incidence on post-thrombotic syndrome, thrombus lysis, and major bleeding in patients with deep vein thrombosis (see chapter 11).

We also asked the authors to base the answers to their questions on evaluations of the scientific literature, in particular focusing on recent, methodologically rigorous systematic reviews of randomized controlled trials (RCTs). If authors did not identify a recent and rigorous systematic review, they were asked to search for RCTs and summarize the findings of these studies to answer their clinical questions. Observational studies were included only if RCTs did not answer the specific question (or did not provide information on a particular outcome). Thus, the search studies we suggested focused on relevant systematic reviews or meta-analyses (a pooled statistical summary of relevant studies) followed by searches for randomized trials and observational studies if systematic reviews did not exist or did not include sufficient information to answer the posed questions. For example, Imrie and Cheung (chapter 42) searched for systematic reviews and randomized trials in the Cochrane Library (2006, Issue 3) and Medline (1966–August 2006,

Table 1.1 Grading recommendations.

Grade of recommendation*	Balance of desirable versus undesirable effects	Methodologic quality of supporting evidence
Strong recommendation High-quality evidence 1A	Desirable effects clearly outweigh undesirable effects or vice versa	Consistent evidence from randomized controlled trials without important limitations or exceptionally strong evidence from observational studies.
Strong recommendation Moderate-quality evidence 1B	Desirable effects clearly outweigh undesirable effects or vice versa	Evidence from randomized controlled trials with important limitations (inconsistent results, methodologic flaws, indirect or imprecise), or very strong evidence from observational studies.
Strong recommendation Low or very low quality evidence 1C	Desirable effects clearly outweigh undesirable effects, or vice versa	Evidence for at least one critical outcome from observational studies, case series, or from randomized controlled trials with serious flaws or indirect evidence.
Weak recommendation High-quality evidence 2A	Desirable effects closely balanced with undesirable effects	Consistent evidence from randomized controlled trials without important limitations or exceptionally strong evidence from observational studies.
Weak recommendation Moderate-quality evidence 2B	Desirable effects closely balanced with undesirable effects	Evidence from randomized controlled trials with important limitations (inconsistent results, methodologic flaws, indirect or imprecise), or very strong evidence from observational studies.
Weak recommendation Low or very low quality evidence 2C	Desirable effects closely balanced with undesirable effects	Evidence for at least one critical outcome from observational studies, case series, or from randomized controlled trials with serious flaws or indirect evidence.

*GRADE (Grading of Recommendations Assessment, Development, and Evaluation Working Group) system suggests the use of the wording "we recommend" for strong (Grade 1) recommendations and "we suggest" for weak (Grade 2) recommendations. This grading system is based on the work on the GRADE Working Group. The categories of low and very low quality that GRADE includes in its four category system are collapsed here into a single category, resulting in three categories of quality of evidence.

week 2) on treatment for lymphoma. They identified an outdated systematic review and six RCTs to answer the questions whether patients with limited stage follicular lymphoma should receive systemic therapy in combination with local radiotherapy to improve disease-free survival. They based their answer, in the format of a clinical recommendation, on a summary of the evidence from the six RCTs.

Evaluating the quality of evidence and making recommendations

Many authors applied the GRADE system for evaluating the quality of evidence and for presenting their recommendations. This approach begins with an initial assessment of the quality of evidence, followed by judgments about the direction (for or against) and strength of recommendations. Since clinicians are most interested in the best course of action, the GRADE system usually presents the strength of the recommendation first as strong (Grade 1) or weak (Grade 2), followed by the quality of the evidence as high (A), moderate (B), low (C), and very low (D). Authors of this book adopted a version of the grading system that combines the low and very low categories, because for many questions in hematology evidence from RCTs is available. Furthermore, we asked authors to phrase recommendations the way that would express their strength. For strong (Grade 1) recommendations, many authors chose the words: "We recommend . . . (for or against a particular course of action)." For weak (Grade 2) recommendations, they used the words: "We suggest . . . (using or not using)" what they believed to be an optimal management approach. They then indicated the methodological quality of the supporting evidence labeling them as A (high quality), B (moderate quality), or C (low or very low quality). Thus, recommendations can fall into the following six categories: 1A, 1B, 1C, 2A, 2B, and 2C (Table 1.1).

Strength of the recommendation

In determining the strength of recommendations, the GRADE system focuses on the degree of confidence in the balance between desirable effects of an intervention on the one hand and undesirable effects on the other (Table 1.1). Desirable effects or benefits include favorable health outcomes, decreased burden of treatment, and decreased resource use (usually measured as costs). Undesirable effects, or downsides, include rare major adverse events, common minor side effects, greater burden of treatment, and more resource consumption. We define burdens as the demands of adhering to a recommendation that patients or caregivers (e.g., family) may dislike, such as taking medication, need for inconvenient laboratory monitoring, or physician visits. If desirable effects of

Table 1.2 Determinants of strength of recommendation.

Factors that influence the strength of a recommendation	Comment
Balance between desirable and undesirable effects	A strong recommendation is more likely as the difference between the desirable and undesirable consequences becomes larger. A weak recommendation is more likely as the net benefit becomes smaller and the certainty around that net benefit decreases.
Quality of the evidence	A strong recommendation becomes more likely with higher quality of evidence.
Values and preferences	A strong recommendation is more likely as the variability of or uncertainty about patient values and preferences decreases. A weak recommendation is more likely as the variability or uncertainty about patient values and preferences increases.
Costs (resource allocation)	A weak recommendation is more likely as the incremental costs of an intervention (more resources consumed) increase.

an intervention outweigh undesirable effects, we recommend that clinicians offer the intervention to typical patients. How close is the balance between desirable and undesirable effects and the uncertainty associated with that balance will determine the strength of recommendations.

Table 1.2 describes the factors GRADE relies on to determine the strength of recommendation.

When chapter authors were confident that the desirable effects of adherence to a recommendation outweighed the undesirable effects or vice versa, they offered a strong recommendation. Such confidence usually requires evidence of high or moderate quality that provides precise estimates of both benefits and downsides, and their clear balance in favor of, or against, one of the management options. The authors offered a weak recommendation when low-quality evidence resulted in appreciable uncertainty about the magnitude of benefits or downsides, or the benefits and downsides were finely balanced. We will describe the factors influencing the quality of evidence in subsequent sections of this chapter. Other reasons for not being confident in the balance between desirable and undesirable effects include: (1) imprecise estimates of benefits or harms, (2) uncertainty or variation in how different individuals value particular outcomes and thus their preferences regarding management alternatives, (3) small benefits, or (4) situations when benefits may not be worth the costs (including the costs of implementing the recommendation). Although the balance between desirable and undesirable effects, and thus the strength of a recommendation, is a continuum, the GRADE system classifies recommendations for or against an intervention into two categories: strong or weak. Categorizing recommendations as "strong" or "weak" is inevitably arbitrary. The GRADE Working Group believes that the simplicity and behavioral implications of this explicit grading outweigh the disadvantages.

For instance, the choice of adjusted-dose warfarin versus aspirin for prevention of stroke in patients with atrial fibrillation exemplifies a number of the factors that influence the strength of a recommendation. A systematic review with meta-analysis found a relative risk reduction (RRR) of 46% in all strokes with warfarin versus aspirin (6). This large effect supports a strong recommendation for warfarin. Furthermore, the fairly narrow 95% confidence interval around this estimate (29% to 57%) suggests that warfarin provides an RRR of at least 29% that further supports strong recommendation. At the same time, warfarin is associated with burdens that include keeping dietary intake of vitamin K constant, monitoring the intensity of anticoagulation with blood tests, and living with the increased risk of bleeding. Most patients, however, are much more stroke averse than they are bleeding averse (7). As a result, most patients with high risk of stroke would choose warfarin, suggesting the appropriateness of a strong recommendation.

A patient's baseline risk of the adverse outcome (also called control risk or control event rate) that an intervention is expected to prevent can be an important issue. Consider another 65-year-old patient with atrial fibrillation and no other risk factors for stroke. This individual's risk for stroke in the next year is approximately 2%. Dose-adjusted warfarin can, relative to aspirin, reduce the risk to approximately 1%. Some stroke-averse patients may consider the downsides of taking warfarin well worth it. Others are likely to consider the benefit not worth the risks and inconvenience. When fully informed patients are likely to make different choices across the range of their values and preferences, guideline panels should offer weak (Grade 2) recommendations.

While the ideal approach for clinicians is to elicit preferences and values from their patients and to recommend obtaining values and preference estimates from population-based studies, such studies are rarely available. When value or preference judgments are crucial for interpreting recommendations, some chapter authors have made statements about the key values underlying their recommendations.

Table 1.3 Implications of strong and weak recommendations.

Implications	Strong recommendation	Weak recommendation
For patients	Most individuals in this situation would want the recommended course of action and only a small proportion would not. Formal decision aids are not likely to be needed to help individuals make decisions consistent with their values and preferences.	The majority of individuals in this situation would want the suggested course of action, but many would not.
For clinicians	Most individuals should receive the intervention. Adherence to this recommendation according to the guideline could be used as a quality criterion or performance indicator.	Recognize that different choices will be appropriate for different patients and that you must help each patient arrive at a management decision consistent with her or his values and preferences. Decision aids can help individuals making decisions consistent with their values and preferences.
For policy makers	The recommendation can be adapted as policy in most situations	Policy making will require substantial debates and involvement of many stakeholders

For instance, McRae and Eikelboom suggested that clinicians not use thrombolytic therapy routinely in patients with deep venous thrombosis (DVT) (Grade 2B) because this recommendation ascribes a high value to the increased risk of bleeding with thrombolytic therapy.

As benefits and risks become more finely balanced or more uncertain, decisions to administer an effective therapy also become more cost sensitive. We have not asked authors to explicitly include cost in the recommendations, but cost will bear on the implementation of many recommendations in clinical practice (8).

Interpreting strong and weak recommendations

Table 1.3 shows suggestions for interpreting strong and weak recommendations. For decisions in which benefits far outweigh downsides or downsides far outweigh benefits, almost all patients will make the same choice, and guideline developers can offer a strong recommendation.

For instance, consistent results from high-quality randomized trials suggest that aspirin reduces the relative risk of death after myocardial infarction by approximately 25%. Depending on age and factors such as the presence of heart failure, typical patients with acute myocardial infarction face risks of death in the first 30 days of between 2% and 40% (9). One can therefore expect a 0.5% absolute reduction in risk (from 2% to 1.5%) in the lowest-risk patients and a 10% reduction (from 40% to 30%) in the highest-risk ones. Aspirin has minimal side effects and is very inexpensive. Because, even in the lowest-risk subgroups, the desirable effects clearly outweigh the undesirable effects, the administration of aspirin is strongly endorsed and widely used. Using letters and numbers to express the quality of the evidence and strength of recommendations (Table 1.1), both low- and high-risk patients would fall within the category of a strong recommendation based on high-quality evidence or Grade 1A ("1" because the desirable effects clearly outweigh the undesirable ones, and "A" because the evidence comes from high-quality, randomized trials that yielded consistent results).

Therefore, for typical patients, strong recommendations provide a mandate for the clinician to explain the intervention along with a suggestion that the patient will benefit from its use. Further elaboration will seldom be necessary. However, when clinicians face weak recommendations, they should consider the benefits, harms, and burden to the patient more carefully and ensure that the decision is consistent with the patient's values and preferences. These situations arise when appreciable numbers of patients would make different choices because of variability in values and preferences.

Consider a 40-year-old man who has suffered an idiopathic DVT followed by treatment with adjusted-dose warfarin for one year to prevent recurrent DVT and pulmonary embolism. Continuing on standard-intensity warfarin beyond this period will reduce his absolute risk for recurrent DVT by more than 7% per year for several years (10). The burdens of treatment include taking a warfarin pill daily, keeping dietary intake of vitamin K constant, monitoring the intensity of anticoagulation with blood tests, and living with the increased risk of bleeding. Patients who are very averse to a recurrent DVT would consider the benefits of avoiding DVT worth the downsides of taking warfarin. Other patients are likely to consider the benefit not worth the potential harms and burden.

Individualization of clinical decision making in the context of weak recommendations remains a challenge. Although clinicians should always consider patients' preferences and values, when they face weak recommendations, they should consider more detailed conversations with patients than for strong recommendations to ensure that the ultimate decision is consistent with the patient's values. A decision aid that presents patients with both benefits and downsides of therapy is likely to improve knowledge, decrease decision-making conflict, and support a decision most consistent with patients' values and preferences (11). Clinicians cannot use decision aids in all patients because of time constraints and the limited availability of decisions aids. For strong recommendations, the use of decision aids is inefficient.

Table 1.4 Categories of quality of evidence.

Underlying methodology*	Quality rating
RCT and observational studies with very large effects	high
Downgraded RCTs or upgraded observational studies	moderate
Observational studies with control groups & RCTs and with major limitations	low

*RCT, randomized controlled trial.

Other ways of interpreting strong and weak recommendations relate to performance or quality indicators. Strong recommendations are candidate performance indicators. For weak recommendations, performance could be measured by monitoring whether clinicians have discussed recommended actions with patients or their surrogates or carefully documented the evaluation of benefits and downsides in the patient's chart.

How methodologic quality of the evidence contributes to strength of recommendation

In the GRADE system, evidence of the highest quality comes from one or more well-designed and well-executed RCTs, yielding consistent and directly applicable results. High-quality evidence can also come from well-done observational studies yielding very large effects (defined as a relative risk reduction of at least 80%) (Table 1.4).

RCTs with important methodologic limitations and well-done observational studies yielding large effects constitute the moderate-quality category. Well-done observational studies yielding modest effects, and RCTs with very serious limitations, will be rated as low-quality evidence. Next, we describe the system of grading the methodologic quality of evidence in more detail.

Factors that decrease the quality of evidence

Table 1.5 shows the limitations may decrease the quality of evidence supporting a recommendation.

1. Limitation of methodology: Our confidence in recommendations decreases if studies suffer from major limitations that are likely to result in a biased assessment of the treatment effect. These methodologic limitations include lack of blinding when subjective outcomes highly susceptible to bias are measured, failure to adhere to an intention-to-treat principle in the analysis of results, a large loss to follow-up, or stopping the study early because of observed benefit.

For instance, a randomized trial suggests that danaparoid sodium is beneficial in treating heparin-induced thrombocytopenia complicated by thrombosis (12). In that trial, however, there was no blinding, and the key outcome trial was the clinicians' subjective judgment on when the thromboembolism had resolved.

2. Inconsistent results (unexplained heterogeneity of results): If studies yield widely differing estimates of the treatment effect (heterogeneity or variability in results), investigators should look for explanations for that heterogeneity. For example, interventions may have larger relative effects in sicker populations or when given in larger doses. When heterogeneity exists, but investigators fail to identify a plausible explanation, the quality of evidence decreases. For example, RCTs of pentoxifylline in patients with intermittent claudication have shown conflicting results that defy explanation (13).

3. Indirectness of evidence (i.e., the question addressed in the recommendation is quite different from the available evidence regarding the population, intervention, comparison, or outcome): Investigators may have undertaken studies in similar, but not identical, populations to those under consideration for a recommendation. For example, many of the antithrombotic therapies rigorously tested in randomized trials in adults are also administered to children. The adult trials provide strong evidence for adult recommendations, but because of indirectness, they represent only moderate- or low-quality evidence for children.

4. Imprecision: If studies include few patients and few events and thus have wide confidence intervals, making recommendations includes judging evidence lower than it otherwise would be because of resulting uncertainty in the results. For instance, a well-designed and rigorously conducted RCT addressed the use of nadroparin, a low-molecular-weight heparin, in patients with cerebral venous sinus thrombosis (14). Of 30 treated patients, 3 had a poor outcome, as did 6 of 29 patients in the control group. The investigators' analysis suggests a 7% risk difference (which, if true, would correspond to a requirement to treat approximately 14 patients to prevent a single poor outcome), but the confidence interval also included not only a 26% absolute difference in favor of treatment but also a 12% difference in favor of placebo.

5. Publication bias: The quality of evidence can be reduced if investigators fail to report outcomes or selective outcome reporting (typically, those that show no effect) or if other reasons lead to withheld results. Unfortunately, it is often required to make guesses about the likelihood of publication bias.

Table 1.5 Factors that may decrease the quality of evidence.

- Limitations in the design and implementation of available RCTs,* suggesting high likelihood of bias
- Inconsistency of results (including problems with subgroup analyses)
- Indirectness of evidence (indirect population, intervention, control, outcomes)
- Imprecision of results (wide confidence intervals)
- High probability of publication bias

*RCT, randomized controlled trial.

Factors that increase the quality of evidence

Observational studies can provide moderate or strong evidence (14). Whereas well-done observational studies usually yield low-quality evidence, there may be unusual circumstances in

Table 1.6 Factors that may increase the quality of evidence.

- Large magnitude of effect (direct evidence, RR > 2 or RR < 0.5 with no plausible confounders; very large with RR > 5 or RR < 0.2 and no threats to validity
- All plausible confounding would reduce a demonstrated effect
- Dose-response gradient

RR, relative risk.

which guideline panels classify such evidence as moderate or even high quality (Table 1.6).

1. On rare occasions when methodologically strong observational studies yield large or very large and consistent estimates of the magnitude of a treatment effect, we may be confident about the results. In those situations, while the observational studies are likely to have provided an overestimate of the true effect, the weak study design may not explain all of the apparent benefit. Thus, despite reservations based on the observational study design, we are confident that the effect exists. Table 1.6 shows how the magnitude of the effect in these studies may move the assigned quality of evidence from low to moderate, or even to high quality. For example, a meta-analysis of 37 observational studies evaluating the impact of warfarin prophylaxis in cardiac valve replacement found that the relative risk for thromboembolism with warfarin was 0.17 (95% CI 0.13–0.24). This very large effect suggests a rating of high-quality evidence (16).

2. On occasion, all plausible biases from observational studies may be working to underestimate an apparent treatment effect. For example, if only sicker patients receive an experimental intervention or exposure, yet they still fare better, it is likely that the actual intervention or exposure effect is larger than the data suggest.

3. The presence of a dose-response gradient may also increase our confidence in the findings of observational studies and thereby enhance the assigned quality of evidence. For example, our confidence in the result of observational studies that show an increased risk of bleeding in patients who have supratherapeutic anticoagulation levels is increased by the observation of a dose-response gradient between higher levels of the international normalized ratio (INR) and the increased risk of bleeding (17).

Interpreting the recommendations

Clinicians, third-party payers, institutional review committees, and the courts should not construe recommendations in this book as absolute. In general, anything other than a Grade 1A recommendation indicates that the chapter authors acknowledge that other interpretations of the evidence, and other clinical policies, may be reasonable and appropriate. Even Grade 1A recommendations will not apply to all patients in all circumstances, and following Grade 1A recommendations will at times not serve the best interests of patients with atypical values or preferences or whose risks differ markedly from the usual patient. For instance, consider patients who find anticoagulant therapy extremely aversive, either because it interferes with their lifestyle (e.g., prevents participation in contact sports) or because monitoring in needed. Clinicians may reasonably conclude that following some Grade 1A recommendations for anticoagulation for either group of patients will be a mistake. The same may be true for patients with particular comorbidities (e.g., a recent gastrointestinal bleed, repeated falls, or an arteriovenous malformation) or other special circumstances (e.g., very advanced age) that put them at unusual risk. No clinician, and nobody charged with evaluating clinician's actions, should attempt to apply the recommendations in rote or blanket fashion.

Summary

The strength of any recommendation for practice depends on two factors: the trade-off between desirable factors and undesirable factors (risks, burden, and cost) and our confidence in estimates of those effects. The GRADE framework, with the minor modifications adopted by the authors of this book, classifies the trade-off between desirable and undesirable effects in two categories; (1) in which the trade-off is clear enough that most patients, despite differences in values, would make the same choice; and (2) in which the trade-off is less clear, and individual patients' values will likely lead to different choices. Three categories of methodologic strength exist: (A) high-quality evidence, usually from RCTs; (B) randomized trials with important limitations or observational studies with large effects; and (C) usually from observational studies. The framework summarized in Table 1.1 therefore generates recommendations from the very strong (1A: desirable and undesirable effects clear, methods high quality) to the very weak (2C: desirable and undesirable effects questionable, methods low quality). Clinicians must use their judgment when applying the recommendations, considering both local and individual patient circumstances and patient values, to help patients make individual decisions. In general, however, clinicians should place progressively greater weight on expert recommendations as they move from 2C to 1A.

References

1 Haynes RB, Devereaux PJ, Guyatt GH. Physicians' and patients' choices in evidence based practice. *BMJ*. 2002;**324**(7350):1350.

2 Atkins D, Best D, Briss PA, et al. Grading quality of evidence and strength of recommendations. *BMJ*. 2004;**328**(7454):1490.

3 Guyatt G, Gutterman D, Baumann M, et al. Grading strength of recommendations and quality of evidence in clinical guidelines. *Chest*. 2006;**129**:174–81.

4 Guyatt G, Vist G, Falck-Ytter Y, et al. An emerging consensus on grading recommendations? (editorial) *ACP J Club*. 2006;**144**(1):A8.

5 Schunemann HJ, Jaeschke R, Cook DJ, et al. An official ATS statement: grading the quality of evidence and strength of recommendations in ATS guidelines and recommendations. *Am J Respir Crit Care Med*. 2006;**174**(5):605–14.

6 van Walraven C, Hart RG, Singer DE, et al. Oral anticoagulants vs aspirin in nonvalvular atrial fibrillation: an individual patient meta-analysis. *JAMA.* 2002;**288**(19):2441–48.

7 Devereaux PJ, Anderson DR, Gardner MJ, et al. Differences between perspectives of physicians and patients on anticoagulation in patients with atrial fibrillation: observational study. *BMJ.* 2001;**323**(7323):1218–22.

8 Guyatt G, Baumann M, Pauker S, et al. Addressing resource allocation issues in recommendations from clinical practice guideline panels: suggestions from an American College of Chest Physicians task force. *Chest.* 2006;**129**(1):182–87.

9 Stevenson R, Ranjadayalan K, Wilkinson P, et al. Short and long term prognosis of acute myocardial infarction since introduction of thrombolysis. *BMJ.* 1993;**307**:349–53.

10 Büller HR, Agnelli G, Hull RD, et al. Antithrombotic therapy for venous thromboembolic disease: the Seventh ACCP Conference on Antithrombotic and Thrombolytic Therapy. *Chest.* 2004;**126**(3 Suppl):401S–28S.

11 O'Connor AM, Stacey D, Entwistle V, et al. Decision aids for people facing health treatment or screening decisions. *Cochrane Database Syst Rev.* 2003(2):CD001431.

12 Chong BH, Gallus AS, Cade JF, et al. Prospective randomised open-label comparison of danaparoid with dextran 70 in the treatment of heparin-induced thrombocytopaenia with thrombosis: a clinical outcome study. *Thromb Haemost.* 2001;**86**(5):1170–75.

13 Clagett GP, Sobel M, Jackson MR, et al. Antithrombotic therapy in peripheral arterial occlusive disease: the Seventh ACCP Conference on Antithrombotic and Thrombolytic Therapy. *Chest.* 2004;**126**(3 Suppl):609S–26S.

14 de Bruijn SF, Stam J. Randomized, placebo-controlled trial of anticoagulant treatment with low-molecular-weight heparin for cerebral sinus thrombosis. *Stroke.* 1999;**30**(3):484–88.

15 Glasziou P, Chalmers I, Rawlins M, et al. When are randomised trials unnecessary? Picking signal from noise. *BMJ.* 2007;**334**(7589): 349–51.

16 Cannegieter SC, Rosendaal FR, Briet E. Thromboembolic and bleeding complications in patients with mechanical heart valve prostheses. *Circulation.* 1994;**89**(2):635–41.

17 Levine MN, Raskob G, Beyth RJ, et al. Hemorrhagic complications of anticoagulant treatment: the Seventh ACCP Conference on Antithrombotic and Thrombolytic Therapy. *Chest.* 2004;**126**(3 Suppl): 287S–310S.

2 An Overview of Systematic Reviews

Martin Prins, Arina ten Cate-Hoek, Pieter Leffers

Introduction: Systematic versus narrative reviews

The introduction of evidence-based medicine has resulted in an increased application of primary research evidence in healthcare practice and decision making. Reviews that summarize research have become mandatory for coping with the increasing amount of evidence. Narrative reviews historically have been an important tool for information transfer in teaching medicine, but their purpose should not focus on making clinical decisions regarding patient care. Such reviews focus on a certain clinical condition or group of conditions, usually sharing a common etiology or group of symptoms, but are not likely to provide unbiased evaluations of management strategies for patient care. Narrative reviews may be useful for introducing learners to any medical subject, as well as for updating clinicians on a (biological) subject of interest. In general, narrative reviews offer a broad view on a subject but are guided by personal interests, opinions, and accents. Therefore, a high degree of bias can be involved. Narrative reviews have no formal rules other than to give an authoritative overview.

A systematic review however is meant to systematically provide the "best available evidence" to answer a focused clinical question. Scientific methods and rules do apply for systematic reviews in order to limit bias. As soon as the subject of a review is focused sufficiently to condense it to a single clinical question, one should apply the technology available to conduct systematic reviews.

Thus, depending on the situation, however, either a narrative review or a systematic review can be the best option. When a more comprehensive overview is needed, for instance, to understand the biological basis of a disease, the scope of a systematic review can be too narrow and preference can be given to a narrative review. Without the knowledge required to write narrative reviews on a subject, it may be impossible to ask the relevant clinical question that underlies a systematic review. Likewise, without this knowledge, it may be impossible to place the result of a systematic review in the context of the usual approach to the condition or disease. The term *meta-analysis* is often misunderstood. Although meta-analysis is sometimes indiscriminately interchanged with *systematic review*, this is not appropriate. Meta-analysis applies a statistical method to data retrieved from multiple studies in order to give a quantitative summary estimate of a (comparative) effect of treatment, for example. Only, if the data retrieved from these studies were the result of an adequately conducted systematic review, one can consider the effect-estimate resulting from this meta-analysis as representing the best available evidence.

So while the focus of this chapter will be on the science of systematic reviews emphasizing the availability of systematic reviews for clinical decision making, we should realize that in medical education and in practice both systematic and narrative reviews have their own appropriate place.

The clinical question

The key element of a systematic review in clinical medicine is the formulation of an answerable clinical question. Ultimately, the relevance of the results of a systematic review is determined by the clinical relevance of the question posed. A clinical question is often referred to by the abbreviation PICO(T) (see chapters 1, 2, and 4) (1,2), which stands for Patient/Population, Intervention, Comparison, Outcome, and Time. Each element should be as specific and realistic as possible. Systematic reviews primarily deal with questions regarding interventions. Research questions on other areas such as etiology, diagnosis, and prognosis can also be the focus of a systematic review (see chapter 6). The framework of PICO(T) still applies but requires modification. A clinically relevant scientific treatment question might thus be the following: "In patients with a carotid stenosis of 50% to 70%, does aspirin,

Evidence-based Hematology. Edited by Mark A. Crowther, Jeff Ginsberg, Holger J. Schünemann, Ralph M. Meyer, and Richard Lottenberg.

in a daily dosage of 30 to 50 mg compared with a dosage of 600 mg or more, reduce the occurrence of any stroke (ischemic, hemorrhagic, or undefined) during treatment periods of one year or longer?"

Structure of a systematic review

Systematic reviews are characterized by a series of steps that should be conducted with a certain methodological rigor. Following the definition of a focused clinical question a comprehensive and exhaustive search of the literature and other sources should then be undertaken to identify potentially relevant data for the systematic review question. Sometimes multiple searches are required to retrieve all available relevant articles or study reports. To minimize selection bias, at least two independent reviewers must assess the scientific quality of the selected studies. All data should be extracted in the same way, and exclusion criteria have to be documented. The validity of combining data should be assessed by looking at possible heterogeneity of outcomes. Homogeneous results can be combined statistically and presented in the form of a meta-analysis. Detailed instructions on how to perform a systematic review are available from a number of sources, in particular the Cochrane Collaboration (www.cochrane.org) (3,4,5). The Cochrane Collaboration, an independent, international not-for-profit organization, is dedicated to making up-to-date, accurate information about the effects of health care readily available worldwide. It produces and disseminates systematic reviews of healthcare interventions and promotes the search for evidence in the form of clinical trials and other studies of interventions. The major product of the collaboration is the *Cochrane Database of Systematic Reviews*, which is published quarterly as part of the Cochrane Library.

Literature search

To identify relevant publications, first search readily available, adequately indexed, and regularly updated databases of medical literature, such as Medline, PubMed, and EMBASE. However, small, negative trials frequently are not published, or they are published only after many perils. Therefore, there is a risk of publication bias, especially if only a limited number of relevant publications can be identified. Publication bias is associated with funnel plot asymmetry. Funnel plots are scatter plots of relative measures of treatment effect (relative risk, odds ratio) plotted on a logarithmic scale on the x-axis and the sample sizes or standard error on the y-axis. In the absence of bias, the plot should resemble an inverted funnel (see Figure 2.1) (6).

In particular, if publication bias is surmised, consider additional sources, such as conference abstracts, experts' personal databases, contact with for-profit and not-for-profit sponsors, and databases of regulatory authorities. A future source will be the databases

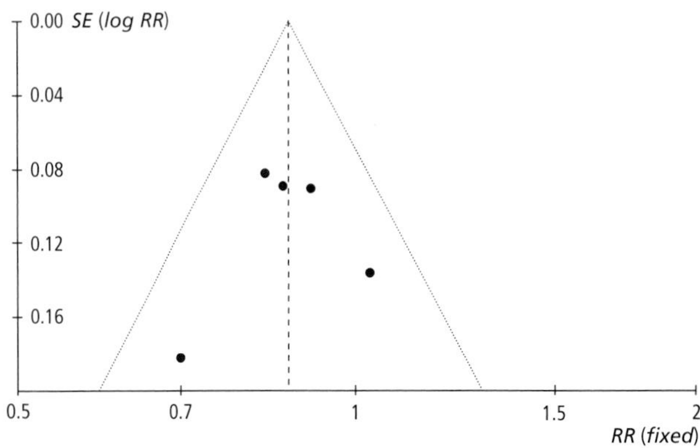

Figure 2.1 Inverted funnel plot for randomized controlled trials of parenteral anticoagulation in cancer patients from (6).

of central medical ethical committees and trial registries, such as www.clinicaltrials.gov.

In searching the databases of medical literature, include terms that identify the clinical question of interest as well as some methodological terms related to the type of clinical question of interest (see chapter 4). It is acceptable to search relatively narrowly to find a "best article" to answer the clinical question because the best articles are likely to be specifically indexed. For a systematic review, a broad search strategy is required because all relevant articles (i.e., bits of evidence) should be identified. The list of obtained references can then be reduced by manually reviewing titles and abstracts of articles for which the full text should be obtained, either because they are obviously relevant or because their irrelevance based on the frequently limited information available from title and abstract cannot be decided. The applied search strategy should be reported in detail. The process of manual review should be carried out by two independent researchers and the results of that process made transparent by reporting as described in the QUOROM statement (7). Box 2.1 reports an example of an adequate search strategy.

Selection of relevant articles

The selection of studies to be included in the final review should be made based on prespecified criteria for inclusion and exclusion. Usually, the inclusion criteria are directly based on the PICO(T), while the exclusion criteria are based on criteria for minimal methodology criteria (e.g., randomization, adequate population, independent assessment, or potential confounding effects). For each excluded study, report the reason for the exclusion.

Naturally, background knowledge of the field can help to adapt the exclusion criteria to an acceptable level. If, for example, the clinical question asked is (expected to be) only addressed in relatively

Box 2.1 Example of an adequate search

We searched electronic databases from 1985 until January 2006. These included MEDLINE, EMBASE, Cochrane Library, Google Scholar, epidemiological research Web sites, abstracts of scientific meetings, and bibliographies of relevant studies. The search terms were compiled from the names of individual drugs, the therapeutic class, mode of activity, cardiovascular and cerebrovascular outcome terms, and study design terms. We also searched on authors' names. Titles and abstracts of articles identified by the searches were reviewed by the authors. Searches were repeated using additional search terms identified from articles considered relevant to the review. From McGettigan P, Henry D. Cardiovascular risk and inhibition of cyclooxygenase: a systematic review of the observational studies of selective and nonselective inhibitors of cyclooxygenase 2. *JAMA*. 2006;**296**:1633–44.

old studies (or as a secondary question), it can be a realistic strategy to allow for clinical controlled trials with a concurrent control group, rather than to limit the acceptance of studies to those "truly randomized with adequate concealment of allocation." The strength of the conclusion and its consequent recommendation should be adapted to the quality of the underlying evidence.

Assessment of quality

An essential part of the result section of a systematic review is the systematic reporting of essential quality elements in the identified eligible studies. The absence of some quality items might also be used as an exclusion criterion. The choice is usually guided by prior knowledge of paucity or abundance of data in the field. For example, for studies on the prevention of deep vein thrombosis in orthopedic elective hip surgery, one could be likely to apply some important methodological criterion (e.g., venography assessed unaware of knowledge of treatment allocation) as an inclusion criterion; whereas for studies on the (secondary) prevention of thrombosis in patients with established heparin-induced thrombocytopenia one might be tempted to accept any evidence at hand. However, the latter policy will result in a weaker conclusion. The overall quality of evidence for the question addressed in the systematic review cannot surpass the quality of the original studies. Nevertheless, the broader, systematically reviewed evidence will better inform decision makers.

For therapeutic studies, important items of quality include, but are not limited to, randomization, adequate concealment of allocation, blinding (at least for assessment of outcomes), intention-to-treat analysis, and reports on all patients.

For diagnostic studies, important items of quality include assessment of the new test, independent of knowledge of the result of the reference test; performance of the reference test in all participants; study performance in an adequate population suspected of disease.

Occasionally, "quality scores" or "quality scales" are used to report on quality of methodology individual studies. These scales usually honor the presence of a quality item or a reporting item with some points. However, missing points could be due to an extremely relevant missing methodological issue (e.g., adequate concealment of allocation prior to randomization) or to one or more much less relevant issues (e.g., not reporting a power analysis and the fate of two patients in a trial of more than 10.000 patients with an outcome frequency of 10%). Hence, it is more important to focus on individual methodology items of high importance than to trust (and compare) overall quality scores. In fact, lack of usefulness of study level quality scores has been shown (4). In any case, if a scoring system is used, the scores for the individual items on the scale should be provided and results with and without the lower-quality studies should be compared.

Usually, two independent researchers assess the quality of individual studies. They discuss any discrepancy in their result (with a third person) to arrive at a consensus conclusion. Extracting data from individual studies follows a similar process.

Presentation of data and summary statistics

A final point is the presentation of the identified data (evidence) and if possible calculation of summary statistics using meta-analysis to assess therapeutic efficacy, harm, or diagnostic accuracy. Next to the table with information on the basic design and methodological quality of the identified studies, a summary presentation showing the results of the individual studies provides important information in a systematic review. In the summary statistics, which pool the results of each individual study (meta-analysis), each study can be seen as an individual data point or experiment. These summary statistics should provide both a point estimate and a 95% confidence interval. Figure 2.2 shows a forest plot, one of the frequently used graphic methods to show results of a meta-analysis (8).

Meta-analysis should only be performed when the results from the identified trials are consistent (7,9). Assessing homogeneity can be done by inspection of the graphical display of the individual studies in a forest plot (see Figure 2.2). If a significant heterogeneity is found (confidence intervals do not overlap), then the results of the studies should not be pooled. The play of chance should be ruled out by the application of a chi-square test or the calculation of I^2. I^2describes the proportion of total variation in study estimates due to heterogeneity rather than sampling error (chance). I^2 ranges from 0% to 100%, and a value greater than 50% may be considered substantial heterogeneity and should be explored (10). Whenever heterogeneity is found to be existent, an explanation for the heterogeneity should be provided. All choices made in a systematic review are based on assumptions and may therefore

Review: Anticoagulation for thrombosis prophylaxis in cancer patients with central venous catheters
Comparison: 03 Any Anticoagulant vs. Control
Outcome: 04 Symptomatic DVT

Study	Treatment n/N	Control n/N	Relative Risk (Random) 95% CI	Weight (%)	Relative Risk (Random) 95% CI
Abdelkefi 2004	1/38	5/36		5.2	0.19 [0.02, 1.54]
Bern 1990	4/54	13/54		17.0	0.31 [0.11, 0.88]
Heaton 2002	2/45	1/43		4.2	1.91 [0.18, 20.32]
Karthaus 2006	10/294	5/145		17.0	0.99 [0.34, 283]
Monreal 1996	1/16	5/13		5.6	0.16 [0.02, 1.22]
Verso 2005	2/155	6/155		8.7	0.33 [0.07, 1.63]
Young 2005	25/408	33/403		42.3	0.75 [0.45, 1.24]
Total (95% CI)	1010	849		100.0	0.56 [0.34, 0.92]

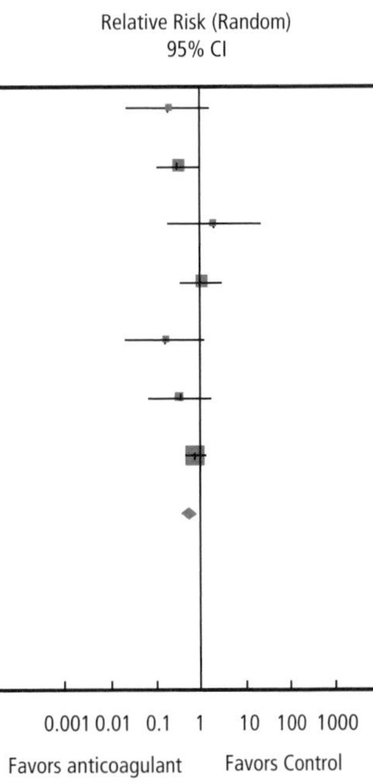

Total events: 45 (Treatment), 68 (Control)
Test for heterogeneity chi-square = 7.40 df = 6 p = 0.29 I^2 = 18.9%
Test for overall effect z = 2.30 p = 0.02

0.001 0.01 0.1 1 10 100 1000

Favors anticoagulant Favors Control

Figure 2.2 Forest plot and meta-analysis results of randomized trials comparing anticoagulant therapy to no therapy for the prevention of deep venous thrombosis related to central venous lines. The plot includes name of the study (identified by the first author and the year of publication), the number of events and patients in the treatment and control group, a graphical representation of the relative risk of each individual study together with the confidence interval, the relative weight of each study contributing to the overall effect measure and the numerical results for each individual study, and the overall estimate of effect. The total number of events and results of tests for heterogeneity are also given (see text). From (8).

influence the results. Sensitivity analysis, that is, performing separate pooled analysis after excluding some of the studies (for instance, those of lower methodological quality) can show that differences in effect exist between relevant studies.

Conclusion

Systematic reviews are essential for informed healthcare decisions and are often quoted as the highest-quality evidence. However, even if a systematic review is conducted according to the highest applicable standards , the evidence included in a systematic review can be weak. Hence, the strength of the conclusion of a systematic review and its use for developing recommendations will have to be based on this underlying quality and consistency of this evidence (see chapter 1). For this reason, it is crucial to understand whether a systematic review fulfills basic methodological criteria and what the quality of the underlying evidence is. Furthermore, the main conclusion of a systematic review should be based on the clinical question addressed in the review. Finally, as with all scientific results, this conclusion should be put into the current clinical perspective.

Glossary

Review The general term for all attempts to synthesize the results and conclusions on a given topic.

The following features of reviews could be distinguished:

Narrative review Authoritative overview on a given topic, based on results and conclusions available in the literature; this category typically does not include a method section and differs from the others in its methodological rigor.

Systematic review When a review strives to identify and track down all the literature following a protocol with detailed inclusion and exclusion criteria. The usual intent of this type of review is to provide complete and, if possible, quantitative information.

Meta-analysis A statistical method to summarize quantitatively evidence from individual studies (most sensible when applied in the context of systematic reviews). Sometimes used as a single term to indicate a quantitative, systematic review that includes a summary statistic as a whole.

References

1 Oxman AD, Sackett DL, Guyatt GH. Users' guides to the medical literature. I. How to get started: the Evidence-Based Medicine Working Group. *JAMA*. 1993;**270**(17):2093–95.

2 McKibbon A, Hunt D, Richardson SW, et al. Finding the evidence. In: Guyatt GH, Rennie D, editors. *Users' guides to the medical literature: a manual for evidence-based clinical practice*. Chicago: JAMA Press; 2002.

3 Higgins JPT, Green S, editors. *Cochrane handbook for systematic reviews of Interventions 4.2.5* [updated May 2005]. Chichester, UK; John Wiley & Sons; 2005. Cochrane Library No. 3.

4 Tallon D, Schneider M, Egger M. Quality of systematic reviews published in high impact general and specialist journals. In Proceedings of 2nd Symposium on Systematic Reviews: Beyond the Basics; Oxford; 1999.

5 Cook DJ, Mulrow CD, Haynes RB. Systematic reviews: synthesis of best evidence for clinical decisions. *Ann Int Med*. 1997;**126**:376–80.

6 Akl E, van Doormaal F, Barba M, et al. Parenteral anticoagulation for prolonging survival in patients with cancer who have no other indication for anticoagulation. *Cochrane Database Syst Rev* and *Chest*. 2007;**3**: CD006652, DOI: 10.1002/14651858, CD006652. *J Exp Clin Cancer Res*. 2007;**26**:175–86.

7 Moher D, Cook DJ, Eastwood S. Improving the quality of reports of meta-analysis of randomized controlled trials: the QUOROM statement. *Lancet*. 1999;**354**:1896–900.

8 Akl E, Karmath G, Yosuico V, et al. Anticoagulation for thrombosis prophylaxis in cancer patients with central venous catheters. *Cochrane Database Syst Rev* [Online]. Article CD006468.

9 Stroup DF, Berlin JA, Morton SC, et al. Meta-analysis of observational studies in epidemiology. The MOOSE guidelines. A proposal for reporting. *JAMA*. 2000;**283**:2008–12.

10 Higgins JP, Thompson SG. Quantifying heterogeneity in a meta-analysis. *Stat Med*. 2002;**21**(11):1539–58.

3 Interpreting Results in Clinical Research

Overview of measures of effect, measures of precision, and measures of diagnostic accuracy for clinicians and researchers

Marcello Di Nisio, Harry R. Büller, Patrick M. M. Bossuyt

Introduction

Judgments about the value of treatment strategies or diagnostic tests are largely based on clinicians' and researchers' critical appraisal of findings from clinical studies integrated with their individual clinical expertise (see chapter 5). Several studies have shown how interpretation of study results can be influenced by their presentation by researchers (1–4). Thus, the same data may lead to different conclusions, depending on what measures of effect or diagnostic accuracy are used (1–4).

The goal of this chapter is to familiarize readers with the most common indicators of treatment effect and diagnostic accuracy they encounter when reading a clinical study. The chapter has two main sections. In the first part, we discuss different ways of presenting and summarizing findings from clinical trials that evaluate a new intervention versus a control treatment. In the second part, we present indexes of diagnostic accuracy commonly used to summarize data from studies evaluating the ability of a diagnostic test to identify subjects with a target condition among those suspected for that condition.

Measures of effect

Relative risk, odds ratio, hazard ratio, and risk difference

One of the notions of risk is the probability of a (future) event, which can be estimated by dividing the number of people with the event by the total number of individuals in the group initially without the event. Odds are an alternative way to describe the possibility of suffering an event relative to those not having the event (Table 3.1).

In clinical trials, one can compare the risk in two groups: a control group receiving standard treatment and another group receiving the new intervention. The effect of the new intervention can be expressed as a relative change in suffering an event given the treatment, that is, either as relative risk (also called risk ratio) or odds ratio. These measures of effect can be expressed through simple mathematical formulas, presenting results in a 2×2 table such as in Tables 3.1 and 3.2 (5).

Table 3.1a shows data from a hypothetical clinical study evaluating thrombolysis versus heparin for the initial treatment in patients with hemodynamically unstable pulmonary embolism who are at high risk for fatal or non-fatal recurrent thrombosis during hospital stay. Thrombolytic treatment is associated with a 10% risk of such an event versus 20% in the group receiving heparin. The effect of thrombolytic treatment corresponds to a relative risk of 0.50 for recurrent venous thromboembolism or death during hospital stay. In other words, thrombolysis decreases the chance of having recurrent thrombosis by 50% relative to heparin.

This reduction is called *relative risk reduction*, which in mathematical terms is expressed by the equation (1–relative risk). The greater the relative risk reduction, the more efficacious the new intervention. The odds ratio for thrombolysis and heparin is 0.44, which indicates a lower chance of having the event with thrombolysis. In general, by convention, if the experimental treatment decreases the risk for an event, the relative risk and odds ratio are both smaller than 1. If it has an effect that is identical to that of the control treatment, the relative risk and the odds ratio are both unity. If it increases the chance of having the event, the relative risk and odds ratio exceed 1. However, this not consistently applied.

When evaluating a new intervention, clinical trials usually report on both the efficacy and safety of the experimental treatment. Table 3.1b shows the distribution of major bleeding events in the study group with hemodynamically unstable pulmonary embolism. The relative risk for major bleeding is 2, which indicates that thrombolysis increases the risk of major bleeding by 100% as compared to heparin. From Table 3.1b one can calculate an odds ratio of 2.25. Because of how they are calculated, odds ratios are farther away from unity than the corresponding relative risks. If the experimental treatment (in the present example thrombolysis) is associated with a lower event rate (recurrent pulmonary embolism

Evidence-based Hematology. Edited by Mark A. Crowther, Jeff Ginsberg, Holger J. Schünemann, Ralph M. Meyer, and Richard Lottenberg.

Table 3.1a Recurrent pulmonary embolism or death during hospital stay in a hypothetical trial in patients with hemodynamically unstable pulmonary embolism randomised to thrombolysis or heparin.

	Pulmonary embolism or death present	Pulmonary embolism or death absent	Total
Thrombolysis	20	180	200
Heparin	80	320	400
	50	550	600

Relative risk: (a/(a + b))/(c/(c + d)) = (20/200)/(80/400) = 0.10/0.20 = 0.50
Relative risk reduction: 1 − [(a/(a + b))/(c/(c + d))] = 1 − 0.50 = 0.50
Odds ratio: (a/b)/(c/d) = ad/bc = 0.44
Risk difference: (a/(a + b)) − (c/(c + d)) = 0.10 − 0.20 = −0.10
Number needed to treat: 1/[(a/(a + b)) − (c/(c + d))] = 1/0.05 = 10

Table 3.1b Major bleeding during hospital stay in a hypothetical trial in patients with hemodynamically unstable pulmonary embolism randomized to thrombolysis or heparin.

	Major bleeding present	Major bleeding absent	Total
Thrombolysis	40	160	200
Heparin	40	360	400
	80	520	600

Relative risk: (a/(a + b))/(c/(c + d)) = (40/200)/(40/400) = 0.20/0.10 = 2
Odds ratio: (a/b)/(c/d) = ad/bc = (40 × 360)/(40 × 160) = 2.25
Risk difference: (a/(a + b)) − (c/(c + d)) = 0.20 − 0.10 = 0.10
Number needed to harm: 1/[(a/(a + b)) − (c/(c + d))] = 1/0.10 = 10

Table 3.2a Recurrent pulmonary embolism or death during hospital stay in a hypothetical trial in patients with hemodynamically stable pulmonary embolism randomized to thrombolysis or heparin.

	Pulmonary embolism or death present	Pulmonary embolism or death absent	Total
Thrombolysis	5	195	200
Heparin	20	380	400
	25	575	600

Relative risk: (a/(a + b))/(c/(c + d)) = (5/200)/(20/400) = 0.025/0.05 = 0.50
Relative risk reduction: 1 − [(a/(a + b))/(c/(c + d))] = 1 − 0.50 = 0.50
Odds ratio: (a/b)/(c/d) = ad/bc = (5 × 380)/(20 × 195) = 0.49
Risk difference: (a/(a + b)) − (c/(c + d)) = 0.025 − 0.05 = −0.025
Number needed to treat: 1/(a/(a + b)) − (c/(c + d)) = 1/0.025 = 40

Table 3.2b Major bleeding during hospital stay in a hypothetical trial in patients with hemodynamically stable pulmonary embolism randomized to thrombolysis or heparin.

	Major bleeding present	Major bleeding absent	Total
Thrombolysis	4	196	200
Heparin	6	394	400
	10	590	600

Relative risk: (a/(a + b))/(c/(c + d)) = (4/200)/(6/400) = 0.02/0.015 = 1.33
Odds ratio: (a/b)/(c/d) = ad/bc = (4 × 394)/(6 × 196) = 1.34
Risk difference reduction: 1 − (a/(a + b))/(c/(c + d)) = 0.02 − 0.015 = 0.005
Number needed to harm: 1/(a/(a + b)) − (c/(c + d)) = 1/0.005 = 200

or death), both the odds ratio and the relative risk will be less than unity, with the former being smaller. Conversely, if the event rate (major bleeding) increases in the treatment group, the odds ratio and relative risk will both be greater than 1, with the odds ratio exceeding relative risk. Odds and relative risk are similar when the event rate is low, and if the risk is below 25%, odds and risks are approximately equal. On the other hand, if events are frequent in either the control or experimental group, odds ratios can sensibly differ from relative risk. Odds and relative risk also tend to be more alike when the treatment effect is small (both close to 1.0) than when the treatment effect is large.

An important limitation of the relative risk and the odds ratio is that results are expressed as a proportion of the control group. Thus, these effect indicators do not immediately determine the actual number of patients who have benefited. They do not distinguish large absolute treatment effects from small ones.

Let us consider a hypothetical trial comparing thrombolysis with heparin in a group at low risk: patients with hemodynamically stable pulmonary embolism (Table 3.2a). In this case, the risk of recurrent pulmonary embolism or death during hospital stay decreases from 5% in the heparin group to 2.5% with thrombolysis, giving a relative risk of 0.50. This relative risk is similar to the one calculated for patients with hemodynamically unstable pulmonary embolism. In this latter group, however, the risk of an event decreased from 20% in the heparin group to 10% with thrombolysis (Table 3.1a). Thus, while thrombolysis halves the risk in both cases, the actual change in number of events is very different.

Given the limitations of relative risk and odds ratio to relate differences in absolute terms, another concept, the difference in risk between two groups, can help clinicians evaluate the benefit or downsides of a treatment. The risk difference is calculated from the risk or event rate in the experimental group minus the risk in the control group. The risk difference is zero if the experimental intervention is associated with an event rate that is identical to that of the control. In the presented examples, the risk difference for thrombolysis versus heparin is 10% (20% minus 10%) in patients with hemodynamically unstable pulmonary embolism and 2.5% (5% minus 2.5%) in those that have hemodynamically stable pulmonary embolism, respectively (Figure 3.1).

Although relative risk and odds ratio might be similar or even identical across different risk groups, risk differences can differ

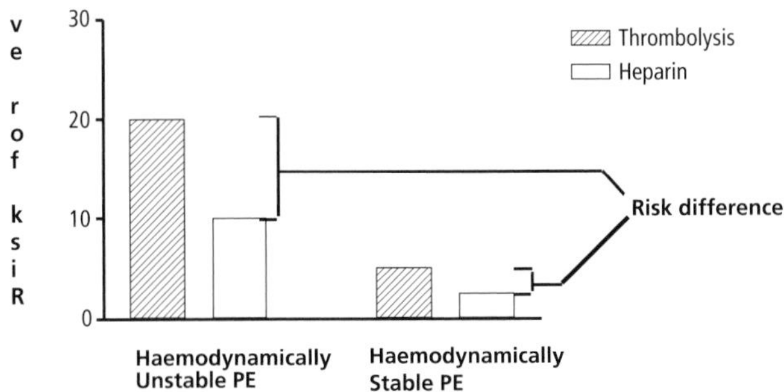

Figure 3.1 The relation between baseline risk and risk difference.

importantly. An intervention tested in high-risk patients may give remarkable results in terms of relative risk, odds reduction, and relative risk reduction, whereas in lower-risk patients despite similar relative risk and odds ratio, the risk difference (and the net benefit) can be substantially lower.

When it is calculated over a period of time, as in survival analysis, risk is better reported as a hazard: the instantaneous rate of the occurring event. The hazard (rate) ratio can then replace the relative risk and odds ratio. The hazard ratio is the risk of the event in the intervention group divided by the risk in the control group over a specific period. A hazard ratio above 1 indicates an increased risk and below 1 a decreased risk for the event in the intervention group as compared to the control group.

Measures of precision

When judging measures of effect, clinicians will encounter two measures related to an estimate's precision: p values and confidence intervals (6). The p value describes the probability of observing an effect as large or larger than that observed in a particular trial when the null hypothesis holds. In most cases, the null hypothesis specifies the absence of a treatment effect. Traditionally, p values less than 0.05 are considered statistically significant: that is, the hypothesis of no effect is judged to be ruled out. This value of 1 in 20 (probability of 0.05) has in fact nothing exclusive. It represents only a widely agreed upon cut-off value beyond which one believes the role of chance plays a much smaller role in evaluating effects and associations.

Returning to the first hypothetical trial on unstable pulmonary embolism, let us suppose that the relative risk of 0.5 is statistically significant, with an associated p value of 0.02. In other terms, if the effect of thrombolysis was identical to that of heparin, we could observe a relative risk of 0.50 or less in 2 out of 100 identical trials by the play of chance alone. The fact that an estimate is statistically significant ($p < 0.05$) does not exclude the play of chance, but it makes chance a much less likely explanation of the observed effect. However, given the cut-off value of 0.05, if a large number of studies on thrombolysis versus heparin in patients with hemodynamically unstable pulmonary embolism are carried out, 1 in 20 can be expected to show statistical significance by the play of chance alone. Thus, statistical significance of an estimate is not the only aspect to consider in interpreting the results of a study.

When deciding which one of two available treatments to use, one needs to know not only which therapy is more effective but also how *much* more effective it is compared to the other treatment. A finding that is statistically significant may be irrelevant to patients because the effect is small. This might happen because small differences of no clinical interest can be statistically significant with high event rates and large sample sizes, whereas patient-important effects might not be statistically significant only because the number of subjects studied was too small, or too few events occurred. p values fail to provide clinicians with the information they most need, that is, the range within which the true treatment effect might plausibly lie when considering trial data. Such information can be obtained from calculating confidence intervals, such as 95% confidence intervals.

Relative risk or odds ratios such as those calculated from Tables 3.1 and 3.2 constitute point estimates of the risk difference between thrombolysis and heparin. However, if the same study was repeated with a different group sampled from the same population, the calculated relative risks or odds ratios would be similar but unlikely identical, just because of the chance variation between samples. However, if one would repeat the study several times, in the long run, 95% of the calculated confidence intervals would include the true value. We can deduce that there is a 95% chance that the confidence interval calculated for a single study includes the true value. Confidence intervals are distinct directly but related to p values in a way that, in general, if $p < 0.05$, the 95% confidence interval for the estimate will not include unity (for relative risk or odds ratio) or zero (for risk difference). Under these circumstances, a study can be considered statistically significant.

In general, larger sample sizes but, more important, a larger number of events gives more precise results, with narrower confidence intervals. Conversely, small studies, in particular those with few events, will produce wide confidence intervals, making the conclusions less reliable. To decide whether confidence intervals are sufficiently narrow to recommend for or against the therapy, clinicians need to think about the smallest amount of benefit for their patient that would justify the new therapy. When a study, such as our hypothetical trial on patients with hemodynamically unstable pulmonary embolism, shows a lower risk with the new intervention, consider the upper boundary of the confidence interval, which represents the smallest plausible treatment effect compatible with the results.

Suppose that the 95% confidence interval of the relative risk for the event ranges from 0.20 to 0.95. The upper boundary of the interval indicates a 5% reduction in relative risk. The fact that it is in the interval implies that it cannot be excluded at a 5% significance level. If the 5% reduction is greater than the smallest benefit considered important for a patient, the conclusions of this trial might be regarded as acceptable. If, on the contrary, 5% is smaller than the smallest benefit considered important for the patient, uncertainty remains about whether the use of thrombolysis in this group of patients is beneficial, and the trial cannot be considered definitive.

For studies showing no significant effect of a new intervention, focus on the lower boundary of the confidence interval representing the largest plausible treatment effect that cannot be excluded at the 0.05 significance level with the trial data. If it falls below the smallest difference considered important for the patient, the findings of the trial can be regarded as negative. Conversely, if the lower boundary exceeds the smallest patient-important difference, then the trial is not conclusive, and more trials with larger sample sizes are needed.

Confidence intervals can be especially valuable in cases in which the estimated treatment effect is small. In these circumstances, confidence intervals indicate where patient-important treatment benefit remains plausible and may prevent clinicians from mistakenly interpreting a lack of evidence of effectiveness as evidence of no effect.

Number needed to treat and number needed to harm

Some studies present their results as number needed to treat (NNT) or the number needed to harm (NNH). The NNT represents the number of patients to whom a clinician has to administer a particular treatment over a given time period to prevent one additional patient from having the event of interest. In mathematical terms, the NNT represents the inverse of the risk difference, which means that if risk difference is large the NNT will be low. If the risk difference is presented as a difference in percentages, the NNT will be 100 divided by the risk difference.

Returning to the hypothetical trial on patients with hemodynamically unstable pulmonary embolism, one can calculate the NNT from the data in Table 3.1A. Since the risk difference is 10%, the NNT is 10 (100/10), which indicates that 10 patients have to be given thrombolysis rather than heparin to prevent one death or pulmonary embolism during hospital stay. In patients with hemodynamically stable pulmonary embolism, the NNT is 40 (100/2.5), indicating that 40 patients need to receive thrombolysis to avoid one additional event in one of them.

Like the risk difference, the NNT might help to identify substantial differences between treatments, when relative risk or odds ratios are similar. To appreciate the relevance of a treatment or prophylactic intervention, the NNT has to be considered with the NNH, which represents the number of patients who would have to receive the treatment over a given time for one of them to experience one additional adverse effect.

Many clinicians are not too familiar with NNT and NNH, and they may find these summary estimates difficult to interpret. It can be challenging to determine the NNT that is acceptable to justify the benefits and risks of a specific therapy. Determinants of such a threshold NNT are related to the NNH, patient preferences, the severity of the outcome that can be prevented, and the costs of the intervention (7). An important issue for applying results is to determine the extent to which the patient who is to receive the intervention is comparable to those included in the study from which NNT was derived.

Measures of diagnostic accuracy

Researchers and clinicians use tests that are usually referred to as "diagnostic"—including imaging and biochemical technologies, pathological and psychological investigations, and signs and symptoms elicited during history taking and physical examination (8) —for purposes other than diagnosis. These purposes include identifying physiological abnormalities, helping establish prognosis, and monitoring progression of illness. This section focuses primarily on the use of tests for diagnoses. To use a diagnostic test in clinical practice, clinicians need to know how well a test helps to determine whether a patient has a suspected disease. An ideal diagnostic test would give negative results in all patients without the disease and would be positive in all patients with the disease. Unfortunately, this is often not the case, and most diagnostic tests cannot definitely distinguish between diseased and not diseased subjects.

To be regarded as clinically useful, a diagnostic test should be able to change the pretest probability of having or not having the disease into a posttest probability that is sufficiently different to help the diagnostic process. Clinicians can deduce pretest clinical probabilities from their own experience with similar clinical cases, although this approach might lead to biases and error. Better estimates can be derived from cohort studies in representative populations, which apply standard reference tests and possibly report the frequency of diagnosis in subgroups with peculiar clinical or laboratory features. If the diagnostic test results do not alter the posttest probabilities to a large extent, further testing might be necessary for the clinician to reach a final diagnosis.

Measures of diagnostic accuracy such as likelihood ratios, sensitivity, specificity, and predictive values can be calculated through simple mathematical formulas from a 2×2 table reporting study results (Table 3.3)(9).

Furthermore, clinicians often administer diagnostic tests as a package. For example, clinicians managing patients with suspected deep vein thrombosis may choose to go directly to high-resolution chest CT or, alternatively, ask the patient to first undergo ultrasound of the legs and D-dimer testing. Testing may involve an implied sequence in which an initial sensitive but nonspecific test, if positive, is followed by a more specific test. Thus, one can often think of evaluating or recommending not a single test but a diagnostic strategy.

Those giving advice to clinicians about the use of diagnostic tests should clearly establish the purpose of the diagnostic test or strategy under consideration. This process should begin with determining the standard diagnostic pathway—or pathways—for the target-patient presentation and identify their associated limitations. Knowing the limitations, the panel can then identify the particular limitations for which the alternative offers a putative

Table 3.3 Diagnostic accuracy of the D-dimer test in patients with suspected venous thromboembolism. Data are taken from reference (9).

	Venous thromboembolism present	Venous thromboembolism absent	Total
D-dimer positive	77	171	248
D-dimer negative	6	193	199
	83	364	447

Sensitivity: $a/(a + c) = 93$
Specificity: $d/(b + d) = 53$
Negative predictive value: $d/(c + d) = 97$
Positive predictive value: $a/(a + b) = 31$
Negative likelihood ratio: (1-sensitivity)/specificity = 0.14
Positive likelihood ratio: sensitivity/(1-specificity) = 2
Prevalence: $(a + c)/(a + b + c + d) = 83/447 = 0.18$

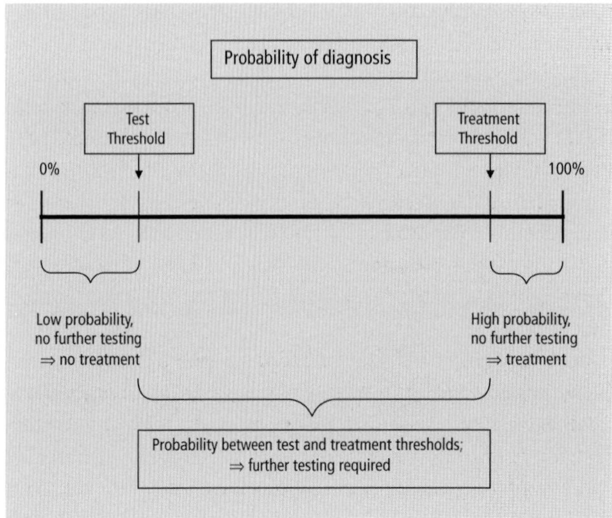

Figure 3.2 Test and treatment thresholds.

remedy (e.g., eliminating a high proportion of false positive or negative results, enhancing availability, decreasing invasiveness, decreasing cost). In doing so, guideline panels should develop sensible clinical questions. Similar to other clinical management problems, questions related to diagnosis have four components: patients, diagnostic intervention, comparison, and the outcomes of interest (5). Box 3.1 shows an example.

Test accuracy is a surrogate for patient important outcomes

Usually, when clinicians think about diagnostic tests, they focus on their accuracy. Investigations can elucidate the tests likelihood ratios, which provide one informative way of moving from pretest to posttest probability. Depending on a patient's pretest probability and the likelihood ratio associated with a test result, each test result generates a particular posttest probability.

That posttest probability will fall into one of three ranges (Figure 3.2) (8). If the posttest probability is high enough, it falls above what we call the treatment threshold, and allows the clinician to make a diagnosis and treat the patient accordingly (Figure 3.2). If the posttest probability is low enough, the result falls below what we call the test threshold, and the clinician rejects the diagnosis and moves on to other possibilities (Figure 3.2). If the posttest probability falls between the test and treatment threshold, further testing is indicated (Figure 3.2).

Box 3.1

In patients suspected of coronary artery disease, does multislice spiral computed tomography of coronary arteries compared with conventional invasive coronary angiography accurately diagnose coronary artery disease and affect patient important outcomes?

Clinicians do not, however, order tests simply to modify probabilities. The underlying assumption is that by getting a better idea of whether a target condition is present or absent, patient management and ultimately patient outcome will improve. If a test accurately moves patients from the mid-range of probability in which further testing is required over either the test or treatment threshold, we anticipate that uncertainty decreases and clinicians can recommend effective treatment or confidently withhold toxic but ineffective treatment. If the test fails to improve accuracy, but decreases morbidity associated with an invasive test it still may be of net benefit.

Finally, a test may benefit patients not by resulting in better use of effective treatment or reducing complications but by decreasing the psychological burden associated with uncertainty. Consider, for instance, genetic testing for Huntington's chorea, which either leaves the patient with huge relief that he will not suffer from the condition, or able to plan for his future knowing that he will sadly fall victim. If these happy results do not follow from use of a test—that is, the test fails to improve patient important outcomes— there would be no reason to use the test, whatever its accuracy.

From an understanding that the real purpose of a test is to improve patient outcomes flows the realization that the ideal way to assess a diagnostic strategy is a controlled trial in which patients are randomized to the experimental or control diagnostic approaches. For example, a randomized trial explored whether additional diagnostic testing can be safely withheld in patients with suspected pulmonary embolism who have negative erythrocyte agglutination D-dimer test results (10). As it turned out, the group randomized to receive no further testing if the D-dimer test result was negative did not have a higher rate of complications.

However, head-to-head comparisons of alternative testing strategies that measure the impact on patient-important outcomes are rarely available. In these situations, assessment of test measurement properties—that is, ideally, their likelihood ratios—and their complications provide indirect evidence concerning the likelihood of patient benefiting.

The greater the accuracy of the test, the greater the probability that it will increase desirable outcomes and decrease undesirable ones. Multilevel likelihood ratios provide the optimal approach to application of diagnostic tests, although the impact of the test will depend on the distribution of pretest probabilities in the target population. Unfortunately, an approach capable of dealing with the complexities of the full distribution of test results is not available, and the possible distributions of pretest probability in the patient population are rarely known. A simplified approach that classifies test results into yielding true positives (patients correctly classified above the treatment threshold; Figure 3.2), false positives (patients incorrectly classified above the treatment threshold), true negatives (patients correctly classified below the treatment threshold), and false negatives (patients incorrectly classified below the treatment threshold) is appropriate.

Inferring from accuracy data that a diagnostic test or strategy improves patient-important outcome requires the availability of efficacious treatment that can be administered to patients above the treatment threshold. Alternatively, evidence of fewer test-related side effects or evidence that exclusion of a disease, its confirmation, or its classification for prognostic purposes improves patient well-being may be adequate to infer benefit.

Likelihood ratios

Likelihood ratios contrast the proportions of patients with and without the target disorder who have a specific diagnostic test result. In other terms, the likelihood ratio expresses the probability that a diagnostic test result can be expected in a patient with the target disorder, relative to those without the target disorder. In practice, likelihood ratios can indicate by how much a given diagnostic test will raise or lower the pretest probability of the target disorder.

Table 3.3 shows data from a study evaluating the use of the D-dimer test in the diagnostic work-up of patients with suspected venous thromboembolism (9). The examples show that a positive D-dimer is found in 93% of patients with venous thromboembolism and 47% patients without the disorder, which means that an abnormal D-dimer result is about two times as likely (93%, 47%) to be seen in someone with venous thromboembolism than in someone without it. This ratio is called *positive likelihood ratio.* Likelihood ratios above 1.0 indicate an increased probability that the disorder is present, the higher the likelihood ratio the greater the increase. Likelihood ratios below 1.0 decrease the probability of the target disorder, and the smaller the likelihood ratio, the greater is the decrease in probability.

The negative likelihood ratio can be calculated in a similar fashion. The D-dimer is normal in 7% of patients with venous thromboembolism and 53% of those without the disease, resulting in a negative likelihood ratio of 0.14. Thus, a normal D-dimer value is approximately 7 times more likely in patients without venous thromboembolism.

Likelihood ratios may also vary with changes in disease severity. Higher likelihood ratios can be observed in later stages of florid disease, and lower likelihood ratios in early, mild stages.

One of the most interesting properties of likelihood ratios is that they can be used to calculate the posttest probability of a target disorder. Once the pretest probability is known, posttest odds can be derived by multiplying pretest odds by the likelihood ratio. An easy way to calculate posttest probability is the use of nomograms (5). An advantage of likelihood ratios is that they can be easily calculated for different levels of a quantitative test result. This makes likelihood ratios efficient measures of diagnostic accuracy when tests have more than two possible results (8). In contrast, sensitivity and specificity require a cut-off point, which is decided often arbitrarily, need to be recalculated for any cut-off point, and most importantly, might discard important information by simply dichotomizing a test result as positive or negative. We will provide a further description of how pretest probability, posttest probability and likelihood ratios help us making decisions in clinical practice in chapter 6 ("Using Evidence to Guide the Diagnosis of Disease").

Sensitivity, specificity, and predictive values

The sensitivity of a diagnostic test is the proportion of patients with the target disorder who have a positive test, whereas specificity is the proportion of patients who do not have the target disorder and who have a negative test result.

In the example in Table 3.3, the sensitivity of the D-dimer test in this population is 93%, which indicates that 93% (77/83) of patients with thrombosis had a positive D-dimer test (true positives), whereas 7% with a confirmed diagnosis of venous thromboembolism had a normal D-dimer result (false negatives). Fifty-three percent of the 364 patients without the event had normal D-dimer test result (true negatives), yielding a specificity of 53%. Forty-seven percent of the patients had a positive test result despite no objective evidence of the target condition (false positives).

When a test has a very high sensitivity, a negative result effectively rules out the diagnosis. Similarly, when a test has a very high specificity, a positive result effectively rules in the diagnosis. With its high sensitivity, the D-dimer test represents in fact an excellent noninvasive tool in patients with suspected venous thromboembolism. A normal D-dimer test in fact excludes the diagnosis in patients at low-clinical probability avoiding further costly imaging testing (11). When interpreting the accuracy of a diagnostic test, the spectrum of disease within a study population needs to be considered because this could affect the test performance. If a clinically inappropriate population has been chosen to evaluate a diagnostic test, the study results will not apply (12). A test can perform better when it is used to evaluate patients with more severe disease than with patients whose disease is less advanced and less obvious. With a relatively more severe form of the disease, the tests used to diagnose it are likely to be relatively more sensitive because of the extension and severity of signs or symptoms.

The main concern for clinicians using a diagnostic test is the meaning they can attribute to positive or negative results of the test or, in other words, the probability that a negative result indicates true absence of the disease and a positive result indicates its true presence. The negative predictive value (NPV) represents the proportion of patients with negative test results who do not have the target disorder, whereas the positive predictive value (PPV) is the proportion of patients with positive test results who have the target disorder. Predictive values are even more strongly influenced by changes in prevalence in the population studied than sensitivity and specificity. Higher prevalence results in a higher proportion of patients with a positive test result who do in fact have the disease for which they are being tested. In general, as prevalence falls, PPV falls along with it, and NPV rises.

In the example above, 97 patients out of 100 with a normal D-dimer result do not have an objectively confirmed diagnosis of venous thrombosis, which gives a NPV of 0.97. Thus, a normal D-dimer test result is quite reliable for excluding the diagnosis. In contrast, the PPV is 0.31, that is, only 31 patients out of 100 with a positive D-dimer have indeed venous thromboembolism, whereas 69 patients with a positive D-dimer do not have the disease. The low PPV might be explained by the fact that several other disorders cause high D-dimer values, which obviously limits the use of the test to rule in the diagnosis (13). Confidence intervals can also be similarly calculated for diagnostic accuracy indexes.

Conclusions

Physicians who strive to practice evidence-based medicine need to become familiar with estimates such as relative risk, risk difference, sensitivity and specificity, predictive values, and likelihood ratios. They will come across these measures in individual studies and in meta-analyses.

We have provided a condensed guide on how to interpret these measures of effect and diagnostic accuracy results in clinical research. For an overall quality judgment of a clinical study and its conclusions, clinicians and researchers need to integrate these notions with a critical appraisal of the methodological aspects of the study (8).

References

1 Forrow L, Taylor WC, Arnold RM. Absolutely relative: how research results are summarized can affect treatment decisions. *Am J Med.* 1992;**2**:121–24.

2 Naylor CD, Chen E, Strauss B. Measured enthusiasm: does the method of reporting trial results alter perceptions of therapeutic effectiveness? *Ann Intern Med.* 1992;**117**(11):916–21.

3 Fahey T, Griffiths S, Peters TJ. Evidence based purchasing: understanding results of clinical trials and systematic reviews. *BMJ.* 1995;**311**: 1056–59.

4 Montori VM, Jaeschke R, Schünemann HJ, et al. Users' guide to detecting misleading claims in clinical research reports. *BMJ.* 2004;**329**:1093–96.

5 Sackett DL, Straus SE, Richardson WS, et al., editors. *Evidence-based medicine: how to practice and teach EBM.* Churchill Livingstone: New York; 2000.

6 Altman DG, Machin D, Bryant TN, et al., editors. *Statistics with confidence.* Bristol: JW Arrowsmith; 2002.

7 Sinclair JC, Cook RJ, Guyatt GH, Pauker SG, Cook DJ. When should an effective treatment be used? Derivation of the threshold number needed to treat and the minimum event rate for treatment. *J Clin Epidemiol.* 2001;**54**(3):253–62.

8 Guyatt GH, Rennie D. *Users' guide to the medical literature: a manual for evidence-based clinical practice.* Chicago: AMA Press; 2002.

9 Di Nisio M, Sohne M, Kamphuisen PW, et al. D-dimer test in cancer patients with suspected acute pulmonary embolism. *J Thromb Haemost.* 2005;**3**(6):1239–42.

10 Kearon C, Ginsberg JS, Douketis J, et al. An evaluation of D-dimer in the diagnosis of pulmonary embolism: a randomized trial. *Ann Intern Med.* 2006;**144**(11):812–21.

11 Wells PS, Owen C, Doucette S, et al. Does this patient have deep vein thrombosis? *JAMA.* 2006;**295**:199–207.

12 Whiting P, Rutjes AWS, Reitsma JB, et al. Sources of variation and bias in studies of diagnostic accuracy: a systematic review. *Ann Intern Med.* 2004;**140**:189–202.

13 Kelly J, Rudd A, Lewis RR, et al. Plasma D-dimers in the diagnosis of venous thromboembolism. *Arch Intern Med.* 2002;**162**:747–56.

Measures of Effect: Definitions

Relative risk:	risk of the event in one group divided by the risk of the event in the other group. If an experimental intervention has an identical effect to the control, the relative risk will be 1. If it reduces the chance of having the event, the relative risk will be less than 1; if it increases the chance of having the event, the relative risk will be bigger than 1.
Relative risk reduction:	(1–relative risk)
Risk difference:	risk in the experimental group minus risk in the control group. If the experimental intervention has an identical effect to the control, the risk difference will be 0. If it reduces the risk, the risk difference will be lower than 0. If it increases the risk, the risk difference will be higher than 0. The risk difference cannot be above 1 or below −1.

(*Continued.*)

Measures of Effect: Definitions	
Odds ratio:	odds of the event occurring in one group divided by the odds of the event occurring in the other group. If an experimental intervention has an identical effect to the control, the odds ratio will be 1. If it reduces the chance of having the event, the odds ratio will be less than 1; if it increases the chance of having the event, the odds ratio will be bigger than 1.
Hazard ratio:	relative risk of an event over a period of time. The hazard ratio above 1 indicates an increased risk and below 1 a decreased risk for the event in the intervention group as compared to the control group.
Number needed to treat:	number of patients who have to be treated with the experimental treatment rather than the control treatment in order to prevent one patient from having an adverse outcome over a predefined period of time. The number needed to treat is the inverse of the risk difference reduction.
Number needed to harm:	the number of patients who have to be treated with the experimental treatment rather than the control treatment in order to cause an adverse event to one patient over a predefined period of time.

Measures of Diagnostic Accuracy: Definitions	
Sensitivity:	proportion of patients with the target disorder who have positive test.
Specificity:	proportion of patients who do not have the target disorder who have negative (normal) test results.
Negative predictive value:	proportion of patients with negative test results who do not have the target disorder.
Positive predictive value:	proportion of patients with positive test results who have the target disorder.
Likelihood ratio:	probability that a given diagnostic test result is seen in a patient with the target disorder, relative to the probability of observing that result in a patient without the target disorder.

4 Finding the Evidence in Hematology

K. Ann McKibbon, Cynthia J. Walker-Dilks, R. Brian Haynes

All clinicians, including hematologists, know firsthand the challenges of implementing evidence-based practice. The areas of leukemia and lymphoma treatment and venous thromboembolism have been studied in high-quality randomized controlled trials, but keeping up with the flow of new studies and their nuances of application can be difficult. Hematologists also treat many conditions that lack a well-developed evidence base for which defining "current best evidence" is problematic. The commonly cited barriers to practicing evidence-based medicine include the time required to find and review literature, duplication of effort by individual hematologists seeking the same information, and lack of relevant studies in common areas of hematology practice (1).

The growth in information resources over the past decade has been both a blessing and a curse—a blessing because an astounding amount of information is online, often freely available, and clinicians can search for what they need from just about anywhere. However, this array of choices can quickly become a curse and recalls the first commonly cited barrier: time. How does one quickly and reliably find the resources really useful to one's own practice? Many resources falsely claim to be "evidence based" or "one-stop shopping." What of the potentially useful resources you don't know about?

We start this chapter with three questions that hematologists often encounter as they care for patients. We then talk about the kinds of resources that potentially could be used to provide evidence to answer them. After this discussion of resources, we then proceed to use examples to find this evidence. The questions are first, a diagnosis question on what is the best way to triage assessment of suspected deep venous thrombosis (DVT). The second and third are treatment questions: Is erythropoietin or darbepoetin effective for anemia related to cancer? Can prophylactic transfusions be stopped in children with sickle cell disease? While reading the following sections, try to think which ones we will choose to provide evidence to help answer the three questions.

Evidence-based Hematology. Edited by Mark A. Crowther, Jeff Ginsberg, Holger J. Schünemann, Ralph M. Meyer, and Richard Lottenberg.
 ISBN: 978-1-4051-5747-6.

We proposed a "4S" model for the organization of evidence-based information services (2) and have recently updated it to a "5S" model (3). The model is hierarchical and begins with original *studies* at the foundation, followed by *syntheses* (that is, systematic reviews such as Cochrane reviews), *synopses* (brief descriptions of original studies and reviews such as appear in evidence-based abstract journals often accompanied by expert commentaries), *summaries* (management options for diseases or conditions arranged by clinical topics as appear in *Clinical Evidence*, PIER, and other evidence-based textbooks), and *systems* (integrated decision support services; Figure 4.1). Information seekers are encouraged to begin their search as high up in the pyramid as possible because this strategy will generally save time and labor. Why try and synthesize several individual studies found in MEDLINE when a chapter on the relevant topic has been done in a dynamic textbook?

With clinical examples, this chapter will follow the "5S" model to explore some resources that are useful to the practice of hematology.

Systems

A system integrates published evidence from high-quality studies and reviews with patient-specific information as found in medical records. Clinicians can call up external evidence while viewing the electronic medical record to assist in understanding a particular patient's situation and in making decisions. Some prototypes are currently available (4), such as systems that assist in anticoagulation dosing. One computer application of dosing adjustment reduced hospital length of stay compared with usual care when warfarin was initiated for hospital inpatients (5). Another program regulated heparin dosing after patients with myocardial infarction were treated with thrombolytics. Patients who received computer dosing had a lower rate of cardiovascular events (6). We are unaware of any systems that cover all areas of hematology, but progress in electronic medical records overall will expedite development in this area.

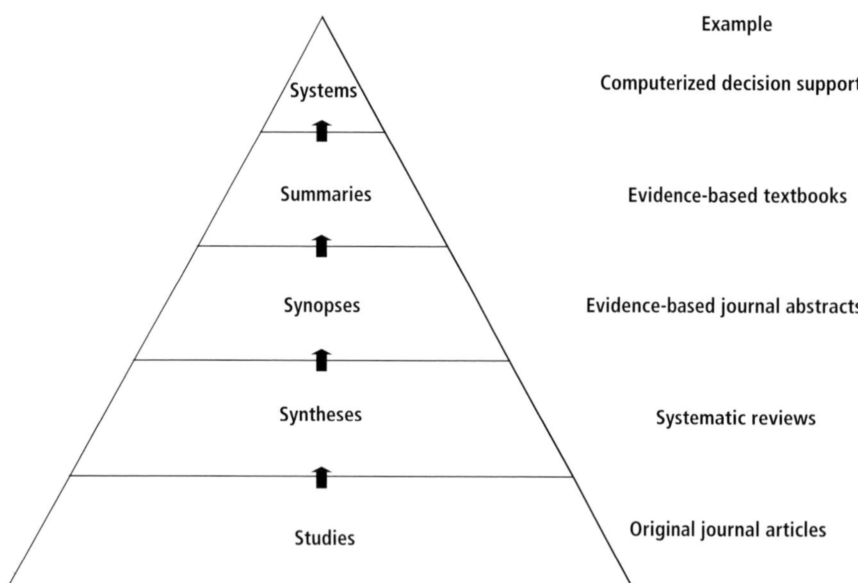

Figure 4.1 The "5S" levels of organization of evidence from healthcare research (3). (Reproduced with permission of the American College of Physicians.)

Summaries

This level of the evidence pyramid summarizes the information around a clinical topic. These may be disease-specific textbooks, such as this one, or *Evidence-Based Endocrinology* (7) or *Evidence-Based Diabetes Care* (8), which are print-based textbooks, often with a CD-ROM version of the book that is searchable. However, unless they have an accompanying Web site that provides updates to the content, textbooks can quickly become out of date. Internet-based textbooks can be useful if they integrate evidence-based information around specific clinical topics and are regularly updated. *Clinical Evidence* (9), from the BMJ Publishing Group, summarizes evidence on benefits and harms of healthcare interventions for selected medical conditions, the evidence being drawn from systematic reviews and original studies. UpToDate (10) is much more comprehensive in its topic coverage, including areas of inquiry beyond treatment and prevention, and makes specific recommendations for patient care according to "quality of evidence," but the review process is not fully explicit or systematic yet. The American College of Physicians Physicians' Information and Education Resource (PIER) (11) is an integrated summary service that provides evidence-based guidance and practice recommendations for clinicians. It is organized into five topic types (diseases, screening and prevention, complementary and alternative medicine, ethical and legal issues, and procedures), with each topic containing several modules, and its authors are supported by an explicit evidence-based process. A popular electronic summary is FIRSTConsult (12), from Elsevier, which delivers updated, evidence-based guidance on patient evaluation, diagnosis, and management directed at primary care clinicians. Information is arranged around the components of differential diagnosis, medical topics, patient education, and procedures. Although it draws on strongly evidence-based sources such as *Cochrane Database of Systematic Reviews* and *Clinical Evidence* to compile its recommendations, levels of evidence or links to supporting evidence do not accompany each recommendation. A feature of FIRSTConsult is that it can be connected to electronic medical records through the iCONSULT clinical decision support system. Two additional collections of information resources to keep in mind are STAT!Ref (13) and MDConsult (14). Both products offer searching across multiple resources from one site that include, but are by no means restricted to, electronic textbooks and journals. Unfortunately, these resources do not provide for explicit evidence processing or updating.

Synopses

The next best place to search for answers to clinical questions is in synopses of systematic reviews and individual studies. Synopses are structured abstracts or brief digests of published studies and reviews that have been screened for methodological soundness. This allows the reader to reap the benefits of a labor-intensive screening process that assesses the rigor of the evidence presented. The studies and reviews selected are usually those felt by the editors to warrant attention and to influence practice. Some of these evidence-based abstract journals that contain studies relevant to hematology include *ACP Journal Club*, *Evidence-Based Medicine*, *Journal Watch*, and *Bandolier*. An important feature is that the synopses are brief and take just a few minutes to read, and most are available on the Web. A list of resources (with hotlinks) from the synopsis level of the pyramid is available at www.ebmny.org/journal.html.

Syntheses

When no synopsis can be found or more detail is needed than a structured abstract contains, systematic reviews provide syntheses of the highest-quality evidence available on a specific clinical question. Systematic reviews detail the sources searched for gathering the evidence (e.g., databases searched, references checked for relevant studies, and meeting proceedings reviewed), the methods followed for including and excluding studies (e.g., randomized placebo-controlled trials with >6 months of follow-up to answer a question about treatment of hemophilia), and methodological and statistical justification for combining (meta-analysis) or not combining studies. As numbers of individual studies grow, so too do systematic reviews. One of the most notable compilations of systematic reviews is the Cochrane Database of Systematic Reviews (CDSR), part of the Cochrane Library (15). The Cochrane Collaboration consists of several review groups that concentrate on specific healthcare areas. The Cochrane Haematological Malignancies Group (www.chmg.de/) prepares and maintains systematic reviews of healthcare interventions in the area of defined hematological malignancies using predominantly randomized controlled trial evidence. As well as developing and updating Cochrane reviews, the Cochrane Library also hosts databases that contain abstracts of other systematic reviews (Database of Abstracts of Reviews of Effects [DARE]), individual clinical trials (Cochrane Central Register of Controlled Trials), technology assessments (Health Technology Assessment Database), and economic evaluations (U.K. NHS Economic Evaluation Database). The Cochrane Collaboration prepares less than half of the world's supply of systematic reviews; Cochrane Reviews and reviews published in journals and by major technology assessment agencies can be accessed through bmjupdates$^+$ (16), a free service, and Ovid's Evidence-Based Medicine Reviews (EBMR) (17), which provides for simultaneous searching across a number of evidence-based resources, including synopses (*ACP Journal Club*), syntheses (CDSR and DARE), and original studies (MEDLINE).

Studies

When none of the upper layers of the pyramid yield an answer to your question, it's time to look for individual studies. Fortunately, this is not as daunting as it once was. Most searching interfaces for bibliographic databases are easy to use, requiring no knowledge of controlled vocabulary, searching protocol, or other knowledge obtained from search manuals or help screens. bmjupdates$^+$ provides access to scientifically sound and relevant studies published in over 120 premier clinical journals. MEDLINE, the largest biomedical database, is accessible through PubMed directly from the producer, the U.S. National Library of Medicine. MEDLINE currently has over 16 million citations, so being able to search efficiently and find what you're looking for is important.

The Clinical Queries screen in PubMed

The Web site www.ncbi.nlm.nih.gov/entrez/query/static/clinical.shtml contains ready-to-use search strategies that filter retrieval for methodologically sound studies on topics of therapy, diagnosis, etiology, prognosis, and clinical prediction (18). There are also filters for systematic reviews, qualitative studies, and health services research topics. Such an interface requires that the searcher only enters basic content information (e.g., leukemia and stem cell), and the methodology "hedge" takes care of the methodological refining.

Another method for finding or keeping up to date with the research literature is to let it come to you. Alerting systems that target articles to individual clinicians according to their clinical discipline include bmjupdates$^+$ (16) and MEDSCAPE Best Evidence alerts (19). By filling in an interest profile, adjusted for how much you want to see, you are sent e-mail alerts about new evidence that contain links to the citation in PubMed and full text if available, plus clinical ratings and comments from other clinicians. Clinicians with interest in a specific clinical problem can also search a continuously updated cumulative bibliographic database of methodologically screened studies and reviews in bmjupdates$^+$. My NCBI (www.ncbi.nlm.nih.gov/books/bv.fcgi?rid=helppubmed.section. pubmedhelp.My_NCBI) provides a similar service, sending you new citations from MEDLINE on clinical areas you value. This service is broader than bmjupdates$^+$ (16), but you will need to critically appraise the evidence yourself.

Clinical Questions

We now move to using some of the resources described above to answer the three clinical questions listed at the start of the chapter.

Question 1. Triage of DVT

You are a general internist who works shifts in the emergency department. You are starting to question your approach to diagnosing symptomatic DVT based on your interactions with the D-dimer test kit salespeople, the new residents, and recent studies you have read. You assign one of the residents to read a new health technology assessment of noninvasive testing strategies for DVT (20) and to be ready to present her findings at the next unit journal club. You looked briefly at the 180-page document and decided that you would like a shorter and more concise summary of the evidence to support the work the resident will present. You go to PIER (11) through your own subscription, although you could have gone through your library's Web interface, and

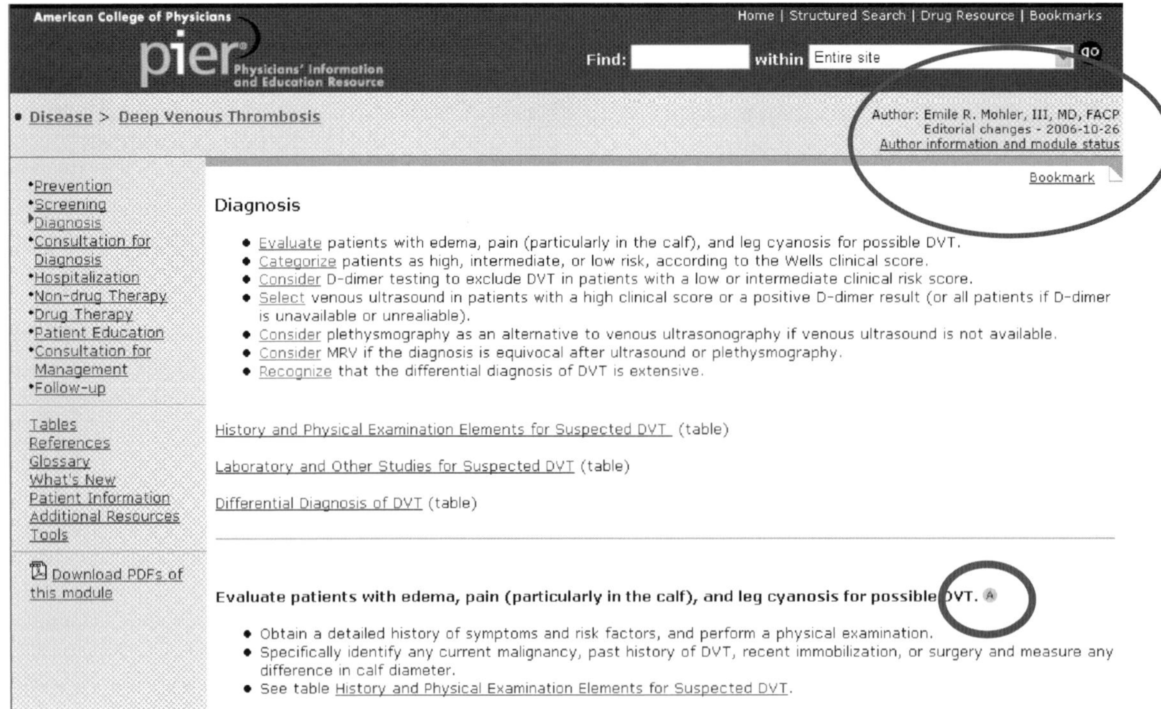

Figure 4.2 PIER results screen. (Reproduced with permission of the American College of Physicians.)

enter the search terms "dvt triage." Clicking on the "Deep Venous Thrombosis—Diagnosis" section you get the chapter listing and links to various tests and approaches, including their tables of evidence for the history and physical elements, laboratory and other related studies, and differential diagnosis (Figure 4.2).

PIER summarizes the evidence on a topic and provides the evidence behind their recommendations. The small oval in Figure 4.2 indicates the strength of the evidence. "A" evidence is defined as "the preponderance of data supporting this statement is derived from level 1 studies, which meet all of the evidence criteria for that study type." In this case, very strong evidence backs their clinical recommendations. In addition, by looking at the larger oval, you can see when the recommendations were reviewed and updated.

UpToDate (10) is another summary service (electronic textbook) that provides a service similar to that of PIER. Figure 4.3 shows the topic breakdown in the section on DVT: "Approach to the Diagnosis and Therapy of Suspected Deep Vein Thrombosis." Searching in UpToDate is best done with very simple words. In this case, we put in only "DVT." Armed with these two resources, you are ready to go the journal club to discuss the best approach to triaging DVT.

Question 2. Erythropoietin or darbepoetin versus transfusions for anemia in cancer

The debate rages on—is erythropoietin or darbepoetin better than transfusions to treat mild anemia in patients with cancer? You are a hematologist who has been asked to present at medical grand rounds about whether erythropoietin or darbepoetin improves quality of life. As usual, you have left things to the last minute so you wonder if you could tap into evidence already compiled by other researchers in systematic reviews and meta-analyses (syntheses level of the 5S pyramid). The librarian in your institution suggests that you search in Ovid's EBMR database (17) to identify systematic reviews from the CDSR and DARE. As an added bonus, the EBMR database collection integrates the *ACP Journal Club* abstracts (synopses). We break our question down into searchable components (Figure 4.4):

What does "you have left things a bit late" mean? You have left things to the last minute?

The drugs: erythropoietin or darbepoetin
The condition: cancer
The outcome: quality of life

Eleven items met the searching criteria, and the third one is a recently updated Cochrane Review on your question (Figure 4.5).

Bohlius and colleagues (21) conclude that erythropoietin and darbepoetin reduce the risk for blood transfusions (number of units transfused) and improve hematologic response for patients with mild anemia. However, the data on quality of life are only "suggestive" of improvements and come from studies with some limitations. Several other reviews in the initial retrieval of 11 documents also look promising for your rounds session so you go back and retrieve them.

Question 3. Stopping transfusions in children with sickle cell anemia

The third question is especially important to one of your patients and his family. The parents would like to stop the routine transfusions for their child with sickle cell anemia because of the potential adverse effects of multiple transfusions and the child's aversion to

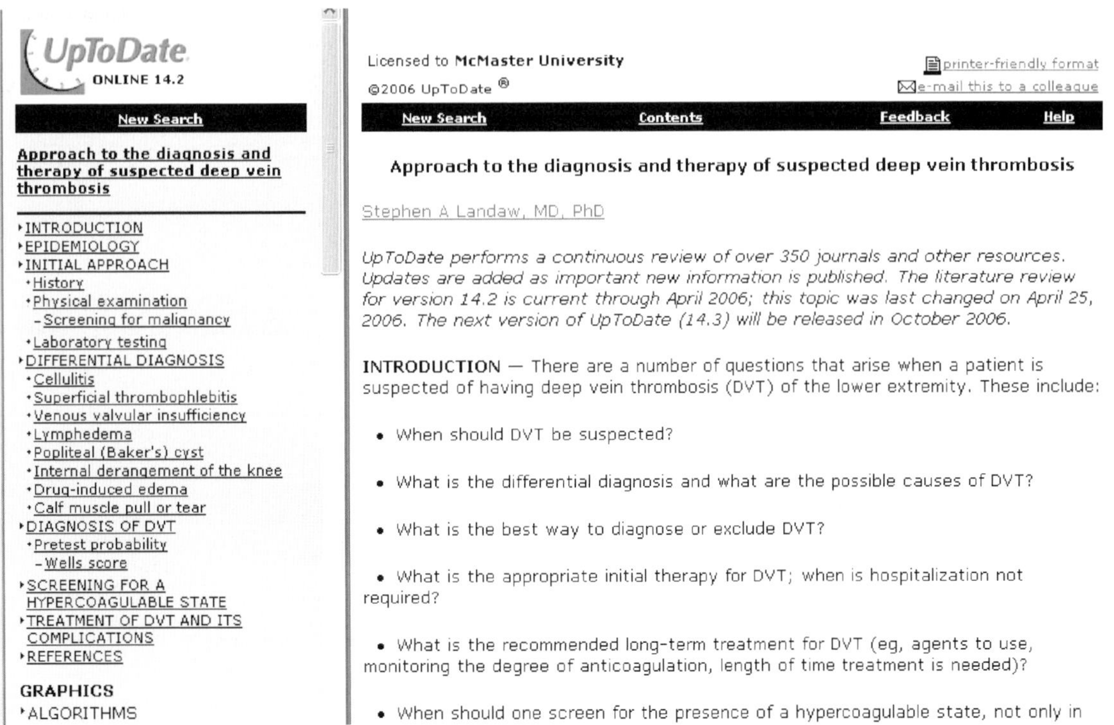

Figure 4.3 UpToDate screen showing the sections of the deep vein thrombosis disease section. The diagnosis section includes the Wells scoring system for triage of DVTs.

receiving them. You feel that this topic might not be as well studied as some other areas of hematology so you decide to go to MEDLINE to determine if any high-quality studies exist. Besides, you remember vaguely that a well-done trial was published in the *New England Journal of Medicine* in the past couple of years, and a MEDLINE search would retrieve this article. You choose to go to PubMed to do your MEDLINE search, even though you could have accessed MEDLINE through your institution's OVID sub-

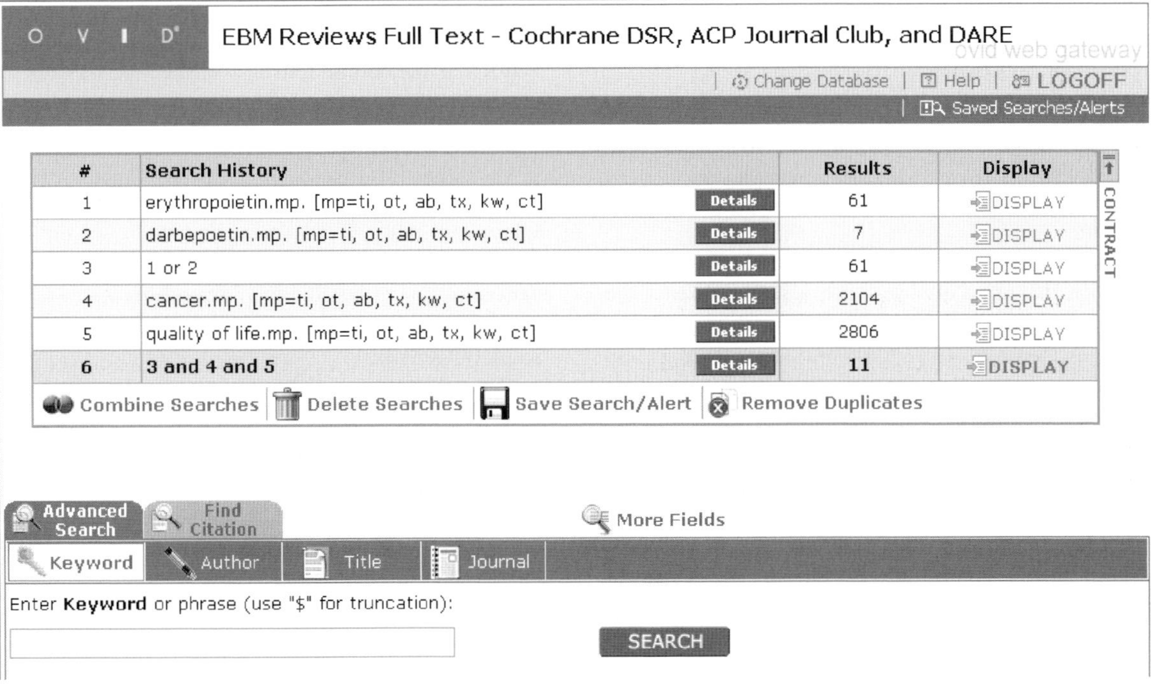

Figure 4.4 Ovid EBMR database collection of Cochrane, DARE, and *ACP Journal Club*.

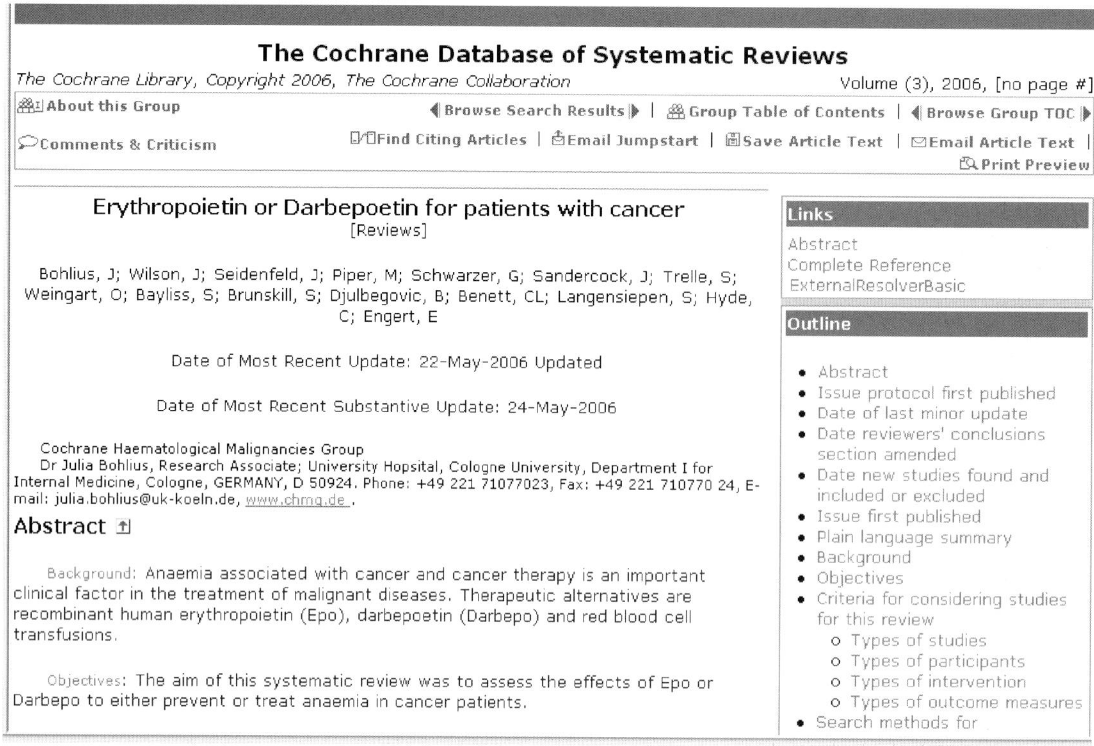

The Cochrane Database of Systematic Reviews

The Cochrane Library, Copyright 2006, The Cochrane Collaboration Volume (3), 2006, [no page #]

About this Group | Browse Search Results | Group Table of Contents | Browse Group TOC

Comments & Criticism | Find Citing Articles | Email Jumpstart | Save Article Text | Email Article Text | Print Preview

Erythropoietin or Darbepoetin for patients with cancer
[Reviews]

Bohlius, J; Wilson, J; Seidenfeld, J; Piper, M; Schwarzer, G; Sandercock, J; Trelle, S; Weingart, O; Bayliss, S; Brunskill, S; Djulbegovic, B; Benett, CL; Langensiepen, S; Hyde, C; Engert, E

Date of Most Recent Update: 22-May-2006 Updated

Date of Most Recent Substantive Update: 24-May-2006

Cochrane Haematological Malignancies Group
Dr Julia Bohlius, Research Associate; University Hopsital, Cologne University, Department I for Internal Medicine, Cologne, GERMANY, D 50924. Phone: +49 221 71077023, Fax: +49 221 710770 24, E-mail: julia.bohlius@uk-koeln.de, www.chmg.de .

Abstract

Background: Anaemia associated with cancer and cancer therapy is an important clinical factor in the treatment of malignant diseases. Therapeutic alternatives are recombinant human erythropoietin (Epo), darbepoetin (Darbepo) and red blood cell transfusions.

Objectives: The aim of this systematic review was to assess the effects of Epo or Darbepo to either prevent or treat anaemia in cancer patients.

Links
Abstract
Complete Reference
ExternalResolverBasic

Outline
- Abstract
- Issue protocol first published
- Date of last minor update
- Date reviewers' conclusions section amended
- Date new studies found and included or excluded
- Issue first published
- Plain language summary
- Background
- Objectives
- Criteria for considering studies for this review
  - Types of studies
  - Types of participants
  - Types of intervention
  - Types of outcome measures
- Search methods for

Figure 4.5 Abstract of a Cochrane Review found in the Ovid EBMR search.

scription. PubMed is designed for clinicians (and scientists) with considerable input from clinicians. It is particularly useful for clinical searches for two reasons. First, you can enter the terms in which you are interested using almost any format and the system will map to synonyms and correct spelling mistakes. Second, PubMed has clinical filters that enrich retrievals with higher-quality articles that have a good probability of being relevant to clinical care.

This question, whether you can discontinue transfusions given prophylactically to children to prevent stroke, has components of

Stroke prevention
Sickle cell anemia
Transfusions
The children who receive the transfusions

You start on the first PubMed search screen and enter the words "stroke prevention children transfusion sickle cell" and get 69 citations (Figure 4.6). This is a lot to read through and you decide that you will try the clinical queries feature to retrieve only those articles with strong methods and potential for clinical importance.

You use the same words only this time you put them into the Clinical Queries filter search box (Figure 4.7) and check that you would like to retrieve only those articles that deal with therapy (i.e., a randomized controlled trial) and that you would like a narrow, specific retrieval (a few high-quality articles). This brings the retrieval down to 15 citations with the *New England Journal of Medicine* article you remembered as the fourth citation (22).

Considering the various methods of searching that we have discussed, you wonder if a Web-based program exists that will pull all of the searching methods together into one easy-to-use site. Two United Kingdom researchers have produced a resource called TRIP (Turning Research into Practice) (23) that searches across 150 evidence-based resources and sorts retrieval into categories that reflect the bottom four of the "5S" levels. Figure 4.8 shows the TRIP search screen with the terms "stroke sickle cell prevention children transfusion" entered. Our retrieval includes the *New England Journal of Medicine* article (22) (Figure 4.9).

The retrievals in a TRIP search are sorted, providing access to summaries, synopses, syntheses, and studies as well as practice guidelines, clinical calculators, clinical questions, images, and patient education materials. Most retrievals are linked to the full text of the documents although some may require a subscription to access full reports.

Conclusion

In this chapter, we have provided you with a framework with which to organize your approach to information searching. Although only a smattering of resources has been discussed, these are examples of different layers of the "5S" pyramid. We have used several of the resources to show you how they work using hematology questions. Many other resources exist that could provide good answers. Discussions with your health sciences librarian will apprise you of

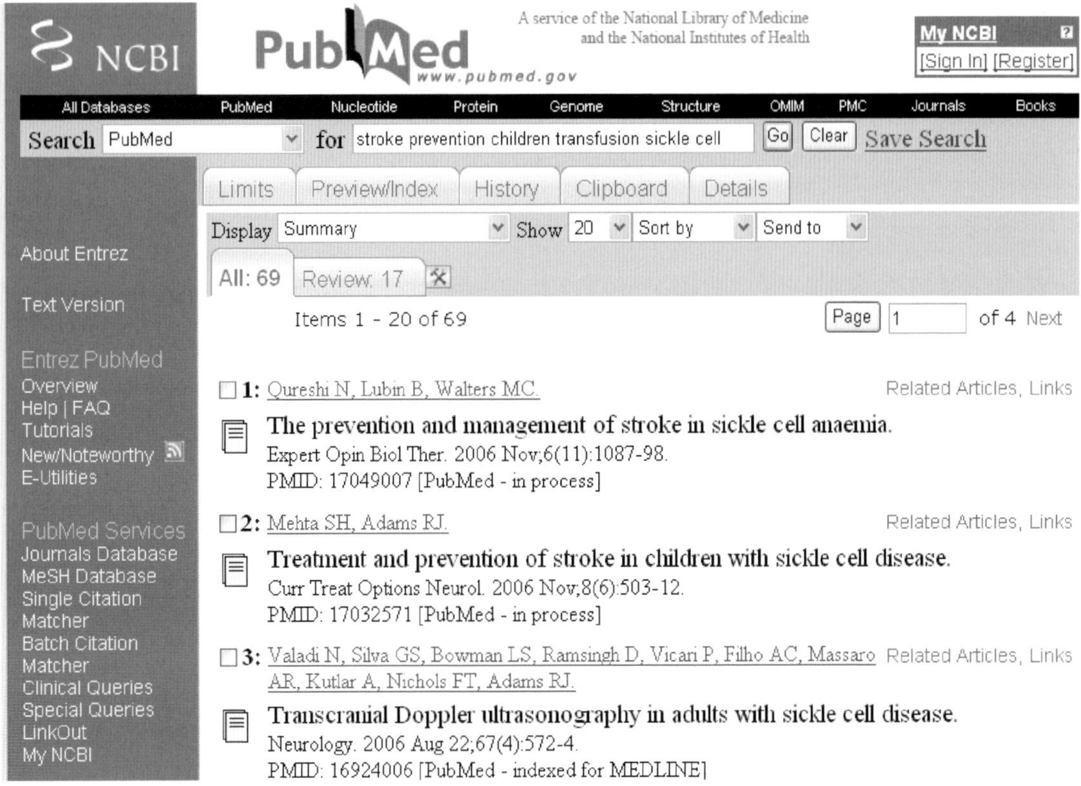

Figure 4.6 PubMed search in all of MEDLINE: 69 citations.

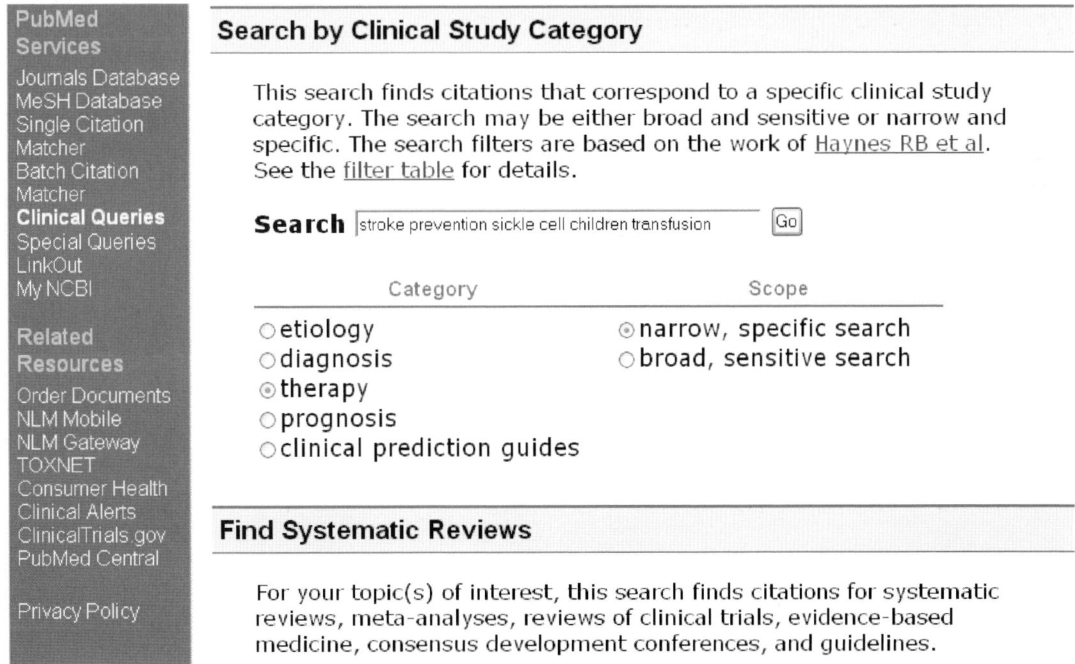

Figure 4.7 Clinical Queries search filter.

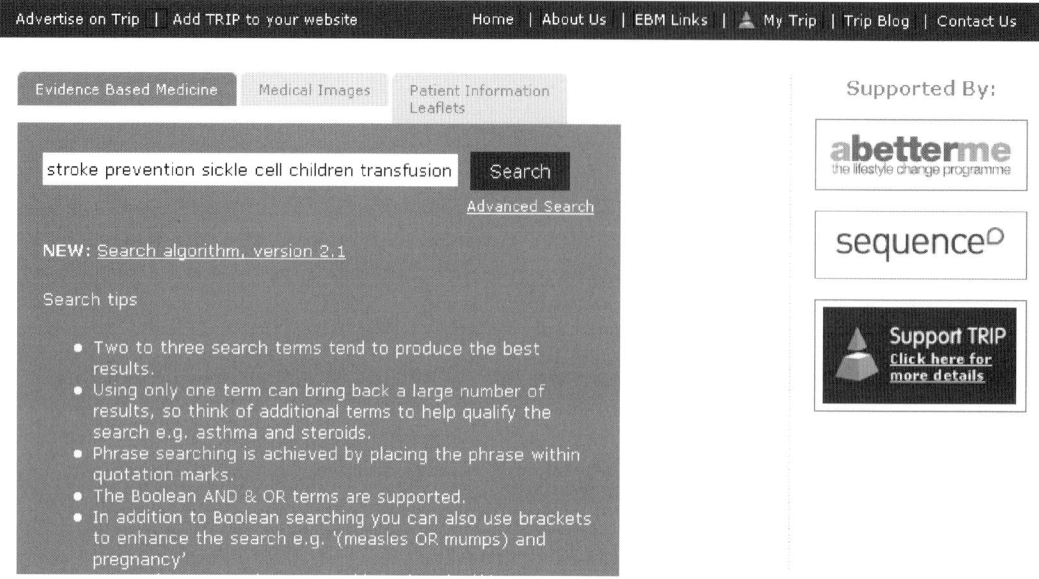

Figure 4.8 Entry of terms into the TRIP search engine.

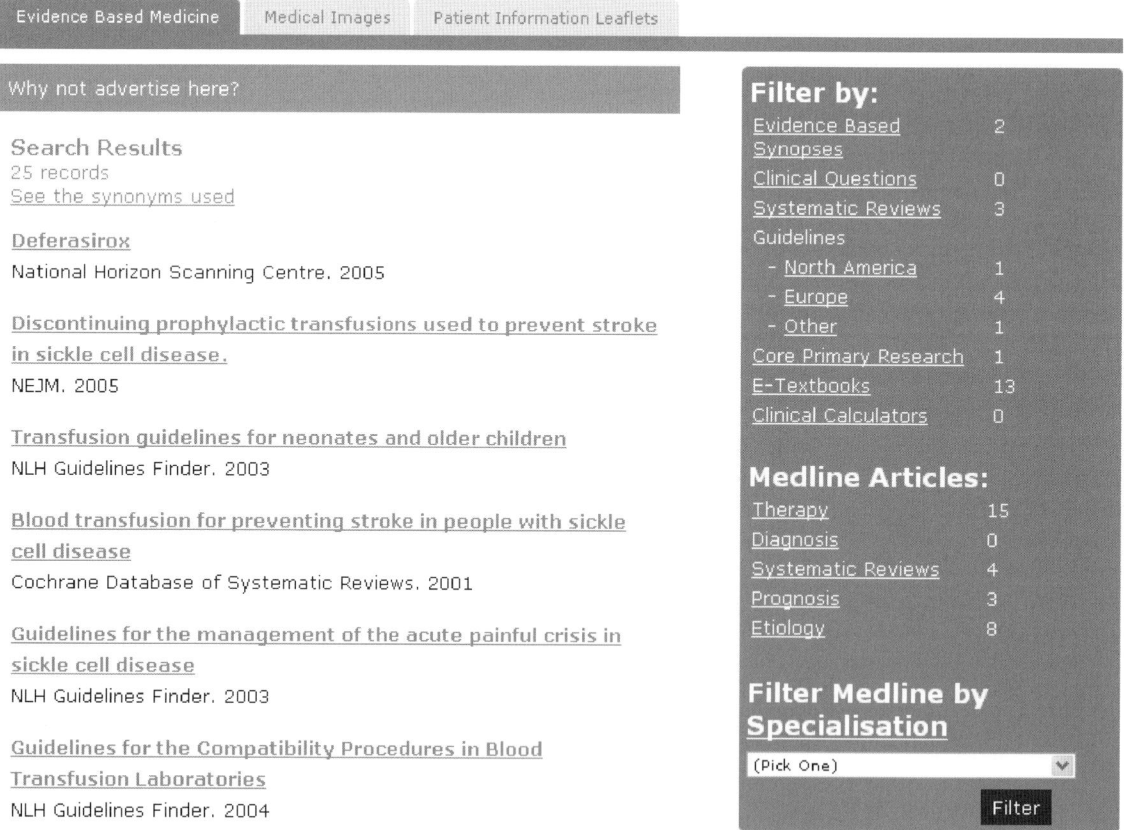

Figure 4.9 TRIP retrieval on stroke prevention in children with sickle cell disease.

new resources that warrant your attention to practice evidence-based hematology with ease.

References

1 Galloway MJ, Reid MM. Is the practice of haematology evidence based? I. Evidence based clinical practice. *J Clin Pathol.* 1998;**51**(5):345–46.

2 Haynes RB. Of studies, syntheses, synopses, and systems: the "4S" evolution of services for finding current best evidence. *ACP J Club.* 2001;**134**(2):A11–13.

3 Haynes RB. Of studies, syntheses, synopses, summaries, and systems: the "5S" evolution of information services for evidence-based healthcare decisions. *ACP J Club.* 2006;**145**(3):A8.

4 Garg AX, Adhikari NK, McDonald H, et al. Effects of computerized clinical decision support systems on practitioner performance and patient outcomes: a systematic review. *JAMA.* 2005;**293**(10):1223–38.

5 White RH, Hong R, Venook AP, et al. Initiation of warfarin therapy: comparison of physician dosing with computer-assisted dosing. *J Gen Intern Med.* 1987;**2**(3):141–48.

6 Mungall DR, Anbe D, Forrester PL, et al. A prospective randomized comparison of the accuracy of computer-assisted versus GUSTO nomogram–directed heparin therapy. *Clin Pharmacol Ther.* 1994;**55**(5):591–96.

7 Montori VM. *Evidence-based endocrinology.* Totowa, NJ: Humana Press; 2005.

8 Gerstein HC, Haynes RB. Evidence-based diabetes care. Hamilton: BC Decker; 2001.

9 BMJ Clinical Evidence [online database]. London: BMJ Publishing Group [2008 Feb 12]. Available at: http://clinicalevidence.bmd.com/ceweb/index.jsp.

10 UpToDate [online database]. Waltham, MA [2008 Feb 12]. Available at: www.uptodate.com/

11 Physicians' Information and Education Resource (PIER) [online database]. Philadelphia: American College of Physicians [2008 Feb 12]. Available at: pier.acponline.org//index.html

12 FIRSTConsult [online database]. Oxford: Elsevier [2008 Feb 12]. Available at: http://www.mdconsult.com/das/pdxmd/lookup/87755889-2

13 STAT!Ref [online database]. Jackson, WY: Teton Data Systems [2008 Feb 12]. Available at: http://www.mdconsult.com/php/87756061-2/homepage

14 MDConsult [online database]. Oxford: Elsevier [2008 Feb 12]. www.mdconsult.com/

15 Cochrane Library [online database]. Oxford: Wiley InterScience. Available at: www3.interscience.wiley.com/cgi-bin/mrwhome/106568753/HOME

16 Haynes RB. bmjupdates+, a new free service for evidence-based clinical practice. *Evid Based Nurs.* 2005;**8**(2):39.

17 OVID Evidence-Based Medicine Reviews [online database]. New York: Ovid Technologies [2008 Feb 12]. Available at: www.ovid.com/site/index.isp

18 Haynes RB, McKibbon KA, Wilczynski NL, et al. Optimal search strategies for retrieving scientifically strong studies of treatment from MEDLINE: analytical survey. *BMJ.* 2005;**330**(7501):1179.

19 MEDSCAPE Best Evidence alerts [online newsletter; 2008 Feb 12]. Available at: https://profreg.medscape.com/px/newsletter.do.

20 Goodacre S, Sampson F, Stevenson M, et al. Measurement of the clinical and cost-effectiveness of non-invasive diagnostic testing strategies for deep vein thrombosis. *Health Technol Assess.* 2006;**10**(15):1–168, iii–iv.

21 Bohlius J, Wilson J, Seidenfeld J, et al. Erythropoietin or darbepoetin for patients with cancer. *Cochrane Database Syst Rev.* 2006;**3**: CD003407.

22 Adams RJ, Brambilla D. Optimizing Primary Stroke Prevention in Sickle Cell Anemia (STOP 2) Trial Investigators. Discontinuing prophylactic transfusions used to prevent stroke in sickle cell disease. *N Engl J Med.* 2005;**353**(26):2769–78.

23 TRIP database [2008 Feb 12]. Available at: www.tripdatabase.com/index.html

5 Applying EBM in Clinical Practice

Alessandro Squizzato, Walter Ageno, Davide Imberti

Introduction

Evidence-based medicine (EBM) aims at solving clinical problems while integrating the best available evidence from clinical research with the expertise of the clinician and patient's values and preferences (1). EBM posits a hierarchy of evidence, from the most valid results of systematic reviews of randomized controlled trials (RCTs) to unsystematic clinical observations that are most prone to bias. EBM provides tools to assess the quality of evidence and to transfer the results of clinical research to daily clinical practice (1,2). Practicing EBM can be time consuming. To support clinicians in applying EBM, sources of preprocessed evidence have been developed, such as systematic reviews and evidence-based clinical practice guidelines. The aim of this chapter is to provide readers with some examples on how different types of evidence can be applied to patient care. However, readers should understand that evidence alone is never sufficient to make a clinical decision. Biological, socioeconomic, and epidemiological factors should always be taken into account, and patient values and preferences are critical to making decisions (1).

Applying an evidence-based guideline in clinical practice

Clinical scenario

You are the hematologist on call, and one of your colleagues, an oncologist, requests your consultation. A 79-year-old man is on chemotherapy for a prostatic adenocarcinoma with bone metastases. The day before the patient underwent compression ultrasound of the veins of the lower limbs because of a sudden onset of pain and edema in the right leg. He was diagnosed with a femoral-popliteal deep vein thrombosis (DVT). His platelet count was above 150,000/mm^3, and creatinine clearance was normal. The patient had no known risk factors for bleeding. Your colleague prescribed therapeutic dose subcutaneous low-molecular weight heparin (LMWH), and he would now like to start the patient on warfarin treatment as soon as possible. Before you go to see the patient, you decide to evaluate what current evidence-based international guidelines on antithrombotic treatment recommend (3).

Clinical question

In cancer patients with recent DVT, does LMWH compared with warfarin reduce the risk of recurrent DVT, and does it have at least the same safety profile?

Finding and appraising the evidence

The guidelines issued by the American College of Chest Physicians (ACCP) Conference on Antithrombotic and Thrombolytic Therapy represent the reference standard for clinical practice. The last edition was published in *Chest* in 2004 (Chest 2004; 126 (Suppl): 163S–696S; http://www.chestjournal.org/content/vol126/3_suppl/). This document fulfils the requirement of an evidence-based guideline, because it was developed with due methodological rigor. It is based on systematic reviews, considering all available treatment options and outcomes for each clinical question, and the recommendations are explicit, transparent, unambiguous, and directly linked to the supporting evidence (4). In addition, the values and preferences of the guideline panel members that were considered while formulating recommendations are clearly stated. The recommendations follow a clear and simple grading system expressing the strength of a recommendation and the quality of evidence supporting it. A recommendation is strong when the guideline developers are certain that benefits do, or do not, outweigh risks, burdens, and costs of a given intervention. Alternatively, a recommendation is weak when they are not certain of the balance between the benefits and the risks, burdens, and costs. In deciding on the quality of supporting evidence, a highest level is assigned to the studies that are least prone to bias—RCTs

Evidence-based Hematology. Edited by Mark A. Crowther, Jeff Ginsberg, Holger J. Schünemann, Ralph M. Meyer, and Richard Lottenberg.

with consistent results and without methodological limitations. RCTs with inconsistent results, or with important methodological limitations, constitute moderate-quality evidence, and observational studies or generalization from one group of patients included in randomized trials to a different, but somewhat similar, group of patients who did not participate in those trials constitute low-quality evidence (5). One criticism of these guidelines relates to the lack of patient representatives on the guideline panel, which could introduce a possible source of bias in choosing the outcomes of interest and judging their relative importance (1). This is a limitation of most clinical practice guidelines. To evaluate fully the quality of a guideline, users may use the AGREE instrument, a validated tool for appraisal of clinical practice guidelines (6).

For the above clinical question, the ACCP guidelines recommend the following: "For patients with DVT and cancer, we recommend LMWH for the first 3 to 6 months of long-term anticoagulant therapy (Grade 1A). For these patients we recommend anticoagulant therapy indefinitely or until the cancer is resolved (Grade 1C)" (3). Given that the cost of treatment with LMWH compared with warfarin greatly varies among countries, any final therapeutic decision should be made with due consideration of local circumstances.

Resolution of the scenario

Once in the oncology department, you learn that the patient is on long-term prednisone therapy for rheumatoid arthritis and that he has a moderate/severe osteoporosis. When you start discussing the benefits and harms of LMWH with the patient, you mention that a lower incidence of osteopenia has been reported with the use of LMWH, when compared with unfractioned heparin. Having been informed of the possible adverse outcomes, the patient values the prevention of complications from DVT higher than the possible complication of osteopenia. He prefers the subcutaneous injections based on their favorable benefit/risk profile and begins taking LMWH.

Applying the results of a systematic review in clinical practice

Clinical scenario

You are the attending physician on duty when a 76-year-old former professor of pulmonary medicine is transferred from the Emergency Department. She was admitted because of dyspnea at rest and bilateral leg edema. She was diagnosed with New York Heart Association (NYHA) class IV congestive heart failure. The chest X-ray confirmed acute pulmonary edema. The ECG showed no significant abnormalities. The patient's medical history was positive for chronic heart failure secondary to arterial hypertension. The body mass index is 31 kg/m^2. Creatinine concentration in serum and creatinine clearance is normal. Because of her age, severe heart failure, and forced bed rest, she is at increased risk of venous thromboembolism (VTE). You plan to administer adequate thromboprophylaxis. The resident on duty suggests the use of LMWH, but he cannot define the real benefits and risks of thromboprophylaxis in this clinical setting. He poses the following clinical question to increase his understanding of the factors that influence the decision.

Clinical question

In an elderly immobilized patient with NYHA class IV congestive heart failure, does anticoagulation, compared with no antithrombotic treatment, reduce the occurrence of VTE with at least the same safety profile, and if so, is LMWH more effective or safer than unfractionated heparin (UFH)?

Finding and appraising the evidence

The fundamentals of methodology for systematic reviews and meta-analyses are described in the chapter 2 by Prins et al. You performed a MEDLINE search and found a systematic review evaluating the efficacy and safety of UFH or LMWH in the prevention of VTE in acutely ill medical patients (7). You quickly appraised the quality of this systematic review. You noticed that the data were pooled from studies done in quite different populations of patients and used different methods for assessing outcomes. You are also aware of three high-quality RCTs that have been published after this systematic review was completed: two compared LMWH with a placebo and one compared fondaparinux with a placebo. All included patients with congestive heart failure (NYHA class III and IV) (8). Authors of the systematic review included seven trials, with a total of 15,095 patients, comparing UFH or LMWH to control and nine trials with a total of 4,669 patients comparing UFH to LMWH. In the trials comparing UFH or LMWH to a placebo, an estimated pooled relative risk (RR) of DVT or pulmonary embolism (PE) was 0.49 (95% confidence interval [CI]: 0.33–0.73) and 0.47 (95% CI: 0.33–0.67), respectively. The RR of major bleeding was 1.57 (95% CI: 0.85–2.88) with active treatment compared with a placebo or no anticoagulation. The authors also reviewed the nine trials with a total of 4,669 patients comparing the efficacy and safety of LMWH to UFH in medical patients. They found a nonsignificant trend toward lower risk of DVT and PE in patients receiving LMWH compared with UFH—RR: 0.83 (95% CI: 0.56–1.24) and RR: 0.74 (95% CI: 0.29–1.80), respectively. The risk of major bleeding was marginally lower with LMWH compared with UFH (RR: 0.48, 95% CI: 0.23–1.0). These results confirmed the efficacy of thromboprophylaxis in this setting, although the estimates of the effect were still not precise enough to answer your second question, whether LMWH was more efficacious than UFH.

Readers can use the *Users' Guides to the Medical Literature* to assess the quality of a systematic review (1). The international Cochrane Collaboration (9), the primary purpose of which is to generate and disseminate high-quality systematic reviews of healthcare interventions, provides an important source of preprocessed evidence. The Cochrane Library (http://www.cochrane.org) contains regularly updated collection of evidence-based medicine resources, including a database of systematic reviews, a register of controlled trials, and a database for economic evaluations. The quality of Cochrane reviews varies, however; on average, Cochrane reviews provide good-quality systematic summary of the literature.

Resolution of the scenario

Your patient has several known risk factors for VTE: NYHA class IV congestive heart failure, immobilization, advanced age, and obesity. There is no apparent increased risk of bleeding. The available evidence strongly supports the use of either unfractionated heparin or low-molecular weight heparin. After reading the systematic review, you decide to offer low-dose LMWH to this patient because, in your setting, the cost of LMWH is less important than the ease of use of LMWH compared with UFH.

Applying the results of a randomized controlled trial in clinical practice

Clinical scenario

You are the thrombosis expert on call. Your colleague, a neurologist, asked you to discuss the optimal long-term secondary prophylaxis in a patient with a recent ischemic stroke. A 62-year-old engineer was admitted to the Stroke Unit after an acute ischemic stroke, and he was treated with intravenous fibrinolytic therapy. The pathogenesis of the cerebrovascular event is atherothrombotic. He is now on low-dose aspirin. The patient read an article in a newspaper suggesting that clopidogrel offers additional protection when added to aspirin in high-risk vascular patients and asked the neurologist whether combined antiplatelet therapy was appropriate in his case. Your colleague knows that the results of a CHARISMA trial have been published (10), and this is the only study addressing this question. For a better discussion on the merits of combined treatment with aspirin and clopidogrel, you print a copy of the article and a copy of its synopsis published in the *ACP Journal Club* (11).

Clinical question

In patients who have experienced a noncardioembolic stroke, does the combination of clopidogrel and aspirin, compared with aspirin alone, reduce the risk of cardiovascular events and does it have at least the same safety profile?

Finding and appraising the evidence

No guideline or systematic review addressed this issue because trials directly comparing the effects of combined treatment with aspirin and clopidogrel appeared only recently. In 2006, the results of the CHARISMA study were published (10). Three steps can be followed in appraising an article reporting the results of a RCT (1). First, you should determine whether the results of the study are valid; second, you should assess the results; and third, you should decide whether the results apply to the patient in your practice. The assessment of study quality is performed to identify possible sources of bias, including the choice of the population, intervention, comparison, and outcomes, as well as the execution of the study (e.g., proper randomization, concealment of allocation, blinding of patients and investigators, analysis of results according to the intention-to-treat principle, and percentage of patients lost to follow-up). The CHARISMA was a properly randomized placebo-controlled trial with concealed allocation. Investigators, patients, and outcome assessors were blinded to the treatment. Data were analyzed according to the intention-to-treat principle with the inclusion of all patients as randomized. You conclude that there is a low risk of bias in the CHARISMA study. This trial enrolled 15,603 patients followed for a median of 28 months. The primary efficacy endpoint (a composite of first occurrence of myocardial infarction, stroke of any cause, or death from cardiovascular causes [including bleeding]) was 6.8% with clopidogrel plus aspirin and 7.3% with aspirin alone (RR: 0.93, 95% CI: 0.83–1.05). The rate of the primary safety endpoint (severe bleeding according to the GUSTO definition) was 1.7% in the combined treatment group and 1.3% in the aspirin alone group (RR: 1.25, 95% CI: 0.97–1.61).

Resolution of the scenario

You discussed the above evidence with your colleague. The addition of clopidogrel to aspirin seems unlikely to provide any additional benefit for this patient compared with aspirin alone and could increase the risk of bleeding. Moreover, you tell him that in the international register of ongoing clinical trials available at http://www.clinicaltrial.gov, two other studies (FASTER and SPS3) explore the effect of clopidogrel and aspirin combination in patients with ischemic stroke, and that this could change the assessment in the future. You also remind your colleague that a recent RCT, the ESPRIT trial, investigated the benefit of adding extended-release dipyridamole to aspirin in patients within six months of a transient ischemic attack or minor stroke of presumed arterial origin and found a considerable benefit of the combined treatment with aspirin and dipyridamole and that this may be another option (12).

Practice of evidence-based medicine in the absence of high-quality evidence

Clinical scenario

You are the resident on call when a 51-year-old primary-school teacher visits the Emergency Department with right hemiparesis and a headache. She was on anticoagulation with warfarin for an apparently idiopathic DVT of the right lower limb complicated with pulmonary embolism that occurred less than two weeks ago. A physical examination reveals a blood pressure of 220/120 mm Hg. An urgent cerebral CT shows that there is a left intraparenchymal hemorrhage. The International Normalized Ratio is 7.6. You decide it is a life-threatening hemorrhage; you choose to treat her with intravenous vitamin K and prothrombin complex concentrates, but you are afraid of recurrent thromboembolism. In the meantime, the attending physician has already called the interventional radiologist to insert a retrievable inferior vena cava filter. While you consider that this could be a reasonable choice, you wonder whether there is evidence supporting this course of action.

Clinical question

In patients with a major hemorrhage during antithrombotic therapy for pulmonary embolism secondary to DVT, does placement of an inferior vena cava filter, in comparison to temporary discontinuation of antithrombotic therapy, reduce recurrent PE, and is at least equally safe?

Finding and appraising the evidence

For rare disorders or complications, RCTs are often not feasible. Other evidence derived from observational studies such as cohort studies, case-control studies, or case series may provide some evidence supporting clinical decisions. When such evidence is also unavailable, unsystematic observations from one's own clinical experience, experience of one's colleagues, or biological rationale may provide the best possible evidence.

For the question above, no RCT is available to provide the answer. The best evidence is very indirect. For example, a randomized trial of 400 patients with symptomatic DVT (all of whom received either UFH or LMWH), showed a lower incidence of PE after 12 days in patients assigned to a placement of an inferior vena cava filter compared with those without such a filter. However, the incidence of recurrent DVT at one year was higher in the patients with filters compared with those without filters (13). The solution to this scenario can be therefore based on pathophysiologic rationale and clinical experience. Both PE and intracerebral hemorrhage are potentially lethal diseases. If left untreated, PE-related mortality is about 30% (14), and more than one-third of patients with intracerebral hemorrhage die within one month after the onset of symptoms (15). In this situation, a prompt normalization of the INR is necessary to limit active bleeding and to allow a rapid neurosurgical intervention, if necessary. Given the absence of evidence on the optimal timing for restarting anticoagulant treatment in a potentially fatal bleeding, a placement of a vena cava filter seems to be a reasonable choice for preventing PE during reversal of warfarin-related coagulopathy.

Resolution of the scenario

The senior physician discusses the potential benefits and downsides of an inferior vena cava filter insertion with the patient. He explains, that the major risks, although infrequent, are related to the insertion of the filter and that a retrievable filter will be removed as soon as possible. Conversely, a filter will protect from the recurrence of PE, giving the clinicians the opportunity to treat the cerebral hemorrhage. The patient consents to the insertion of a retrievable inferior vena cava filter.

Choosing the best diagnostic strategy

Clinical scenario

You are the hematologist on call when a 51-year-old neurosurgeon working at your hospital presents to your Thrombosis Unit with a suspected DVT. He has pain and mild edema of the right calf that began 10 days ago. Two days ago, he has started self-injecting a low-dose LMWH. Before performing any diagnostic test, you assessed his probability of having a DVT (pretest probability) with a well-validated clinical prediction rule developed by Wells and colleagues (16). The Wells score was 3, which meant a high pretest probability of DVT. Meanwhile, your colleague showed you the result of an ELISA D-dimer test, performed that morning, that was negative (<500 ng/mL). This result had reassured him then, but you were still not convinced. Given the high pretest clinical probability, you explained that a negative d-dimer result is probably not sufficient to exclude DVT.

Clinical question

In outpatients with a high clinical suspicion of deep venous thrombosis, what is the diagnostic accuracy of D-dimer testing?

Finding and appraising the evidence

Nearly all clinicians intuitively use a Bayesian approach in their reasoning when making a diagnosis (2). This means that the clinician usually has some notion of the probability of certain disease in a patient even before performing any diagnostic tests. This initial probability is called *pretest probability*. If a patient has no additional risk or prognostic factors, then pretest probability is simply the prevalence of this disease in a similar population. Performing a diagnostic test changes the probability of this disease in this patient. Probability of a disease increases, if the test is positive and decreases, if it is negative. The ability of a diagnostic test to change the probability of a given disease is described by a likelihood ratio, which is the ratio of likelihood of a given test result (positive or negative) in patients with a disease and the likelihood of the same test result in patients without this disease. Every diagnostic test has an associated likelihood ratio of a positive and of a negative result. Knowledge of a likelihood ratio associated with a diagnostic test in the investigation of a given disease helps clinicians to choose which test might be more suitable for the patient. Knowing (broadly) the pretest probability of a given disease in a patient, one may determine the posttest probability using a likelihood ratio nomogram (see chapter 6 on diagnosis).

The Wells score has been developed to assess pretest probability of DVT (i.e., the probability before performing additional diagnostic tests, but the Wells score may be considered a diagnostic tool allowing a clinician to determine the "post-Wells score" probability of DVT). This score classifies the risk of DVT as low, intermediate, or high (16). Our patient has a high pretest probability of DVT, which means more than 30%. A recent systematic review with meta-analysis confirmed that the D-dimer test has a high sensitivity and a high likelihood ratio of a negative result, and therefore it is useful in excluding a disease (17). For a rapid ELISA D-dimer, the negative likelihood ratio is 0.09, which roughly means that a likelihood of a negative test result in patients with DVT is 10 times lower that the likelihood of the negative test result in patients without DVT. A negative D-dimer result in a patient with a low risk of DVT allows us then to be quite certain that the patient does not have DVT. A negative D-dimer result in a patient with a high pretest probability of DVT means that posttest probability of DVT is still at least 3%, and additional tests to confirm or exclude the presence of DVT seem warranted. Even if D-dimer has a high sensitivity in diagnosis of DVT, a false-negative test result can occur (18). In our patient, two well-recognized reasons of a false-negative result of a D-dimer test are present: treatment with heparin and a time lag between the onset of symptoms and performing a test.

Resolution of the scenario

You explain to your colleague that in outpatients with a high pretest probability of DVT, a compression ultrasound is warranted. Testing for D-dimer levels is probably of no further benefit in these patients because even with a negative result posttest probability still does not allow the exclusion of a fairly high probability of DVT (i.e., at least 3%) (19). The results of the compression ultrasound of the leg reveal partial thrombosis of the popliteal vein.

Conclusion

In this chapter, we provided examples on how to apply results of clinical research in medical practice. In particular, we suggest how to apply different types of evidence to clinical problems. Knowing the tools of evidence-based practice is helpful but never sufficient for providing the highest quality of patient care (1). Clinical decisions must always include consideration of (a) clinical circumstances, for example, the presence of concomitant diseases and the availability of diagnostic and therapeutic options; (b) best research evidence; (c) patient's values and preferences; and (d) clinical expertise that is needed to bring these considerations together and help the patient to make a decision (20,21).

References

1 The Evidence-Based Medicine Working Group. *Users' guides to the medical literature: a manual for evidence-based clinical practice.* 2nd ed. Chicago: AMA Press; 2006.

2 Straus SE, Richardson WS, Glasziou P, et al. *Evidence-based medicine: How to practice and teach EBM.* 3rd ed. Edinburgh: Elsevier; 2005.

3 Büller H, Agnelli G, Hull RD, et al. Antithrombotic therapy for venous thromboembolic disease. The Seventh ACCP Conference on Antithrombotic and Thrombolytic Therapy. *Chest.* 2004;**126**:401S–28S.

4 Schünemann HJ, Munger H, Brower S, et al. Developing evidence-based guidelines for the ACCP Conference on Antithrombotic and Thrombolytic Therapy. *Chest.* 2004;**126**:174S–78S.

5 Hirsh J, Guyatt G, Albers G, et al. The Seventh ACCP Conference on Antithrombotic and Thrombolytic Therapy. Evidence-Based Guidelines. *Chest.* 2004;**126**:172S–73S.

6 AGREE Collaboration. Development and validation of an international appraisal instrument for assessing the quality of clinical practice guidelines: the AGREE project. *Qual Saf Health Care.* 2003;**12**:18–23.

7 Mismetti P, Laporte-Simitsidis S, Tardy B, et al. Prevention of venous thromboembolism in internal medicine with unfractioned or low-molecular-weight heparins: a meta-analysis of ransomised clinical trials. *Thromb Haemost.* 2000;**83**:14–19.

8 Leizorovicz A, Mismetti P. Preventing venous thromboembolism in medical patients. *Circulation.* 2004;**110**(Suppl IV):IV-13–IV-19.

9 Bero L, Rennie D. The Cochrane Collaboration: preparing, maintaining, and disseminating systematic reviews of the effects of health care. *JAMA.* 1995;**274**:1935–38.

10 Bhatt DL, Fox KAA, Hacke W, et al. (for the CHARISMA Investigators). Clopidogrel and aspirin versus aspirin alone for the prevention of atherothrombotic events. *N Engl J Med.* 2006;**354**:1706–17.

11 Ballew KA. Clopidogrel plus aspirin did not differ from aspirin alone for reducing MI, stroke, and CV death in high-risk atherothrombosis. *ACP J Club.* 2006;**145**:33.

12 The ESPRIT Study Group. Aspirin plus dipyridamole versus aspirin alone after cerebral ischaemia of arterial origin (ESPRIT): randomised controlled trial. *Lancet.* 2006;**367**:1665–73.

13 Decousus H, Leizorovicz A, Parent F, et al. A clinical trial of vena caval filters in the prevention of pulmonary embolism in patients with proximal deep-vein thrombosis. *N Engl J Med* 1998;**338**:409–16.

14 Barritt DW, Jordan SC. Anticoagulant drugs in the treatment of pulmonary embolism: a controlled trial. *Lancet.* 1960;**1**:1309–12.

15 Broderick JP, Adams HP Jr, Barsan W, et al. Primary intracerebral hemorrhage in the Oxfordshire Community Stroke Project. 2. Prognosis. *Cerebrovasc Dis.* 1995;**5**:26–34.

16 Wells PS, Anderson DR, Bormanis J, et al. Value of assessment of pretest probability of deep-vein thrombosis in clinical management. *Lancet.* 1997;**350**:1795–98.

17 Stein PD, Hull RD, Patel KC, et al. D-dimer for the exclusion of acute venous thrombosis and pulmonary embolism. *Ann Intern Med.* 2004;**140**:589–602.

18 Pauker SG, Kassirer JP. The threshold approach to clinical decision-making. *N Engl J Med.* 1980;**302**:1109.

19 Wells PS, Anderson DR, Rodger M, et al. Evaluation of D-dimer in the diagnosis of suspected deep-vein thrombosis. *N Engl J Med.* 2003;**349**:1227–35.

20 Haynes RB, Devereaux PJ. Physicians' and patients' choices in evidence based practice: evidence does not make decisions, people do. *BMJ.* 2002;**324**:1350.

21 McCormick J. Death of the personal doctor. *Lancet.* 1996;**348**:667–8.

6 Using Evidence to Guide the Diagnosis of Disease

Lucas M. Bachmann, Holger J. Schünemann

Diagnosis—its role in clinical care

Clinicians use diagnostic tests routinely to identify, screen for, stage, and monitor illnesses. The means to achieve these tasks comprise a multitude of sources, including imaging and biochemical technologies, pathological and psychological investigations, and signs and symptoms elicited during history taking and clinical examinations (1). The results of tests, however, generally do not fully discriminate between the presence and absence of the illness at issue; tests generally are inconclusive in this respect, so that diagnosis can only be uncertain or probabilistic. Thus, the essence of diagnosis is the probability with which a clinician takes that illness to be present (see chapter 3).

If the diagnostic probability for a particular illness is set high enough, it is said to constitute a (practical) rule-in diagnosis of that illness; and conversely, if it is set low enough, it is equivalent to a practical rule-out diagnosis. Ancient Egyptian medical papyri (1550 BC) already emphasized diagnosis by physical examination as the cornerstone of the decision to treat or not to treat an ailment (2). In clinical practice, tests are commonly combined in diagnostic sequences, and disease probabilities are usually estimated in a hierarchical manner first combining information from history and examination followed by additional information obtained from technically advanced (and often invasive) tests. The information about the likelihood of a diagnosis comes from a combination of tests.

For clinicians, however, assimilating information from published literature on the value of tests is fraught with difficulties. This is in part due to variation in the type of diagnostic research designs (3,4) and in part due to exaggeration of claims about accuracy by authors (5). Moreover, clinicians themselves misinterpret diagnostic evidence (6,7). This is in stark contrast to the framework that clinicians can neither diagnose nor prognosticate correctly without accurate tests. An inaccurate diagnosis can harm patients by exposing them to inadequate therapy, while correct diagnosis of disease allows timely use of effective therapy, correct information, or reassurance. Collation of evidence from individual research studies on tests in systematic reviews can help, but it presents challenges due to concerns about the poor quality of many studies (8–10), reporting bias and other related biases (11), unrealistic assumptions about consistency of accuracy measures (sensitivity, specificity, and likelihood ratios) across disease spectra (12,13), and methodological challenges in statistically pooling results (14–17).

Scientific diagnosis

Despite the crucial importance of an appropriate use of diagnostic and screening tests in clinical decision making, many tests, clinical findings, and items from medical history have not been subjected to rigorous evaluation in studies following modern standards of clinical epidemiology. Widely disseminated, sophisticated, and expensive tests may prove to have marginal clinical value or economic benefit once critically evaluated. Well-known examples include the carcinoembryonic antigen test in the diagnosis of colon cancer (18), iodine 125-labled fibrinogen scans in the diagnosis of deep venous thrombi (19), or rapid magnetic resonance imaging in the management of patients with low back pain (20).

Whereas considerable progress has been made to build a systematically assembled and critically appraised evidence base for the evaluation of efficacy and cost-effectiveness of therapeutic and preventive interventions, the diagnostic process is underresearched, the relevant literature is scattered and difficult to access, and the studies found are often of inadequate methodological quality or uncertain applicability (9).

Studies of diagnostic test evaluation (description)

In studies of diagnostic accuracy, the outcomes from one or more tests under evaluation are compared with outcomes from the reference standard, both measured in individuals who are suspected of having the condition of interest. The term *test* refers to any method

Evidence-based Hematology. Edited by Mark A. Crowther, Jeff Ginsberg, Holger J. Schünemann, Ralph M. Meyer, and Richard Lottenberg.
 ISBN: 978-1-4051-5747-6.

Table 6.1 Definitions of measures of diagnostic accuracy.

		Target condition	
		Present	Absent
Test result	+	a	b
	−	c	d

Sensitivity	$a/(a+c)$ Proportion of true positives that are correctly identified by the test
Specificity	$d/(b+d)$ Proportion of true negatives that are correctly identified by the test
Likelihood ratio (LR)	Describes how may times a person with disease is more likely to receive a particular test result than a person without disease. A likelihood ratio greater than one indicates that the test result is associated with the presence of disease, a likelihood ratio less than one that it is associated with the absence of disease. Likelihood ratio for positive result (LR+) $= [a/(a+c)]/[b/(b+d)] =$ sensitivity /(1− specificity) Likelihood ratio for negative result (LR −) $= [c/(a+c)]/[d/(b+d)] =$ (1− sensitivity) / specificity
Predictive value	Positive predictive value: proportion of patients with positive test results who are correctly diagnosed Positive predictive value (PPV) $= a/(a+b)$ Negative predictive value: proportion of patients with negative test results who are correctly diagnosed Negative predictive value (NPV) $= d(c+d)$ Predictive values depend on disease prevalence, the more common a disease is, the more likely it is that a positive test result is right and a negative result is wrong. They can also be calculated by using the likelihood ratios to transform the pretest probability of disease: PPV = Posttest odds for positive test /(1+ Posttest odds for positive test) NPV = Posttest odds for negative test /(1+ Posttest odds for negative test) Posttest odds for positive test = Pretest odds × LR + Posttest odds for negative test = Pretest odds × LR − Pretest odds = Pretest probability of disease (prevalence) / (1 − pretest probability of disease)
Diagnostic odds ratio (DOR)	Used as an overall (single indicator) measure of the diagnostic accuracy of a diagnostic test. It is calculated as the odds of positivity among diseased persons, divided by the odds of positivity among nondiseased. When a test provides no diagnostic evidence, then the DOR is 1.0. DOR $= [a/c]/[b/d]$ = [sensitivity / (1 –specificity)] / [(1 – sensitivity) / specificity] = LR + ve / LR − ve $= ad/bc$

for obtaining additional information on a patient's health status. It includes information from history and physical examination, laboratory tests, imaging tests, function tests, and histopathology. The condition of interest or target condition can refer to a particular disease or to any other identifiable condition that may prompt clinical actions, such as further diagnostic testing, or the initiation, modification, or termination of treatment. In this framework, the reference, or "gold," standard is considered to be the best-available method for establishing the presence or absence of the condition of interest. The reference standard can be a single method, or a combination of methods, to establish the presence of the target condition. It can include laboratory tests, imaging tests, and pathology but also dedicated clinical follow-up of participants. The term *accuracy* refers to the amount of agreement between the information from the test under evaluation, referred to as the index test, and the reference standard. Diagnostic accuracy can be expressed in many ways, including sensitivity and specificity, likelihood ratios, diagnostic odds ratio, and the area under a receiver operator characteristic (ROC) curve (see Table 6.1).

In 2003, the Standards for Reporting of Diagnostic Accuracy (STARD) developed a checklist and a generic flow diagram for studies of diagnostic accuracy (21). The purpose of the STARD initiative is to improve the quality of reporting of diagnostic studies. The guiding principle in the development of the checklist was to select items that would help readers to judge the potential for bias in the study and to appraise the applicability of the findings. It contains 25 items covering salient issues in respect to design, conduct, and analysis of test accuracy studies. Follow-up work has resulted in a validated tool, the QUADAS (Quality Assessment of Studies of Diagnostic Accuracy included in Systematic Reviews) tool (22).

Measures of test properties and interpretation of results

Several related diagnostic accuracy parameters exist (see chapter 3). Perhaps the most well known are *sensitivity* (the proportion of patients with an abnormal test result among those who test positive on the reference standard) and *specificity* (the proportion of patients with a normal test result among those who test negative on the reference standard). The *likelihood ratio* is defined as the proportion of patients with a particular test result among those who test positive on the reference standard divided by the proportion of patients with that particular test result among those who test negative on the reference standard. The disadvantage of sensitivity, specificity, and likelihood ratios is that they produce at least two parameters of test performance. The *odds ratio* and the closely related area under the ROC curve compress the information into a single quantity. The odds ratio is defined as the likelihood ratio for a particular test result divided by the likelihood ratio for a negative test result. The area under the ROC curve quantifies the ability of the test to classify correctly individuals with and without the disease. It is particularly helpful if the test gives results on an ordinal or interval scale. A perfect test has an area of 1.0; a test that does not discriminate beyond chance has an area of 0.5.

Beyond single test evaluations

Over the past two decades, several authors increasingly recognized the importance of a rigorous evaluation process of diagnostic tests before introducing these tests into clinical practice (3,23,24). Studies to determine the diagnostic accuracy as described are an early and important part in this evaluation process (3,23–25); however, more upstream investigations particularly those including diagnostic algorithms are also mandatory. The early evaluations allow identifying promising tests with the potential to be useful in clinical practice, whereas the more sophisticated assessments provide empirical justification for clinical use. New diagnostic technologies should pass all these evaluations before they are implemented in practice.

Systematic reviews of test evaluation studies

History/current activities

There also is growing acknowledgment of the need for systematic reviews of studies evaluating the accuracy of diagnostic and screening tests. The number of such published reviews has increased in recent years: the Database of Abstracts of Reviews of Effects (DARE) maintained by the Centre for Reviews and Dissemination at the University of York includes 27 diagnostic test accuracy reviews for 1998, increasing to 49 in 2003. The Cochrane Collaboration is planning to include reviews of test accuracy studies. There has also been an increase in methodological work in this area (1,26–31). However, considerable uncertainty remains about the best way to formally synthesize test accuracy studies, and statistical methodology is much more varied than in meta-analysis of therapeutic interventions.

Meta-analytic methods

A number of different measures of diagnostic test accuracy, as shown in Table 6.1 and a variety of ways of meta-analyzing them exist. For example, recent reviews published in the *Annals of Internal Medicine* have chosen to perform fixed- or random-effects meta-analysis of positive and negative likelihood ratios (32,33) or of sensitivity and specificity (27,34,35), to pool patients across studies to calculate sensitivity and specificity (33), or to derive summary receiver operating characteristic (SROC) curves (34,35). A recent survey of reviews of diagnostic accuracy that were included in the Centre for Reviews and Dissemination's Database of Abstract of Reviews of Effects (DARE) up to 2002 (36) found that of 133 reviews in which meta-analysis was performed, 52% computed one or more summary measures of accuracy, 18% conducted only SROC analyses, and 30% did both. Of the 109 reviews that computed summary measures of accuracy, 89% used sensitivity or specificity, 24% used likelihood ratios, and 10% used predictive

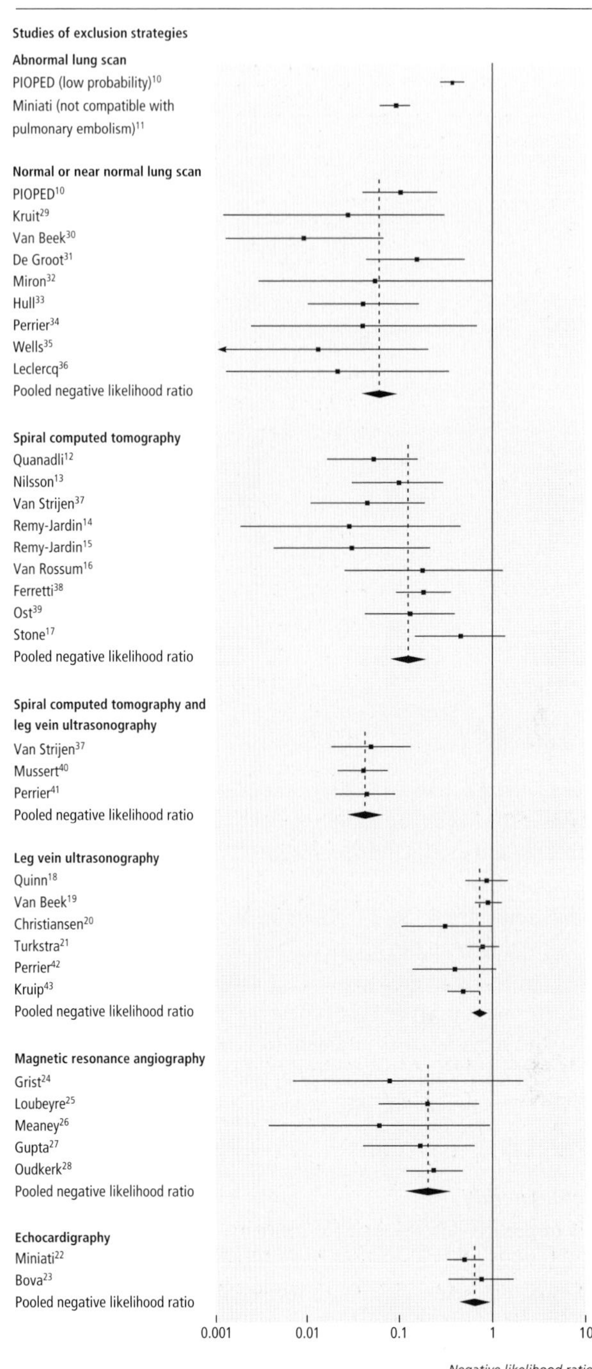

Figure 6.1 Summary plot of negative likelihood ratios (squares) and 95% confidence intervals for strategies used to exclude a diagnosis of pulmonary embolism. The size of squares relate to the variance of the study. The broken line represents pooled negative likelihood ratio, and limits of diamond represents 95% confidence intervals of pooled ratios. From (59).

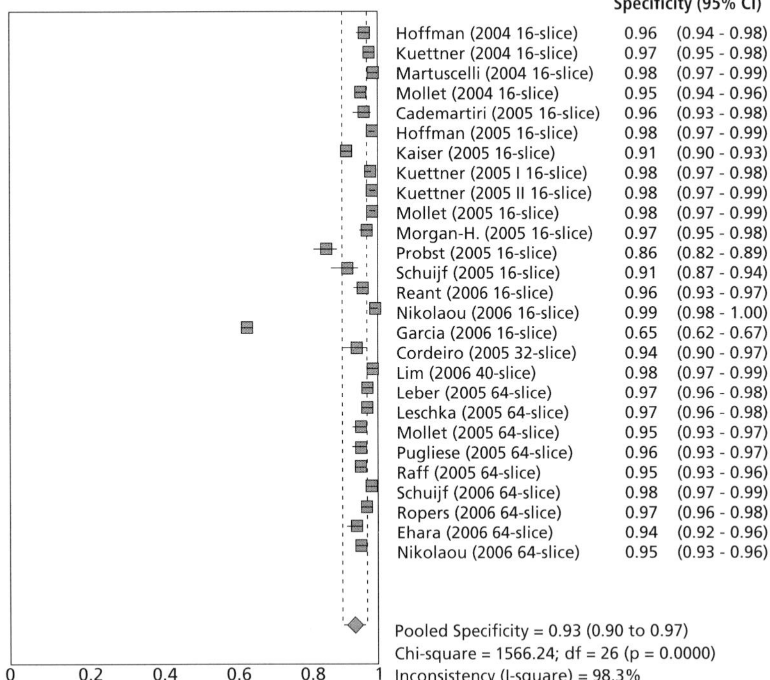

Figure 6.2 Summary plot and pooled estimate of specificity of multislice CT compared with coronary angiogram (adapted from reference (37)).

values. Figure 6.1 and 6.2 show examples of the use of summary measures for likelihood ratios related to D-dimer diagnostic test properties and specificity of multislice CT compared with coronary angiogram based on a systematic review of 27 diagnostic accuracy studies, respectively (36, 37). There are also several alternative ways of computing both SROC curves and summary measures of accuracy, differing in the weighting given to each study or whether a transformation is used (38). Because the use of systematic reviews and meta-analysis in diagnosis is becoming more popular, we describe the most commonly applied meta-analytic methods and their advantages and disadvantages and refer readers for more details to other texts (39).

Simple pooling

This approach derives a single summary 2 × 2 table by adding the numbers of true positives, false positives, true negatives, and false negatives across all studies. Test sensitivity and specificity can then be estimated as though all the data came from a single study. This can be thought of as a form of fixed-effect meta-analysis of sensitivity and specificity, ignoring any correlation between them and assuming no between-study heterogeneity (that is, differences in results between the studies) (1).

Separate random-effects meta-analysis of sensitivity and specificity

This approach (shown in Figure 6.2) allows for between-study heterogeneity in sensitivity and specificity but again ignores their correlation. Logit (log odds) transforms of sensitivity and specificity are used, as the assumption of a normal distribution between studies is more reasonable on the logit scale. In addition to summary points and confidence intervals for these points, summary ROC curves can be obtained from this method using the estimated between-study variances (26).

Separate meta-analysis of positive and negative likelihood ratios

Likelihood ratios are ratios of probabilities and so positive and negative likelihood ratios can be separately meta-analyzed using the same mathematical methods and software as risk ratios, based on either fixed-effect or random-effects models (see Figure 6.1) (1). This ignores the correlation between positive and negative likelihood ratios.

Littenberg-Moses summary ROC curve

The Littenberg-Moses summary ROC curve approach again uses the logit-transforms of sensitivity and specificity and is based on simple linear regression of their sum (the log of the diagnostic odds ratio) on their difference (25). The fitted regression line can then be used to give a summary ROC curve. This method allows for the correlation between sensitivity and specificity, but the method has other shortcomings, making it less statistically rigorous (28–30).

Bivariate random-effects meta-analysis

This approach, which represents an extension of separate random-effects meta-analyses of logit-transformed sensitivity and specificity, is statistically more rigorous in that it allows for the negative correlation between sensitivity and specificity and for the underlying binomial distributions as well as between-study heterogeneity (26). Its main advantages are that in addition to summary estimates of average sensitivity and specificity across studies, it can be used to provide a 95% confidence region for this summary point and prediction regions within which we expect the sensitivity and specificity of 95% of future studies to lie.

Hierarchical summary ROC curve (HSROC) analysis

In this approach, the relationship between logit-transformed sensitivity and specificity in each study is expressed in terms of key test characteristics: accuracy (quantified by the log of the diagnostic odds ratio) and threshold. The method allows for between-study variation, as well as for a parameter that determines the shape of the summary ROC curve. The results of this type of analysis are usually expressed as a summary ROC curve. Harbord et al. have shown elsewhere that in many circumstances, in particular when no covariates are added to the model, this method is statistically identical to bivariate random-effects meta-analysis (40). It follows that each can be used to derive the same summary estimates of sensitivity and specificity, 95% confidence and prediction regions, and summary ROC curves.

Interpretation of results

The barriers to the optimal use and appropriate interpretation of test evaluation data in clinical practice remain ill understood. From the point of view of decision-making theory (41), prediction rules that allow the calculation of posttest probabilities should overcome many of the cognitive biases that are known to affect diagnostic problem solving, including, for example, "compression error" (common conditions are underweighted, rare conditions are overweighted), the confusion of posttest probability with sensitivity, the "conjunction fallacy" (the erroneous assumption that a joint event is more probable than the probability of individual events alone), and "conservatism" (the hesitation to revise probabilities as new information becomes available) (42). Informal methods of opinion revision still dominate in practice (43). Furthermore, from a problem-solving perspective (44), it is unclear whether other factors, such as the failure to generate the correct hypothesis, are more important than the errors in estimating and revising probabilities emphasized by decision theory. Factors such as the experience of the health professional ordering tests, their propensity for risk taking, and the nature and levels of stress experienced may also be important. The attitudes of patients toward testing and their views on the value of results will often influence decisions, as indicated by the survey on the use of the ankle rules. Finally, many ways how to convey probabilistic information exist (e.g., natural frequencies, translation into everyday risks), but it is unclear what measures are used and useful in practice and how they are best synthesized and presented to primary care physicians.

Grading the quality of evidence and strength of recommendations for diagnostic recommendations

Those making recommendations regarding diagnostic test or strategies, such as a guideline panel, should begin by establishing its purpose. We emphasized in the preceding sections that a panel would have to determine the diagnostic standard for the target patient and the associated limitations of the standard. It should then identify the particular limitations for which the new test offers a putative remedy (e.g., eliminating a high proportion of false positive or negative results, enhancing availability, decreasing invasiveness or cost). This process will lead to the identification of sensible clinical questions, similar to that for other clinical management problems, with four components: patients, diagnostic intervention, comparison, and the outcomes of interest (45). Based on these criteria, a complete process to making recommendations about diagnostic tests includes the conduct or identification of a high-quality systematic review for the diagnostic test or strategy in question.

Test accuracy is a surrogate for patient-important outcomes

When clinicians think about diagnostic tests, they usually focus on their accuracy (i.e., how well does the test classify patients correctly as diseased or nondiseased or, in other words, sensitivity and specificity). Their underlying assumption is, however, that their obtaining a better idea of whether a target condition is present or absent will result in better patient management and outcomes. Another common rationale for a new test is avoiding complications associated with a more invasive alternative or limiting resources spent on expensive procedures (46). A new noninvasive and less expensive test that limits possible adverse consequences and increased resource use of more invasive tests would be considered superior. In this situation, a new test only needs to replicate the sensitivity and specificity of the reference standard to demonstrate superiority.

However, if a test fails to improve important outcomes, there is no reason to apply it, whatever its accuracy. Consider genetic testing for a rare, not-treatable, and life-shortening hematological disease that provides either welcome reassurance that a patient will not suffer from the condition or ability to plan for the future knowing that he will sadly fall victim. If the test will not lead to an outcome that is in some form beneficial to the patient, there is no need to test.

Thus, since the primary purpose of a test is to improve patient-important outcomes, the highest standard to assess a diagnostic strategy is a controlled trial in which investigators randomize patients to experimental or control diagnostic approaches and measure morbidity, mortality, symptoms, and quality of life (including psychological well-being). For example, Kearon and coworkers randomized 456 patients with negative erythrocyte agglutination D-dimer test results, categorized into low- and moderate- to high-risk groups, to different diagnostic management strategies (47). The authors evaluated patient-important outcomes (symptomatic venous thromboembolism) during six months of follow-up. They found that in patients with a low probability of pulmonary embolism who have negative D-dimer results, additional diagnostic testing can be withheld without increasing the frequency of venous thromboembolism during follow-up. In situations for which such trial evidence exists, the quality of evidence and the balance of desirable and undesirable effects should be evaluated using the framework described in chapter 1. However, such trials are rarely available. The few examples in the hematology literature include the use of D-dimer and other tests for the diagnosis of deep venous thrombosis and pulmonary embolism (47–49).

Thus, if randomized controlled trials are not feasible or available, those making recommendations must focus on studies of test accuracy and make inferences about the likely impact on patient-important outcomes. With this approach to any new test or strategy, the key questions are (i) whether there will be a reduction in false negatives (cases missed) or false positives (cases erroneously labeled as disease present), (ii) how these previous false negatives and false positives are similar or different to the usual spectrum, and (iii) what outcomes both those labeled as cases and those labeled as not having disease experience.

Using indirect evidence to make inferences about impact on patient-important outcomes

A recommendation associated with a diagnostic question depends on the balance between desirable and undesirable consequences of the diagnostic test or strategy. We described that greater accuracy of a test (superior sensitivity or specificity) improves the probability that it will increase desirable outcomes and decrease undesirable ones if there is a strong relation between accuracy data and patient-important outcomes. In this chapter, we are using the simplified approach that classifies test results into yielding true positives (patients correctly classified above the treatment threshold; see chapter 3), false positives (patients incorrectly classified above the treatment threshold), true negatives (patients correctly classified below the treatment threshold), and false negatives (patients incorrectly classified below the treatment threshold). However, inferring from accuracy data that a diagnostic test or strategy improves patient-important outcome often requires the availability of effective treatment (50). Alternatively, even without an effective treatment, a test may be beneficial if it reduces test-related adverse effects; if it leads to exclusion of a disease and reduction in anxiety; or if confirming a diagnosis improves patient well-being from the prognostic information it imparts such as in our example of genetic testing for hematological disease.

Situations in which the consequences of false-positives and false-negative results are less clear will result in weaker inferences about the balance between desirable and undesirable consequences. Having provided a rationale for the focus on patient-important outcomes, we will now describe the factors that influence the judgments about the balance of desirable and undesirable effects using the framework of the Grading of Recommendations Assessment, Development, and Evaluation (GRADE) Working Group (31).

Judgment about the quality of the underlying evidence for diagnostic questions

GRADE's four categories of quality of evidence of the system imply a gradient of confidence in estimates of the effect of a diagnostic test or strategy on patient-important outcomes (50). Randomized controlled trials involving direct comparison of the impact of alternative diagnostic strategies on patient-important outcomes, such as the randomized trial of strategies for the management of suspected venous thromboembolism, in the absence of limitations in design and conduct, imprecision, inconsistency, indirectness, and reporting bias, represents high-quality evidence (51–53).

Evidence will likely be lower quality if only studies of diagnostic accuracy are available. While valid accuracy studies start as high quality in the GRADE diagnostic framework, such studies are vulnerable to limitations as a result of the indirect evidence they may provide regarding impact on patient-important outcomes and are usually downgraded (31). Table 6.2 describes how GRADE deals with the challenges of assessing the quality of evidence regarding desirable and undesirable consequences of alternative diagnostic strategies.

Table 6.2 also highlights how judgment about quality differs when panels must rely on diagnostic accuracy studies to judge the impact of alternative diagnostic strategies. We will now comment further on three of the important differences: how GRADE views study design, limitations in planning and execution, and directness (31).

Study design

Studies focusing on accuracy allow only indirect evidence about the important consequences of alternative testing strategies. Panels making recommendations often face challenging judgments about the appropriate inferences from this indirect evidence.

Study limitations of diagnostic accuracy studies

GRADE considers the following factors (a) consecutive patients with an uncertain diagnosis who are representative of the target population should be included; (b) a comparison between the test or tests under consideration and an appropriate reference standard is included; (c) those who conduct or interpret the test must be unaware of the gold standard, or vice versa (both test and reference standard interpretations should be blind to one another). In general, these criteria are in agreement with existing instruments to evaluate the validity of the studies evaluating diagnostic test accuracy (54–57).

Directness

Judging directness (i.e., the question being addressed is quite different from the available evidence in regards to the population, diagnostic test or strategy, or intervention, comparison, or outcome) is perhaps the greatest challenge for those making recommendations for use or against use of diagnostic tests. If a new test, that may be much more expensive than what currently exists, reduces false positives and false negatives, to what extent will that reduction lead to improvement in patient-important outcomes? Alternatively, a new test may be simpler to perform with lower risk and cost but produce false positives and false negatives.

Consider the example of D-dimer testing instead of ultrasonography for the diagnosis of deep venous thrombosis. True-positive results will lead to the administration of therapies of known

Table 6.2 Factors that decrease the quality of evidence for studies of diagnostic accuracy and how they differ from evidence for other interventions.*

Factors that may decrease the quality of evidence	Explanations and how the factor may differ from the quality of evidence for other interventions
Indirectness	Additional quality criteria Panels assessing diagnostic tests often face an absence of direct evidence about impact on patient-important outcomes. They must therefore make deductions from diagnostic test studies about the likelihood that reduction in false positives or false negatives will benefit patients in important ways. Therefore, most accuracy studies suffer from indirectness.
Serious limitations in design or execution of the study	Different quality criteria for accuracy studies Consecutive patients recruited as a single cohort and not classified by disease state where the selection and referral process is clearly described (49). Test performed in all patients Same patient population for test and well described reference standard
Important inconsistency in study results	Similar quality criteria Similar judgments but, for accuracy studies, inconsistency in sensitivity, specificity, or likelihood ratios rather than relative risk or mean differences
Imprecise evidence	Similar quality criteria Similar judgments, but for accuracy studies wide confidence intervals, but now around estimates of test accuracy, or true and false positive and negatives
High probability of reporting bias	Similar-quality criteria Similar judgments

*Valid accuracy studies are cross-sectional or cohort studies in patients with diagnostic uncertainty and direct comparison of test results with an appropriate reference standard. These studies are considered high quality and can move to moderate, low, or very low, depending on other limitations.

effectiveness (anticoagulants); false-positive results will lead to adverse effects (unnecessary drugs and complications, interventions, and burden, including the possibility of follow-up visits) without possible benefit; true-negative results will spare patients the possible adverse effects of the reference standard test or the burden of more testing; and false negatives will result in patients not receiving the benefits of available interventions leading to a greater risk of thromboembolic complications. Thus, inferences that minimizing false positives and false negatives will benefit patients—and increasing them will have a negative impact on patient-important outcomes—are strong. As for outcomes in treatment studies, the degree of importance of these consequences for patients varies and should be addressed when balancing desirable and undesirable consequences (i.e., pulmonary embolism will be more important than postthrombotic syndrome).

The impact of inconclusive test results is less clear, but they are clearly undesirable, in that they are likely to induce anxiety, and may lead to unnecessary intervention or delay the application of effective treatment. Because our knowledge of the consequences of the false positive, false negative, inconclusive results, and complication rates with the alternative diagnostic strategies are secure, and those outcomes are important, we can make strong inferences concerning the relative impact of D-dimer testing and ultrasonography on patient-important outcomes.

Situations in which the consequences of the false-positive and false-negative results are less clear will result in weaker inferences about the balance between desirable and undesirable consequences (18,58,59).

Arriving at a recommendation for diagnostic tests and strategies

Similar to making a decision regarding treatment, the balance of desirable (true positives, true negatives, and reduced cost) and undesirable (false positives, false negatives, complications, and higher cost) consequences of a test and the relation to patient-important outcomes determine whether a panel recommends for or against applying a specific test. Other factors influencing the strength of a recommendation are the uncertainty or variation in values and preferences associated with the tests and outcomes. Users of recommendations on diagnostic tests should bear in mind that the likelihood of the disease (prevalence) in the patient before them has important consequences for the probability of a true and false positive in that patient.

Conclusions

This chapter described the use of systematic methods to evaluated and summarize the evidence regarding diagnostic tests and strategies. Encouraging examples of well-done randomized comparisons of diagnostic strategies exist in the hematology literature. In most situations, however, clinicians and other decision makers must rely on accuracy studies that are prone to limitations. Systematic reviews and meta-analyses of diagnostic test outcome measures is playing an increasing role in clinical medicine but bears methodological challenges as a consequence of complicated study design issues. Nevertheless, systematic reviews of the available evidence should form the basis of formal recommendations for diagnostic tests and strategies. The GRADE Working Group has developed a framework that those making recommendations can apply to make judgments about the quality of evidence of diagnostic research and the balance of desirable and undesirable effects related to diagnostic tests and strategies (29).

References

1 Deeks JJ. Systematic reviews in health care: systematic reviews of evaluations of diagnostic and screening tests. *BMJ.* 2001;**323**(7305): 157–62.

2 Nunn JF. *The medical papyri: ancient Egyptian medicine.* London: British Museum Press; 1996:24–41.

3 Fryback DG, Thornbury JR. The efficacy of diagnostic imaging. *Med Decis Making.* 1991;**11**(2):88–94.

4 Guyatt GH, Tugwell PX, Feeny DH, et al. A framework for clinical evaluation of diagnostic technologies. *CMAJ.* 1986 **15**;134(6):587–94.

5 Khan KS, Khan SF, Nwosu CR, et al. Misleading authors' inferences in obstetric diagnostic test literature. *Am J Obstet Gynecol.* 1999;**181**(1):112–15.

6 Hoffrage U, Lindsey S, Hertwig R, et al. Communicating statistical information. *Science.* 2000;**290**(5500):2261–62.

7 Steurer J, Fischer JE, Bachmann LM, et al. Communicating accuracy of tests to general practitioners: a controlled study. *BMJ.* 2002;**324**(7341):824–26.

8 Lijmer JG, Mol BW, Heisterkamp S, et al. Empirical evidence of design-related bias in studies of diagnostic tests. *JAMA.* 1999;**282**(11):1061–66.

9 Reid MC, Lachs MS, Feinstein AR. Use of methodological standards in diagnostic test research: getting better but still not good. *JAMA.* 1995;**274**(8):645–51.

10 Sheps SB, Schechter MT. The assessment of diagnostic tests: a survey of current medical research. *JAMA.* 1984;**252**(17):2418–22.

11 Song F, Khan KS, Dinnes J, Sutton AJ. Asymmetric funnel plots and publication bias in meta-analyses of diagnostic accuracy. *Int J Epidemiol.* 2002;**31**(1):88–95.

12 Mulherin SA, Miller WC. Spectrum bias or spectrum effect? Subgroup variation in diagnostic test evaluation. *Ann Intern Med.* 2002;**137**(7):598–602.

13 Ransohoff DF, Feinstein AR. Problems of spectrum and bias in evaluating the efficacy of diagnostic tests. *N Engl J Med.* 1978;**299**(17):926–30.

14 Irwig L, Macaskill P, Glasziou P, et al. Meta-analytic methods for diagnostic test accuracy. *J Clin Epidemiol.* 1995;**48**(1):119–30; discussion 31–32.

15 Midgette AS, Stukel TA, Littenberg B. A meta-analytic method for summarizing diagnostic test performances: receiver-operating-characteristic-summary point estimates. *Med Decis Making.* 1993;**13**(3): 253–57.

16 Shapiro DE. Issues in combining independent estimates of the sensitivity and specificity of a diagnostic test. *Acad Radiol.* 1995;**2** Suppl 1:S37–S47; discussion S65–S69, S83.

17 Vamvakas EC. Meta-analyses of studies of the diagnostic accuracy of laboratory tests: a review of the concepts and methods. *Arch Pathol Lab Med.* 1998;**122**(8):675–86.

18 Fletcher RH. Carcinoembryonic antigen. *Ann Intern Med.* 1986;**104**(1):66–73.

19 Lensing AW, Hirsh J. 125I-fibrinogen leg scanning: reassessment of its role for the diagnosis of venous thrombosis in post-operative patients. *Thromb Haemost.* 1993;**69**(1):2–7.

20 Jarvik JG, Hollingworth W, Martin B, et al. Rapid magnetic resonance imaging vs radiographs for patients with low back pain: a randomized controlled trial. *JAMA.* 2003;**289**(21):2810.

21 STARD checklist [cited 16 Jan 2002]. Available at: http://www.consort-statement.org/stardstatement.htm.

22 Whiting P, Rutjes AWS, Reitsma JB, et al. The development of QUADAS: a tool for the quality assessment of studies of diagnostic accuracy included in systematic reviews. *BMC Med Res Method.* 2003;**3**:25.

23 Gluud C, Gluud LL. Evidence based diagnostics. *BMJ.* 2005;**330**(7493):724–26.

24 Guyatt G, Drummond M, Feeny D, et al. Guidelines for the clinical and economic evaluation of health care technologies. *Soc Sci Med.* 1986;**22**(4):393–408.

25 Kent DL, Larson EB. Disease, level of impact, and quality of research methods. Three dimensions of clinical efficacy assessment applied to magnetic resonance imaging. *Invest Radiol.* 1992;**27**(3):245–54.

26 Moses LE, Shapiro D, Littenberg B. Combining independent studies of a diagnostic test into a summary ROC curve: data-analytic approaches and some additional considerations. *Stat Med.* 1993;**12**(14):1293–316.

27 Cook RL, Hutchison SL, Ostergaard L, et al. Systematic review: noninvasive testing for *Chlamydia trachomatis* and *Neisseria gonorrhoeae. Ann Intern Med.* 2005;**142**(11):914–25.

28 Reitsma JB, Glas AS, Rutjes AW, et al. Bivariate analysis of sensitivity and specificity produces informative summary measures in diagnostic reviews. *J Clin Epidemiol.* 2005;**58**(10):982–90.

29 Rutter CM, Gatsonis CA. A hierarchical regression approach to meta-analysis of diagnostic test accuracy evaluations. *Stat Med.* 2001;**20**(19):2865–84.

30 Rutter CM, Gatsonis CA. Regression methods for meta-analysis of diagnostic test data. *Acad Radiol.* 1995;**2** Suppl 1:S48–S56; discussion S65–S67, S70–71.

31 Schunemann HJ, Oxman AD, Brozek J, et al. GRADEing the quality of evidence and strength of recommendations for diagnostic tests and strategies. *BMJ.* (in press).

32 Marx A, Pewsner D, Egger M, et al. Meta-analysis: accuracy of rapid tests for malaria in travelers returning from endemic areas. *Ann Intern Med.* 2005;**142**(10):836–46.

33 Terasawa T, Blackmore CC, Bent S, et al. Systematic review: computed tomography and ultrasonography to detect acute appendicitis in adults and adolescents. *Ann Intern Med.* 2004;**141**(7):537–46.

34 Safdar N, Fine JP, Maki DG. Meta-analysis: methods for diagnosing intravascular device-related bloodstream infection. *Ann Intern Med.* 2005;**142**(6):451–66.

35 Karassa FB, Matsagas MI, Schmidt WA, et al. Meta-analysis: test performance of ultrasonography for giant-cell arteritis. *Ann Intern Med.* 2005;**142**(5):359–69.

36 Dinnes J, Deeks J, Kirby J, et al. A methodological review of how heterogeneity has been examined in systematic reviews of diagnostic test accuracy. *Health Technol Assess.* 2005;**9**(12):1–113, iii.

37 Hamon M, Biondi-Zoccai GG, Malagutti P, et al. Diagnostic performance of multislice spiral computed tomography of coronary arteries as compared with conventional invasive coronary angiography: a meta-analysis. *J Am Coll Cardiol.* 2006;**48**(9):1896–910.

38 Riley RD, Abrams KR, Sutton AJ, et al. Bivariate random-effects meta-analysis and the estimation of between-study correlation. *BMC Med Res Methodol.* 2007;**7**:3.

39 Macaskill P. Empirical Bayes estimates generated in a hierarchical summary ROC analysis agreed closely with those of a full Bayesian analysis. *J Clin Epidemiol.* 2004;**57**(9):925–32.

40 Harbord RM, Deeks JJ, Egger M, et al. A unification of models for meta-analysis of diagnostic accuracy studies. *Biostatistics.* 2007;**8**(2): 239–51.

41 Sox HC, Blatt MA, Hinggins MC, et al. Medical decision making. Butterworth-Heinemann: Boston; 1987.

42 Elstein AS. Heuristics and biases: selected errors in clinical reasoning. *Acad Med.* 1999;**74**(7):791–94.

43 Elstein AS, Schwarz A. Clinical problem solving and diagnostic decision making: selective review of the cognitive literature. *BMJ.* 2002;**324**(7339):729–32.

44 Schmidt HG, Norman GR, Boshuizen HP. A cognitive perspective on medical expertise: theory and implication. *Acad Med.* 1990;**65**(10):611–21.

45 Oxman AD, Guyatt GH. Guidelines for reading literature reviews. *CMAJ.* 1988;**138**(8):697–703.

46 Bossuyt PM, Irwig L, Craig J, et al. Comparative accuracy: assessing new tests against existing diagnostic pathways. *BMJ.* 2006;**332**(7549):1089–92.

47 Kearon C, Ginsberg JS, Douketis J, et al. An evaluation of D-dimer in the diagnosis of pulmonary embolism: a randomized trial. *Ann Intern Med.* 2006;**144**(11):812–21.

48 Kearon C, Ginsberg JS, Douketis J, et al. A randomized trial of diagnostic strategies after normal proximal vein ultrasonography for suspected deep venous thrombosis: D-dimer testing compared with repeated ultrasonography. *Ann Intern Med.* 2005;**142**(7):490–96.

49 Rathbun SW, Whitsett TL, Raskob GE. Negative D-dimer result to exclude recurrent deep venous thrombosis: a management trial. *Ann Intern Med.* 2004;**141**(11):839–45.

50 Deeks JJ. Systematic reviews in health care: systematic reviews of evaluations of diagnostic and screening tests. *BMJ.* 2001;**323**(7305):157–62.

51 Guyatt G, Oxman AD, Kunz R, et al. What is "quality of evidence" and why is it important to clinicians? *BMJ.* (in press).

52 Atkins D, Best D, Briss PA, et al. Grading quality of evidence and strength of recommendations. *BMJ.* 2004;**328**(7454):1490.

53 Schünemann HJ, Jaeschke R, Cook DJ, et al. An official ATS statement: grading the quality of evidence and strength of recommendations in ATS guidelines and recommendations. *Am J Respir Crit Care Med.* 2006;**174**(5):605–14.

54 Bossuyt PM, Reitsma JB, Bruns DE, et al. Towards complete and accurate reporting of studies of diagnostic accuracy: the STARD Initiative. *Ann Intern Med.* 2003;**138**(1):40–44.

55 Bossuyt PM, Reitsma JB, Bruns DE, et al. The STARD statement for reporting studies of diagnostic accuracy: explanation and elaboration. *Ann Intern Med.* 2003;**138**(1):W1–12.

56 Whiting P, Rutjes AW, Reitsma JB, et al. The development of QUADAS: a tool for the quality assessment of studies of diagnostic accuracy included in systematic reviews. *BMC Med Res Methodol.* 2003;**3**:25.

57 Whiting PF, Weswood ME, Rutjes AW, et al. Evaluation of QUADAS, a tool for the quality assessment of diagnostic accuracy studies. *BMC Med Res Methodol.* 2006;**6**:9.

58 Hlatky MA, Pryor DB, Harrell FE Jr, et al. Factors affecting sensitivity and specificity of exercise electrocardiography. Multivariable analysis. *Am J Med.* 1984;**77**(1):64–71.

59 Levy D, Labib SB, Anderson KM, et al. Determinants of sensitivity and specificity of electrocardiographic criteria for left ventricular hypertrophy. *Circulation.* 1990;**81**(3):815–20.

60 Roy P-M, Colombet I, Durieux P, et al. Systematic review and meta-analysis of strategies for the diagnosis of suspected pulmonary embolism. *BMJ.* 2005;**331**(7511):259–68.

2 Hemostasis and Thrombosis

Jeff Ginsberg

7 Diagnosis of Deep Vein Thrombosis

Lori-Ann Linkins

Deep vein thrombosis (DVT) has an estimated incidence of 48 per 100,000 person-years in the United States (1). The incidence of DVT increases with age and the presence of additional risk factors (e.g., thrombophilia, surgery, malignancy) (2). Patients with DVT who do not receive anticoagulant therapy are at high risk for developing pulmonary embolism (PE), a potentially fatal complication. Even with adequate treatment, 0.4% of patients with DVT will die from fatal PE (3) and an estimated 20%–50% will develop post-thrombotic syndrome, a chronic condition that is both debilitating for patients and costly for the healthcare system (4).

This chapter will provide an overview of the methods used to diagnose DVT and provide the author's opinion on the quality of evidence. Grading of the quality of evidence and strengths of recommendations in this chapter are based on the guidelines proposed by the international Grading of Recommendations Assessment, Development, and Evaluation Working Group (GRADE) adopting the modification used by the American College of Chest Physicians that merges the very low and low categories of quality of evidence (see chapter 1). Clinical studies were identified from a MEDLINE search using the following terms (MeSH and free text): *venous thrombosis, diagnosis, ultrasonography, venography, magnetic resonance, CT venography, D-dimer, clinical model, clinical trial.* High-quality meta-analyses are referenced rather than individual studies where possible. Diagnosis of recurrent DVT and DVT during pregnancy will be addressed separately at the end of the chapter.

Diagnosis of first acute deep vein thrombosis

Why is objective testing needed to diagnose DVT?

The signs and symptoms most commonly associated with DVT include edema, pain, tenderness, and erythema. Unfortunately, these features are nonspecific and 3 out of 4 ambulatory patients who are suspected to have DVT will have an alternative explanation for their symptoms (e.g., muscle cramp, Baker's cyst, cellulitis, and others). Failure to diagnose DVT exposes patients to the risk of fatal PE (1 out of 20 pulmonary emboli are fatal) (4). However, inappropriate use of anticoagulant therapy exposes patients to the risk of serious complications, including fatal hemorrhage (1 out of 11 anticoagulant-related major bleeds are fatal) (5). Because clinical assessment alone is unreliable, objective testing to confirm the diagnosis is crucial when DVT is suspected.

Evidence-based Hematology. Edited by Mark A. Crowther, Jeff Ginsberg, Holger J. Schünemann, Ralph M. Meyer, and Richard Lottenberg.

Which imaging modalities can be used to diagnose DVT?

Compression ultrasonography

Compression ultrasonography is considered the first-line imaging test for DVT because it is accurate, safe, and noninvasive (Grade 1A). Using the method described by Lensing et al. (6), the common femoral vein and popliteal vein are imaged in real time and compressed with an ultrasound transducer probe. Inability to fully compress the vein is diagnostic of venous thrombosis. Most centers currently evaluate compression at 1-cm intervals from the common femoral vein to the calf trifurcation. Accuracy studies comparing compression ultrasound with venography, the reference standard test for DVT, showed compression ultrasound to have a sensitivity of 97% and a specificity of 94% for symptomatic proximal DVT (7). Management studies using serial compression ultrasonography (i.e., a repeat ultrasound is performed one week after an initial negative ultrasound) have shown that it is safe to withhold anticoagulant therapy in patients with suspected DVT who have negative serial ultrasounds (i.e., 1%–2% of these patients developed venous thromboembolism (VTE) during six months of follow-up) (7).

Unlike the case with proximal DVT, the utility of compression ultrasonography for diagnosing isolated calf vein thrombosis is controversial (Grade 2C). The sensitivity of this method for isolated calf vein thrombosis is significantly lower than for proximal DVT (50%–75%) and the number of indeterminate exams is higher (7). Visualization of the calf veins is limited by patient position, presence of edema or hematomas, and operator skill. Furthermore, the clinical value of detecting isolated calf vein thrombosis is debatable. Studies have suggested that only 13% of DVT are isolated to the calf (8,9) and only 20% of these will extend into the proximal veins if left untreated (10). The previously mentioned management studies for diagnosing DVT using serial compression ultrasonography showed a low incidence of VTE in follow-up even though all ultrasound examinations were restricted to the proximal veins.

Some investigators have proposed a single complete compression ultrasound that includes examination of the calf veins as an alternative to time-consuming serial ultrasounds in patients with suspected DVT (Grade 2B). Studies using this method have reported an incidence of VTE of 0.5% after three months follow-up (11–13). However, there is concern that this method has the potential to diagnose calf DVT that would have safely resolved without treatment, thereby exposing patients to the risk of bleeding due to anticoagulant therapy without clear benefit. A randomized controlled trial that compares ultrasonography restricted to the proximal veins with single complete ultrasonography (withholding anticoagulant therapy for negative ultrasounds in both groups) would help address this issue.

Ultrasonography has also been proposed as an alternative to venography for screening patients for asymptomatic DVT, particularly following orthopedic surgery (Grade 2B). A meta-analysis of methodologically high-quality studies comparing screening ultrasonography with venography reported sensitivity of 62%, specificity of 97%, and positive predictive value of 66% of ultrasonography for asymptomatic proximal DVT (14). A more recent meta-analysis reported similar results with respect to pooled sensitivity and specificity but based on using an alternative summary method (diagnostic odds ratio) concluded that ultrasound screening was accurate for asymptomatic DVT in the proximal veins (15). Translating diagnostic odds ratios into clinical practice, however, is more problematic than pooled sensitivity/specificity; therefore, the accuracy of ultrasonography for diagnosing asymptomatic DVT is still questionable. (Impedance plethysmography is another validated, noninvasive test for DVT, but because it has been replaced by ultrasonography and is no longer being manufactured, it will not be reviewed here.)

Contrast venography

Contrast venography is recognized as the reference standard imaging test for deep vein thrombosis (16) (Grade 1A). This method allows direct visualization of the veins from the calf to the vena cava after injection of contrast into a superficial vein on the dorsum of the foot. An intraluminal filling defect seen in two views is considered diagnostic for thrombosis. Unfortunately, venography is invasive, operator-dependent, and expensive. In addition, the use of contrast exposes patients to the risk of allergic reactions and contrast-induced nephropathy. Because of these drawbacks, the role of contrast venography has been restricted to (i) surrogate marker for VTE in studies evaluating new anticoagulants; (ii) confirmatory test in cases where suspicion of DVT is high, but a compression ultrasound is nondiagnostic; and (iii) diagnosis of recurrent DVT.

Contrast venography and magnetic resonance venography

The limitations of compression ultrasound in diagnosing DVT in certain clinical settings (e.g., obese patients, patients with plaster casts, patients with isolated pelvic vein thrombosis) have led to evaluation of other imaging modalities, such as CT venography and magnetic resonance venography.

Contrast venography has been used in combination with CT pulmonary angiography in patients with suspected PE. This approach offers the advantage of imaging for DVT and PE in one examination as well as potentially identifying nonthrombogenic pathology (e.g., cancer). However, combining both imaging tests requires a larger bolus of contrast and is still subject to difficulties in interpretation (e.g. due to streak artifacts, poor opacification). One small study with methodological limitations compared the accuracy of CT venography with conventional venography for diagnosing acute DVT (6 patients with suspected PE without DVT were included) and reported sensitivity of 100% and specificity of 92% (17). The sensitivity and specificity of CT venography has been reported between 89% to 100% and 94% to 100%, respectively, when compared with ultrasonography in one review (18), but the majority of the studies included in these estimates were case series. Given the cost, exposure to radiation, and limited availability, it is highly unlikely that CT venography will ever replace ultrasonography as the first-line imaging test for first acute DVT.

Magnetic resonance venography can be performed with injection of gadolinium or without any contrast (MR direct thrombus imaging). Gadolinium-enhanced MR venography is performed by injecting contrast into either a vein in the foot or as a single peripheral bolus with imaging timed to record filling of the veins of the lower limb. As with conventional venography, the presence of an intraluminal filling defect is diagnostic of DVT. MRDTI is performed without contrast so diagnosis of thrombus is based on detection of a high signal against a suppressed background. A recent meta-analysis of studies comparing MR venography with conventional venography reported a pooled sensitivity of 92% and specificity of 95% of MR venography for proximal DVT (19). The authors noted that there was significant heterogeneity between the studies, which means the pooled estimates should be interpreted with caution. Potential explanations for the heterogeneity included differences in MR technique, operator skill, and study type (one study used ultrasound as the reference standard and two studies enrolled asymptomatic patients; Grade 1B). MRDTI has only been evaluated in a single accuracy study to date (included in the meta-analysis described above) (20).

How can clinical pretest probability be used to diagnose DVT?

The clinical features of DVT alone cannot be used to either confirm or exclude the diagnosis of DVT. However, structured clinical prediction models based on the presence or absence of risk factors, typical signs and symptoms of DVT, and alternative explanations for symptoms can be used to stratify patients into categories based on the probability of DVT (e.g., high, intermediate, or low). Such categorization is useful in streamlining further investigations for DVT (Grade 1A).

Several clinical prediction models have been developed with the Wells model being the most widely validated (21). The Wells model divides patients into low-, moderate-, or high-probability categories for DVT with a prevalence of DVT of greater than 10%, 25%, and 60%, respectively. Management studies have shown that outpatients in the low-probability group who have one other negative diagnostic test (i.e., ultrasound or D-dimer assay) require no further investigation and have a low rate of confirmed VTE at three months (Grade 1A). The most recent version of the Wells score includes an additional item (previously documented DVT) and uses only two categories for patients: DVT likely or DVT unlikely (22). Studies have shown that empirical assessment of clinical pretest probability is also useful for stratifying patients, but results in fewer patients being classified as "low" when compared with the Wells model, which reduces clinical utility (23).

How can D-dimer assays be used to diagnose DVT?

D-dimer is formed when cross-linked fibrin is broken down by plasmin. D-dimer levels are typically elevated in patients with acute DVT; therefore, a negative D-dimer assay helps to exclude this diagnosis (high negative predictive value). A positive D-dimer assay may be due to DVT, or it may be due to inflammation, trauma, pregnancy, malignancy, or surgery (low positive predictive value). Consequently, a negative D-dimer is helpful in excluding the diagnosis of DVT, but a positive D-dimer does not confirm the diagnosis of DVT.

There are several different types of D-dimer assay available for clinical use: enzyme-linked immunosorbent assays (ELISA), quantitative rapid ELISA, semiquantitative rapid ELISA, qualitative rapid ELISA, quantitative latex, semiquantitative latex, and whole blood (24). These assays differ markedly with respect to their diagnostic properties for DVT. The assays with the highest sensitivity for DVT are the traditional, time-consuming ELISA and quantitative rapid ELISAs (e.g., VIDAS). However, the high sensitivity of these assays comes at the price of lower specificity. Thus, these assays can be used as a stand-alone test to exclude the diagnosis of DVT (Grade 1A), but they produce a high number of false-positive results, which reduces their clinical utility (25). Less-sensitive D-dimer assays (e.g., SimpliRED) have better specificity but must be combined with another diagnostic test to exclude the diagnosis of DVT (i.e., clinical pretest probability, ultrasound examination; Grade 1A).

The combination of clinical pretest probability and D-dimer was compared with the combination of clinical pretest probability and ultrasound in one randomized trial (22). The thromboembolic event rate in the patients who had DVT excluded based on clinical pretest probability and ultrasound was 1.4% compared with an event rate of 0.4% in the patients who had DVT excluded based on clinical pretest probability and D-dimer ($p = 0.16$). Consequently, while both diagnostic strategies were shown to be safe, the use of the D-dimer significantly reduced the number of ultrasounds that were required (Table 7.1).

Diagnosis of Recurrent DVT

Which imaging modalities can be used to diagnose recurrent DVT?

Diagnosing recurrent DVT is more problematic than diagnosing first acute DVT. To begin with, the signs and symptoms experienced by patients with recurrent DVT are also seen in patients with postthrombotic syndrome, a condition that affects approximately 20% to 50% of patients with previous DVT (4). Differentiating between these two conditions is important because postthrombotic syndrome does not require treatment with anticoagulant therapy, whereas recurrent DVT that remains untreated places patients at risk for fatal PE. Unfortunately, to date, there is no reference standard noninvasive test that has been shown to diagnose recurrent DVT accurately.

Compression ultrasonography is commonly used as the first-line diagnostic test for patients with suspected recurrent DVT. In patients with a recent ultrasound that demonstrated either limited extent of their previous DVT or complete resolution, the presence of a new noncompressible segment on ultrasound examination is accepted as diagnostic for recurrent DVT (Grade 1B). Unfortunately, persistent abnormalities of the deep veins on ultrasound examination are common following first acute DVT despite adequate treatment. Heijboer and colleagues (26) reported that 50% of patients with lower-limb DVT will still have abnormal compression on ultrasound examination one year after diagnosis. Consequently, the presence of incomplete compression on ultrasound examination of a previously affected limb is rarely diagnostic of recurrent DVT.

Other ultrasound parameters such as residual vein diameter, Doppler flow, and thrombus echogenicity have been used to diagnose recurrent DVT, but the evidence to support these methods is very limited. Measurement of residual vein diameter is the only one of these parameters that has been systematically evaluated for diagnosing recurrent DVT (27). In their management study of patients with suspected recurrent DVT, Prandoni and colleagues (27) reported that it was safe to withhold anticoagulant therapy in patients who had less than a 4-mm increase in residual vein diameter between two compression ultrasound examinations (Grade 1C). A drawback of this method is that a recent ultrasound, prior to the episode of suspected recurrence, is required for comparison. In addition, there is some evidence to suggest that the reproducibility of this measurement is only moderate (28). The evidence for use of Doppler flow or thrombus echogenicity for diagnosis of recurrent DVT is even more limited with no large accuracy or management trials using these parameters published to date (28) (Grade 2C). Change in thrombus length on ultrasound examination using anatomical landmarks as reference points has been proposed as an ultrasound parameter that could be used to

Table 7.1 Summary of Diagnostic Tests for First Acute DVT (with ACCP category 1 recommendation): strategies for diagnosis of first acute DVT according to patient population.

Diagnostic test	Criteria	Confirms DVT	Excludes DVT	Evidence grade
Symptomatic outpatients				
Compression US*	Noncompressible proximal veins (no history of DVT in same leg)	X		1A
Contrast venography	Intraluminal filling defect on 2 views	X		1A
PTP and D-dimer	Low PTP and negative D-dimer (sensitivity ≥85% and specificity ≥70%)		X	1A
PTP and Compression US	Low PTP and normal US (all proximal veins fully compressible)		X	1A
D-dimer and Compression US	Negative D-dimer (sensitivity ≥ 85% and specificity ≥ 70%) and normal US		X	1A
PTP and serial compression US	Moderate PTP and normal US at presentation and on serial testing in 5 to 7 days		X	1A
D-dimer	Negative D-dimer (sensitivity ≥ 98% and specificity ≥ 40%)		X	1A
Contrast venography	All deep veins visualized and no intralulminal filling defects seen		X	1A
CT Venography or Magnetic Resonance Venography	All proximal veins visualized and no intraluminal filling defects seen		X	1B
Symptomatic inpatients				
Compression US*	Noncompressible proximal veins (no history of DVT in same leg)	X		1A
Contrast venography	Intraluminal filling defect on 2 views	X		1A
PTP and compression US	Low PTP and normal US (all proximal veins fully compressible)		X	1B
PTP and serial compression US	Moderate PTP and normal US at presentation and on serial testing in 5 to 7 days		X	1B
Contrast venography	All deep veins visualized and no intralulminal filling defects seen		X	1A
Asymptomatic patients				
Contrast venography	Intraluminal filling defect on 2 views	X		1A
Contrast venography	All deep veins visualized and no intralulminal filling defects seen		X	1A

*From common femoral vein to calf trifurcation only. US, ultrasound; PTP. pretest probability.

diagnose recurrent DVT, but has not been validated in a clinical trial (29).

Contrast venography is considered the reference standard diagnostic imaging test for recurrent DVT. As with first acute DVT, a new intraluminal defect seen in two views confirms the diagnosis of recurrence. However, venography is frequently nondiagnostic in patients with suspected recurrent DVT due to nonfilling of previously affected venous segments. Because it is not dependent on contrast flow, MR direct thrombus imaging may offer an alternative imaging test for recurrent DVT, but further studies are needed before it can be recommended for this indication (20).

How can clinical pretest probability be used to diagnose recurrent DVT?

As with first acute DVT, clinical features alone cannot be used to either confirm or exclude the diagnosis of recurrent DVT. As

Table 7.2 Summary of diagnostic tests for recurrent DVT and DVT during pregnancy.

Diagnostic Test	Criteria	Confirms DVT	Excludes DVT	Evidence grade
Suspected recurrent DVT				
Compression US*	New noncompressible proximal vein with recent normal US (or US showing limited extent of previous DVT) for comparison	X		1B
Contrast venography	Intraluminal filling defect on 2 views	X		1A
Compression US	Difference in residual vein diameter ≥ 4 mm when compared with recent US	X		1C
Contrast venography	All deep veins visualized and no intralulminal filling defects seen		X	1A
Compression US	Less than 1-mm increase in residual vein diameter when compared with recent US and remains unchanged on repeat US testing at 2 and 7 days		X	1C
D-dimer	Negative D-dimer (sensitivity ≥ 98% and specificity ≥ 40%)		X	1C
Pregnant patients				
Compression US	Noncompressible proximal veins (no history of DVT in same leg)	X		1B
Compression US	Normal US at presentation and with repeat testing in 7 days		X	1C

*From common femoral vein to calf trifurcation only. US, ultrasound; PTP, pretest probability.

previously mentioned, Wells and colleagues most recent version of a clinical prediction model for DVT includes allocation of a point to "previously documented deep-vein thrombosis" (22). In their study comparing two noninvasive diagnostic strategies for DVT, 36% of patients had a history of previous ipsilateral DVT, but the results for these patients were not reported separately. Further validation of this model for patients with suspected recurrent DVT is required.

Using the data from an ongoing prospective cohort study evaluating D-dimer for the diagnosis of recurrent DVT, Bates and colleagues (30) developed a clinical prediction model for recurrent DVT. Patients are categorized as low (<10% prevalence), moderate (10%–60% prevalence), and high (>60% prevalence) probability of recurrence using the following predictors: recent risk factors for DVT, greater than two previous episodes of VTE, absence of therapeutic anticoagulation, previous VTE unprovoked or associated with an ongoing risk factor, and no alternative diagnosis more likely. Prospective validation of this model is pending.

How can D-dimer assays be used to diagnose recurrent DVT?

The safety of using a negative D-dimer assay to exclude the diagnosis of recurrence in patients with suspected recurrent DVT is less studied than with first acute DVT. Rathbun and colleagues (31) evaluated the STA-Liatest D-dimer assay in a cohort study of patients with suspected recurrent DVT using compression ultrasound as the reference standard test. Anticoagulant therapy was withheld from patients who had a negative D-dimer. Patients with a positive D-dimer underwent a compression ultrasound examination; recurrence was confirmed if there was a greater than 4-mm increase in residual vein diameter when a previous ultrasound examination and the study ultrasound examination were compared. The incidence of recurrent VTE during three months of follow-up in patients with a negative D-dimer (45% of patients) was 0.75%. Ultrasound confirmed recurrence in 33% of patients with a positive D-dimer, in each case, based on new noncompressibility of a venous segment. Using this approach, the investigators were able to safely exclude recurrent VTE in 42% of patients, but investigations remained inconclusive in 5 patients with a negative D-dimer and 33 patients with a positive D-dimer. Consequently, it appears that a negative D-dimer helps to rule out the diagnosis of recurrent DVT, but a reliable reference standard test for confirming the diagnosis of recurrent DVT is still needed (Grade 1C). A cohort study using the MDA D-dimer to exclude recurrent DVT is under way.

The primary focus of recent research has been whether the result of a D-dimer assay can be used to predict which patients are at the highest risk of recurrence and therefore should remain on anticoagulant therapy indefinitely (Table 7.2).

Diagnosis of DVT during pregnancy

Which diagnostic tests can be used to diagnose DVT during pregnancy?

The incidence of VTE is increased by two- to fourfold during pregnancy (32). However, leg edema with or without calf pain is common in pregnant women, especially in the third trimester. Consequently, only 8% of pregnant women presenting with suspected DVT will have this diagnosis confirmed on objective testing (33). Studies have also shown that pregnant women are far more likely to have left leg DVT than right leg DVT. Explanations for this finding include compression of the left iliac vein by the right iliac artery, and a decrease in the velocity of blood flow when a pregnant women lies in the supine position. Clearly, the risk to both mother and fetus if a diagnosis of venous thrombosis is missed or if anticoagulant therapy is used when it is not needed, emphasizes the importance of objective testing in this patient population (34).

Serial compression ultrasonography is the first-line diagnostic test for DVT during pregnancy although it is not well-validated in this population (Grade 1B). The accuracy of this test for proximal DVT is likely comparable to its performance in nonpregnant females. However, isolated iliac vein thrombosis is believed to be more common in pregnant females and cannot be detected by compression ultrasound. Magnetic resonance imaging has been used to diagnose isolated iliac vein thrombosis in a small cohort of patients but has not been formally evaluated in pregnant patients. The natural history of calf vein thrombosis is also less certain in pregnant females so the safety of serial ultrasonography is unclear.

Venography is the reference standard diagnostic test for DVT during pregnancy. However, concern about exposure of the fetus to ionizing radiation is a major barrier to its use. Case-control studies suggest that exposure to radiation in utero may cause a small increase in the relative risk of childhood cancer. Unilateral venography exposes the fetus to approximately 0.314 rads compared with less than 0.001 rads exposure during a chest radiograph (35). Use of abdominal shielding during venography reduces fetal exposure.

No large studies using D-dimer levels to diagnose DVT during pregnancy have been published to date. D-dimer levels are known to increase with gestational age and some complications of pregnancy therefore the clinical utility of these assays is likely to be less than in the nonpregnant population (36). Studies addressing this issue are ongoing.

The Future

Extensive research has led to the development of a number of validated diagnostic tests to confirm and exclude first acute DVT. Current development for these patients is focused on streamlining the diagnostic approach to reduce the time and expense required to arrive at a diagnosis. The areas where challenges remain include (i) diagnosis of asymptomatic DVT in high-risk patients who cannot receive thromboprophylaxis, (ii) diagnosis of recurrent ipsilateral DVT, and (iii) diagnosis of DVT during pregnancy. As imaging technology continues to evolve, it will be interesting to see how it contributes to progress in these areas.

References

1 Silverstein MD, Heit JA, Mohr DN, et al. Trends in the incidence of deep vein thrombosis and pulmonary embolism: a 25-year population-based study. *Arch Intern Med.* 1998;**158**:585–93.

2 Heit JA. Venous thromboembolism: disease burden, outcomes, and risk factors. *J Thromb Haemost.* 2005;**3**:1611–17.

3 Douketis JD, Kearon C, Bates S, et al. Risk of fatal pulmonary embolism in patients with treated venous thromboembolism. *JAMA.* 1998;**279**:458–62.

4 Kahn SR, Ginsberg JS. Relationship between deep venous thrombosis and the postthrombotic syndrome. *Arch Intern Med.* 2004;**164**:17–26.

5 Linkins L, Choi PT, Douketis JD. Clinical impact of bleeding in patients taking oral anticoagulant therapy for venous thromboembolism: a meta-analysis. *Ann Intern Med.* 2003;**139**:893–900.

6 Lensing AW, Prandoni P, Brandjes D, et al. Detection of deep-vein thrombosis by real-time B-mode ultrasonography. *N Engl J Med.* 1989;**320**:342–45.

7 Kearon C, Julian JA, Newman TE, et al. Noninvasive diagnosis of deep venous thrombosis. McMaster diagnostic imaging practice guidelines initiative. *Ann Intern Med.* 1998;**128**:663–77.

8 Hull R, Hirsh J, Sackett DL, et al. Combined use of leg scanning and impedance plethysmography in suspected venous thrombosis. An alternative to venography. *N Engl J Med.* 1977;**296**:1497–500.

9 Hull R, Hirsh J, Sackett DL, et al. Replacement of venography in suspected venous thrombosis by impedance plethysmography and 125I-fibrinogen leg scanning: a less invasive approach. *Ann Intern Med.* 1981;**94**: 12–15.

10 Kakkar VV, Howe CT, Flanc C, et al. Natural history of postoperative deep-vein thrombosis. *Lancet.* 1969;**2**:230–32.

11 Stevens SM, Elliott C, Chan KJ, et al. Withholding anticoagulation after a negative result on duplex ultrasonography for suspected symptomatic deep venous thrombosis. *Ann Intern Med.* 2004;**140**:985–91.

12 Elias A, Mallard L, Elias M, et al. A single complete ultrasound investigation of the venous network for the diagnostic management of patients with a clinically suspected first episode of deep venous thrombosis of the lower limbs. *Thromb Haemost.* 2003;**89**:221–27.

13 Schellong S, Schwarz T, Halbritter K, et al. Complete compression ultrasonography of the leg veins as a single test for the diagnosis of deep vein thrombosis. *Thromb Haemost.* 2003;**89**:228–34.

14 Wells PS, Lensing AW, Davidson BL, et al. Accuracy of ultrasound for the diagnosis of deep venous thrombosis in asymptomatic patients after orthopedic surgery: a meta-analysis. *Ann Intern Med.* 1995;**122**: 47–53.

15 Kassai B, Boissel JP, Cucherat M, et al. A systematic review of the accuracy of ultrasound in the diagnosis of deep venous thrombosis in asymptomatic patients. *Thromb Haemost.* 2004;**91**:655–66.

16 de Valois JC, van Schaik CC, Verzijlbergen F, et al. Contrast venography: from gold standard to 'golden backup' in clinically suspected deep vein thrombosis. *Eur J Radiol.* 1990;**11**:131–37.

17 Baldt MM, Zontsich T, Stumpflen A, et al. Deep venous thrombosis of the lower extremity: efficacy of spiral CT venography compared with conventional venography in diagnosis. *Radiology.* 1996;**200**:423–28.

18 Kanne JP, Lalani TA. Role of computed tomography and magnetic resonance imaging for deep venous thrombosis and pulmonary embolism. *Circulation.* 2004;**109**(12 Suppl 1):I15–I21.

19 Sampson FC, Goodacre SW, Thomas SM, et al. The accuracy of MRI in diagnosis of suspected deep vein thrombosis: systematic review and meta-analysis. *Eur Radiol.* 2007;7:**17**:175–81.

20 Fraser DG, Moody AR, Morgan PS, et al. Diagnosis of lower-limb deep venous thrombosis: a prospective blinded study of magnetic resonance direct thrombus imaging. *Ann Intern Med.* 2002;**136**:89–98.

21 Wells PS, Anderson DR, Bormains J, et al. Value of assessment of pretest probability of deep-vein thrombosis in clinical management. *Lancet.* 1997;**350**:1795–98.

22 Wells PS, Anderson DR, Rodgers M, et al. Evaluation of D-dimer in the diagnosis of suspected deep-vein thrombosis. *N Engl J Med.* 2003;**349**:1227–35.

23 Kelly J, Hunt BJ. The utility of pretest probability assessment in patients with clinically suspected venous thromboembolism. *J Thromb Haemost.* 2003;**1**:1888–96.

24 Stein PD. D-dimer for the exclusion of acute venous thrombosis and pulmonary embolism: a systematic review. *Ann Intern Med.* 2004;**140**:589–602.

25 Perrier A, Desmarais S, Miron MJ, et al. Non-invasive diagnosis of venous thromboembolism in outpatients. *Lancet.* 1999;**353**:190–95.

26 Heijboer H, Jongbloets LM, Buller HR, et al. Clinical utility of real-time compression ultrasonography for diagnostic management of patients with recurrent venous thrombosis. *Acta Radiol.* 1992;**33**:297–300.

27 Prandoni P, Lensing AW, Bernardi E, et al. The diagnostic value of compression ultrasonography in patients with suspected recurrent deep vein thrombosis. *Thromb Haemost.* 2002;**88**(3):402–6.

28 Linkins LA, Stretton R, Probyn L, et al. Interobserver agreement on ultrasound measurements of residual vein diameter, thrombus echogenicity, and Doppler venous flow in patients with previous venous thrombosis. *Thromb Res.* 2006;**117**:241–47.

29 Linkins L, Pasquale P, Paterson S, et al. Change in thrombus length on venous ultrasound and recurrent deep vein thrombosis. *Arch Intern Med.* 2004;**164**:1793–96.

30 Bates SM, Julian J, Kearon C, et al. Derivation of a clinical model to predict the likelihood of recurrent deep vein thrombosis. *J Thromb Haemost* [abstract]. 2005;**3**(Suppl 1):P2237.

31 Rathbun SW, Whitsett TL, Raskob GE. Negative D-dimer result to exclude recurrent deep venous thrombosis: a management trial. *Ann Intern Med.* 2004;**141**:839-45.

32 Bates SM, Ginsberg JS. Pregnancy and deep vein thrombosis. *Semin Vasc Med.* 2001;**1**:97–104.

33 Hull R, Hirsh J, Carter CJ. Diagnostic efficacy of impedance plethysmography for clinically suspected deep vein thrombosis. *Ann Intern Med.* 1985;**102**:21–28.

34 Bates SM, Ginsberg JS. How we manage venous thromboembolism during pregnancy. *Blood.* 2002;**100**:3470–78.

35 Ginsberg JS, Hirsh J, Rainbow AJ, et al. Risks to the fetus of radiologic procedures used in the diagnosis of maternal venous thromboembolic disease. *Thromb Haemost.* 1989;**61**:189–96.

36 Nolan TE, Smith RP, Devoe LD. Maternal plasma D-dimer levels in normal and complicated pregnancies. *Obstet Gynecol.* 1993;**81**:235–38.

8 The Diagnosis of Acute Pulmonary Embolism

Victor F. Tapson

Background and purpose

Pulmonary embolism (PE) is a common disease associated with unacceptable morbidity and mortality if untreated. The goal of this chapter is to review various diagnostic strategies for confirming or excluding PE and to make evidence-based recommendations.

Data Sources, study selection, and analysis

PubMed was searched through October 2006 (using keywords pertaining to PE diagnosis) together with a hand search of key journals after 2004. Articles in the English language were reviewed. Data were collected that evaluated presence or absence of acute PE based on a defined gold standard and those that evaluated outcome. Large systematic reviews were included. All relevant publications could not be included but appropriate representative studies were referenced. Abstracts and subanalyses of previously published studies were excluded. Recommendations were graded based on the American College of Chest Physicians' modification of the Grading of Recommendations, Assessment, Development, and Evaluation (GRADE) system (1,2). The recommendations offered in this chapter center around the following questions involving the diagnostic approach to suspected acute PE:

1. Which risk factors should steer the clinician in the direction of possible PE?
2. Should a clinical prediction rule be utilized?
3. How should D-dimer testing be incorporated in the diagnostic evaluation?
4. When can ventilation-perfusion (VQ) scanning be considered diagnostic, and when are ancillary tests necessary?
5. How has computed tomographic angiography (CTA) technology changed, and how has this affected its usefulness?
6. When can CTA scanning be considered diagnostic, and when are ancillary tests necessary?
7. What are appropriate approaches to the diagnosis of suspected PE in the pregnant patient?

Evidence-based Hematology. Edited by Mark A. Crowther, Jeff Ginsberg, Holger J. Schünemann, Ralph M. Meyer, and Richard Lottenberg.
 ISBN: 978-1-4051-5747-6.

Introduction

Venous thromboembolism (VTE) encompasses the spectrum of deep venous thrombosis (DVT) and pulmonary embolism (PE). The diagnosis of PE is often delayed (2) and autopsy studies have repeatedly documented the high frequency with which PE has gone unsuspected and thus, undetected (3,4), emphasizing the need for appropriate prophylactic and diagnostic approaches. Treatment of acute PE has a substantial impact on reducing mortality.

The diagnostic approach generally depends on whether DVT or PE first results in symptoms. Symptoms and signs are neither sensitive nor specific, so when PE is suspected, further testing is required. The presence of specific risk factors both guide prophylaxis and raise the index of suspicion for acute PE (Table 8.1). Clinical probability should be assessed based on knowledge and experience, and one of several validated clinical prediction scores can be used. Many recent studies use clinical outcome (symptomatic VTE in long-term [>3 months] follow-up), as the primary outcome measure, rather than the sensitivity and specificity of diagnostic tests.

Clinical manifestations: risk factors, symptoms, and signs

Whereas the symptomatic presentation of DVT and PE may depend on the thromboembolic burden, very large thrombi may evolve silently and present first as symptomatic or fatal PE. Symptoms and signs are neither sensitive nor specific for DVT or PE (5,6). Dyspnea and chest pain are often sudden in onset. Pleuritic chest pain and hemoptysis are more common with pulmonary *infarction* due to smaller, peripheral emboli. Cough, palpitations, anxiety, lightheadedness, and syncope are nonspecific and may also result from other diseases. Symptoms of DVT should be evaluated. Tachypnea and tachycardia are common but

Table 8.1 Risk factors for acute venous thromboembolism.

Prolonged immobility or reduced mobility
Previous venous thromboembolism
Surgery
Trauma
Spinal cord injury
Cancer
Prolonged air or ground travel
Advanced age
Obesity
Thrombophilias
Oral contraceptives
Pregnancy/postpartum
Varicose veins
Intravascular access
Acute medical illness
Myocardial infarction
Stroke
Pneumonia
Congestive heart failure
Chronic obstructive lung disease exacerbation
Infection

nonspecific. Other physical findings include fever, wheezing, rales, a pleural rub, a loud pulmonic component of the second heart sound, a right-sided gallop, and a right ventricular lift, as well as signs compatible with acute DVT. Symptoms and signs compatible with VTE should be particularly heeded in the setting of risk factors.

Dyspnea or chest pain from PE can be mistaken for a flare of chronic obstructive lung disease, pneumothorax, acute bronchitis or pneumonia, anxiety with hyperventilation, heart failure, angina or myocardial infarction, musculoskeletal pain, rib fracture, pericarditis, herpes zoster, intrathoracic cancer, and occasionally even an intra-abdominal process, such as acute cholecystitis. Acute PE may be masked when there is concomitant cardiopulmonary disease.

Electrocardiography and chest radiography

Electrocardiographic abnormalities are present in the majority of patients with acute PE (6). While ST-segment abnormalities, T-wave changes, and left- or right-axis deviation are common, they are nonspecific. Only one-third of patients with massive or submassive emboli have manifestations of acute cor pulmonale, such as the S1 Q3 T3 pattern, right bundle branch block, P-wave pulmonale, or right-axis deviation. Electrocardiography in suspected acute PE may be useful in establishing or excluding alternative diagnoses, such as acute myocardial infarction.

The chest radiograph is often abnormal in acute PE but nonspecific. Common findings include atelectasis, pleural effusion, pulmonary infiltrates, and mild elevation of a hemidiaphragm (6). Classic findings of pulmonary infarction, such as Hampton's hump or central pulmonary prominence with decreased peripheral vascularity (Westermark's sign), are suggestive but are infrequent. A chest radiograph is recommended when PE is suspected, and may offer an alternative diagnosis.

Blood tests

Arterial blood gas analysis

While acute PE is most commonly associated with hypoxemia, some patients may have a normal arterial oxygen tension (PaO_2) and even rarely a normal alveolar-arterial difference (6). A sudden or unexplained decrease in the PaO_2 or oxygen saturation should raise concern for acute PE. Hypocapnia and hypoxemia are included in the original Geneva clinical prediction rule (7).

Cardiac troponins

Cardiac troponin T and troponin I levels have been found to be elevated in acute PE (8). Troponin is specific for cardiac myocyte damage, and the right ventricle appears to be the source of this enzyme, usually with more massive embolism with myocyte injury due to right ventricular strain (9). It is most commonly used in prognosticating in established PE and is not sensitive for acute PE. However, an unexplained, elevated troponin in a patient with symptoms compatible with acute PE should be investigated further.

D-dimer Assays

Plasma measurements of circulating D-dimer (a specific derivative of cross-linked fibrin) in patients with suspected acute VTE have been extensively evaluated and they have variable sensitivity and specificity (10–12). Cover-slide semiquantitative latex tests rely on visual interpretation and have proven less useful (13). The conventional D-dimer enzyme-linked immunosorbent assay method (ELISA) has shown outstanding negative predictive values but is time consuming (10). Excellent results have been obtained with both the new rapid ELISA (14) and the turbidimetric D-dimer tests (15). Rapid erythrocyte agglutination D-dimer assays have been used effectively when combined with low clinical probability in outcome studies (12,16).

A positive D-dimer means that DVT or PE is possible, but it is nonspecific. For example, when the ELISA D-dimer level cutoff is 500 μg/L, the sensitivity for PE may be as high as 96% to 98%, but the specificity is much lower; limiting the use of D-dimer in hospitalized patients with infection, cancer, trauma, and other settings in which a positive assay is common. Although it has been suggested that a negative result on a quantitative rapid ELISA is as diagnostically useful as a normal lung scan and may serve as a "stand-alone" test in suspected acute PE (10), a clinical probability assessment is advised (see The Canadian and Swiss Clinical Scores) and a high-clinical probability should not be ignored (17). Patients with previous VTE who present with suspected acute PE are less likely to have a negative D-dimer test and thus are more likely to need imaging (18). D-dimer testing should be considered in the low or moderate clinical probability setting, as discussed in more detail in the sections on clinical probability and imaging.

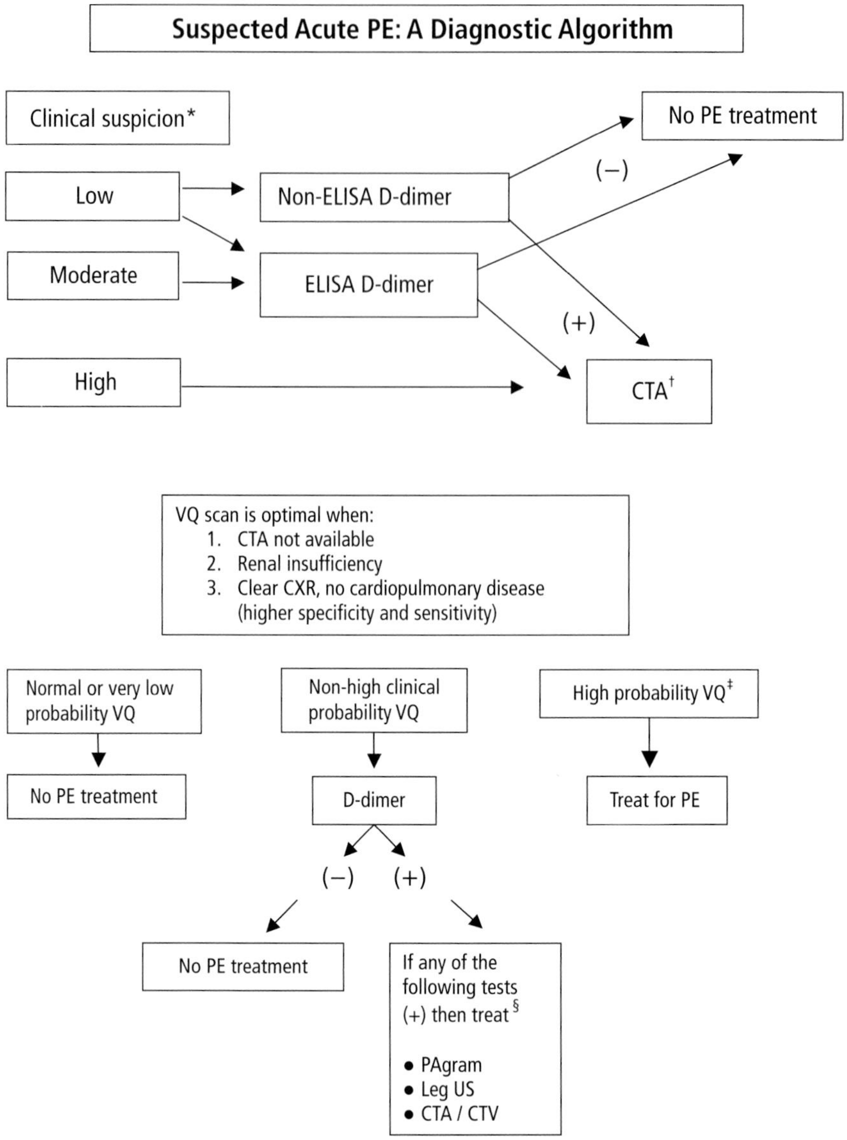

Figure 8.1 Suspected acute pulmonary embolism: A diagnostic algorithm. This algorithm is based on initial clinical probability assessment and D-dimer testing. At most institutions, computed tomographic angiography (CTA) is the initial imaging study.

Brain natriuretic peptide

Brain natriuretic peptide (BNP) assays have been studied as markers that might predict acute PE (19) and increases with ventricular stretching from any cause. While use of the pro-BNP assay together with D-dimer testing has proven to increase the specificity for acute PE, it is not specific enough clinical use (19). Like troponin, its best use may be in prognosticating. An algorithm for the approach to suspected acute PE is provided in Figure 8.1.

Using clinical probability assessment in the diagnostic approach

When PE is suspected, a careful clinical assessment should be based on the history, physical exam, assessment of risk factors, and consideration of additional studies, such as arterial blood gas analysis, D-dimer, and chest radiography. A validated clinical prediction rule is appropriate to consider (Grade 1A) (5,20,21). The above assessment, together with imaging or other studies, then follows. Graded recommendations for the diagnostic approach to suspected acute PE appear in Table 8.2.

The Canadian and Swiss Clinical Scores

Of the clinical prediction scores for suspected PE studied to date, two have dominated the evidence-based literature. The Geneva is based on eight variables (Table 8.3) (7) and was subsequently modified to include active malignancy, hemoptysis, unilateral leg pain, tenderness or edema, with deletion of the arterial blood gas and chest radiograph parameters. The modified score has undergone internal and external validation and now awaits outcome data (22).

Table 8.2 Summary: recommendations for the diagnostic approach to suspected acute pulmonary embolism.*

In patients with suspected acute PE
1. A careful clinical assessment based on the history, physical exam, assessment of risk factors, and consideration of additional studies such as arterial blood gas analysis, D-dimer, and chest radiography is appropriate. A validated clinical prediction rule is appropriate to consider (Grade 1A) (5,7,16,20,21).
2. In a patient with a negative ELISA D-dimer assay, no additional testing or treatment is needed, except when there is high pretest probability (Grade 1A) (10,27–29).
3. In a patient with low clinical probability and a negative, less sensitive D-dimer assay (e.g., red cell agglutination), no additional testing or treatment is needed. (Grade 1A) (10,12,16,27,31).
4. D-dimer testing is nonspecific and a decision to treat cannot be made based on a positive D-dimer, without imaging studies (Grade 1A) (10,27,31).
5. A normal perfusion lung scan effectively rules out acute PE (Grade 1A) (5,30,33,34).
6. Except when there is a history of prior PE, without prior scans available for review, a high-probability VQ scan should be considered diagnostic of acute PE (Grade 1A) (If no other parenchymal lung disease is present (e.g., sarcoidosis), a high-probability scan may occasionally not reflect PE, and additional testing may be needed).
7. The diagnosis of PE should be rigorously pursued even when the VQ scan is low or intermediate probability if the clinical probability is high (Grade 1A) (5).
8. After a nondiagnostic VQ scan, pulmonary arteriography can be performed. When negative, PE is excluded and when positive, it is ruled in (Grade 1A) (5,35). Another option in this setting when clinical probability is low or moderate is to perform serial leg ultrasonography; a negative result precludes the need for therapy (Grade 1C) (23). While excellent outcome has been demonstrated, this benefit is outweighed by the relative inconvenience.
9. After a nondiagnostic perfusion scan, with low clinical probability or normal D-dimer testing and moderate probability, no additional testing or therapy are indicated (Grade 1C) (5, 30,34).
10. A normal pulmonary arteriogram excludes acute PE and a positive study rules in acute PE (Grade 1A) (5).
11. A negative single-detector spiral CT, together with low to moderate clinical probability, and a negative leg ultrasound, requires no additional testing or treatment (Grade 1B) (47).
12. In the setting of a negative multidetector CTA result, no additional testing or treatment is required, regardless of pretest probability, or D-dimer results. (Grade 1B) (20).
13. If a single or multidetector CTA is positive for acute PE, treatment should be instituted (Grade 1A) (57,44–46).
14. Negative thoracic MR resonance imaging appears to safely rule out acute PE, although no large randomized trials have been completed (Grade 1C) (56).
15. In the setting of suspected PE in pregnancy, a noninvasive approach is favored, but either CTA or VQ scanning should be considered if thoracic imaging is required Grade 1B) (62). Large, well-designed outcome studies have not included pregnant patients (20,21), but data can very likely be extrapolated from these trials.

*Supportive data for many of the recommendations are based predominantly on patients presenting in the outpatient setting, although inpatients are also included in some of them. Based on this, the quality of the evidence could be considered for downgrading in some instances. The primary concern is simply that increased complexity and comorbidity in inpatients would frequently render D-dimer tests positive and thus not helpful in a high percentage of cases as well as potentially affecting the quality of imaging studies, limiting the usefulness of the strategies. CTA, computed tomographic angiography; PE, pulmonary embolism; VQ, ventilation-perfusion.

The Canadian (Wells) scoring system was developed based on very simple and easily obtained parameters (23) and has been studied extensively (Table 8.2). A prospective observational study performed in a cohort of 607 patients with suspected PE demonstrated that the predictive value of the Wells score is derived primarily from its subjective component (24). More recently, the score has been dichotomized (Table 8.2) (25) and used with multidetector CTA (20). Both the Canadian and Swiss scoring systems have proven useful in prospective clinical trials.

Using D-dimer testing with clinical probability assessment

Clinical probability should be incorporated in the evaluation for suspected PE (26). Most evidence-based studies have used one of the clinical prediction rules, rather than a nonscored clinical judgment to estimate clinical probability. The prediction rules are useful when probability is low or moderate and the D-dimer is negative. Although the ELISA has been touted as the most sensitive assay to use and has been validated in both low and moderate probability patients, excellent results have been obtained with certain non-ELISA assays, such as the erythrocyte agglutination assay, when coupled together with low clinical probability (16).

In a patient with a negative ELISA D-dimer assay, no additional testing or treatment is needed, except when there is high pretest probability (Grade 1A) (10,27–29). In a patient with low clinical probability and a negative, less-sensitive assay (e.g., red cell agglutination), no additional testing or treatment is needed (Grade 1A) (10,12,16,27,30,31). D-dimer testing is nonspecific and a decision to treat cannot be made based on a positive D-dimer, without imaging studies (Grade 1A) (10,27,31).

Many of the outcome studies have been neither randomized nor blinded and usually include predominantly outpatients. At least one recent, large randomized, nonblinded outcome study included inpatients and served as further evidence that, in patients with a low clinical probability of PE and a negative erythrocyte agglutination D-dimer assay, no additional diagnostic testing was needed (12). Another large, well-designed study incorporated alveolar dead-space fraction into a diagnostic approach together with the Wells score and D-dimer testing, which proved as safe as a standard strategy of starting with VQ scanning (32). Further discussion

Table 8.3 Clinical prediction scores for suspected acute pulmonary embolism.

Variable	Points
A. The Canadian (Wells) Prediction Score	
DVT symptoms/signs	3.0
PE as or more likely than an alternative diagnosis*	3.0
Heart rate > 100 beats/min	1.5
Immobilization/surgery previous 4 weeks	1.5
Previous DVT or PE	1.5
Hemoptysis	1.0
Malignancy	1.0
Total score	**Pretest Probability**[†]
<2.0	Low
2.0 to 6.0	Moderate
>6.0	High
Dichotomized Wells Score[‡]	
≤4 PE unlikely	
>4 PE likely	
B. The Original Geneva (Wicki) Score[§]	
Age 60–79 years	1
≥80	2
Previous DVT or PE	2
Recent surgery	3
Pulse >100/minute	1
pCO_2 < 4.8 kPa (<36.2 mm Hg)	2
4.8–5.19 kPa (36.2–38.9 mm Hg)	1
pO_2 < 6.5 kPa (<48.8 mm Hg)	4
6.5–7.99 kPa (48.8–59.9 mm Hg)	3
8.0–9.49 kPa (60–71.2 mm Hg)	2
9.5–10.99 (71.2–82.4 mm Hg)	1
Chest radiograph	
Plate-like atelectasis	1
Elevation of hemidiaphragm	1
C. The Modified Geneva Score[‖]	
Age > 65 years	1
Previous DVT or PE	3
Surgery or fracture in previous month	2
Active cancer	2
Unilateral lower limb pain	3
Hemoptysis	2
Heart rate 75–94 bpm	3
≥95 bpm	5
Pain on leg palpation/unilateral edema	4

* Physicians used clinical information, chest radiography, electrocardiography, and lab results.

[†] The pretest probability of PE was low, moderate, and high in 527, 339, and 64 patients (1.3%, 16.2%, and 37.5% had PE), respectively. Of the 437 patients with a negative D-dimer result and low clinical probability, only one developed PE during follow-up; thus, the negative predictive value for the combined strategy of using the clinical model with D-dimer testing in these patients was 99.5% (16).

[‡] In the Christopher investigators study, PE was classified as unlikely in 2,206 patients (66.7%). The combination of PE unlikely and a normal D-dimer test result occurred in 1,057 patients (32.0%), of whom 1028 were not treated with anticoagulants; subsequent nonfatal VTE occurred in 5 patients; 0.5% (95% confidence interval 0.2%–1.1%) (20,25).

[§] Results were based on 986 patients (7). A probability score ranging from 0 to 16 was calculated by adding points assigned to these variables. A cutoff score of 4 best identified patients with low probability of PE. A total of 486 patients (49%) had a low clinical probability of PE (score ≤ 4), of which 50 (10.3%) had a proven PE. The prevalence of PE was 38% in the 437 patients with an intermediate probability (score of 5–8; n = 437) and 81% in the 63 patients with a high probability (score ≥ 9). Other scoring systems have evolved from this one to help identify patients at low-risk of having PE (22).

[‖] The score consisted of 8 entirely clinically based variables with points assigned. In the validation set, the prevalence of PE was 8% in the low-probability category (0 to 3 points), 28% in the intermediate-probability category (4 to 10 points), and 74% in the high-probability category (≥11 points). The prediction score has been internally and externally validated and awaits testing for clinical usefulness in an outcome study (22).

of these clinical prediction rules is offered under the subsequent sections on imaging.

Imaging studies for acute pulmonary embolism

Because of the lack of specificity of D-dimer testing, and the high clinical probability setting, imaging is frequently necessary. The choice of imaging depends on availability and specific patient characteristics.

Ventilation-perfusion scanning

While CTA is being used increasingly, the VQ scan offers useful results, particularly when normal or high probability. Furthermore, with renal insufficiency, CTA cannot be performed. In the Prospective Investigation of Pulmonary Embolism Diagnosis (PIOPED), when clinical suspicion was considered very high, PE was present in 96% of patients with high-probability scans, in 66% of patients with intermediate scans, and in 40% with low-probability scans (5). Without cardiopulmonary disease, the VQ scan is more likely to be diagnostic (5). A normal perfusion lung scan effectively rules out acute PE (Grade 1A) (5,33,34). Except when there is a history of prior PE, without previous scans to review, a high-probability VQ scan should be considered diagnostic of acute PE (Grade 1A) (5,33,34). If other parenchymal lung disease is present (e.g., sarcoidosis), a high-probability scan may occasionally not reflect PE, and further testing may be needed.

The diagnosis of PE should be rigorously pursued even when the VQ scan is low or intermediate probability if the clinical setting suggests the diagnosis (Grade 1A) (5). After a nondiagnostic lung scan, several options are possible. Pulmonary arteriography can be performed. When negative, PE is excluded and when positive, it is ruled in (Grade 1A) (5,35). Another option, when clinical probability is low or moderate, is to perform serial leg ultrasonography; while inconvenient, a negative result precludes the need for therapy (Grade 1C) (23). Other, more sensitive leg studies could be considered after a nondiagnostic VQ scan, such as magnetic resonance (MR) imaging or venography, but less outcome data are available. While it has been suggested that after a nondiagnostic VQ scan, negative single-detector CTA does not definitively rule out acute PE (36), more recent multidetector CTA data, albeit not evaluated with the same study design, appears to be more definitive (20). After a nondiagnostic perfusion scan, with low clinical probability or normal D-dimer testing and moderate probability, no additional testing or therapy are indicated (Grade 1C) (5,30,34).

Pulmonary arteriography

Pulmonary arteriography has remained the accepted gold-standard technique for the diagnosis of acute PE, though it is rarely necessary. It is extremely sensitive, specific, and safe. However, multidetector CTA, is less invasive, very specific, a negative study is associated with excellent outcome, and it is more likely to offer an alternative diagnosis. Complications of pulmonary arteriography are rare (37). A normal pulmonary arteriogram excludes acute PE and a positive study rules it in (Grade 1A) (5).

Spiral (helical) computed tomographic arteriography

Computed tomographic arteriography has the greatest sensitivity and specificity for emboli in the main, lobar, or segmental pulmonary arteries. Early studies suggested that segmental and subsegmental PE were often missed (38) although the importance of subsegmental emboli has been questioned (39). The use of multidetector CT has led to decreased section thickness, reduced scanning times, and markedly improved visualization of segmental and subsegmental vessels (40). Visualization of these smaller pulmonary arteries is superior with four-detector spiral CTA and thin collimation (1.25 mm) when compared with single-detector CTA (41). Sensitivity for PE with four-detector CTA has been reported to be 96% (42) and 100% (43) with respective specificities of 98% and 89%. Advantages of CTA over VQ scanning include the rapidity of scanning, the ability to define nonvascular structures, and the ability to evaluate for DVT. Significant renal insufficiency is a contraindication.

Perhaps more important than the accuracy of a diagnostic test compared with a gold-standard, may be determining who is likely to subsequently suffer from recurrent VTE or fatal PE in the absence of therapy. Large systematic reviews have included outcome studies in which patients with negative CTA are not treated (44–46). While they overlap in terms of studies included, all indicate that recurrent VTE is rare when CTA is negative. In the three largest prospective trials included in the Moores analysis (44), anticoagulation was withheld only when both CTA and ultrasonography of the legs were negative (47–49). When the prevalence of DVT detected by ultrasonography in patients with negative CTA results could be calculated, it was quite low (0.8%) in one study (49) but significantly higher in two others (8.4% and 6.3%, respectively) (47,50) and reached 18.8% in a study of 117 hospitalized patients (51). Most outcome studies utilizing 4- or 16-detector CTA have used additional testing to rule out PE (48). A negative single-detector spiral CT, together with low to moderate clinical probability, and a negative leg ultrasound, requires no further testing or treatment (Grade 1B) (47).

Clinical probability should be considered. If it is low or intermediate, meta-analyses suggest that PE can be ruled out with a normal single-detector CTA (45). Two recent large, prospective clinical trials used clinical probability, D-dimer testing, and CTA to determine outcome. Perrier and colleagues (21), demonstrated that in patients with a low or intermediate probability Geneva score, and an ELISA D-dimer <500 μg/L, no further studies were needed and outcome was excellent. With high clinical probability, or when the ELISA was >500 μg/L, multidetector CTA was performed. When CTA and leg ultrasound were both negative, outcome was excellent, but even without ultrasound, the three-month risk of VTE in would have been only 1.5% (95% confidence interval [CI], 0.8 to 3.0). Thus, while multidetector CTA did not appear to require the addition of leg studies, the authors advised a larger study (21).

The Christopher investigators' study enrolled 3,306 patients and is a true management study because all clinical decisions were based on a decision rule (dichotomized Wells score), D-dimer testing, and CTA (20). Only two quantitative (ELISA and turbidometric) D-dimer assays were permitted. When PE was "unlikely" and D-dimer testing negative, treatment was withheld. If PE was "likely" or if the D-dimer was positive, CTA was performed. Computed tomography excluded PE in 1,505 patients, of whom 1,436 patients were not treated with anticoagulants; in these, the three-month incidence of VTE was 1.3% (95% CI, 0.7%–2.0%). The algorithm was completed and allowed a management decision in 97.9% of patients. In patients classified as "PE likely" in whom CTA still excluded PE, no anticoagulation was administered and the three-month thromboembolic risk was 12 of 619 patients (1.9%; 95% CI, 1.1%–3.4%), compatible with VTE risk after a negative pulmonary angiogram. Based on this study, in the setting of negative multidetector CTA, no further diagnostic studies or treatment are necessary, regardless of pretest probability or D-dimer results (Grade 1B) (20). Although the large sample size and the narrow confidence intervals are quite convincing, it is a single outcome study, hence the Grade 1B recommendation. When acute PE is suspected and either single or multidetector CTA are positive, the specificity is such that treatment should be instituted (Grade 1A) (20,21,44–46).

Because of the potential importance of the presence of DVT in clinical outcome, CTA has been studied together with computed tomographic venography (CTV). Several prospective trials support an increased yield of VTE when CTV is combined with (51–54). The PIOPED II trial evaluated multidetector CTA alone and combined with CTV in suspected acute PE (54). Spiral CTA alone had a sensitivity of 83%, while CTA-CTV increased the sensitivity to 90%. Specificity was about 95% for both approaches. The predictive value of either CTA or CTA-CTV was very high with a concordant clinical assessment, but additional testing was suggested when clinical probability was inconsistent with imaging results. While the outcome results described for CTA alone suggest CTV may not be necessary (20), it can be considered in individualized settings.

Other diagnostic tests

Magnetic Resonance Imaging

Magnetic resonance imaging has been used in suspected PE, but at present the excellent sensitivity and specificity for the diagnosis of DVT is its main advantage (55). Despite the potential to evaluate the legs, lungs, and heart with MR imaging, CTA is much faster and far less claustrophobic. In a large prospective study, 221 consecutive patients with suspected PE underwent thoracic MRI followed by MR venography and 17% more cases of VTE were diagnosed compared with separate examinations (56). No comparator or outcome data were available. While negative thoracic MR resonance imaging is very accurate in experienced hands and may safely rule out acute PE (Grade 1C) (56,57), no large randomized trials or large outcome studies have been completed. Prospective trials are under way (58). Experienced centers appear to find it the most useful.

Echocardiography in acute pulmonary embolism

Echocardiography, can be obtained rapidly and may reveal findings that strongly support hemodynamically significant pulmonary embolism (59). Imaging or Doppler abnormalities of right ventricular size or function may suggest the diagnosis. Unfortunately, particularly with underlying cardiopulmonary disease, neither right ventricular dilation nor hypokinesis can be relied on even as indirect evidence of PE. Transesophageal echocardiography may have potential advantages over the transthoracic approach. Actual emboli may occasionally be imaged. Intravascular ultrasound imaging has been shown to adequately image large emboli and may be performed at the bedside (60), but no prospective randomized or outcome studies are available.

Cost–benefit in suspected acute PE

Evidence-based protocols using less diagnostic imaging have proven cost-effective (61). CT has proven to be a cost-effective alternative to VQ scanning, particularly when the sensitivity is high (45). Determining clinical probability and utilizing D-dimer testing in low or moderate probability patients helps to minimizes cost (29).

The approach to suspected acute PE in the pregnant patient

The risk of acute VTE is increased in pregnancy and particularly in the postpartum period (62). Many of the common diagnostic tests used for acute PE have not been appropriately validated in pregnancy, and systematic reviews indicate that strong evidence-based recommendations cannot be made (63). Although clinical trials have been conducted (64), additional research is needed. The issues involving the diagnostic approach to suspected PE during pregnancy are as follows: The D-dimer concentration increases in normal pregnancy and in many pregnancy-related complications, such as pre-eclampsia, but a normal value is clinically helpful (65). Ultrasonography of both legs has a relatively low yield, but a positive study is specific for DVT. Ventilation perfusion imaging is associated with a higher radiation dose to the fetus but a lower radiation dose to the mother/breast than CTA (66,67). A half-dose perfusion scan can be performed without a ventilation scan unless a perfusion defect is present (68). The radiation doses to breast or fetus are below the thresholds estimated to be associated with significant risk. The safety of withholding anticoagulation in patients with a low or indeterminate probability VQ scan has not been validated in a large controlled study (64).

With CTA, the risk of iodinated contrast to the fetus is not clear. The patient should be given information explaining the risks of fetal and maternal radiation and risks to the mother and child of failing to accurately diagnose PE. The CTA protocol should be modified to minimize the radiation dose (62). While noninvasive/nonimaging modalities are advised when possible, concern regarding radiation should not deter the clinician from using CTA or VQ scanning when necessary. In the setting of suspected PE in pregnancy, either CTA or VQ scanning should be considered if thoracic imaging is required (Grade 1B). While the large outcome studies involving CTA have not included pregnant patients (20,21), extrapolation from these trials regarding outcome would appear reasonable.

Conclusions

When it is untreated, the mortality from PE is high. Symptoms and signs are neither sensitive nor specific for the disease, so that when PE is suspected, further testing is required. Risk factors should be considered. Clinical probability should be assessed, either with very careful empiric clinical assessment, or with one of several validated clinical prediction scores; together with D-dimer testing, imaging can sometimes be avoided. Chest CTA has the advantage of offering alternative or concomitant diagnoses, and negative multidetector CTA is associated with excellent outcome. A normal VQ scan is among the most sensitive tests to rule out acute PE, but is uncommon. Pulmonary angiography is rarely needed. “As in antiquity, clinical judgment retains a prominent role in medical practice, but unlike the physicians of that time, we have the tools to be better at it” (69, p. 141).

References

1 Guyatt G, Gutterman D, Baumann MH, et al. Grading strength of recommendations and quality of evidence in clinical guidelines: report from an American College of Chest Physicians Task Force. *Chest.* 2006;**129**:174–81.

2 Guyatt G, Vist G, Falck-Yttr Y, et al. An emerging consensus on grading recommendations? *ACP J Club.* 2006;**144**:A8–A9.

3 Elliott CG, Goldhaber SZ, Jensen RL. Delays in diagnosis of deep vein thrombosis and pulmonary embolism. *Chest.* 2005;**128**:3372–76.

4 Stein PD, Henry JW. Prevalence of acute pulmonary embolism among patients in a general hospital and at autopsy. *Chest.* 1995;**108**:978–81.

5 The PIOPED Investigators. Value of the ventilation/perfusion scan in acute pulmonary embolism: results of the prospective investigation of pulmonary embolism diagnosis. *JAMA.* 1990;**263**:2753–59.

6 Stein PD, Terrin ML, Hales CA, et al. Clinical, laboratory, roentgenographic, and electrocardiographic findings in patients with acute pulmonary embolism and no pre-existing cardiac or pulmonary disease. *Chest.* 1991;**100**:598–603.

7 Wicki J, Perneger TV, Junod AF, et al. Assessing clinical probability of pulmonary embolism in the emergency ward: a simple score. *Arch Intern Med.* 2001;**161**:92–97.

8 Douketis JD, Crowther MA, Stanton EB, et al. Elevated cardiac troponin levels in patients with submassive pulmonary embolism. *Arch Intern Med.* 2002;**162**:79–81.

9 Tapson VF. Diagnosing and managing acute pulmonary embolism: role of cardiac troponins. *Am Heart J.* 2003;**145**:751–53.

10 Stein PD, Hull RD, Patel KC, et al. D-dimer for the exclusion of acute venous thrombosis and pulmonary embolism: a systematic review. *Ann Intern Med.* 2004;**140**:589–602.

11 Kline JA, MS Runyon, Webb WB, et al. Prospective study of the diagnostic accuracy of the simplify D-dimer assay for pulmonary embolism in emergency department patients. *Chest.* 2006;**129**:1417–23.

12 Kearon CJ, Ginsberg JS, Douketis J, et al. An evaluation of D-dimer in the diagnosis of pulmonary embolism: A randomized trial. *Ann Intern Med.* 2006;**144**:812–21.

13 Reber G, de Moerloose P. D-dimer assays and the exclusion of venous thromboembolism. *Semin Thromb Hemost.* 2000; **26**:619–24.

14 Engelhardt W, Palareti G, Legnani C, et al. Comparative evaluation of D-dimer assays for exclusion of deep venous thrombosis in symptomatic outpatients. *Thromb Res.* 2003;**112**:25–32.

15 Brown MD, Lau J, Nelson RD, Kline JA. Turbidimetric D-dimer test in the diagnosis of pulmonary embolism: a meta-analysis. *Clin Chem.* 2003;**49**:1846–53.

16 Wells PS, Anderson DR, Rodger M, et al. Excluding pulmonary embolism at the bedside without diagnostic imaging: management of patients with suspected pulmonary embolism presenting to the emergency department by using a simple clinical model and D-dimer. *Ann Intern Med.* 2001;**135**:98–107.

17 Righini M, Aujesky D, Roy P-M, et al. Clinical usefulness of D-dimer depending on clinical probability and cutoff value in outpatients with suspected pulmonary embolism. *Arch Intern Med.* 2004;**164**: 2483–87.

18 Le Gal G, Righini M, Roy P-M, et al. Value of D-dimer testing for the exclusion of pulmonary embolism in patients with previous venous thromboembolism. *Arch Intern Med.* 2006;**166**:176–80.

19 Melanson SE, Laposata M, Camargo CA Jr., et al. Combination of D-dimer and amino-terminal pro-B-type natriuretic peptide testing for the evaluation of dyspneic patients with and without acute pulmonary embolism. *Arch Pathol Lab Med.* 2006;**130**:1326–29.

20 Christopher Study Investigators. Effectiveness of managing suspected pulmonary embolism using an algorithm combining clinical probability, D-dimer testing, and computed tomography. *JAMA.* 2006;**295**:172–79.

21 Perrier A, Roy P-M, Sanchez O, et al. Multidetector-row computed tomography in suspected pulmonary embolism. *N Engl J Med.* 2005;**352**:1760–68.

22 Le Gal G, Righini M, Roy P-M, et al. Prediction of pulmonary embolism in the emergency department: the Revised Geneva Score. *Ann Intern Med.* 2006;**144**:165–71.

23 Wells PS, Ginsberg JS, Anderson DR, et al. Use of a clinical model for safe management of patients with suspected pulmonary embolism. *Ann Intern Med.* 1998;**129**:997–1005.

24 Kabrhel C, McAfee AT, Goldhaber SZ. The contribution of the subjective component of the Canadian pulmonary embolism score to the overall score in emergency department patients. *Acad Emerg Med.* 2005;**12**:915–20.

25 Wells PS, Anderson DR, Rodger M, et al. Derivation of a simple clinical model to categorize patients probability of pulmonary embolism: increasing the models utility with the SimpliRED D-dimer. *Thromb Haemost.* 2000;**83**:416–20.

26 Stein PD, Woodard PK, Weg JG, et al. Diagnostic pathways in acute pulmonary embolism: recommendations of the PIOPED II Investigators. *Radiology.* 2007;**242**:15–21.

27 Kruip MJ, Leclercq MG, van der Heul C, et al. Diagnostic strategies for excluding pulmonary embolism in clinical outcome studies: a systematic review. *Ann Intern Med.* 2003;**138**:941–51.

28 Perrier A, Desmarais S, Miron MJ, et al. Non-invasive diagnosis of venous thromboembolism in outpatients. *Lancet.* 1999;**353**:190–95.

29 Perrier A, Nendaz MR, Sarasin FP, et al. Cost-effectiveness analysis of diagnostic strategies for suspected pulmonary embolism including helical computed tomography. *Am J Respir Crit Care Med.* 2003;**167**: 39–44.

30 de Groot MR, van Marwijk Kooy M, et al. The use of a rapid D-dimer blood test in the diagnostic work-up for pulmonary embolism: a management study. *Thromb Haemost.* 1999;**82**:1588–92.

31 Roy P-M, Colombet I, Durieux P, et al. Systematic review and meta-analysis of strategies for the diagnosis of suspected pulmonary embolism. *Brit Med J.* 2005;**331**:259.

32 Rodger MA, Bredeson CN, Jones G, et al. The bedside investigation of pulmonary embolism diagnosis study: A double-blind randomized controlled trial comparing combinations of 3 bedside tests vs ventilation-perfusion scan for the initial investigation of suspected pulmonary embolism. *Arch Intern Med.* 2006; **166**:181–87.

33 ten Wolde M, Hagen PJ, Macgillavry MR, et al. Non-invasive diagnostic work-up of patients with clinically suspected pulmonary embolism; results of a management study. *J Thromb Haemost.* 2004;**2**:1110–17.

34 Perrier A, Bounameaux H, Morabia A, et al. Diagnosis of pulmonary embolism by a decision analysis-based strategy including clinical probability, D-dimer levels, and ultrasonography: a management study. *Arch Intern Med.* 1996;**156**:531–36.

35 Van Beek EJ, Reekers JA, Batchelor DA, et al. Feasibility, safety and clinical utility of angiography in patients with suspected pulmonary embolism. *Eur Radiol.* 1996;**6**:415–19.

36 Van Strijen MJL, de Monye W, Kieft GJ, et al. Accuracy of single-detector spiral CT in the diagnosis of pulmonary embolism: a prospective multicenter cohort study of consecutive patients with abnormal perfusion scintigraphy. *J Thromb Haemost.* 2005;**3**:17–25.

37 Stein PD, Athanasoulis C, Alavi A, et al. Complications and validity of pulmonary angiography in acute pulmonary embolism. *Circulation.* 1992;**85**:462–68.

38 Remy-Jardin M, Remy J, Wattinne L, et al. Central pulmonary thromboembolism: diagnosis with spiral volumetric CT with the single-breath-hold technique. Comparison with pulmonary angiography. *Radiology.* 1992;**185**:381–87.

39 Egermayer P, Town GI, Turner JG, et al. Usefulness of D-dimer, blood gas, and respiratory rate measurements for excluding pulmonary embolism. *Thorax.* 1998;**53**:830–34.

40 Schoepf U, Holzknecht N, Helmberger TK, et al. Subsegmental pulmonary emboli: improved detection with thin-collimation multidetector-row spiral CT. *Radiology.* 2002;**222**:483–90.

41 Raptopoulos V, Boiselle PM. Multi-detector row spiral CT pulmonary angiography: comparison with single-detector row spiral CT. *Radiology.* 2001;**221**:606–13.

42 Coche E, Verschuren F, Keyeux A, et al. Diagnosis of acute pulmonary embolism in outpatients: comparison of thin-collimation multi-detector row spiral CT and planar ventilation-perfusion scintigraphy. *Radiology.* 2003;**229**:757–65 [Erratum, *Radiology.* 2004;**232**:627–28].

43 Winer-Muram HT, Boone JM, Brown HL, et al. Pulmonary embolism in pregnant patients: fetal radiation dose with helical CT. *Radiology.* 2002;**224**:487–92.

44 Moores LK, Jackson WL Jr, Shorr AF, et al. Meta-analysis: outcomes in patients with suspected pulmonary embolism managed with computed tomographic pulmonary angiography. *Ann Intern Med.* 2004;**141**:866–74.

45 Quiroz R, Kucher N, Zou KH, et al. Clinical validity of a negative computed tomography scan in patients with suspected pulmonary embolism: a systematic review. *JAMA.* 2005;**293**:2012–17.

46 Hogg K, Brown G, Dunning J, et al. Diagnosis of pulmonary embolism with CT pulmonary angiography: a systematic review *Emerg Med J.* 2006;**23**:172–78.

47 Musset D, Parent F, Meyer G, et al. Diagnostic strategy for patients with suspected pulmonary embolism: a prospective multicentre outcome study. *Lancet.* 2002;**360**:1914–20.

48 Perrier A, Roy P-M, Aujesky D, et al. Diagnosing pulmonary embolism in outpatients with clinical assessment, D-dimer measurement, venous ultrasound, and helical computed tomography: a multicenter management study. *Am J Med.* 2004;**116**:291–99.

49 van Strijen MJ, de Monye W, Schiereck J, et al. Single-detector helical computed tomography as the primary diagnostic test in suspected pulmonary embolism: a multicenter clinical management study of 510 patients. *Ann Intern Med.* 2003;**138**:307–14.

50 Perrier A, Howarth N, Didier D, et al. Performance of helical computed tomography in unselected outpatients with suspected pulmonary embolism. *Ann Intern Med.* 2001;**135**:88–97.

51 Loud PA, Katz DS, Bruce DA, Klippenstein DL, Grossman ZD. Deep venous thrombosis with suspected pulmonary embolism: detection with combined CT venography and pulmonary angiography. *Radiology.* 2001;**219**:498–502.

52 Cham MD, Yankelevitz DF, Henschke CI. Thromboembolic disease detection at indirect CT venography versus CT pulmonary angiography. *Radiology.* 2005;**234**:591–94.

53 Richman PB, Wood J, Kasper DM, et al. Contribution of indirect computed tomography venography to computed tomography angiography of the chest for the diagnosis of thromboembolic disease in two United States emergency departments. *J Thromb Haemost.* 2003;**1**:652–57.

54 Stein PD, Fowler SE, Goodman LR, et al. Multidetector computed tomography for acute pulmonary embolism. *N Engl J Med.* 2006;**354**:2317–27.

55 Tapson VF. Pulmonary embolism—new diagnostic approaches. *N Engl J Med.* 1997;**336**:1449–51.

56 Kluge A, Mueller C, Strunk J, et al. Experience in 207 combined MRI examinations for acute pulmonary embolism and deep vein thrombosis. *Am J Roentgenol.* 2006;**186**:1686–96.

57 Tapson VF, Carroll BA, Davidson BL, et al. The diagnostic approach to acute venous thromboembolism: clinical practice guideline. *Am J Respir Crit Care Med.* 1999;**160**:1043–1066.

58 http://www.clinicaltrials.gov/show/NCT00241826

59 Goldhaber SZ, Haire WD, Feldstein ML, et al. Alteplase versus heparin in acute pulmonary embolism: randomized trial assessing right ventricular function and pulmonary perfusion. *Lancet.* 1993;**341**:507–10.

60 Tapson VF, Davidson CJ, Kisslo KB, et al. Rapid visualization of massive pulmonary emboli utilizing intravascular ultrasound. *Chest.* 1994;**105**:888–90.

61 Gospodarevskaya EV, Goergen SK, Harris AH, et al. Economic evaluation of a clinical protocol for diagnosing emergency patients with suspected pulmonary embolism. *Cost Eff Resour Alloc.* 2006;**4**:12.

62 Matthews S. Imaging pulmonary embolism in pregnancy: what is the most appropriate imaging protocol? *Brit J Radiol.* 2006;**79**:441–44.

63 Nijkeuter M, Ginsberg JS, Huisman MV. Diagnosis of deep vein thrombosis and pulmonary embolism in pregnancy: a systematic review. *J Thromb Haemost.* 2006;**4**:496–500.

64 Chan WS, Ray JG, Murray S, et al. Suspected pulmonary embolism in pregnancy: clinical presentation, results of lung scanning, and subsequent maternal and pediatric outcomes. *Arch Intern Med.* 2002;**162**:1170–75.

65 Epiney M, Boehlen F, Boulvain M, et al. D-dimer levels during delivery and the postpartum. *J Thromb Haemost.* 2005;**3**:268–71.

66 Groves AM, Yates SJ, Win T, et al. CT pulmonary angiography versus ventilation-perfusion scintigraphy in pregnancy: implications from a UK survey of doctors' knowledge of radiation exposure. *Radiology.* 2006;**240**:765–70.

67 Parker MS, Hui FK, Camacho MA, et al. Female breast radiation exposure during CT pulmonary angiography. *Am J Roentgenol.* 2005;**185**:1228–33.

68 Balan KK, Critchley M, Vedavathy KK, et al. The value of ventilation-perfusion imaging in pregnancy. *Br J Radiol.* 1997;**70**:338–40.

69 Douketis JD. Use of a clinical prediction score in patients with suspected deep venous thrombosis: two steps forward, one step back? *Ann Intern Med.* 2005;**143**:141.

9 Initial Therapy of Deep Vein Thrombosis and Pulmonary Embolism

Sam Schulman

Introduction

1. Is anticoagulant treatment necessary in deep vein thrombosis?
2. What is the most effective and safe anticoagulant drug for the initial treatment of the majority of patients with deep vein thrombosis?
3. What is the most effective and safe anticoagulant drug for the initial treatment of the majority of patients with pulmonary embolism?
4. What is the optimal regimen for heparin?
5. When does this regimen have to be modified and in what way?
6. When and how should secondary prophylaxis with vitamin K antagonists be initiated?
7. Can patients with VTE be treated at home?
8. What is the role of early mobilization, compression stockings, and other treatments in venous thromboembolism?

This chapter will discuss the initial anticoagulant treatment of venous thromboembolism (VTE). Thrombolytic therapy and mechanical removal of the thrombus or embolus is discussed in chapter 11, and interruption of vena cava in chapter 12. The typical population with VTE will be discussed first, and thereafter the different subgroups will be addressed, except for pregnant women (chapter 13) or children with VTE (chapter 14). The search for literature was performed in MEDLINE and EMBASE without restriction regarding language or year of publication. Only studies where VTE was objectively confirmed were included.

Grading of the quality of evidence and strengths of recommendations in this chapter are based on the guidelines proposed by the international Grading of Recommendations Assessment, Development, and Evaluation Working Group (GRADE) adopting the modification used by the American College of Chest Physicians that merges the very low and low categories of quality of evidence (see chapter 1).

Evidence-based Hematology. Edited by Mark A. Crowther, Jeff Ginsberg, Holger J. Schünemann, Ralph M. Meyer, and Richard Lottenberg.
 ISBN: 978-1-4051-5747-6.

1. Is anticoagulant treatment necessary in deep vein thrombosis?

The first question to be posed is actually whether initial treatment with an anticoagulant agent is needed at all for patients with deep vein thrombosis (DVT). The anticoagulant drug does not dissolve the thrombus, and it may cause bleeding complications. Therefore, in theory, secondary prophylaxis against progression or recurrence with vitamin K antagonists could suffice. In three studies, patients with DVT were randomized to initial treatment with heparin or saline intravenously (1–3). Two of the studies were published in Danish, one of those only as an abstract. In both studies, the control group did not receive active secondary prophylaxis either. The smallest study only included 23 patients and the rate of the recurrence was 42%–45% in both groups (2). The two larger studies showed a clear benefit from active treatment with a significant reduction of recurrent DVT (Table 9.1). Indirect evidence from trials with inadequate anticoagulation associated with progression of the DVT also supports the recommendation that symptomatic DVT should be treated with anticoagulation (Grade 1A).

From this discussion follows the question whether a DVT confined to the calf (distal DVT) also requires anticoagulant therapy. In a review of the topic, Righini et al. (4) identified five studies of patients with symptomatic calf vein thrombosis, to whom no treatment was given and who were examined for proximal progression with venography or compression ultrasonography. This occurred in 25 cases of 353 patients (7%).

One randomized controlled trial has been published, specifically addressing the need for anticoagulation for distal DVT (5). In this study, 196 patients were randomized to receive (a) oral anticoagulation alone (international normalized ratio [INR] target, 2.5), (b) unfractionated heparin (UFH) 5,000 U twice daily, or (c) 12,500 U once daily or control. Treatment was given for eight weeks and all patients were treated with elastic stockings. In the comparison of ultrasonograms from baseline and at eight weeks, progression of the thrombus was seen in 11%, 11%, 7%, and 78%, respectively.

Table 9.1 Characteristics and results of studies on active initial treatment versus placebo in patients with deep vein thrombosis.*

Ref	Year	Design	Diagnostic methods	Treatment	Number	Follow up (w)	Recurrence No. (%)	ARR (95% CI)	NNT
3	1968	RCT, DB	Not reported	Heparin	70	3	5 (7)	15 (3, 27)	7
				Saline	64	3	14 (22)		
2	1988	RCT, DB	Venography	Heparin	11	13	5 (45)		
				Saline	12	13	5 (42)		
1	1992	RCT, DB	Venography	Heparin	60	24	4 (6.7)	13 (2, 24)	7
				Placebo	60	24	12 (20)		

*ARR, absolute risk reduction; NNT, number need to treat; RCT, randomized controlled trial; DB, double blind; CI, confidence interval.

At the end of follow-up at 24 weeks, progression was seen in 2.3%, 2.3%, 0%, and 25%, respectively. There were no cases with pulmonary embolism (PE), but one patient in the control group had a clinically important progression to the femoral and iliac veins. In conclusion, for patients with distal DVT serial ultrasonography is impractical, and many centers recommend treatment in case of symptoms since the risk or burden of a limited duration of therapy is very small (Grade 1B).

2. What is the most effective and safe anticoagulant drug for the initial treatment of the majority of patients with deep vein thrombosis?

Until recently, the only alternatives for the initial anticoagulant treatment were UFH and low-molecular-weight heparin (LMWH). The half-life of LMWH is longer than that of UFH, 3–6 hours versus 30–60 minutes, and the bioavailability of LMWH is better—close to 100% after subcutaneous injection—with a lower interindividual variability than with UFH. These advantages of LMWH can all be related to the decreased binding to cells and proteins.

Twenty-three randomized controlled studies were identified, where treatment with UFH, dose-adjusted according to activated partial thromboplastin time (APTT), was compared with a fixed subcutaneous dose of LMWH and with identical secondary prophylaxis. Twenty-two of these studies were included in a critical review with calculation of odds ratios for recurrence, major hemorrhage, and death (Table 9.2) (6). Thirteen of the studies consisted of patients with DVT without symptoms of PE. In nine studies, only patients with proximal DVT were enrolled, and among these, recurrent VTE occurred in 3.6% treated with LMWH versus 6.3% treated with UFH by the end of follow-up, major bleeding occurred in 1.0% and 2.1%, respectively, by the end of the initial treatment period, and the mortality at the end of follow-up was 3.3% and 5.3%, respectively. All differences were statistically significant. Therefore, LMWH at a fixed dose is more effective and safer than adjusted dose UFH in the treatment of proximal DVT (Grade 1A).

Adjustment of the dose of UFH requires repeated venipunctures for APTT tests, and treatment with UFH thus appears inferior from several aspects. However, in a study published after this critical review, UFH, adjusted to body weight and thereafter given at a fixed dose subcutaneously twice daily without APTT monitoring, compared well with LMWH (7). There was no significant difference in recurrence, major bleeding, or death between the treatments. The study was discontinued prematurely because of slow recruitment, and confirmation of the results in another study would be desirable.

Recently, a pentasaccharide containing the smallest glycosaminoglycan sequence with affinity to antithrombin, has been synthesized. Advantages with this pentasaccharide, fondaparinux, are that it is a homogenous substance, not of animal origin and

Table 9.2 Outcomes in meta-analysis of trials comparing fixed dose LMWH with adjusted dose UFH for the treatment of VTE.*

Outcome	Studies	Odds ratio	95% confidence interval
VTE overall			
Recurrence			
During initial treatment period	15	0.68	0.48–0.97
At 3 months	13	0.68	0.53–0.88
At 6 months	6	0.68	0.48–0.96
At end of follow-up	18	0.68	0.55–0.84
Major hemorrhage	19	0.57	0.39–0.83
Death at end of follow-up	18	0.76	0.62–0.92
Proximal DVT alone			
Recurrence at end of follow-up	9	0.57	0.44–0.75
Major hemorrhage	8	0.50	0.29–0.85
Death	8	0.62	0.46–0.84
PE alone			
Recurrence at end of follow-up	4	0.88	0.48–1.63

*DVT, deep vein thrombosis; LMWH, low-molecular-weight heparin; UFH, unfractionated heparin; VTE, venous thromboembolism.

Table 9.3 Dose recommendations for the initial anticoagulant treatment of venous thromboembolism.

Treatment	Deep vein thrombosis	Submassive pulmonary embolism*
UFH		
Intravenously†	According to APTT‡	According to APTT†
Subcutaneously	According to APTT‡	Not recommended
LMWH (all subcutaneously)		
Dalteparin	200 IU/kg once daily	As DVT or 120 IU/kg bid
Enoxaparin	1.5 mg/kg once daily	As DVT or 1 mg/kg bid
Tinzaparin	175 IU/kg once daily	As DVT
Nadroparin	171 IU/kg once daily	85 IU/kg bid
Fondaparinux (subcutaneously)		
	7.5 mg once daily§	7.5 mg once daily§

*Patients who are hemodynamically stable.
† Continuous infusion.
‡ APTT (activated partial thromboplastin time) range corresponding to anti-Xa levels 0.3–0.7 IU/ml. Starting dose is with intravenous bolus of 80 U/kg, followed by 18 U/kg/h intravenously or with 17,500 U bid subcutaneously.
§ 5 mg for patients with body weight <50 kg; 10 mg for patients with body weight >100 kg.

without any clinically significant cross-reactivity against platelets. Fondaparinux, has been compared with LWMH for the initial treatment of DVT in 2,205 patients (8). Both drugs were given by subcutaneous injection, fondaparinux at a dose of 7.5 mg (5 mg for patients with a body weight below 50 kg and 10 mg for those above 100 kg) and enoxaparin at a dose of 1 mg per kg twice daily. There were no significant differences in recurrence, bleeding, or mortality between the drugs. The results regarding efficacy are supported by a dose-ranging trial in patients with DVT (9) as well as by a large study on pulmonary embolism. Fondaparinux is therefore an alternative to LMWH for the initial treatment of DVT (Grade 1A).

The recommended doses for initial treatment of DVT are shown in Table 9.3. These conclusions pertain to the vast majority of patients with DVT. Exceptions are those with limb-threatening DVT (*phlegmasia coerulea dolens, phlegmasia alba dolens*) or young patients with extensive although not limb-threatening DVT, for whom thrombolytic therapy or thrombectomy should be primarily considered (chapter 11).

3. What is the most effective and safe anticoagulant drug for the initial treatment of the majority of patients with pulmonary embolism?

The only study in which active treatment was compared with control for patients with pulmonary embolism is the classical study by Barritt and Jordan from 1960 (10). Twenty-six percent each of the patients in the control group had recurring nonfatal or fatal PE. Although the methodology of this trial was suboptimal, with mainly clinical diagnosis of the initial event and lack of blinding, it is considered unethical to repeat this study. Together with the evidence from studies on DVT, anticoagulant treatment of symptomatic PE is generally considered a Grade 1A recommendation. Patients with massive PE and who are hemodynamically unstable should be considered for thrombolytic therapy (chapter 11).

In the critical review of adjusted dose UFH versus fixed dose LMWH by van Dongen et al. (6), there were four studies that provided results on patients with symptomatic PE without symptomatic DVT (Table 9.2). The reduction of recurrent VTE events treated with LMWH was not statistically significant. The convenience of subcutaneous injections of LMWH without monitoring and the lower risk of bleeding compared with UFH in a large number of trials on VTE support treatment of PE with LMWH. Both LMWH and UFH are Grade 1A recommendations. Fondaparinux, given subcutaneously in the same doses as for DVT (see Question 2), has been compared with UFH in intravenous infusion in 2,213 patients with symptomatic PE (11). There were no statistically significant differences in recurrence, major bleeding, or death. However, since there is only a single study on this indication, the recommendation is at Grade 1B level. Dose recommendations are given in Table 9.3.

4. What is the optimal regimen for heparin?

The mode of administration of UFH has been compared in a large number of trials. In older trials, regular intravenous bolus injections were used. This generates high-peak concentrations of heparin and a higher risk of bleeding (than UFH given by other regimens) and is not recommended. Eight studies were identified in which a continuous intravenous infusion was compared with subcutaneous injections twice daily of UFH. One study was not a randomized trial and another had incomplete follow-up. The remaining six studies with 783 patients were included in a meta-analysis by Hommes et al. (12). Progression of the VTE occurred in 10.3% of patients with intravenous infusion and in 7.4% of patients with subcutaneous injections (odds ratio 0.62, 95% confidence interval (CI), 0.39–0.98). There was no statistically significant difference in the risk of bleeding. The blood sample for APTT should be obtained six hours after the morning injection. Based on the results of these studies, subcutaneous injection twice daily of UFH is at least as effective and as safe as continuous intravenous infusion (Grade 1A), and it allows for easier mobilization of the patient.

In clinical practice, most patients who are hospitalized and not eligible for LMWH receive UFH by continuous intravenous infusion. This choice is probably related to concern about bleeding in this subset of patients and the wish to be able to stop treatment abruptly in case of bleeding. Raschke et al. (13) demonstrated in a randomized controlled trial that by using a weight-based nomogram, the time to APTT prolongation of 1.5 times the control or the time to reach the therapeutic range (APTT, 1.5–2.3 times the control) was significantly shorter than with a fixed dose of UFH. This weight-based dose was an initial bolus of 80 U/kg followed by infusion of 18 U/kg/h. However, it is not entirely clear that early recurrence of VTE is associated with a subtherapeutic APTT compared with a therapeutic APTT during the first 24 hours (odds ratio 1.30, 95% CI 0.64–2.63) or the first 48 hours of treatment (odds ratio 1.32, 95% CI 0.51–3.44), according to a pooled analysis of three studies with data from the group treated with UFH intravenously (14).

Determination of the intravenous maintenance dose of UFH may be more optimal if age and plasma volume are taken into account instead of the body weight (15).

LMWH has a longer half-life than UFH, allowing for once daily injection. Six studies were identified with a comparison of once versus twice daily-injection of the same LMWH within each study. The total daily dose was the same with the two regimens in only three of these studies. A meta-analysis and a Cochrane review with five of these studies and a total of 1,508 patients with symptomatic DVT have been published (16,19). There was no statistically significant difference in recurrence, major bleeding, or death, and therefore once daily injection of LMWH can be recommended in patients with DVT (Grade 1A).

5. When does this regimen have to be modified and in what way?

In patients with extreme obesity, the dosing of many medications is problematic. It is unclear whether the dose of UFH or LMWH should be increased linearly according to the body weight or capped, since these patients have been excluded from many trials. No randomized controlled trials were identified. Pharmacokinetic studies with measurement of anti-Xa levels in patients or volunteers with body weight up to 190 kg have provided conflicting results. Two studies with LMWH (dalteparin and tinzaparin) failed to demonstrate any influence of body weight on anti-Xa levels (18,19), whereas two other studies showed that the anti-Xa response was about 1.4 times greater in obese patients receiving dalteparin or nadroparin (20,21). It is thus unclear how heparin should be dosed optimally in morbidly obese patients (Grade 2C).

Renal failure has no significant influence on the clearance of UFH, which at therapeutic doses is cleared via adhesion to endothelial cells and macrophages, with subsequent internalization and depolymerization. With decreasing molecular weight, the clearance via renal excretion becomes more important. In a systematic review of studies with prospective analysis of pharmacokinetics of LMWH in nondialyzed patients with renal impairment, Nagge et al. (22) concluded that the antifactor Xa activity accumulates when the renal function is impaired. However, with tinzaparin, which has a higher mean molecular weight than the other LMWHs, there was no accumulation observed at creatinine clearances down to 20 mL/min (22). With the other LMWHs, a reduction of the dose should be considered in patients with renal impairment, but there is no evidence-based formula for calculation of the optimal dose. Thus, for patients with renal failure, treatment with UFH is preferable or, alternatively, with LMWH and dose adjustments according to anti-Xa levels (Grade 1C).

The requirements for UFH are higher in some patients with antithrombin deficiency, or high-circulating levels of FVIII or of proteins that bind heparin, creating a "heparin-resistant state." In a randomized trial in patients with VTE, requiring more than 35,000 U per 24 hours of UFH, dose adjustments according to anti-Xa levels (targeted range, 0.35–0.67 IU/mL) or APTT (targeted range, 60–85 s) were compared (23). Monitoring the anti-Xa levels allowed for significantly lower daily dose of heparin without any noticeable loss of efficacy, although the study was not dimensioned to determine noninferiority of the clinical endpoint (Grade 1B).

6. When and how should secondary prophylaxis with vitamin K antagonists be initiated?

The question can be reformulated, "Is there a need to give initial treatment with heparin for 10–14 days to halt the coagulation process and avoid progression—or will the number of days needed to allow a vitamin K antagonist (VKA) to become effective suffice?" Four randomized studies were identified, in which the VKA was started early (days 1–3) or late (days 4–10) (24–27). The characteristics and results are summarized in Table 9.4. There were no statistically significant differences regarding recurrence, major bleeding, or death in any of the studies. If the results are pooled, with a total of 807 patients, the odds ratio (and 95% CI) for early versus late start of VKA is for recurrence 0.95 (0.43–2.1), major bleeding 1.4 (0.65–3.0), and death 1.1 (0.71–1.8). It can therefore be concluded that early or essentially concomitant start of UFH/LMWH and VKA is as effective and safe (Grade 1A) and allows for shorter treatment with heparin. The latter is important since the risk of heparin-induced thrombocytopenia thereby becomes minimal.

Another question that has been addressed is whether the VKA should be started with a high "bolus" dose in an attempt to shorten the time until the therapeutic range is achieved or with a lower, estimated maintenance dose. Six randomized trials were identified, all with warfarin as the VKA, but in one of the studies, the recruited patients were started on warfarin as primary prophylaxis after open heart surgery (28). Four of the studies compared two fixed starting doses (29–32), whereas one compared a fixed dose (5 mg) with an individually calculated dose based on age, weight, serum albumin, and presence of malignancy (mean 7.7 mg) (33) (Table 9.5). The studies had an open design, and the follow-up was usually only until the therapeutic range of INR had been achieved. The patient population was purely with the diagnosis of VTE in two of the studies and with mixed diagnoses in the other three. In general, the risk of bleeding was low in these populations. The clinical endpoints recurrence, bleeding, and death were only reported in three of the trials, and bleeding was reported in one additional

Table 9.4 Characteristics and results of studies on early or late initiation of vitamin K antagonist.

Ref	Year	Design*	Diagnostic methods*	Treatment start	Number	Follow up (w)	Recurrence No. (%)	Bleeding No. (%)	Death No. (%)
(24)	1986	RCT	Venography	Day 1–3	139	13–26	4(2.8)	3(2.2)	30(22)
		open	lung scan	Day 7	127	13–26	2(1.6)	2(1.6)	30(24)
(25)	1990	RCT, DB	Venography	Day 1	99	12	7(7.1)	7(7.1)	8(8.1)
				Day 5	100	12	7(7.0)	6(6.0)	2(2.0)
(27)	1992	RCT	Ultrasound	Day 1–2	63	26	1(2)	1(2)	0
		open	lung scan†	Day >4	56	26	2(4)	1(2)	3(5)
(26)	1998	RCT	Venography	Day 1	112	26	0	5(5)	5(5)
		open		Day 10	111	26	1(1)	2(2)	2(2)

*RCT, randomized controlled trials; DB, double blind.
†Forty patients with left ventricle thrombus, diagnosed with two-dimensional echocardiogram were also included.

trial, with few events and no differences. The surrogate efficacy endpoint varied between studies but was achieved better with the lower dose in one and better with the higher dose in three. Thus, starting with a higher dose of warfarin in patients with a low risk of bleeding may lead to faster achievement of therapeutic INR without any effect on clinical outcome (Grade 2B).

7. Can patients with VTE be treated at home?

The transition from treatment with UFH in continuous infusion to more recent subcutaneous injection of LMWH or UFH without monitoring of coagulation tests has made it feasible to discharge patients early from the ward or to avoid admission completely. Most trials addressing this issue have compared two different treatment regimens, for example, UFH in hospital with LMWH at home. Schraibman et al. (34) performed a Cochrane review and identified only two published trials that fulfilled the criteria, but they also had access to preliminary data from a third trial. In this study, all patients were treated with LMWH, but 102 were hospitalized for 10 days, and 99 were treated entirely at home (35). In the other two studies, many patients in the experimental arm received part of their treatment in the hospital. There was no difference in the clinical outcomes for PE, extension of DVT, death, or other serious complications. There is, however, a substantial health economic benefit of treatment in the outpatient setting,

Table 9.5 Characteristics and results of randomized studies on low versus high starting dose of warfarin.*

Ref	Year	Population	Starting Dose (mg)	Number	Surrogate endpoint	Result	Comment
(32)	1984	DVT, PE	15–7.5–7.5	62/20	Time to INR >2	4.3/4.7 d	The study had
			15 until INR		(days on	(6.0/5.4 d)	two parts
			>1.87	67/20	heparin)	3.3/3.4	
						(5.0/4.4)	
(30)	1997	Mainly	5	24	Proportion with	19 (79%)	Vitamin K given
		VTE	10	25	INR 2–3 at 84 h	15 (60%)	at INR >4.5: 1 vs 4
(29)	1999	Mainly	5	31	INR 2–3, but not	21(66%)	$p < 0.003$
		VTE	10	21	>3 for 2 d during	5(24%)	
					day 3–5		
(31)	2003	VTE	5	97	Therapeutic INR	83%	$p < 0.001$
			10	104	day 5	46%	
(33)	2003	VTE, a-fib	5	46	Time to thera-	5.0	$p = 0.007$
			Per regression	44	peutic INR	4.2	
			formula, mean 7.7				

*INR, international normalized ratio; PE, pulmonary embolism; VTE, venous thromboembolism. DVT, deep vein thrombosis.

Table 9.6 Characteristics and results of studies on DVT with or without early mobilization.*

Ref	Year	Design	Diagnostic methods	Mobilization start	Number	Follow up (d)	PE No. (%)	Death No. (%)	DVT No. (%)
(39)	1999	RCT	Lung scan	Day 1	64	8	14(22)	0	
		open		Day 9	62	8	10(16)	0	
(38)	2000	RCT	Lung scan,	Day 1, nonelastic compr	15	9	2(13)	0	4(27)
		open	Ultrasound	Day 1, elastic compr	15	9	1(7)	0	1(7)
				Day 9, no compr	15	9	1(7)	0	4(27)
(37)	2001	RCT	Lung scan/	Day 1	69	4/90†	10(14)	3(4)	2(3)
		open	clinical	Day 5	60	4/90†	6(10)	2(3)	1(2)

*DVT, deep venous thrombosis; PE, pulmonary embolism; RCT: randomized controlled trials. †Follow-up with lung scan and clinically, respectively.

estimated in one of the studies to provide 56% reduction of costs. The majority of patients probably prefer this alternative, and it enhances physical activity and social functioning.

In the Columbus Investigator's study, 271 patients (27%) had PE initially, and they were also randomized to UFH or LMWH, the latter given predominantly at home (36). Eight patients (5.9%) in each group had a recurrence. Additional studies on the feasibility of home treatment for PE were uncontrolled. Taken together, outpatient treatment is possible in the majority of patients with DVT and is safe and effective (Grade 1A), but very limited data exist for pulmonary embolism and this strategy should only be considered for minimally symptomatic patients with submassive PE (Grade 1B).

8. What is the role of early mobilization, compression stockings, and other treatments in venous thromboembolism?

Immobilization was a major part of the treatment of DVT before effective anticoagulants became available. The fear of detachment and embolization of thrombus fragment maintained this routine, but physical activity is known to increase the release of tissue plasminogen activator from the endothelium and thereby improve fibrinolysis. Three studies were identified in which patients with DVT were randomized to bed rest or early mobilization (Table 9.6) (37–39). The studies were small and not dimensioned to demonstrate noninferiority regarding any endpoint. There was no statistically significant increase in new pulmonary perfusion defects, progression of DVT, or deaths with early mobilization, which therefore should be encouraged (Grade 1B).

Compression therapy is intuitively beneficial to reduce swelling and improve venous return, especially via the deep veins. Three randomized studies were identified, that compared graduated compression stockings (30–40 mm Hg) with no intervention (40,41) or with placebo stockings (42). The two larger studies showed a significant risk reduction of the postthrombotic syndrome after 2 years. Overall, the odds ratio when comparing compression with no compression was 0.31 (95% CI, 0.20–0.48) for any form of postthrombotic syndrome, and 0.39 (95% CI, 0.20–0.76) for the severe form. However, it may be too early to measure for compression stockings during the initial treatment period if the leg is very swollen. Improvement after discharge may require new stockings after a few weeks. In that case, the patient can be provided with provisional, simple elastic stockings for the first few weeks. In conclusion, graduated compression stockings are effective for the reduction of postthrombotic syndrome (Grade 1A).

Finally, a Cochrane review analyzed the effect of nonsteroidal anti-inflammatory drugs (NSAIDs) compared with UFH in the initial treatment of VTE (43). Two randomized trials with significant heterogeneity were identified. Both studies were small with insufficient power to evaluate clinically relevant endpoints. The authors concluded that in view of the vast and positive experience of UFH and LMWH in the treatment of VTE a large trial to determine the effect of NSAIDs would not be ethically justified (Grade 2C).

References

1 Brandjes DP, Heijboer H, Buller HR, et al. Acenocoumarol and heparin compared with acenocoumarol alone in the initial treatment of proximal-vein thrombosis. *N Engl J Med.* 1992;**327**:1485–89.

2 Ott P, Eldrup E, Oxholm P. [Value of anticoagulant therapy in deep venous thrombosis in the lower limb in elderly, mobilized patients. A double-blind placebo controlled study with open therapeutic guidance]. *Ugeskr Laeger.* 1988;**150**:218–21.

3 Rosenbeck-Hansen JV, Valdorf-Hansen F, Dige-Petersen H, et al. En kontrolleret undersøgelse af antikoagulationsbehandlingens effekt ved dyb venetrombose og lungeemboli. *Nord Med.* 1968;**80**: 1305–6.

4 Righini M, Paris S, Le Gal G, et al. Clinical relevance of distal deep vein thrombosis: review of literature data. *Thromb Haemost.* 2006;**95**: 56–64.

5 Belcaro G, Laurora G, Cesarone MR, et al. Prevention of the extension of distal deep venous thrombosis: a randomized controlled trial with a 6-month follow-up. *Minerva Med.* 1997;**88**:507–14.

6 van Dongen CJJ, van der Belt AGM, Prins MH, et al. Fixed dose subcutaneous low molecular weight heparins versus adjusted dose unfractionated heparin for venous thromboembolism. *Cochrane Database Syst Rev.* 2004:CD001100.

7 Kearon C, Ginsberg JS, Julian JA, et al. Comparison of fixed-dose weight-adjusted unfractionated heparin and low-molecular-weight heparin for acute treatment of venous thromboembolism. *JAMA.* 2006;**296**: 935–42.

8 Büller HR, Davidson BL, Decousus H, et al. Fondaparinux or enoxaparin for the initial treatment of symptomatic deep venous thrombosis: a randomized trial. *Ann Intern Med.* 2001;**140**:867–73.

9 Treatment of proximal deep vein thrombosis with a novel synthetic compound (SR90107A/ORG31540) with pure anti-factor Xa activity: A phase II evaluation. The Rembrandt Investigators. *Circulation.* 2000;**102**:2726–31.

10 Barritt DW, Jordan SC. Anticoagulant drugs in the treatment of pulmonary embolism. *Lancet.* 1960;**1**:1309–12.

11 Büller HR, Davidson BL, Decousus H, et al. Subcutaneous fondaparinux versus intravenous unfractionated heparin in the initial treatment of pulmonary embolism. *N Engl J Med.* 2003;**349**:1695–1702.

12 Hommes DW, Bura A, Mazzolai L, et al. Subcutaneous heparin compared with continuous intravenous heparin administration in the initial treatment of deep vein thrombosis: a meta- analysis. *Ann Intern Med.* 1992;**116**:279–84.

13 Raschke RA, Reilly BM, Guidry JR, et al. The weight-based heparin dosing nomogram compared with a "standard care" nomogram: a randomized controlled trial. *Ann Intern Med.* 1993;**119**:874–81.

14 Anand SS, Bates S, Ginsberg JS, et al. Recurrent venous thrombosis and heparin therapy: an evaluation of the importance of early activated partial thromboplastin times. *Arch Intern Med.* 1999;**159**:2029–32.

15 Rosborough TK. In unfractionated heparin dosing, the combination of patient age and estimated plasma volume predicts initial antifactor Xa activity better than patient weight alone. *Pharmacotherapy.* 1998;**18**:1217–23.

16 van Dongen CJ, MacGillavry MR, Prins MH. Once versus twice daily LMWH for the initial treatment of venous thromboembolism. *Cochrane Database Syst Rev.* 2005:CD003074.

17 Couturaud F, Julian JA, Kearon C. Low molecular weight heparin administered once versus twice daily in patients with venous thromboembolism: a meta-analysis. *Thromb Haemost.* 2001;**86**:980–84.

18 Hainer JW, Barrett JS, Assaid CA, et al. Dosing in heavy-weight/obese patients with the LMWH, tinzaparin: a pharmacodynamic study. *Thromb Haemost.* 2002;**87**:817–23.

19 Wilson SJ, Wilbur K, Burton E, et al. Effect of patient weight on the anticoagulant response to adjusted therapeutic dosage of low-molecular-weight heparin for the treatment of venous thromboembolism. *Haemostasis.* 2001;**31**:42–8.

20 Heizmann M, Baerlocher GM, Steinmann F, et al. Anti-Xa activity in obese patients after double standard dose of nadroparin for prophylaxis. *Thromb Res.* 2002;**106**:179–81.

21 Yee JY, Duffull SB. The effect of body weight on dalteparin pharmacokinetics: a preliminary study. *Eur J Clin Pharmacol.* 2000;**56**:293–97.

22 Nagge J, Crowther M, Hirsh J. Is impaired renal function a contraindication to the use of low-molecular-weight heparin? *Arch Intern Med.* 2002;**162**:2605–9.

23 Levine MN, Hirsh J, Gent M, et al. A randomized trial comparing activated thromboplastin time with heparin assay in patients with acute venous thromboembolism requiring large daily doses of heparin. *Arch Intern Med.* 1994;**154**:49–56.

24 Gallus A, Jackaman J, Tillett J, et al. Safety and efficacy of warfarin started early after submassive venous thrombosis or pulmonary embolism. *Lancet.* 1986;**2**:1293–96.

25 Hull RD, Raskob GE, Rosenbloom D, et al. Heparin for 5 days as compared with 10 days in the initial treatment of proximal venous thrombosis. *N Engl J Med.* 1990;**322**:1260–64.

26 Leroyer C, Bressollette L, Oger E, et al. Early versus delayed introduction of oral vitamin K antagonists in combination with low-molecular-weight heparin in the treatment of deep vein thrombosis: a randomized clinical trial. The ANTENOX Study Group. *Haemostasis.* 1998;**28**:70–77.

27 Mohiuddin SM, Hilleman DE, Destache CJ, et al. Efficacy and safety of early versus late initiation of warfarin during heparin therapy in acute thromboembolism. *Am Heart J.* 1992;**123**:729–32.

28 Ageno W, Turpie AG, Steidl L, et al. Comparison of a daily fixed 2.5-mg warfarin dose with a 5-mg, international normalized ratio adjusted, warfarin dose initially following heart valve replacement. *Am J Cardiol.* 2001;**88**:40–4.

29 Crowther MA, Ginsberg JB, Kearon C, et al. A randomized trial comparing 5-mg and 10-mg warfarin loading doses. *Arch Intern Med.* 1999;**159**:46–8.

30 Harrison L, Johnston M, Massicotte MP, et al. Comparison of 5-mg and 10-mg loading doses in initiation of warfarin therapy. *Ann Intern Med.* 1997;**126**:133–36.

31 Kovacs MJ, Rodger M, Anderson DR, et al. Comparison of 10-mg and 5-mg warfarin initiation nomograms together with low-molecular-weight heparin for outpatient treatment of acute venous thromboembolism. A randomized, double-blind, controlled trial. *Ann Intern Med.* 2003;**138**:714–19.

32 Schulman S, Lockner D, Bergström K, et al. Intensive initial oral anticoagulation and shorter heparin treatment in deep vein thrombosis. *Thromb Haemost.* 1984;**52**:276–80.

33 Shine D, Patel J, Kumar J, et al. A randomized trial of initial warfarin dosing based on simple clinical criteria. *Thromb Haemost.* 2003;**89**:297–304.

34 Schraibman IG, Milne AA, Royle EM. Home versus in-patient treatment for deep vein thrombosis. *Cochrane Database Syst Rev.* 2001: CD003076.

35 Boccalon H, Elias A, Chale JJ, et al. Clinical outcome and cost of hospital vs home treatment of proximal deep vein thrombosis with a low-molecular-weight heparin: the Vascular Midi-Pyrenees study. *Arch Intern Med.* 2000;**160**:1769–73.

36 The Columbus Investigators. Low molecular weight heparin is an effective and safe treatment for deep-vein thrombosis and pulmonary embolism. *N Engl J Med.* 1997;**337**:657–62.

37 Aschwanden M, Labs KH, Engel H, et al. Acute deep vein thrombosis: early mobilization does not increase the frequency of pulmonary embolism. *Thromb Haemost.* 2001;**85**:42–6.

38 Partsch H, Blättler W. Compression and walking versus bed rest in the treatment of proximal deep venous thrombosis with low molecular weight heparin. *J Vasc Surg.* 2000;**32**:861–69.
39 Schellong SM, Schwarz T, Kropp J, et al. Bed rest in deep vein thrombosis and the incidence of scintigraphic pulmonary embolism. *Thromb Haemost.* 1999;**82**:127–29.
40 Brandjes DP, Buller HR, Heijboer H, et al. Randomised trial of effect of compression stockings in patients with symptomatic proximal-vein thrombosis. *Lancet.* 1997;**349**:759–62.
41 Prandoni P, Lensing AW, Prins MH, et al. Below-knee elastic compression stockings to prevent the post-thrombotic syndrome: a randomized, controlled trial. *Ann Intern Med.* 2004;**141**:249–56.
42 Ginsberg JS, Hirsh J, Julian J, et al. Prevention and treatment of postphlebitic syndrome: results of a 3-part study. *Arch Intern Med.* 2001;**161**:2105–9.
43 Cundiff DK, Manyemba J, Pezzullo JC. Anticoagulants versus nonsteroidal anti-inflammatories or placebo for treatment of venous thromboembolism. *Cochrane Database Syst Rev.* 2006:CD003746.

10 Long-Term Anticoagulation in Venous Thromboembolism

Clive Kearon

Long-term treatment of venous thromboembolism (VTE) refers to treatments that are continued after initial therapy, such as with heparin or thrombolytic agents, has been completed. Long-term treatment of VTE is usually with a vitamin K antagonist (VKA) and less commonly with a low-molecular weight-heparin (LMWH). Long-term therapy has two goals that overlap in timing: (1) to complete treatment of the acute episode of VTE (predominantly the first three months) and (2) to prevent new episodes of VTE that are not directly related to the acute event (predominately after the first months).

Is long-term anticoagulanion necessary? The need for long-term therapy of VTE after an initial 5- to 10-day course of therapeutic-dose heparin has been established by trials that have shown that long-term therapy with VKA markedly reduced recurrent VTE in patients with (1) symptomatic isolated distal deep vein thrombosis (DVT) compared with controls who did not received long-term therapy (0/23 versus 8/28 [29%] at 3 months; $p < 0.01$) (1) and (2) proximal DVT compared with low-dose (5,000 U twice daily) subcutaneous heparin (0/17 versus 9/19 [47%] at 3 months; $p < 0.001$) (2). High rates of recurrent VTE in patients who are only treated with four or six weeks of VKA compared with those who are treated for three or six months further supports the need for long-term therapy (3–5).

Management of vitamin K antagonist therapy

Initiation of VKA

When? Studies that showed that about five days of heparin therapy (VKA started on first or second day) was as effective as 10 to 14 days of heparin therapy (VKA started after about five days) also established that VKA could be started the same day as heparin (6,7).

What dose? Two trials in hospitalized patients showed that starting warfarin at a dose of 5 mg, compared with 10 mg, is associated with less excessive anticoagulation and does not meaningfully delay onset of anticoagulation (8,9). However, a similar study in outpatients with acute VTE found that starting with 10 mg of warfarin was superior to starting with 5 mg (10). Observational studies have shown that lower VKA maintenance doses are required in older patients, women, and those with impaired nutrition and vitamin K deficiency (11,12). Taken together, these data suggest that warfarin can usually be started at a first dose of 10 mg in younger (e.g., less than 60 years) otherwise healthy outpatients, and at a first dose of 5 mg in older patients and those who are hospitalized. The previously noted studies published nomograms to guide the first days of warfarin dosing (9,10).

Long-term monitoring and adjustment of VKA

Many factors modify the anticoagulant response to VKA therapy and, therefore, there are marked differences in the dose of VKA required to achieve an international normalized ratio (INR) of 2.0 to 3.0, both among patients and in the same patient over time (11). Consequently, VKA dosing needs to be adjusted in response to ongoing INR measurements to maximize the proportion of time that patients are in the target INR range. Good anticoagulant control is important as (1) subtherapeutic anticoagulation (particularly below INR 1.5) increases recurrent VTE; (2) supratherapeutic anticoagulation (particularly over INR 5.0) increases bleeding; and (3) poor anticoagulant control increases the burden of anticoagulant therapy and discourages patients and healthcare providers from continuing VKA therapy when it is indicated (11). Principles and management strategies that facilitate optimal long-term anticoagulation are summarized in Table 10.1.

Optimal intensity of Vitamin K antagonist therapy

VKA inhibits two enzymes (vitamin K epoxide reductase and vitamin K reductase) that convert vitamin K epoxide, via vitamin K, to hydroquinone (vitamin KH_2). In turn, deficiency of hydroquinone results in defective carboxylation, and reduced functional levels, of coagulation factors II, VII, IX, and X, thereby achieving

Evidence-based Hematology. Edited by Mark A. Crowther, Jeff Ginsberg, Holger J. Schünemann, Ralph M. Meyer, and Richard Lottenberg.

Table 10.1 Principles and recommendations for maintenance vitamin K antagonist therapy.

Interval between INR measurements

- Gradually increase interval from every 2–3 days in the first week to every 2–4 weeks (e.g., after 6 weeks) (11)
- Decrease interval between testing if the patient becomes ill or if a medication is added or stopped (11,110)
- Decrease interval if INR results become unstable

Dosing of warfarin

- Average daily warfarin dose is about 6 mg at age 50 and about 3.5 mg at age 80 (12)
- If warfarin maintenance dose needs to be increased or decreased, steps of 10% are usually suitable. This can be done by calculating the total dose of warfarin given in the preceding week, and adjusting the next week(s) total dose by 10%; this often translates into a change in the total week's dose of 2.5 to 5.0 mg of warfarin (11).
- If INR $>$ 5.0, 1 or 2 doses of warfarin should be withheld in addition to reducing the maintenance warfarin dose. If INR $>$5.0 and the patient has risk factors of bleeding, or INR $>$10.0, 1 to 2.5 mg of oral vitamin K should also be given (11,111,112).

Method of anticoagulant monitoring

- A systematic process for monitoring VKA should be used that includes patient education, and explicit patient and healthcare provider responsibility for each stage of the process (e.g., patient attends a designated laboratory for INR testing; INR results are communicated to healthcare providers at prespecified time (e.g., same or following day); INR results are recorded in the patient's anticoagulation record; VKA dose is selected; VKA dose and timing of next INR measurement are communicated to the patient) (11).
- Use of a dedicated anticoagulant service can improve delivery of VKA therapy (11).
- Self-testing, or self-dosing, is appropriate in selected well education and motivated patients (11,113).
- Computer programs can facilitate selection of warfarin dose, tracking of INR and VKA dosing, and communication of VKA dosing to patients (e.g., via mail) (11).

Interruption of VKA

- After one month, and particularly after 3 months, of VKA therapy for VTE, short interruptions of VKA (e.g., 5 days) are well tolerated (i.e., associated with a low risk of recurrence) provided patients have not undergone a procedure that is associated with VTE (11,62).
- Patients who have had a procedure that is associated with VTE (e.g., surgery with general anesthetic) should receive supplemental VTE prophylaxis (e.g., a heparin preparation) until their INR increases, or is expected to have increased (e.g., ~3 days), to above INR 1.5 (11;114).

INR, international normalized ratio; VKA, vitamin K antagonist; VTE, venous thromboembolism.

anticoagulation. The degree, or intensity, of resultant anticoagulation is measured as a prothrombin time ratio, usually expressed in a standardized form as the International Normalized Ratio (INR) (11). Hull and colleagues (14,15) established that acute treatment of VTE (i.e., first 3 months) with a target INR of 2.5 (range 2.0–3.0) was similarly effective but caused less bleeding than treatment with a target INR of 3.5 (range 3.0–4.0) (13). In patients with an antiphospholipid antibody and mostly VTE, two studies have shown that targeting an INR of 2.5 is as effective as targeting an INR target of 3.5 (14,15).

The observation in two trials (3,16) that there were no episodes of recurrent VTE among patients who remained on extended-duration VKA targeted to an INR of ~2.5 (3,16) (Table 10.3) suggested that lowering the intensity of anticoagulation to a target INR of ~1.75 after the first three months of conventional intensity therapy might reduce bleeding without loss of efficacy. When this hypothesis was subsequently tested in a double-blind trial of patients with unprovoked VTE, the lower intensity of anticoagulation was less effective at preventing recurrent VTE (intention-to-treat analysis: 1.9% versus 0.7% per patient-year; hazard radio 2.8 [95% confidence interval (CI), 1.1 to 7.0]) and was associated with the same frequency of major bleeding (1.1% versus 0.9% per patient-year; hazard ratio 1.2 [95% CI 0.4 to 3.0]) as conventional intensity therapy (Table 10.3) (17). As noted later in this chapter, after the first three months of conventional intensity VKA therapy, low-intensity anticoagulation (target INR 1.75) has been shown to reduce the risk of recurrent VTE by about two-thirds and is compatible with less frequent INR testing than is usual with conventional intensity anticoagulation (Table 10.3) (18).

Based on these studies, a target INR of 2.5 (range 2.0–3.0) is recommended as the optimal intensity of anticoagulation for both acute and long-term treatment of VTE.

Duration of Anticoagulant Therapy

Anticoagulant therapy for VTE should be continued until (1) its benefits (reduction of recurrent VTE) no longer clearly outweigh its risks (increase in bleeding) or (2) patient preference to stop treatment even if continuing treatment is expected to be of net benefit. In patients with an average risk of bleeding while on anticoagulant therapy, therefore, the decision to stop or continue therapy is dominated by the risk of recurrent VTE if treatment is stopped. Current evidence suggests that the risk of recurrence after stopping therapy is largely determined by two factors: (1) whether the acute episode of VTE has been effectively treated and (2) the patient's intrinsic risk of having a new episode of VTE (i.e., not arising directly from the episode of thrombosis for which patients have been receiving treatment). If therapy is stopped before the acute episode of thrombosis is adequately treated, the risk of recurrent VTE will be higher than if treatment was stopped after a longer course of anticoagulation. If patients have a persistently

Table 10.2 Risk factors for recurrent VTE after stopping anticoagulant therapy.

Variable	Relative risk
Transient risk factor (4,5,24,26,28,29,31,42,58)	≤0.5
Persistent risk factor (4,5,24,26,28,29,42)	≥2
Unprovoked VTE (4,5,16,26,28,31)	≥2
Protein C, protein S, and antithrombin deficiencies (24,31,52,58)	~1.5
Heterozygous for factor V Leiden or the G20210A prothrombin gene (16,18,42,55)	~1.5
Homozygous for factor V Leiden (42,56–58)	1.5–2
Heterozygous for both factor V Leiden and G20210A prothrombin gene (56,58,115–117)	1.5–2
Factor VIII level >150 IU/dL (54,58,65)	~1.4
Antiphospholipid antibodies (16,36,42,59)	1.5–4
Mild hyperhomocysteinemia (68,118)	1.5–2.5
D-dimer elevation after stopping therapy (35,52–54)	~2.5
Family history of VTE (28,56,72)	~1
Cancer (23–26)	~3
Metastatic vs. non–metastatic (23)	~3
Chemotherapy (25)	~2
Discontinuation of estrogen (25,58,119–125)	~0.5
Proximal DVT vs. PE (16;28;38)	~1
Distal DVT vs. proximal DVT or PE (28;30)	~0.5
Residual thrombosis (4,16,22,28,34,62,126)	1–2
Vena caval filter (38,63,64,127)	1–1.5
Second vs. first episode of VTE (3,18,38,39)	1.5–2
Age (16,25,38,56)	~1
Male sex (60)	~1.5
Asian (38)	~0.8

high intrinsic risk for thrombosis, even if the acute episode of thrombosis has effectively been treated, they will have a high risk of recurrence once anticoagulant therapy is stopped; if this risk is high enough relative to the patient's increased risk of bleeding on anticoagulants, indefinite therapy will be indicated. As patients' intrinsic risk of recurrent VTE has influenced which patients have been enrolled in trials that have compared durations of anticoagulant therapy, and needs to be considered in the interpretation of such studies, risk factors for recurrent VTE in individual patients will be considered before reviewing the studies that have compared different durations of VKA in patients with VTE.

Patient-related risk factors for recurrent VTE after stopping anticoagulant therapy

Cancer. Cancer is associated with about a threefold increased risk of recurrent VTE both during (19–23) and after (22,24–26) anticoagulant therapy, and among patients with cancer, the risk of recurrence is about threefold higher in those with metastatic disease (23) (Table 10.2). The risk of recurrent VTE after stopping anticoagulant therapy is expected to be high (i.e., 10% to 20% in the first year) in patients with cancer, particularly if there is progressive or metastatic disease, poor mobility, or ongoing chemotherapy (25–27). The risk of recurrence is uncertain but likely to be lower if the cancer has responded to therapy or if the initial VTE was provoked by an additional reversible risk factor, such as surgery or chemotherapy (see below). Because cancer is considered to be such a strong risk factor for recurrent VTE, there is widespread agreement that most patients with VTE and cancer require long-term anticoagulant therapy, and these patients have generally been excluded from the randomized trials that have compared different durations of anticoagulant therapy.

Reversibility of risk factors for VTE. Patients with VTE provoked by a major reversible risk factor, such as surgery, have a low risk of recurrence (i.e., about 3% in the first year) after three or more months of anticoagulant therapy, whereas this risk is high (i.e., about 10% in the first year) in patients with an unprovoked (also termed *idiopathic*) VTE and in those who have a persistent risk factor for thrombosis (Table 10.2) (4,5,18,26–31). If VTE was provoked by a minor reversible risk factor, such as leg trauma, estrogen therapy, or prolonged air travel (e.g., a flight of over eight hours), there is an intermediate risk of recurrent VTE after stopping anticoagulant therapy (i.e., approximately 5% in the first year) (25,31,32). Because of this difference in risk of recurrence, many recent trials selectively enrolled patients with unprovoked VTE and compared longer durations of therapy (16–18,33–35), or enrolled patients with VTE that was provoked by a reversible risk factor and compared shorter durations of therapy (36) (Table 10.3).

Isolated calf DVT versus proximal DVT. Patients with DVT that is confined to the distal veins (often called *isolated calf* DVT) have about half the risk of recurrence as patients who have DVT that involves the proximal veins (i.e., popliteal or more proximal veins) (28,30,37). If ultrasound rather than venography is used to diagnose distal DVT, the risk of recurrence after distal DVT may be even lower as a higher proportion of such patients may have false-positive findings or may have thrombosis of the muscular rather than of the deep veins. Many studies that compared durations of anticoagulation excluded patients with isolated distal DVT (4,20,34,35).

Second versus first episode of VTE. After a second or subsequent episode of VTE, the risk of recurrence appears to be about 1.5-fold higher than after a first episode (18,38,39). Many studies that compared durations of anticoagulation excluded patients if their VTE was not a first episode (28,30,33–35).

Pulmonary embolism versus deep vein thrombosis. Patients who present with pulmonary embolism (PE) appear to have the same risk of recurrent VTE as those who present with proximal DVT (25,28,38,40). However, after a PE, about 60% of recurrent episodes of VTE are also PE, whereas only about 20% of recurrent episodes of VTE are a PE after an initial DVT (33,34,38,40–42). This pattern of recurrence, with about a threefold higher risk of PE after an initial PE than after an initial DVT, appears to persist long term (38,41,42). About 10% of symptomatic PE are thought to be rapidly fatal (43–45), and another 5% of patients whose PE is diagnosed and treated also die from PE (38,41,46–50). Thus,

Table 10.3 Comparisons of durations and intensities of anticoagulant therapy for DVT and PE.*

First author/year (acronym)	Intervention	Blinding	# Pts analyzed	Length follow-up	Recurrent DVT or PE	Major bleeding	Total mortality	Comments
Short (4 or 6 weeks) versus Intermediate (3 or 6 months) durations of anticoagulation								
Kearon 2004 (36) (SOFAST)	VKA stopped (placebo)	Allocation: Yes Patients: Yes Caregivers: Yes	84/84	11 mo	5/84 (6%)	0/84	0/84	Population: First DVT or PE. Treated for 1 mo. VTE was asymptomatic in 9%, and isolated calf DVT in 18%. One VTE occurred while on warfarin.
	VKA (INR 2.0–3.0) For 2 more mo	Adjudications: Yes Data analysts: Yes	81/81	11 mo	3/81 (4%) RR 0.6 (0.1, 2.5)	0/81 RR 1.0 (0.0, 51.6)	1/81 (1%) RR 0.1, 74	
Pinede 2001 (30) (DOT AVK)	VKA (INR 2.0–3.0) for 1.5 mo	Allocation: Yes Patients: No Caregivers: No	105/105	15 mo	2/105 (2%)	1/105 (1%)	Not specified	Population: First isolated calf DVT.
	VKA (INR 2.0–3.0) for 3 mo	Adjudications: Yes Data analysts: Unlikely	92/92		3/92 RR 1.7 (0.3, 10.0)	3/92 RR 3.4 (0.4, 33)		
Schulman 1995 (28) DURAC (1)	VKA (INR2.0–2.85) for 1.5 mo	Allocation: Yes Patients: No Caregivers: No	443/443	2 y	80/443 (18%)	1/443	22/443 (5%)	First VTE: DVT (distal or proximal) or PE. Only asked about bleeding while on VKAs.
	VKA (INR 2.0–2.85) for 6 mo	Adjudications: VTE, yes other, unlikely Data analysts: Unlikely	454/454		43/454 (9%) RR 0.5 (0.4, 0.7)	5/454 (1%) RR 4.9 (0.6, 42)	17/454 (4%) RR (0.7, 1.4)	
Levine 1995 (4)	VKA stopped (Placebo)	Allocation: Yes Patients: No Caregivers: No	105/107	9 mo	12/105 (11%)	0/105	9/105 (9%)	Proximal DVT (first episode in 91%). Cancer in 21%.
	VKA (INR 2.0–3.0) for 2 more mo	Adjudications: VTE, yes Data analysts: Unlikely	109/113		7/109 (6%) RR 0.6 (0.2, 1.4)	1/109 (1%) RR 2.9 (0.1, 70.2) (within 2 mo of randomization)	9/109 (8%) RR 1.0 (0.4, 2.5)	
British Thoracic Society (5)	VKA (INR 2.0–3.0) For 1 mo	Allocation: Yes Patients: No Caregivers: No	358/358	1 y	28/358 (11%)	5/358 (1%)	26/358 (7%)	Population: DVT or PE; only 71% objectively diagnosed; proportion with a previous VTE not known.
	VKA (INR 2.0–3.0) for 3 mo	Adjudications: No Data analysts: Unlikely	354/354	1 y	14/354 (4%) RR 0.5 (0.3, 0.9)	4/354 (1%) RR 0.8 (0.2, 3.0)	28/354 (8) RR 1.1 (0.6, 1.8)	All bleeds were on VKA. Only 1 recurrent VTE among 116 pts with postoperative VTE.
Summary			2198		RR 0.53 (0.40,0.70)	RR 1.84 (0.76, 4.50)	RR 1.04 (0.74, 1.48)	For all analyses, $p = > 0.1$ for heterogeneity. SOFAST (36) not included in estimate for major bleeding as no events in either group.

Different Intermediate durations (6 or 12 months versus 3 months) of anticoagulation								
Campbell 2004 (74)	VKA (INR 20–3.5) for 3 mo	Allocation: Yes Patients: No Caregivers: No	369/396	1 y	31/369 (8%)	0/369 (during 3 mo treatment)	15/369 (4%)	Population: DVT or PE; proportion with calf DVT not known.
	VKA (INR 2.0–3.5) for 6 mo	Adjudications: No Data analysts: Unlikely	380/414	1 y	29/380 (8%) RR0.9 (0.6, 1.5)	8/380 (2%) (during 6 mo treatment) RR 16.5 (1.0, 285)	19/369 (5%) RR 1.3 (0.6, 2.5)	Only bleeding during treatment is reported. 20% of VTE outcomes were not objectively verified.
Agnelli 2003 (34) (WODIT-PE)	VKA stopped VKA (INR 2.0–3.0) for 9 more mo	Allocation: Yes Patients: No Caregivers: No	91/91 90/90	2.6 y (mean) 2.9 y (mean)	11/91 (12%) 11.90 (12%) RR 1.0 (0.5–2.2)	1/91 (1%) 2/90 (2%) RR 2.0 (0.5–21.9)	7/91 (8%) 8/90 (9%) RR 1.16 (0.4–3.0)	Population: First unprovoked PE. Treated for ≥ 3 mo. Among the 4 groups, only 1 recurrent VTE while on VKA.
	VKA stopped VKA (INR 2.0–3.0) for 3 more mo	Adjudications: Yes Data analysts: Unlikely	70/70 75/75	2.8 y (mean) 2.9 y (mean)	7/70 (10%) 4/75 (5%) RR 0.5 (0.2–1.7)	0/70 (0%) 1/75 (1%) RR 1.9 (0.1–56)	0/70 (0%) 4/75 (5%) RR 8.4 (0.5–153)	Population: First provoked PE. Treated for ≥ 3 mo (see above).
Agnelli 2001 (33) (WODIT-DVT)	VKA stopped	Allocation: Yes Patients: No Caregivers: No	133/133	3.2 y (mean)	21/133 (16%)	2/133 (2%)	7/133 (5%)	Population: First unprovoked proximal DVT treated for 3 mo One patient had recurrent VTE on VKA. Bleeding in the intervention group was while on VKA.
	VKA (INR 2.0–3.0) for 9 mo	Adjudications: Yes Data analysts: Unlikely	134/134	3.1 y (mean)	21/134 (16%) RR 1.0 (0.6, 1.7)	4/134 (3%) RR 2.0 (0.4, 10.7)	7/134 (5%) RR 1.0 (0.4, 2.8)	
Pinede 2001 (30) (DOT AVK)	VKA (INR 2.0–3.0) for 3 mo &	Allocation: Yes Patients: No Caregivers: No	270/270	15 mo	21/270 (8%)	5/270 (2%)	Not specified	Population: First proximal DVT or PE. Recurrent VTE occurred after VKA in 26/28 of the short duration groups and 21/27 of the long duration groups.
	VKA (INR 1.0–3.0) for 6 mo	Adjudications: Yes Data analysts: Unlikely	269/269		23/269 (9%) RR 1.1 (0.6, 1.9)	7/269 (3%)) RR 1.4 (0.4, 4.4)		
Summary			1881		RR 0.95 (0.72, 1.26)	RR 2.53 (1.18, 5.46)	RR 1.3 (0.82, 2.08)	For all analyses, $p \geq 0.1$ for heterogeneity.

Table 10.3 *(Continued.)*

First author/year (acronym)	Intervention	Blinding	# Pts analyzed	Length follow-up	Recurrent DVT or PE	Major bleeding	Total mortality	Comments
Indefinite versus Intermediate durations of anticoagulation (INR ~20–3.0)								
Palereti 2006 (35) (PROLONG)	Remain aff (stop) VKA	Allocation: Yes Patients: No Caregivers: No	103/105	1.4 y (mean) (max 1.5 y)	18/103 (17%)	0/103	1/103 (1%)	Population: First unprovoked proximal DVT or PE. Treated for ≥ 3 mo. VKA stopped & D-dimer positive 1 mo later.
	Restart Indefinitely VKA (INR 2.0–3.0) (not blinded)	Adjudications: Yes Data analysts: Unlikely	120/122		2/120 (2%) RR 0.1 (0.0, 0.4)	1/120 (1%) RR 2.6 (0.1, 62.6)	1/120 (1%) RR 0.9 (0.1, 14)	8 control pts. Restarted VKA, some after superficial phlebitis. 1 recurrent VTE in VKA group after VKA stopped.
Kearon 1999 (16) (LAFIT)	VKA stopped (Placebo)	Allocation: Yes Patients: Yes Caregivers: Yes	83/83	10 mo (mean (max 2 y)	17/83 (20%)	0/83	3/83 (4%)	Population: First unprovoked proximal DVT or PE (5%) had previous provoked VTE). The recurrent VTE in the VKA patient was after stopping VKA.
	VKA (INR 2.0–3.0) for 2 more years	Adjudications: Yes Data Analysts: Yes	79/79		1/79 (1%) RR 0.1 (0.0, 0.5)	3/79 (4%) RR 7.4 (0.4, 140)	1/79 (1%) RR 0.3 (0.0, 3.3)	
Schulman 1997 (3) (DURAC 2)	VKA (INR 2.0–2.85) for 6 mo	Allocation: Yes Patients: No Caregivers: No	111/111	4 y	23/111 (2%)	3/111 (3%)	16/111 (14%)	Second VTE: DVT (distal or proximal) or PE. All recurrent VTE in the indefinite VKA group were after stopping VKAs.
	VKA (INR 2.0–2.85) Indefinitely	Adjudications: VTE, yes other, unlikely Data analysts: Unlikely	116/116		3/116 (3%) RR 0.1 (0.0, 0.4)	10/116 (9%) RR 3.2 (0.9, 11.3)	10/116 (9%) RR 0.6 (0.3, 1.3)	Bleeding during the first 6 mo of VKA in 1 of 6 mo group and 6 of indefinite group (only asked about bleeding while on VKAs).
Summary					RR 0.1 (0.04, 0.22)	RR 3.61 (1.22, 10.7)	RR 0.58 (0.29, 1.14)	For all analyses, $p \geq 0.1$ for heterogeneity.
Indefinite versus Intermediate durations of anticoagulation (INR ~1.5–2.0 after initial INR 2.0–3.0 in both groups)								
Ridker 2003 (18) (PREVENT)	VKA stopped or not restarted (Placebo)	Allocation: Yes Patients: Yes Caregivers: Yes	253/253	2.1 y (mean) (max 4.3 y)	37/253 (15%)	2/253 (1%)	8/253 (3%)	Population: Unprovoked DVT (distal or proximal) or PE (first episode in 38%) 8 recurrent VTE in the VKA group after stopping VKAs.
	VKA INR 1.5–2.0	Adjudications: Yes Data analysts: Yes	255/255		14/255 (5%) RR 0.4 (0.2, 0.7)	5/255 (2%) RR 2.5 (0.5, 12.7)	4/255 (2%) RR 0.5 (0.1, 1.6)	
Low Intensity (INR 1.5–1.9) versus Conventional intensity (INR 2.0–3.0)								
Kearon 2003 (17) (ELATE)	VKA INR 1.5–1.9	Allocation: Yes Patients: Yes Caregivers: Yes	369/369	2.4 y (mean)	16/369 (4%)	9/369 (2%)	16/369 (4%)	Population: Unprovoked proximal DVT or PE (first episode in 31%). Treated for ≥ 3 mo VKA (INR 2.0–3.0) (mean 12 mo) 5 recurrent VTE in INR 1.5–1.9 and 3 in the INR 2.0–3.0 group after stopping VKAs.
	VKA INR 2.0–3.0 (blinded)	Adjudications: Yes Data Analysts: Yes	369/369		6/369 (2%) RR 0.4 (0.1, 0.9)	8/369 (2%) RR 0.9 (0.3, 2.3)	8/369 (2%) RR 0.5 (0.2, 1.2)	

DVT, deep vein thrombosis; INR, international normalized ratio; PE, pulmonary embolism; RR, relative risk; VKA, vitamin K antagonist.

after three or more months of treatment for DVT or PE, recurrent VTE that presents as PE probably has a case-fatality of about 15%. The risk of dying from acute DVT, because of early subsequent PE or other complications (e.g., bleeding, precipitation of myocardial infarction), appears to be 2% or less (24,38,41,47,50,51). Based on these estimates, the case-fatality associated with late-recurrent VTE after a preceding PE is expected to be about 10%, whereas that after a preceding DVT case-fatality is expected to be about 5%. Consistent with the latter estimate, an overview of randomized trials calculated a 5.1% case-fatality for recurrent VTE in patients with DVT who had completed three months of treatment (40). Therefore, although the risk of a recurrence is the same after PE and proximal DVT, the case-fatality for a recurrence is expected to be twofold higher after PE than after DVT.

D-dimer level after withdrawal of treatment. A negative D-dimer test one month after withdrawal of VKA appears to identify patients with a substantially reduced risk of recurrent VTE (relative risk [RR] ~0.4) (35,52–54).

Hereditary thrombophilias. A recent meta-analysis estimated that the risk of recurrent VTE associated with heterozygous factor V Leiden was 1.4 (95% CI 1.1–1.8) and for prothrombin G20210A was 1.7 (1.3–2.3), with heterogeneity of these estimates among studies (55). Among five large prospective studies that included a total of 2,691 patients with a first episode of VTE (provoked and unprovoked), and of whom 117 (4.3%) had homozygous factor V Leiden, homozygous prothrombin gene G20210A, double heterozygous states for these two mutations, or deficiency of protein C, protein S, or antithrombin, the overall odds ratio for recurrent VTE associated with these major thrombophilias was 1.5 (95% CI, 0.9–2.4) (31,52,56–58).

Antiphospholipid antibodies. Schulman et al. found that an anticardiolipin antibody was associated with recurrent VTE in the first four years after a first VTE (59) but was no longer predictive of recurrence at the end of 10 years (42). Kearon found that an anticardiolipin antibody or lupus anticoagulant was associated with recurrent VTE after an unprovoked VTE (hazard ratio 4.0, 95% CI 1.2–13) (16) but not after a provoked VTE (hazard ratio 1.3, 95% CI 0.2–11) (36).

Sex. A recent meta-analysis estimated that the risk of recurrent VTE is higher in males than in females (RR 1.6, 95% CI 1.2–2.0), with heterogeneity of this association among studies (60).

Residual deep vein thrombosis. An association between the presence of residual DVT on ultrasound and risk of recurrent VTE has been reported (22,61). However, a number of other studies has not found that residual DVT is an independent predictor of recurrence (16,34,36,62), and why residual DVT should be associated with DVT in the contralateral leg is unexplained (61).

Vena caval filter. In patients who have a vena caval filter inserted and then receive standard anticoagulant therapy there is a trend to a higher risk of a new episode of DVT (RR 1.3; 95% CI 0.9–1.8), a lower risk of PE (RR 0.4; 95% CI 0.2–0.9), and no difference is the risk of VTE (DVT or PE; RR 1.0; 95% CI 0.7–1.4) after eight years of follow-up (63,64).

Other markers for recurrence. Factor VIII (54,58,65,66), factor IX (58), factor XI (58,67), homocysteine (58,68,69), thrombin generation (70), the activated partial thromboplastin time (71), family history of VTE (72), age at diagnosis (25,38) have been evaluated, but the evidence that they are clinically important risk factors for recurrent VTE is generally weak.

Comparisons of different durations of anticoagulation therapy for venous thromboembolism

Trials that have evaluated different durations of anticoagulant therapy in patients with VTE can be divided into three categories according to the durations of therapy that were compared: (1) short versus intermediate durations; (2) different intermediate durations; and (3) indefinite therapy versus intermediate durations. Within each of these categories, studies that included heterogeneous (i.e., less selected) patients with VTE will be considered first, followed by studies that enrolled subgroups of (i.e., selected) patients who were expected to have either a lower (e.g., associated with reversible risk factors) or a higher (e.g., unprovoked, or second episodes of, VTE) risk of recurrence.

Short (4 or 6 weeks) versus intermediate (3 or 6 months) durations of therapy

Five trials have evaluated shortening the duration of oral anticoagulant therapy from three or six months to four or six weeks in patients with mostly first episodes of VTE (Table 10.3) (4,5,28,30). The first three studies (British Thoracic Society, Levine, DURAC 1; Table 10.3), which mainly enrolled unselected patients with proximal DVT or PE, found that shortening the duration of anticoagulation was associated with about double the frequency of recurrent VTE during follow-up of one to two years (an absolute risk increase of ~5%) (4,5,28). Major bleeding was uncommon during the incremental period of anticoagulation in these three studies (estimated at seven episodes among 1,009 patients during 259 patient-years of additional treatment [2.7% per year]) (4,5,28). Therefore, the main finding of these studies was that anticoagulant therapy should not be shortened to four or six weeks in patients with VTE.

Subgroup analyses of one of these studies (DURAC 1) suggest that isolated distal DVT provoked by a major transient risk factor can safely be treated with only six weeks of therapy (28). A subsequent study (component of DOTAVK), which compared 6 versus 12 weeks of therapy in patients with isolated calf DVT (unprovoked or provoked; mostly diagnosed by ultrasound), found no suggestion that shortening therapy increased the risk of recurrence (RR 0.6; 95% CI, 0.01–3.4), and, in general, observed a low frequency of recurrent VTE with isolated calf DVT (~2% in the first year) compared with proximal DVT or PE (~6% in the first year) (30). These findings suggest that if anticoagulants need to be stopped after six weeks of therapy in patients with isolated distal DVT the subsequent risk of recurrence is not expected to be excessive. The fifth of these studies enrolled only patients with VTE associated with a major reversible risk factor (SOFAST; Table 10.3); however, because only 165 patients were enrolled, its findings were not definitive (36). A meta-analysis of five studies (retrospective identification of the patient's subgroup in four studies [4,5,28,73]; selective enrollment of patients in one study [36] that compared four or six weeks with three or six months of treatment among 725 patients with VTE provoked by a reversible risk factor found that the shorter durations of therapy were associated with more than double the risk of recurrent VTE during the next year (odds ratio 2.9; 95% CI 1.2 to 6.9; absolute increase of ~3.4%) (36).

Different intermediate durations of therapy (6 or 12 months versus 3 months)

Two studies have compared six versus three months of anticoagulant therapy in patients with predominantly first episodes of DVT or PE (unprovoked, or provoked by a reversible risk factor) (DOTAVK, Campbell; Table 10.3) (30;74). There was no difference in the risk of recurrence during follow-up in both studies, and one study (74) reported a lower risk of bleeding in the three-month group (Campbell; Table 10.3).

Agnelli and colleagues compared stopping anticoagulant therapy at three months with continuing it for another nine months after a first episode of unprovoked proximal DVT (WODIT-DVT; Table 10.3) (33). At the end of the first year, recurrent VTE was less frequent in the group that remained on anticoagulant therapy (3.0% versus 8.3%), but this benefit was lost two years after these patients stopped anticoagulant therapy (RR 1.0; 95% CI, 0.6–1.7). The same investigators obtained similar results in a comparable study of patients with unprovoked PE (WODIT PE; Table 10.3) (34).

Based on the findings of these five studies (including the two components of WODIT-PE) (30;33;34;74), anticoagulants are very effective at preventing recurrence while patients are receiving therapy, but, at the end of extended follow-up after stopping treatment, a similar risk of recurrence is expected if anticoagulants are stopped at 6 or 12 months compared to at 3 months (RR for the five studies 0.95; 95% CI 0.72–1.26; Table 10.3) (30,33,34,74), including among patients with unprovoked proximal DVT or PE.

Indefinite therapy versus intermediate durations of anticoagulant therapy

Four trials have compared indefinite (i.e., extended therapy without scheduled stopping of treatment and subsequent follow-up) anticoagulation (target INR of 2.0–2.85 [3], 2.0–3.0 [16,35], 1.5–2.0 [18]) with stopping therapy in patients with VTE who were believed to have a high risk of recurrence because thrombosis was a second episode (3), unprovoked (16,18), or was unprovoked and had a positive D-dimer result one month after stopping therapy (35) (DURAC2, LAFIT, PREVENT, PROLONG; Table 10.3). The results indicate that randomization to indefinite treatment with conventional-intensity VKA (target INR 2.5) reduces recurrent VTE by about 90% (RR for the three studies 0.10; 95%CI 0.04–0.22; Table 10.3) (3,16,35), and randomization to low-intensity therapy (target INR 1.75) reduces VTE by 64% (95% CI for HR, 23%–81%) (18) (Table 10.3; both risk reduction are appreciably greater among patients who remain on VKA therapy).

Bleeding during long-term anticoagulant therapy

A meta-analysis of seven studies (4,16,18,33,39,75,76) that compared durations of conventional-intensity anticoagulant therapy for VTE (not all patients had unprovoked VTE) estimated the rate of major bleeding to be 1.1% per patient-year (18 episodes in 1,571 years) during the extended phase of anticoagulation compared with 0.6% per patient-year (nine episodes during 1,497 years) without anticoagulation (RR of 1.80; 95% CI 0.72–4.51) (77). Similar low rates on major bleeding were observed during long-term treatment of unprovoked VTE in the more recent ELATE and PROLONG studies (Table 10.3) (17,74).

Of factors that have been evaluated as risk factors for major bleeding during anticoagulant therapy, the following appear to have the greatest potential to be clinically useful markers of increased risk: older age, particularly after 75 years; previous gastrointestinal bleeding, particularly if not associated with a reversible cause; previous noncardioembolic stroke; chronic renal or hepatic disease; concomitant antiplatelet therapy (to be avoided if possible); other serious acute or chronic illness; poor anticoagulant control; suboptimal monitoring of anticoagulant therapy (17,78–85).

Balancing reduction of VTE with increase of bleeding during long-term therapy

The likelihood of dying from recurrent VTE depends on whether the recurrence is a PE or a DVT, with PE being much more common after an initial PE than after an initial DVT. After completing three or more months of initial anticoagulant therapy, case-fatality for recurrent VTE is expected to be about 10% after an initial PE and 5% after an initial DVT (see above). Case-fatality with major bleeding during long-term anticoagulant therapy for VTE is about 10% (86). Comparison of associated case-fatalities suggests that the consequence of a major bleed during long-term anticoagulation is similar to that of a recurrent episode of VTE that occurs after a PE and about twice as severe as the consequences of a recurrent episode of VTE that occurs after a DVT. Therefore, given a relative risk of recurrent VTE of over 90%, and a relative risk of bleeding of 2.5, with long-term anticoagulation, if the annual rate of major bleeding on anticoagulant therapy is 2%, the annual risk of recurrent VTE needs to exceed 1.2% after a PE and 2.4% after a DVT just to offset the increase fatal bleeding.

Patient preferences and the burden of anticoagulation

The perceived burden associated with being on VKA therapy differs markedly among patients. For example, Locadia and colleagues identified that being on VKA was associated with a median utility of 0.92 (where 0 is equivalent to death and 1.0 is equivalent to perfect health) by 124 patients who had a recent or remote VTE; however, the associated utility was 0.77 or lower for a quarter of patients and was 0.98 or higher for another quarter of patients (i.e., rated more highly that the median utility of 0.96 associated with not being on VKA). Consistent with these large differences in patients' perception of the burden of VKA therapy, irrespective of whether the risk of recurrence was assumed to be high or low after stopping therapy, 25% of surveyed patients always opted to stop therapy, and 23% always opted to stay on therapy. There were also marked difference in how bad patients' perceptions were of having an episode of bleeding or VTE (87).

Alternatives to vitamin K antagonists

Subcutaneous unfractionated heparin. Adjusted-dose subcutaneous unfractionated heparin (UFH) is an effective approach for the long-term treatment of DVT (88), whereas low-dose UFH (5,000 U twice daily) is inadequate for this purpose (2,89). In a study of 80 patients with DVT and contraindications to VKA therapy that compared 10,000 U UFH with 5,000 IU dalteparin, each administered subcutaneously twice daily for three months, there was a similar low frequency of recurrent VTE and bleeding in both groups but less frequent spinal fracture in the LMWH group (90).

Subcutaneous low-molecular-weight-heparin. Fourteen randomized trials have compared VKA (INR of 2.0–3.0) with widely differing regimens of five LMWH preparations (dalteparin [91–93], enoxaparin [29,94–98], nadroparin [99, 100], tinzaparin [101,102], bemiparin [103]). In these studies, the daily LMWH dose was as low as 4,000 IU (29,94) to as high as 200 IU/kg (93,100); approximately a 3.5-fold difference. Two meta-analyses of studies that compared LMWH with vitamin K antagonist, each given for three months after initial heparin therapy, have been performed (104,105). In the analysis by Iorio and colleagues, which includes seven studies (29,91,94,95,99–101) and a total of 1,379 patients, there were trends toward less recurrent VTE (odds ratio 0.66; 95% CI, 0.41–1.07) and less major bleeding (odds ratio 0.45; 95% CI, 0.18 –1.11) with three months of LMWH compared with VKA (105). Compared with outcomes in patients who received VKA therapy, between study differences of mean daily dose of LMWH had little effect on efficacy but did appear to influence the risk of major bleeding (odds ratio of about 0.2 with ~4,000 IU/day to about 0.7 with 12,000 IU/day, relative to the VKA groups [$p = 0.03$]) (105). Three subsequent studies that selectively enrolled a total of 1,019 patients with VTE in association with active cancer found that, compared with VKA therapy, three (96,106) or six (93) months of therapeutic-dose LMWH was associated with less recurrent VTE in one study (93) and less bleeding in another (96) (Table 10.4) (RR for the three studies: recurrent VTE 0.56 [95% CI 0.38–0.82]; major bleeding 1.01 [95% CI 0.62–1.64]; mortality 0.92 [95% CI 0.78–1.10]; Table 10.4) (96,105,106). Randomized trials have not evaluated approaches to anticoagulant therapy after the first six months of VKA or LMWH therapy in patients with VTE and cancer, either to assess duration of therapy or to compare extended therapy with VKA or LMWH. Observational studies suggest that the risk of recurrent VTE is unacceptably high in patients with active cancer who stop anticoagulant therapy (24–26,38).

New anticoagulants. Ximelagatran, an oral direct thrombin inhibitor, has been shown to be as effective for the initial and long-term treatment of VTE but has been withdrawn because of hepatic toxicity (39,107). Idraparinux, the synthetic long-acting pentasaccharide, was recently reported to be as effective and as safe as VKA for the first three or six months of treatment of DVT but less effective than VKA in patients with PE (108). After six months of treatment of VTE with idraparinux or VKA, compared with placebo, idraparinux reduced recurrence but was associated with increased bleeding (109).

Recommended duration of anticoagulation in individual patients

Based largely on the preceding analysis of risk factors for recurrent thrombosis and bleeding, and on the findings of studies that compared different durations and intensities of anticoagulation, an approach to selecting duration of anticoagulation for individual patients with VTE is outlined in Table 10.5. Because the presence of a reversible risk factor for VTE, lack of a provoking factor, or cancer, at the time of thrombosis has the greatest prognostic influence on the risk of recurrence, this assessment carries most weight.

For patients whose VTE is associated with a major reversible risk factor, such as recent surgery, stopping anticoagulant therapy after three months of treatment is expected to be associated with a subsequent risk of recurrent VTE of about 3% in the first year and about 10% over five years (4,5,18,24,26,29,30,34,39). For patients whose VTE is associated with a lesser reversible risk factor, such as a soft tissue injury to the leg or a prolonged flight, stopping anticoagulant therapy after three months of treatment is expected to be associated with a subsequent risk of recurrent VTE of about 5% in the first year and about 15% over 5 years (31). These rates of VTE are not high enough to justify treatment for longer than three months.

Table 10.4 LMWH versus VKA for long-term treatment of VTE in patients with active cancer.*

First author (acronym)	Interventions	Blinding	Pts analyzed	ength of follow-up	Recurrent DVT or PE	Major bleeding	Total mortality	Comments
Meyer 2002 (96)	VKA (INR 2.0–3.0) for 3 mo after initial enoxaparin	Allocation: Likely Patients: No Caregivers: No	75/75	3 mo	3/75 (4%)	12/75 (16%)	17/75 (23%)	Population: DVT (proportion with calf DVT not known) or PE and active cancer.
	Enoxaparin 1.5 mg/kg OD for 3 mo	Adjudications: Yes Data analysts: Unlikely	71/71	3 mo	2/71 (3%) RR 0.7 (0.1, 4.1)	5/71 (7%) RR 0.4 (0.2, 1.2)	8/71 (11%) RR 0.5 (0.2, 1.1)	All fatal bleeding (n=6) were in VKA group.
Lee 2003 (93) (CLOT)	VKA (INR 2.0–3.0) for 6 mo after initial dalteparin	Allocation: Yes Patients: No Caregivers: No	336/338	6 mo	53/336 (16%)	12/335 (4%)	136/336 (40%)	Population: Proximal DVT or PE and active cancer.
	Dalteparin 200U/kg OD for 1 mo followed by 150 U/kg for 5 mo	Adjudications: Yes Data analysts: Likely	336/338	6 mo	27/336 (8%) RR 0.5 (0.3, 0.8)	19/338 (6%) RR 1.6 (0.8, 3.2)	130/336 (37%) RR 1.0 (0.8, 1.2)	Difference in efficacy mainly due to recurrent DVT (14 vs. 37 episodes).
Hull 2006 (106) (Main LITE-cancer)	VKA (INR2.0–3.0) for 3 mo after initial IV UFH	Allocation: Likely Patients: No Caregivers: No	100/100	3 mo	10/100 (10%)	7/100 (7%)	19/100 (19%)	Population: Proximal DVT and active cancer.
	Tinzaparin 175mg/kg OD for 3 mo.	Adjudications: Yes Data Analysts: Likely	100/100	3 mo	6/100 (6%) RR 0.6 (0.2, 1.6)	7/100 (7%) RR 1.0 (0.4, 2.8)	20/100 (20%) RR1.0 (0.6, 1.9)	Prespecified, stratification, subgroup within a larger trial. Outcomes at 12 mo were also reported.
Summary			1,019		RR 0.7 (0.4, 0.8)	RR 1.0 (0.6, 1.6)	RR 0.9 (0.8, 1.1)	Heterogeneity p <0.1 for all estimates.

*LMWH, low-molecular weight-heparin; PE, pulmonary embolism; RR, relative risk; UFH, unfractionated heparin; VKA, vitamin K antagonist; VTE, venous thromboembolism.

Table 10.5 Recommendations for duration of anticoagulant therapy for VTE

Risk factor for VTE	Durations of treatment (target INR 2.5, range 2.0–3.0)
Transient risk factor*	3 months
Unprovoked	Indefinite†
If also:	
isolated distal DVT; or a first proximal DVT or PE and a moderate or higher risk of bleeding;§ or an informed patient's preference is to stop therapy	*3 months*
Uncontrolled malignancy	Indefinite
If also:	(preferably with low-molecular weight-heparin for at least the first 3 months)
*a very high risk of bleeding;§ isolated distal DVT; or an additional major reversible provoking risk factor for VTE.**	*consider stopping therapy at 3 months or when cancer becomes inactive*

*Transient risk factors include major factors, such as surgery with general anesthesia, plaster cast immobilization of a leg, or hospitalization, all within the past month; and minor factors, such as estrogen therapy, pregnancy, prolonged travel (e.g., longer than 8 hours), less marked leg injury, or the previously noted "major factors" when they occur 1 to 3 months before diagnosis of venous thromboembolism (VTE).

†Decision should be reviewed annually to consider if the patient's risk of bleeding has increased, or if patient preference had changed. Additional factors favoring indefinite therapy include more than one episode of unprovoked VTE; pulmonary embolism (PE) versus proximal deep vein thrombosis (DVT) at presentation; male sex; antiphospholipid antibodies; hereditary thrombophilia.

§ Risk factors for bleeding include age 65 years or older, particularly after 75 years; previous noncardioembolic stoke; previous bleeding (e.g., gastrointestinal), particularly if there was not a reversible cause; active peptic ulcer disease; renal impairment; anemia; thrombocytopenia; liver disease; diabetes mellitus; use of antiplatelet therapy (to be avoided); poor patient compliance; poor control of anticoagulation; structural lesion (including tumor) expected to be associated with bleeding. One or 2 risk factors suggests a moderate risk, and 3 or more risk factors suggests a high risk of bleeding.

For patients with unprovoked VTE, stopping anticoagulant therapy after three or more months of treatment is expected to be associated with a subsequent risk of recurrent VTE of about 10% in the first year and about 30% over five years (26,28,30,33). This rate is high enough to justify long-term anticoagulation in the majority of patients. The argument favoring long-term therapy is stronger if the unprovoked episode of VTE was a second or subsequent episode of unprovoked VTE, was a PE, occurred in a male, or was associated with an antiphospholipid antibody or a hereditary thrombophilia.

Patients with active cancer generally should remain on long-term anticoagulant therapy (LMWH or VKA) because the risk of recurrent VTE is expected to be higher than 10% within a year of stopping treatment.

If anticoagulant therapy is expected to be associated with a high risk of bleeding because of risk factors for bleeding or lack of access to appropriate anticoagulant monitoring, longer than three months of treatment generally should be avoided in patients with a first unprovoked VTE. Annual review is recommended for patients on long-term therapy to ensure that the benefits of continuing therapy are likely to exceed the risks (e.g., that contraindications have not developed).

References

1 Lagerstedt CI, Olsson CG, Fagher BO, et al. Need for long-term anticoagulant treatment in symptomatic calf-vein thrombosis. *Lancet.* 1985;**2**:515–18.

2 Hull R, Delmore T, Genton E, et al. Warfarin sodium versus low-dose heparin in the long-term treatment of venous thrombosis. *N Engl J Med.* 1979;**301**:855–58.

3 Schulman S, Granqvist S, Holmstrom M, et al. The duration of oral anticoagulant therapy after a second episode of venous thromboembolism. *N Engl J Med.* 1997;**336**:393–98.

4 Levine MN, Hirsh J, Gent M, et al. Optimal duration of oral anticoagulant therapy: a randomized trial comparing four weeks with three months of warfarin in patients with proximal deep vein thrombosis. *Thromb Haemost.* 1995;**74**:606–11.

5 Research Committee of the British Thoracic Society. Optimum duration of anticoagulation for deep-vein thrombosis and pulmonary embolism. *Lancet.* 1992;**340**:873–76.

6 Gallus AS, Jackaman J, Tillett J, et al. Safety and efficacy of warfarin started early after submassive venous thrombosis or pulmonary embolism. *Lancet.* 1986;**2**:1293–96.

7 Hull RD, Raskob GE, Rosenbloom D, et al. Heparin for 5 days as compared with 10 days in the initial treatment of proximal venous thrombosis. *N Engl J Med.* 1990;**322**:1260–64.

8 Harrison L, Johnston M, Massicotte MP, et al. Comparison of 5-mg and 10-mg loading doses in initiation of warfarin therapy. *Ann Intern Med.* 1997;**126**:133–36.

9 Crowther MA, Ginsberg JS, Kearon C, et al. A randomized trial comparing 5 mg and 10 mg warfarin loading doses. *Arch Intern Med.* 1999;**159**:46–8.

10 Kovacs MJ, Rodger M, Anderson DR, et al. Comparison of 10-mg and 5-mg warfarin initiation nomograms together with low-molecular-weight heparin for outpatient treatment of acute venous thromboembolism. A randomized, double-blind, controlled trial. *Ann Intern Med.* 2003;**138**:714–19.

11 Ansell J, Hirsh J, Poller L, et al. The pharmacology and management of the vitamin K antagonists: the Seventh ACCP Conference

on Antithrombotic and Thrombolytic Therapy. *Chest.* 2004;**126**: 204S–33S.

12 Garcia D, Regan S, Crowther M, et al. Warfarin maintenance dosing patterns in clinical practice: implications for safer anticoagulation in the elderly population. *Chest.* 2005;**127**:2049–56.

13 Hull R, Hirsh J, Jay R, et al. Different intensities of oral anticoagulant therapy in the treatment of proximal-vein thrombosis. *N Engl J Med.* 1982;**307**:1676–81.

14 Crowther MA, Ginsberg JS, Julian J, et al. A comparison of two intensities of warfarin for prevention of recurrent thrombosis in patients with antiphospholipid antibody syndrome. *N Eng J Med.* 2003;**349**: 1133–38.

15 Finazzi G, Marchioli R, Brancaccio V, et al. A randomized clinical trial of high-intensity warfarin vs. conventional antithrombotic therapy for the prevention of recurrent thrombosis in patients with the antiphospholipid syndrome (WAPS). *J Thromb Haemost.* 2005;**3**:848–53.

16 Kearon C, Gent M, Hirsh J, et al. A comparison of three months of anticoagulation with extended anticoagulation for a first episode of idiopathic venous thromboembolism. *N Engl J Med.* 1999;**340**:901–7.

17 Kearon C, Ginsberg JS, Kovacs MJ, et al. Comparison of low-intensity warfarin therapy with conventional-intensity warfarin therapy for long-term prevention of recurrent venous thromboembolism. *N Eng J Med.* 2003;**349**:631–39.

18 Ridker PM, Goldhaber SZ, Danielson E, et al. Long-term, low-intensity warfarin therapy for prevention of recurrent venous thromboembolism. *N Eng J Med.* 2003;**348**:1425–34.

19 Hutten BA, Prins M, Gent M, et al. Incidence of recurrent thromboembolic and bleeding complications among patients with venous thromboembolism in relation to both malignancy and achieved international normalized ratio: a retrospective analysis. *J Clin Oncol.* 2000;**18**:3078–83.

20 Merli G, Spiro TE, Olsson CG, et al. Subcutaneous enoxaparin once or twice daily compared with intravenous unfractionated heparin for treatment of venous thromboembolic disease. *Ann Intern Med.* 2001;**134**:191–202.

21 Palareti G, Legnani C, Lee A, et al. A comparison of the safety and efficacy of oral anticoagulation for the treatment of venous thromboembolic disease in patients with or without malignancy. *Thromb Haemost.* 2000;):805–10.

22 Piovella F, Crippa L, Barone M, et al. Normalization rates of compression ultrasonography in patients with a first episode of deep vein thrombosis of the lower limbs: association with recurrence and new thrombosis. *Haematologica.* 2002;**87**:515–22.

23 Prandoni P, Lensing AW, Piccioli A, et al. Recurrent venous thromboembolism and bleeding complications during anticoagulant treatment in patients with cancer and venous thrombosis. *Blood.* 2002;**100**:3484–88.

24 Prandoni P, Lensing AWA, Cogo A, et al. The long-term clinical course of acute deep venous thrombosis. *Ann Intern Med.* 1996;**125**:1–7.

25 Heit JA, Mohr DN, Silverstein MD, Petterson TM, O'Fallon WM, Melton LJ III. Predictors of recurrence after deep vein thrombosis and pulmonary embolism: a population-based cohort study. *Arch Intern Med.* 2000;**160**:761–68.

26 Palareti G, Legnani C, Cosmi B, et al. Risk of venous thromboembolism recurrence: high negative predictive value of D-dimer performed after oral anticoagulation is stopped. *Thromb Haemost.* 2002;**87**:7–12.

27 Prandoni P, Lensing AWA, Büller HR, et al. Deep-vein thrombosis and the incidence of subsequent symptomatic cancer. *N Engl J Med.* 1992;**327**:1128–33.

28 Schulman S, Rhedin A-S, Lindmarker P, et al. A comparison of six weeks with six months of oral anticoagulant therapy after a first episode of venous thromboembolism. *N Engl J Med.* 1995;**332**:1661–65.

29 Pini M, Aiello S, Manotti C, et al. Low molecular weight heparin versus warfarin the prevention of recurrence after deep vein thrombosis. *Thromb Haemost.* 1994;**72**(2):191–97.

30 Pinede L, Ninet J, Duhaut P, et al. Comparison of 3 and 6 months of oral anticoagulant therapy after a first episode of proximal deep vein thrombosis or pulmonary embolism and comparison of 6 and 12 weeks of therapy after isolated calf deep vein thrombosis. *Circulation.* 2001;**103**:2453–60.

31 Baglin T, Luddington R, Brown K, et al. Incidence of recurrent venous thromboembolism in relation to clinical and thrombophilic risk factors: prospective cohort study. *Lancet.* 2003;**362**:523–26.

32 Spiezia L, Bernardi E, Tormene D, et al. Recurrent thromboembolism in fertile women with venous thrombosis: incidence and risk factors. *Thromb Haemost.* 2003;**90**:964–66.

33 Agnelli G, Prandoni P, Santamaria MG, et al. Three months versus one year of oral anticoagulant therapy for idiopathic deep vein thrombosis. *N Eng J Med.* 2001;**345**:165–69.

34 Agnelli G, Prandoni P, Becattini C, et al. Extended oral anticoagulant therapy after a first episode of pulmonary embolism. *Ann Intern Med.* 2003;**139**:19–25.

35 Palareti G, Cosmi B, Legnani C, et al. D-dimer testing to determine the duration of anticoagulation therapy. *N Engl J Med.* 2006;**355**:1780–89.

36 Kearon C, Ginsberg JS, Anderson DR, et al. Comparison of 1 month with 3 months of anticoagulation for a first episode of venous thromboembolism associated with a transient risk factor. *J Thromb Haemost.* 2004;**2**:743–49.

37 Hansson PO, Sorbo J, Eriksson H. Recurrent venous thromboembolism after deep vein thrombosis: incidence and risk factors. *Arch Intern Med.* 2000;**160**:769–74.

38 Murin S, Romano PS, White RH. Comparison of outcomes after hospitalization for deep vein thrombosis or pulmonary embolism. *Thromb Haemost.* 2002;**88**:407–14.

39 Schulman S, Wahlander K, Lundström T, et al. Secondary prevention of venous thromboembolism with the oral direct thrombin inhibitor ximelagatran. *N Eng J Med.* 2003;**349**:1713–21.

40 Douketis JD, Kearon C, Bates S, et al. Risk of fatal pulmonary embolism in patients with treated venous thromboembolism. *JAMA.* 1998;**279**:458–62.

41 Kniffin WD Jr, Baron JA, Barrett J, et al. The epidemiology of diagnosed pulmonary embolism and deep venous thrombosis in the elderly. *Arch Intern Med.* 1994;**154**:861–66.

42 Schulman S, Lindmarker P, Holmstrom M, et al. Post-thrombotic syndrome, recurrence, and death 10 years after the first episode of venous thromboembolism treated with warfarin for 6 weeks or 6 months. *J Thromb Haemost.* 2006;**4**:734–42.

43 Bell WR, Simon TL. Current status of pulmonary embolic disease: pathophysiology, diagnosis, prevention, and treatment. *Am Heart J.* 1982;**103**:239–61.

44 Stein PD, Henry JW. Prevalence of acute pulmonary embolism among patients in a general hospital and at autopsy. *Chest.* 1995;**108**:978–81.

45 Kearon C. Natural history of venous thromboembolism. *Circulation.* 2003;**107**:I-22–1-30.

46 Goldhaber SZ, Visni L, De Rosa M. Acute pulmonary embolism: clinical outcomes in the International Cooperative Pulmonary Embolism Registry (ICOPER). *Lancet.* 1999;**353**:1386–89.

47 Heit JA, Silverstein MD, Mohr DN, et al. Predictors of survival after deep vein thrombosis and pulmonary embolism: a population-based, cohort study. *Arch Intern Med.* 1999;**159**:445–53.

48 Ribeiro A, Lindmarker P, Juhlin-Dannfelt A, et al. Echocardiography doppler in pulmonary embolism: right ventricular dysfunction as a predictor of mortality rate. *Am Heart J.* 1997;**134**:479–87.

49 Bell CM, Redelmeier DA. Mortality among patients admitted to hospitals on weekends as compared with weekdays. *N Eng J Med.* 2002;**345**:663–68.

50 Naess IA, Christiansen SC, Romundstad P, et al. Incidence and mortality of venous thrombosis: a population-based study. *J Thromb Haemost.* 2007;**5**:692–99.

51 Beyth RJ, Cohen AM, Landefeld CS. Long-term outcomes of deep-vein thrombosis. *Arch Intern Med.* 1995;**155**:1031–37.

52 Palareti G, Legnani C, Cosmi B, et al. Predictive value of D-dimer test for recurrent venous thromboembolism after anticoagulation withdrawal in subjects with a previous idiopathic event and in carriers of congenital thrombophilia. *Circulation.* 2003;**108**:313–18.

53 Eichinger S, Minar E, Bialonczyk C, et al. D-dimer levels and risk of recurrent venous thromboembolism. *JAMA.* 2003;**290**:1071–74.

54 Shrivastava S, Ridker PM, Glynn RJ, Goldhaber SZ, Moll S, Bounameaux H et al. D-dimer, factor VIII coagulant activity, low-intensity warfarin and the risk of recurrent venous thromboembolism. *J Thromb Haemost.* 2006;**4**:1208–14.

55 Ho WK, Hankey GJ, Quinlan DJ, et al. Risk of recurrent venous thromboembolism in patients with common thrombophilia: a systematic review. *Arch Intern Med.* 2006;**166**:729–36.

56 Lindmarker P, Schulman S, Sten-Linder M, et al. The risk of recurrent venous thromboembolism in carriers and non-carriers of the G1691A Allele in the coagulation factor V gene and the G20210A Allele in the prothrombin gene. *Thromb Haemost.* 1999;**81**:684–89.

57 Eichinger S, Pabinger I, Stumpflen A, et al. The risk of recurrent venous thromboembolism in patients with and without Factor V Leiden. *Thromb Haemost.* 1997;**77**(4):624–28.

58 Christiansen SC, Cannegieter SC, Koster T, et al. Thrombophilia, clinical factors, and recurrent venous thrombotic events. *JAMA.* 2005;**293**:2352–61.

59 Schulman S, Svenungsson E, Granqvist S. Anticardiolipin antibodies predict early recurrence of thromboembolism and death among patients with venous thromboembolism following anticoagulant therapy. *Am J Med.* 1998;**104**:332–38.

60 McRae S, Tran H, Schulman S, et al. Effect of patient's sex on risk of recurrent venous thromboembolism: a meta-analysis. *Lancet.* 2006;**368**:371-78.

61 Prandoni P, Lensing AW, Prins MH, et al. Residual venous thrombosis as a predictive factor of recurrent venous thromboembolism. *Ann Intern Med.* 2002;**137**:955–60.

62 Cosmi B, Legnani C, Cini M, et al. D-dimer levels in combination with residual venous obstruction and the risk of recurrence after anticoagulation withdrawal for a first idiopathic deep vein thrombosis. *Thromb Haemost.* 2005;**94**:969–74.

63 Decousus H, Leizorovicz A, Parent F, et al. A clinical trial of vena caval filters in the prevention of pulmonary embolism in patients with proximal deep-vein thrombosis. *N Engl J Med.* 1998;**338**:409–15.

64 Eight-year follow-up of patients with permanent vena cava filters in the prevention of pulmonary embolism: the PREPIC (Prevention du Risque d'Embolie Pulmonaire par Interruption Cave) randomized study. *Circulation.* 2005;**112**:416–22.

65 Kryle P, Minar E, Hirschl M, et al. High plasma levels of factor VIII and the risk of recurrent venous thromboembolism. *N Eng J Med.* 2000;**343**:457–62.

66 Kraaijenhagen RA, in't Anker PS, Koopman MM, et al. High plasma concentration of factor VIIIc is a major risk factor for venous thromboembolism [see comments]. *Thromb Haemost.* 2000;**83**:5–9.

67 Weltermann A, Eichinger S, Bialonczyk C, et al. The risk of recurrent venous thromboembolism among patients with high factor IX levels. *J Thromb Haemost.* 2003;**1**:28–32.

68 Eichinger S, Stumpflen A, Hirschl M, et al. Hyperhomocysteinemia is a risk factor of recurrent venous thromboembolism. *Thromb Haemost.* 1998;80:566–69.

69 Den Heijer M, Willems HP, Blom HJ, et al. Homocysteine lowering by B vitamins and the prevention of secondary deep vein thrombosis and pulmonary embolism: a randomized, placebo-controlled, double-blind trial. *J Thromb Haemost*. 2003(Suppl 1):OC161.

70 Hron G, Kollars M, Binder BR, et al. Identification of patients at low risk for recurrent venous thromboembolism by measuring thrombin generation. *JAMA.* 2006;**296**:397–402.

71 Hron G, Eichinger S, Weltermann A, et al. Prediction of recurrent venous thromboembolism by the activated partial thromboplastin time. *J Thromb Haemost.* 2006;**4**:752–56.

72 Hron G, Eichinger S, Weltermann A, et al. Family history for venous thromboembolism and the risk for recurrence. *Am J Med.* 2006;**119**:50–53.

73 Schulman S, Lockner D, Juhlin-Dannfelt A. The duration of oral anticoagulation after deep vein thrombosis. *Acta Med Scand.* 1985;**217**:547–52.

74 Campbell IA, Bentley DP, Prescott RJ, et al. Anticoagulation for three versus six months in patients with deep vein thrombosis or pulmonary embolism, or both: randomised trial. *Br Med J.* 2007.

75 Schweizer J, Elix H, Altmann E, et al. Comparative results of thrombolysis treatment with rt-PA and urokinase: a pilot study. *Vasa.* 1998;**27**:167–71.

76 Holmgren K, Andersson G, Fagrell B, et al. One-month versus six-month therapy with oral anticoagulants after symptomatic deep vein thrombosis. *Acta Med Scand.* 1985;**218**:279–84.

77 Ost D, Tepper J, Mihara H, et al. Duration of anticoagulation following venous thromboembolism: a meta-analysis. *JAMA.* 2005;**294**: 706–15.

78 Palareti G, Leali N, Coccheri S, et al. Bleeding complications of oral anticoagulant treatment: an inception-cohort, prospective collaborative study (ISCOAT). *Lancet.* 1996;**348**:423–28.

79 Beyth RJ, Quinn LM, Landefeld S. Prospective evaluation of an index for predicting the risk of major bleeding in outpatients treated with warfarin. *Am J Med.* 1998;**105**:91–9.

80 Kuijer PMM, Hutten BA, Prins MH, et al. Prediction of the risk of bleeding during anticoagulant treatment for venous thromboembolism. *Arch Intern Med.* 1999;**159**:457–60.

81 Pengo V, Legnani C, Noventa F, et al. Oral anticoagulant therapy in patients with nonrheumatic atrial fibrillation and risk of bleeding. a Multicenter Inception Cohort Study. *Thromb Haemost.* 2001;**85**:418–22.

82 Beyth RJ, Quinn L, Landefeld CS. A multicomponent intervention to prevent major bleeding complications in older patients receiving warfarin: a randomized, controlled trial. *Ann Intern Med.* 2000;**133**: 687–95.

83 Dentali F, Douketis JD, Lim W, et al. Combined aspirin-oral anticoagulant therapy compared with oral anticoagulant therapy alone among

patients at risk for cardiovascular disease: a meta-analysis of randomized trials. *Arch Intern Med.* 2007;**167**:117–24.

84 Schulman S, Beyth RJ, Kearon C, et al. Hemorrhagic complications of anticoagulant and thrombolytic treatment. *Chest.* 2007;x:x.

85 Gage BF, Yan Y, Milligan PE, et al. Clinical classification schemes for predicting hemorrhage: results from the National Registry of Atrial Fibrillation (NRAF). *Am Heart J.* 2006;**151**:713–19.

86 Linkins L, Choi PT, Douketis JD. Clinical impact of bleeding in patients taking oral anticoagulant therapy for venous thromboembolism: a meta-analysis. *Ann Intern Med.* 2003;**139**:893–900.

87 Locadia M, Bossuyt PM, Stalmeier PF, et al. Treatment of venous thromboembolism with vitamin K antagonists: patients' health state valuations and treatment preferences. *Thromb Haemost.* 2004;**92**: 1336–41.

88 Hull R, Delmore T, Carter C, et al. Adjusted subcutaneous heparin versus warfarin sodium in the long-term treatment of venous thrombosis. *N Engl J Med.* 1982;**306**:189–94.

89 Bynum LJ, Wilson Je. Low-dose heparin therapy in the long-term management of venous thromboembolism. *Am J Med.* 1979;**67**: 553–56.

90 Monreal M, Lafoz E, Olive A. Comparison of subcutaneous unfractionated heparin with a low molecular weight heparin (fragmin) in patients with venous thromboembolism and contraindications to coumarin. *Thromb Haemost.* 1994;**71**(1):7–11.

91 Das SK, Cohen AT, Edmondson RA, et al. Low-molecular-weight heparin versus warfarin for prevention of recurrent venous thromboembolism: a randomized trial. *World J Surg.* 1996;**20**:521–27.

92 Hamann H. Rezidivprophylaxe nach phlebothrombose—orale antikoagulation oder niedermolelulares heparin subkutan. *Vasomed.* 1998;**10**:133–36.

93 Lee AY, Levine MN, Baker RI, et al. Low-molecular-weight heparin versus a coumarin for the prevention of recurrent venous thromboembolism in patients with cancer. *N Engl J Med.* 2003;**349**:146–53.

94 Gonzalez-Fajardo JA, Arreba E, Castrodeza J, et al. Venographic comparison of subcutaneous low-molecular weight heparin with oral anticoagulant therapy in the long-term treatment of deep venous thrombosis. *J Vasc Surg.* 1999;**30**:283–92.

95 Veiga F, Escriba A, Maluenda MP, et al. Low molecular weight heparin (enoxaparin) versus oral anticoagulant therapy (acenocoumarol) in the long-term treatment of deep venous thrombosis in the elderly: a randomized trial. *Thromb Haemost.* 2000;**84**:559–64.

96 Meyer G, Marjanovic Z, Valcke J, et al. Comparison of low-molecular-weight heparin and warfarin for the secondary prevention of venous thromboembolism in patients with cancer: a randomized controlled study. *Arch Intern Med.* 2002;**162**:1729–35.

97 Beckman JA, Dunn K, Sasahara AA, et al. Enoxaparin monotherapy without oral anticoagulation to treat acute symptomatic pulmonary embolism. *Thromb Haemost.* 2003;**89**:953–58.

98 Kucher N, Quiroz R, McKean S, et al. Extended enoxaparin monotherapy for acute symptomatic pulmonary embolism. *Vasc Med.* 2005;**10**:251–56.

99 Lopaciuk S, Bielska-Falda H, Noszczyk W, et al. Low molecular weight heparin versus acenocoumarol in the secondary prophylaxis of deep vein thrombosis. *Thromb Haemost.* 1999;**81**:26–31.

100 Lopez-Beret P, Orgaz A, Fontcuberta J, et al. Low molecular weight heparin versus oral anticoagulants in the long- term treatment of deep venous thrombosis. *J Vasc Surg.* 2001;**33**:77–90.

101 Hull R, Pineo G, Mah A, et al. Long-term low molecular weight heparin treatment versus oral anticoagulant therapy for proximal deep vein thrombosis. *Blood.* 2000;**96**:449a.

102 Hull RD, Pineo GF, Brant RF, et al. Self-managed long-term low-molecular-weight heparin therapy: the balance of benefits and harms. *Am J Med.* 2007;**120**:72–82.

103 Kakkar V, Gebska M, Kadziola Z, et al. Low-molecular-weight heparin in the acute and long-term treatment of deep vein thrombosis. *Thromb Haemost.* 2003;**89**:674–80.

104 van der Heijden JF, Hutten BA, Büller HR, et al. Vitamin K antagonists or low molecular weight heparin for the long term treatment of symptomatic venous thromboembolism (Cochrane Review). *Cochrane Libr.* 2002;Issue 4 Oxford:Update Software.

105 Iorio A, Guercini F, Pini M. Low-molecular-weight heparin for the long-term treatment of symptomatic venous thromboembolism: meta-analysis of the randomized comparisons with oral anticoagulants. *J Thromb Haemost.* 2003;**1**:1906–13.

106 Hull RD, Pineo GF, Brant RF, et al. Long-term low-molecular-weight heparin versus usual care in proximal-vein thrombosis patients with cancer. *Am J Med.* 2006;**119**:1062–72.

107 Fiessinger JN, Huisman MV, Davidson BL, et al. Ximelagatran vs low-molecular-weight heparin and warfarin for the treatment of deep vein thrombosis: a randomized trial. *JAMA.* 2005;**293**:681–89.

108 Büller HR, on behalf of the Van Gogh Investigators. Evaluation of once weekly subcutaneous idraparinux versus standard therapy with heparin and vitamin K antagonists in the treatment of deep-vein thrombosis or pulmonary embolism [abstract]. *Blood.* 2006;**108**:6.

109 Büller HR, on behalf of the Van Gogh Investigators. Once weekly subcutaneous idraparinux versus placebo in the extended treatment of deep-vein thrombosis or pulmonary embolism [abstract]. *Blood.* 2006;**108**:571.

110 Holbrook AM, Pereira JA, Labiris R, et al. Systematic overview of warfarin and its drug and food interactions. *Arch Intern Med.* 2005;**165**:1095–106.

111 Dentali F, Ageno W, Crowther M. Treatment of coumarin-associated coagulopathy: a systematic review and proposed treatment algorithms. *J Thromb Haemost.* 2006;**4**:1853–63.

112 Dezee KJ, Shimeall WT, Douglas KM, et al. Treatment of excessive anticoagulation with phytonadione (vitamin K): a meta-analysis. *Arch Intern Med.* 2006;**166**:391–97.

113 Heneghan C, Alonso-Coello P, Garcia-Alamino JM,. Self-monitoring of oral anticoagulation: a systematic review and meta-analysis. *Lancet.* 2006;**367**:404–11.

114 O'Donnell M, Kearon C. Perioperative management of oral anticoagulation. *Clin Geriatr Med.* 2006;**22**:199–213, xi.

115 Margaglione, M., Brancaccio, V., Giuliani, N., et al. Increased risk for venous thrombosis in carriers of the prothrombin G—a 20210 gene variant. *Ann Intern Med.* 1998;**129**:89–93.

116 DeStefano V, Martinelli I, Mannucci PM, et al. The risk of recurrent deep venous thrombosis among heterozygous carriers of both factor V Leiden and the G20210A prothrombin mutation [see comments]. *N Engl J Med.* 1999;**341**:801–6.

117 Miles JS, Miletich JP, Goldhaber SZ, et al. G20210A mutation in the prothrombin gene and the risk of recurrent venous thromboembolism. *J Am Coll Cardiol.* 2001;**37**:215–18.

118 Den Heijer M, Willems HP, Blom HJ, et al. Homocysteine lowering by B vitamins and the secondary prevention of deep vein thrombosis and

pulmonary embolism: a randomized, placebo-controlled, double-blind trial. *Blood.* 2007;**109**:139–44.

119 Grady D, Wenger NK, Herrington D, et al. Postmenopausal hormone therapy increases risk for venous thromboembolic disease: the Heart and Estrogen/Progestin Replacement Study. *Ann Intern Med.* 2000;**132**:689–96.

120 Hoibraaten E, Qvigstad E, Arnesen H, et al. Increased risk of recurrent venous thromboembolism during hormone replacement therapy—results of the randomized, double-blind, placebo- controlled estrogen in venous thromboembolism trial (EVTET). *Thromb Haemost.* 2000;**84**:961–67.

121 Rossouw JE, Anderson GL, Prentice RL, et al. Risks and benefits of estrogen plus progestin in healthy postmenopausal women: principal results from the Women's Health Initiative randomized controlled trial. *JAMA.* 2002;**288**:321–33.

122 Hulley S, Furberg C, Barrett-Connor E, et al. Noncardiovascular disease outcomes during 6.8 years of hormone therapy: Heart and Estrogen/Progestin Replacement Study follow-up (HERS II). *JAMA.* 2002;**288**:58–66.

123 Baglin T, Luddington R, Brown K, et al. High risk of recurrent venous thromboembolism in men. *J Thromb Haemost.* 2004;**2**:2152–55.

124 Cushman M, Glynn RJ, Goldhaber SZ, et al. Hormonal factors and risk of recurrent venous thrombosis: the prevention of recurrent venous thromboembolism trial. *J Thromb Haemost.* 2006;**4**:2199–203.

125 Kyrle PA, Minar E, Bialonczyk C,. The risk of recurrent venous thromboembolism in men and women. *N Engl J Med.* 2004;**350**: 2558–63.

126 Lindmarker P, Schulman S. The risk of ipsilateral versus contralateral recurrent deep vein thrombosis in the leg. The DURAC Trial Study Group. *J Intern Med.* 2000;**247**:601–6.

127 White RH, Zhou H, Kim J, et al. A population-based study of the effectiveness of inferior vena cava filter use among patients with venous thromboembolism. *Arch Intern Med.* 2000;**160**:2033–41.

11 Thrombolytic Therapy for Deep Vein Thrombosis and Pulmonary Embolism

Simon J. McRae, John W. Eikelboom

Introduction

Venous thromboembolism (VTE), consisting of deep vein thrombosis (DVT) and pulmonary embolism (PE), is a potentially fatal condition with an annual incidence in Caucasian populations of 0.1% (1). Standard treatment for VTE is anticoagulation, initially with low-molecular-weight (LMWH) or unfractionated heparin (UFH) or fondaparinux for at least 5 days, followed by warfarin, usually for a minimum of three to six months (2). The justification for the use of anticoagulant therapy stems from landmark trials demonstrating its effectiveness for preventing recurrent thrombosis and reducing mortality in patients with symptomatic PE (3), and for limiting thrombus extension and preventing recurrent thrombosis in patients with DVT (4,5).

Despite the routine use of anticoagulant therapy however, a substantial proportion of patients with acute VTE experience adverse outcomes. The rate of fatal PE during anticoagulant therapy is ~0.4% in patients presenting with DVT and ~1.5% in patients presenting with symptomatic PE (6). A further 3%–5% of patients presenting with VTE will develop nonfatal extension or recurrence of thrombosis during anticoagulant treatment (7). Long-term complications of VTE include the postthrombotic syndrome (PTS), which occurs in 30% to 50% of patients presenting with symptomatic DVT and results in chronic pain, swelling, and skin changes in the affected limb (8), and the less frequent but potentially fatal complication, chronic thromboembolic pulmonary hypertension, which occurs in up to 1.0% of patients presenting with symptomatic PE. Additional or alternative treatments that reduce the incidence and severity of the above complications in patients with acute VTE are thus highly desirable.

Evidence-based Hematology. Edited by Mark A. Crowther, Jeff Ginsberg, Holger J. Schünemann, Ralph M. Meyer, and Richard Lottenberg.
 ISBN: 978-1-4051-5747-6.

Rationale for the use of thrombolytic therapy in the initial treatment of VTE

Anticoagulants work by blocking thrombin generation or thrombin activity, thereby preventing new thrombus formation. Anticoagulants do not directly lyse thrombus but facilitate clearance of thrombus by the endogenous fibrinolytic system. Incomplete resolution of thrombus is common in patients with VTE who are treated with anticoagulation; up to 70% of patients who present with acute DVT have evidence of residual thrombus on compression ultrasonography one year after diagnosis (9). As many as 87% of patients who present with acute PE have evidence of residual pulmonary thrombus detected by noninvasive imaging at eight days after diagnosis, and 52% have residual pulmonary thrombus at 11 months after diagnosis (10).

Unlike anticoagulant therapy, thrombolytic drugs directly activate the fibrinolytic system and thus have the potential to increase both the rate and extent of thrombus clearance in patients with VTE. In patients with DVT, more rapid and complete restoration of vein patency may improve venous return and limit valvular damage. As these factors are thought to be central to the development of PTS (8), thrombolytic therapy has the potential to reduce the incidence of PTS. In patients with PE, obstruction to right ventricular outflow by thrombus can lead to increased pulmonary vascular resistance, right ventricular dysfunction, reduced cardiac output, hemodynamic instability and, in severe cases, death (11). The severity of hemodynamic compromise is dependent on the size and location of the embolus as well as the presence of coexisting cardiopulmonary disease. As most patients with fatal pulmonary embolism die within the first few hours of the acute event, rapid lysis of pulmonary thrombus with thrombolytic therapy has the potential to prevent death by restoring pulmonary blood flow and reversing right heart dysfunction. More complete clot lysis may also reduce the risk of recurrent venous thromboembolism and pulmonary hypertension (11).

This chapter reviews the evidence for the use of thrombolytic therapy in patients with acute VTE, focusing specifically on the questions listed in Table 11.1. Grading of the quality of evidence and strengths of recommendations in this chapter are based on

Table 11.1 Clinical questions.*

Deep vein thrombosis

1. What is the efficacy (degree of thrombus lysis, incidence of the postthrombotic syndrome, recurrent venous thrombosis, and death) and safety (major bleeding) of thrombolysis compared with anticoagulant therapy for the initial treatment of deep vein thrombosis?
2. What is the role of thrombolysis in the initial treatment of extensive iliofemoral vein thrombosis?
3. What is the most effective and safest route of administration of thrombolytic therapy for deep vein thrombosis?

Pulmonary embolism

1. What is the efficacy (thrombus resolution, recurrent venous thromboembolism, and death) and safety (bleeding) of systemic thrombolysis compared with standard anticoagulant therapy for the initial treatment of pulmonary embolism?
2. What is the efficacy and safety of systemic thrombolysis compared with standard anticoagulant therapy in patients for the initial treatment of patients with hemodynamically unstable pulmonary embolism?
3. What is the efficacy and safety of systemic thrombolysis compared with standard anticoagulant therapy in patients for the initial treatment of patients with pulmonary embolism and right ventricular dysfunction at presentation?
4. What is the most effective route of administration of thrombolytic therapy for pulmonary embolism?

the guidelines proposed by the international Grading of Recommendations Assessment, Development, and Evaluation Working Group (GRADE), adopting the modification used by the American College of Chest Physicians that merges the very low and low categories of quality of evidence (see chapter 1) (12,13).

Search strategy, study selection criteria, and statistical methods

Potentially relevant studies were identified by a computerized search, restricted to the English-language literature, of the MEDLINE electronic database (source PUBMED, 1966 to November 2006) using relevant text and key words in combination, as follows: (*tissue plasminogen activator OR urokinase OR streptokinase OR thrombolytic OR fibrinolysis*)*AND* (*venous thrombosis OR thromboembolism OR deep vein thrombosis OR pulmonary embolism*)*AND* (*randomized controlled trial OR controlled trial OR random*). Reference lists of retrieved eligible articles were hand-searched to identify additional relevant articles.

Studies were selected for inclusion if they were properly randomized controlled trials that enrolled patients with acute VTE in which at least one treatment arm received thrombolytic therapy.

Pooled estimates for efficacy and safety outcomes in patients treated with thrombolysis compared with anticoagulation were calculated by combining the data from all the eligible studies using the DerSimonian-Laird random-effects model (14), and Review Manager (RevMan) software, version 4.2.7 for Windows (the Cochrane Collaboration, Oxford, United Kingdom). A two-sided probability value of less than 0.05 was considered statistically significant for all analyses.

Thrombolytic therapy for the initial treatment of deep vein thrombosis

A. Clinical question

What is the efficacy (degree of thrombus lysis, incidence of the postthrombotic syndrome, recurrent venous thrombosis, and death) and safety (major bleeding) of thrombolytic therapy compared with anticoagulant therapy for the initial treatment of deep vein thrombosis?

Trials included

We identified 15 randomized trials enrolling 839 patients that compared thrombolytic therapy with anticoagulation for the initial treatment of DVT. The characteristics of the studies are summarized in Table 11.2. Only one trial involved more than 100 patients (23). Nine trials evaluated streptokinase (15–22,24), two trials evaluated urokinase (25,26), and three trials evaluated recombinant tissue plasminogen activator (rTPA) (27–29). All three thrombolytic drugs were evaluated in the remaining study (23). In most of the trials, thrombolysis was given systemically by intravenous infusion (15–17,19–22,25–29); two trials administered the thrombolysis via a peripheral cannula into a loco-regional vein (18,23). One randomized trial used catheter-directed thrombolysis (CDT) via a multiholed catheter to infuse the thrombolytic agent directly onto the clot, advancing the catheter intermittently as required (24). All the trials used UFH as the anticoagulant in the comparator arm. Various dosing regimens were used for UFH (Table 11.2), and several trials used a starting dose of UFH that is less than the currently recommended minimum starting dose of 30,000 U over a 24-hour period (2).

Most patients enrolled in the trials presented with proximal DVT (defined as thrombosis involving the popliteal vein and above), but at least three trials also enrolled patients with isolated calf vein thrombosis (16,17,22), and one trial restricted inclusion to patients with calf vein thrombosis (22). Patients with upper extremity thrombosis were enrolled in at least two trials (21,26). The randomization sequence was considered to be adequate in the six trials (16,18,20,22,28) that used sealed envelopes. The method of randomization was inadequately described in the other studies (15,17,21,23,24,29).

The data from six trials that reported long-term follow-up (ranging from 6 months to 14 years of follow-up) were used to evaluate the effect of thrombolysis compared with UFH on the development of PTS (22–23,30–32).

We excluded randomized trials comparing thrombolysis with anticoagulation in which the diagnosis of DVT was not objectively confirmed (33), trials in which patients were not properly randomized (34–36) and a trial in which outcomes of interest were not reported (37).

Table 11.2 Trials comparing thrombolytic therapy with anticoagulation for DVT treatment.*

Trial, year	Eligibility	n	Thrombolytic regime	UFH regime	Outcomes	Time endpoints
Streptokinase						
Robertson et al. 1968 (15)	DVT leg <4 days symptoms	16	Twice titrated dose then 100,000 U/h for 1 day	7,500 U bolus then 42,500/24 hrs, then sc	Thrombus lysis, PE, major bleeding	Day 5–6
Kakkar et al. 1969 (16)	DVT leg <4 days symptoms	20	500,000 U bolus then 900,000 U 6 hourly for 5 days	10,000 U bolus then 12,500 U 6 hrly adjusted to TCT	Thrombus lysis, mortality, PE, major bleeding	Day 5
Robertson et al. 1970 (17)	DVT leg <4 days symptoms	16	Twice titrated dose then 100,000 U/h for 3 days	7,500 U bolus then 17,500 U for 10 h, then 25,000 U 12 hrly	Thrombus lysis	Day 6–8
Tsapogas et al. 1973 (18)	DVT leg <5 days symptoms	34	100–500,000 U bolus then 100,000 U/h up to 3 days	7,000 U bolus then 1,500 U/h adjusted to APTT 2.0–2.5	Thrombus lysis	Day 3
Porter et al. 1975 (19)	DVT <14 days symptoms	50	250,000 U bolus then 100,000 U/h for 3 days	Bolus 150 U/kg then adjusted to APTT 2.0 to 2.5	Thrombus lysis, mortality, PE, major bleeding	Day 10
Arnesen et al. 1978 (20)	Proximal DVT <5 days symptoms	42	250,000 U bolus then 100,000/h for 3–4 days	15,000 U bolus then 30,000 u /24hrs	Thrombus lysis, mortality, PE, major bleeding	Day 3–6
Elliot et al. 1979 (21)	DVT <8 days symptoms	51	600,000 U bolus then 100,000 U/h for 3 days	10,000 U bolus then 10,000 6 hrly	Thrombus lysis, mortality, PE, major bleeding, PTS	Day 5, 6 mo
Schulman et al. 1986 (22)	Calf vein DVT <7 days symptoms	36	50,000 U bolus then 10,000 U/h for 7 days	5,000 U bolus then adjusted to APTT 2–3×	PE, major bleeding, PTS	Day 5, 60 mo
Schweizer et al. 2000 (23)	Proximal DVT<9 days symptoms	250	3,000,000 U daily over 6 h for up to 7 days	1,000 U/h adjusted to APTT 2.0 to 3.0	Thrombus lysis, mortality, PE, major bleeding, PTS	Day 4–7, 12 mo
Elsharawy et al. 2002 (24)	Iliofemoral venous thrombosis	35	1,000,000 U in first hour then 100,000 U until lysis, no progress†	1,000 U/h adjusted to APTT 2.0	Thrombus lysis, PE, major bleeding	Day 7
Urokinase						
Kiil et al. 1981 (25)	DVT <3 days symptoms	20	200,000 U over 24 h	40,000 U/24 h	Thrombus lysis, mortality, PE, bleeding	Day 6
Goldhaber et al. 1996 (26)	Proximal DVT <14 days symptoms	17	1,000,000 U bolus 8 hrly × 3	5–10,000 U bolus then adjusted APTT 60–80 sec	Thrombus lysis, PE, major bleeding	Day 6–7
Schweizer et al. 2000 (23)	Proximal DVT <9 days symptoms	250	5,000,000 U/d up to 7 days or 100,000 U daily for 7 days*	1,000 IU/h adjusted to APTT 2.0 to 3.0	Thrombus lysis, mortality, PE, major bleeding, PTS	Day 4–7, 12 mo
Recombinant TPA						
Verhaeghe et al. 1989 (27)	Proximal DVT <10 days symptoms	32	100 mg/dL then 50 mg D or 50 mg D1+2	5,000 U bolus then 1,000 U/h up to 72 hrs	Thrombus lysis, bleeding	Day 3
Goldhaber et al. 1990 (28)	Popliteal or more proximal DVT <14 days symptoms	65	0.05 mg/kg/h for 24 h to a dose of 150 mg	100 U/kg bolus then 1,000 U /h adjusted to APTT 1.5 to 2.5	Thrombus lysis, major bleeding	36 hours
Turpie et al. 1990 (29)	Proximal DVT <7 days symptoms	83	0.5 mg/kg over 4 h or 0.5 mg/kg over 8 h d 1 + 2	5,000 U bolus then 30,000/d adjusted to APTT 1.5 to 2.0	Thrombus lysis, major bleeding, PTS	Day 1–2, 3 years
Schweizer et al. 2000 (23)	Proximal DVT <9 days symptoms	250	20 mg/d over 4 h for 4–7 days*	1,000 IU/h adjusted to APTT 2.0 to 3.0	Thrombus lysis, mortality, PE, major bleeding, PTS	Day 4–7, 12 mo

*Administered by loco-regional infusion. APTT, activated partial thromboplastin time; DVT, deep vein thrombosis; PE, pulmonary embolism; PTS, postthrombotic syndrome.
† Catheter directed thrombolysis.

Table 11.3 Comparison of thrombus lysis.

	Significant thrombolysis n/N (%)	
Trial, year	**Thrombolysis**	**Anticoagulation**
Streptokinase		
Robertson et al. 1968 (15)	5/8 (63)	1/8 (13)
Kakkar et al. 1969 (16)	7/10 (70)	2/10 (20)
Robertson et al. 1970 (17)	5/9 (56)	1/7 (14)
Tsapogas et al. 1973 (18)	10/19 (53)	1/15 (7)
Porter et al. 1975 (19)	13/24 (54)	8/26 (31)
Arnesen et al. 1978 (20)	11/21 (52)	2/21 (10)
Elliot et al. 1979 (21)	17/26 (65)	0/25 (0)
Schweizer et al. 2000 (23)	27/50 (54)	3/50 (6)
Urokinase		
Kiil et al. 1981 (25)	1/11 (9)	1/9 (11)
Goldhaber et al. 1996 (26)	1/8 (13)	1/9 (11)
Schweizer et al. 2000 (23)	46/100 (46)	3/50 (6)
Recombinant TPA*		
Goldhaber et al. 1990 (28)	15/53 (28)	0/12 (0)
Turpie et al. 1990 (29)	6/29 (32)	2/30 (5)
Schweizer et al. 2000 (23)	17/50 (34)	3/50 (6)
Catheter directed thrombolysis		
Elsharawy et al. 2002 (24)	11/18 (61)	0/17 (0)

*TPA, tissue plasminogen activator.

Outcomes

Thrombus lysis

In 13 trials, venography was performed before and after treatment, thereby enabling a quantitative or semiquantitative assessment of the degree of thrombus lysis (Table 11.3). For the purpose of this analysis, lysis was defined as "significant" if >50% of the thrombus was lysed (18,21,23,26,28,29) or the degree of lysis was described as good (15,17,20), substantial (16,19), or significant (25). The rate of significant lysis in patients receiving thrombolytic therapy ranged from 9% to 70%, and was greater than 50% in 9 of 13 studies, compared with 0% to 31% significant lysis in patients treated with UFH.

Pooled data from the 13 trials indicate that systemic or loco-regional thrombolysis compared with anticoagulation was associated with a relative risk (RR) of achieving significant lysis of 3.9 (95% confidence interval [CI] 2.3 to 6.6). The effect of thrombolytic therapy on significant thrombus lysis was similar irrespective of whether patients received streptokinase (RR 4.6, 95% CI 2.4–9.2) or rTPA (5.3, 95% CI 2.3–12.2). The RR was somewhat lower in patients receiving urokinase (RR 2.8, 95% CI 0.6–13.9), but the confidence intervals were wide (25). In the only trial in which catheter-directed thrombolysis was used, the rate of complete lysis at one week in patients receiving thrombolysis was 61% vs. 0% in patients receiving anticoagulation ($p < 0.001$).

In summary, the data from individual trials as well as the pooled data indicate that thrombolytic therapy increases the rate of significant thrombus lysis in patients with acute DVT.

Postthrombotic syndrome

For a trial to be included in this analysis, the assessment of the presence or absence of the PTS had to be based on clinical symptoms and signs. Six trials examined the effect of thrombolytic therapy compared with anticoagulation on PTS, with follow-up periods ranging from 6 months to 14 years (21,22,30–31). Two trials required the presence of moderate to severe symptoms or physical signs for patients to be classified as having the PTS, while the remaining trials required the presence of any clinical feature of the syndrome. One trial only enrolled patients with isolated calf vein DVT (22), and a small number of patients that were not part of the original randomized trial were included in another trial report (32). Compression stockings were worn throughout follow-up in the majority of patients in one study (23), but the use of stockings was limited (22), or not clearly described (21,30–31), in the remaining trials.

The results of the studies are summarized in Table 11.4. The incidence of the PTS in thrombolyzed patients ranged from 24% to 81% and was less than 50% in three trials, whereas the incidence of PTS in patients receiving anticoagulant therapy ranged from 50% to 91%.

Pooling the data from the trials, the RR of developing the PTS in patients receiving thrombolytic therapy in comparison to patients receiving anticoagulation was 0.7 (95% CI 0.5–0.9, $p = 0.02$). Although this estimate of treatment effect appears to suggest that thrombolytic therapy reduces the incidence of PTS, the diagnosis of PTS in most of the studies was made by persons who were not blinded to treatment allocation, and there was a high rate of loss to follow-up, limiting the reliability of this conclusion.

Mortality

Six trials reported early mortality (up to 30 days) (16,19,20,21, 24,25). There were only three early deaths in the 283 patients receiving thrombolysis, and four deaths in the 132 patients treated with anticoagulation, a difference that was not statistically significant (RR 0.8, 95% CI 0.2–3.2, $p = 0.8$).

PE

Nine trials reported the incidence of PE after randomization (15–16,18–24). PE occurred in 11 of 343 patients treated with thrombolytic therapy and in 5 of 190 patients receiving anticoagulation, a difference that was not statistically significant (RR 0.7, 95% CI 0.2–2.4, $p = 0.64$).

Recurrent VTE

There were insufficient data concerning the incidence of recurrent VTE during follow-up to draw any conclusion about whether thrombolysis reduces the risk of recurrent thrombosis.

Table 11.4 Effect on the incidence of the postthrombotic syndrome.

Trial, year	Duration FU	Loss to FU*	Incidence of PTS n/N (%)	
			Thrombolysis	Anticoagulation
Streptokinase				
Common et al. 1976 (30)	7 mo	46%	5/15 (33)	6/12 (50)
Johansson et al. 1979 (31)	8 to 14 y	20%	10/14 (71)	4/6 (66)
Elliot et al. 1979 (21)	6 mo	20%	8/21 (38)	18/20 (90)
Arnesen et al. 1982 (32)	6.5 y	17%	4/17 (24)	12/18 (66)
Schulman et al. 1986 (22)	60 mo	3%	11/18 (61)	11/17 (65)
Schweizer et al. 2000 (23)	12 mo	10%	23/45 (51)	41/45 (91)
Urokinase				
Schweizer et al. 2000 (23)	12 mo	10%	69/96 (72)	41/45 (91)
Recombinant TPA†				
Schweizer et al. 2000 (23)	12 mo	10%	39/48 (81)	41/45 (91)

*% of patients from original treatment trial lost to follow-up (FU) at time of assessment of postthrombotic syndrome (PTS).
†TPA, tissue plasminogen activator.

Major hemorrhage

Major hemorrhage was most commonly defined as any clinically overt bleed, resulting in transfusion, cessation of treatment, or a fall in hemoglobin of ≥2g/dL, or bleeding that was intracerebral, intra-articular, intraocular, retroperitoneal, or gastrointestinal in location. In the 13 trials that compared systemic or loco-regional thrombolysis with anticoagulation (15,16,18–23,25–29) (Table 11.5), the incidence of major bleeding in patients receiving thrombolysis was 8% (35 of 463) compared with 5% in patients treated with anticoagulation (12 of 252), yielding a relative risk of bleeding of 1.51 (95% CI 0.7–3.1). The incidence of major bleeding with thrombolytic therapy varied widely among trials (0%–32%), likely reflecting differences in patient characteristics and dose intensity of thrombolytic therapy. Only two episodes of

Table 11.5 Bleeding in trials comparing thrombolysis with anticoagulation for deep vein thrombosis.

Trial, year	Major bleeding n/N (%)		All bleeding n/N (%)	
	Thrombolysis	Anticoagulation	Thrombolysis	Anticoagulation
Streptokinase				
Robertson et al. 1968 (15)	2/8 (25)	1/8 (13)	2/8 (25)	1/8 (13)
Kakkar et al. 1969 (16)	0/10 (20)	2/10 (20)	3/10 (30)	2/10 (20)
Tsapogas et al. 1973 (18)	0/19 (0)	0/14 (0)	4/19 (21)	0/14 ()
Porter et al. 1975 (19)	4/24 (17)	1/26 (4)	4/24 (17)	1/26 (4)
Arnesen et al. 1978 (20)	2/21 (10)	2/21 (10)	3/21 (14)	3/21 (14)
Elliot et al. 1979 (21)	2/26 (8)	0/25 (0)	3/26 (12)	0/25 (0)
Schulman et al. 1986 (22)	3/17 (18)	1/19 (5.3)	5/17 (29)	2/19 (11)
Schweizer et al. 2000 (23)	5/50 (10)	0/50 (0)	5/50 (10)	0/50 (0)
Elsharawy et al. 2002 (24)	0/18 (0)	0/17 (0)	0/18 (0)	0/17 (0)
Urokinase				
Kiil et al. 1981 (25)	0/11 (0)	3/9 (33)	3/11 (27)	4/9(44)
Goldhaber et al. 1996 (26)	0/8 (0)	1/9 (11)	0/8 (0)	1/9 (11)
Schweizer et al. 2000 (23)	5/100 (5)	0/50 (0)	5/100 (5)	0/50 (0)
Recombinant TPA*				
Verhaeghe et al. 1989 (17)	8/25 (32)	0/7 (0)	8/25 (32)	0/7 (0)
Goldhaber et al. 1990 (26)	1/53 (2)	0/12 (0)	13/53 ()	0/12 (0)
Turpie et al. 1990 (24)	1/41 (2)	1/42 (2)	3/41 (7)	1/42 (2)
Schweizer et al. 2000 (27)	2/50 (4)	0/50 (0)	2/50 (4)	0/50 (0)

*TPA, tissue plasminogen activator.

intracerebral hemorrhage were reported, both in patients receiving thrombolytic therapy. In the single small trial using CDT, no bleeding complications were reported (24).

All hemorrhage
When all episodes of hemorrhage were considered, the incidence of bleeding was significantly increased in patients receiving thrombolysis (61/463, 13%) compared with anticoagulation (14/252, 6%; RR 1.8, 95% CI 1.0–3.2, $p = 0.04$) (15–16,18–23,25–29).

B. Clinical question

What is the role of thrombolysis in the initial treatment of extensive iliofemoral vein thrombosis?

Phlegmasia caerulea dolens, usually resulting from extensive iliofemoral thrombosis, is a severe form of DVT that has a high risk of progressing to irreversible venous gangrene (38). Although there are no randomized trials that have compared thrombolytic therapy with anticoagulation in patients with iliofemoral thrombosis, it is plausible to assume that the benefit-to-risk ratio of thrombolytic therapy will be highest in these patients. In a small series of eight patients presenting with iliofemoral vein thrombosis who were treated with either streptokinase (250,000 U bolus followed by 100,000 U for 48 hours) or rTPA (0.5 to 0.7 mg/kg for 4 hours), no patient went onto develop venous gangrene, and there were no episodes of major hemorrhage (39). These data suggest that it is reasonable to consider thrombolytic therapy in patients presenting with iliofemoral vein thrombosis.

C. Clinical question

What is the most effective and safe route of administration of thrombolytic therapy for deep vein thrombosis?

Eligible trials
Two randomized trials directly compared systemic with loco-regional administration of thrombolytic therapy (23,40). No trials were identified that directly compared CDT with other routes of administration of thrombolytic therapy.

Outcomes
Method of administration
Schweider and colleagues randomized 137 patients with proximal leg DVT to receive 20 mg of rTPA over four hours, daily for four to seven days, administered via either a dorsal pedal (loco-regional) or cubital (systemic) vein (40). No difference was observed in the proportion of patients with ≥50% thrombus lysis (loco-regional 21/69 [30%] vs. systemic 22/68 [32%]; RR 0.94, 95% CI 0.6–1.5). Major hemorrhage was significantly more common in patients receiving loco-regional thrombolysis (15/69, 22%) compared with systemic thrombolysis (6/68, 9%; RR 2.4, 95% CI 1.0–6.0). In a subsequent trial, 250 patients were randomized to receive either loco-regional (via a dorsal pedal vein) rTPA or urokinase, systemic urokinase or streptokinase, or UFH (23). The proportion of patients with ≥50% thrombus lysis was significantly reduced in those receiving loco-regional (36/100) compared with systemic (54/100) thrombolysis (RR 0.67, 95% CI 0.5–0.9). A nonsignificant trend toward a lower incidence of bleeding was seen in patients treated with loco-regional therapy (3/100 vs. 9/100; RR 0.33, 95% CI 0.1–1.2).

CDT has not been directly compared with other methods of thrombolytic administration. Previous reviews that pooled data from nonrandomized studies reported rates of significant or complete initial thrombus resolution with CDT of up to 80% (41,42). However, there are no data on the impact of CDT on the long-term incidence of PTS, and in one review, the pooled incidence of major bleeding in patients treated with CDT was 13% (41), which is comparable to rates seen with systemic thrombolytic administration.

In summary, there is currently no evidence that loco-regional thrombolysis or CDT offer any advantages over systemic administration of thrombolytic therapy for DVT.

D. Authors' Conclusions

Thrombolytic therapy compared with anticoagulation results in more rapid and complete lysis of thrombus in patients presenting with symptomatic DVT. Thrombolytic therapy may also reduce the risk of PTS, but the quality of the trials on which this conclusion is based is limited. There is no evidence that thrombolytic therapy for DVT reduces the risk of recurrent VTE or death. Furthermore, any potential benefits of thrombolytic therapy for DVT should be balanced against an increased risk of bleeding complications, including major bleeding. Most of the trials on which these conclusions are based included highly selected young patients (median age 40 years) who were at low risk of bleeding (23). The risk of bleeding with thrombolytic therapy is likely to be significantly higher in unselected patients.

In summary, the currently available randomized data comparing thrombolytic therapy with anticoagulation for the initial treatment of DVT are limited and provide no convincing evidence for a benefit of thrombolytic therapy. If thrombolytic therapy is to be used in preference to anticoagulation for the initial treatment of DVT, it should probably be reserved for young patients with extensive iliofemoral vein thrombosis or patients with *Phlegmasia caerulea dolens*.

E. Recommendations

1. In patients with DVT, we suggest against the routine use of thrombolytic therapy. (Grade 2B).
Underlying values and preferences. This recommendation ascribes a high value to the increased risk of bleeding with thrombolytic therapy.
2. In patients at risk of limb gangrene secondary to venous occlusion, we suggest thrombolysis (Grade 2C).
3. In patients with DVT who are treated with thrombolytic therapy, we recommend the systemic route of administration (Grade 1B).

Table 11.6 Trials comparing thrombolytic therapy with anticoagulation for treatment of pulmonary embolism (PE).

Trial year	Eligibility	n	Thrombolytic regime	Follow up
Urokinase				
UPET trial 1973 (43)	Acute PE, symptoms <5days	160	2,000 U/lb bolus, then 2000 U/lb for 12 h	14 days
Marini 1988 (44)	Acute PE, symptoms ≤7 days	30	800,000 U/12 h for 3 days or 3,300,000/12 h	7 days
Streptokinase				
Tibbutt 1974 (45)	Acute life-threatening PE*	30	600,000 U bolus then 100,000 /h for 72 h	3 days
Ly 1978 (46)	Acute major PE, symptoms <5 days	25	250,000 U loading dose then 100,000 U/h for 72 h	10 days
Dotter 1979 (47)	Acute PE	31	Infusion for 18–72 h	
Jerjes-Sanchez 1995 (48)	Acute massive PE, symptoms ≤ 14 days	8	1,500,000 U/1 h	In hospital
RTPA				
Levine 1990 (49)	Acute PE, symptoms ≤14 days	58	0.6 mg/kg bolus over 2 min	10 days
PIOPED 1990 (50)	Acute PE, symptoms ≤7 days	13	40–80 mg at 1 mg/min	7 days
Dalla-Volta 1992 (51)	Acute PE, symptoms ≤10 days	36	100 mg (10 mg bolus then 50 mg in 1 h, then 40 mg in 2 h)	7–30 days
Goldhaber 1993 (52)	Acute PE, symptoms ≤14 days	101	100 mg over 2 hours	In hospital or 14 days
Konstantinides 2002 (53)	Acute PE, symptoms ≤4 days	256	100 mg (10 mg bolus then 90 mg over 2 h)	In hospital or 30 days

*Thrombolytic and anticoagulant therapy were administered by direct infusion into the main pulmonary artery.

Thrombolytic therapy for the initial treatment of pulmonary embolism

A. Clinical question

What is the efficacy (thrombus resolution, recurrent VTE, and death) and safety (bleeding) of thrombolytic therapy compared with anticoagulant therapy for the initial treatment of pulmonary embolism?

Eligible trials

We identified 11 randomized trials that compared thrombolytic therapy with anticoagulant therapy for the initial treatment of PE and reported relevant clinical or radiographic endpoints (43–53). Data on hemodynamic and radiographic outcomes were also obtained from an earlier report of one of the above trials (54). The characteristics of the studies are summarized in Table 11.6. Two trials evaluated urokinase (45–48), four trials evaluated streptokinase (43,44), and five trials evaluated rTPA (49–53). Thrombolytic therapy was administered by systemic intravenous infusion in all but one trial in which it was administered by direct infusion into the main pulmonary artery (45). All trials used UFH as the anticoagulant in the comparator arm.

All trials enrolled patients with acute PE. Patients with major PE (defined here as PE with hemodynamic instability) were eligible for inclusion in only five trials (43,45–48). Only five trials provided information on the proper concealment of treatment allocation (43,45,46,48,53), and both patients and investigators were blinded to treatment in only three trials (49,50,52). No trials reported the number of patients lost to follow-up.

We excluded trials in which patients were not properly randomized (55) or that reported data that had been previously published or were subsequently published in more detail (56–60).

Outcomes

Thrombus resolution

Three eligible trials that assessed the degree of thrombus resolution by performing pulmonary angiography pre- and posttreatment were identified. In one trial, which used the Miller index to assess the angiographic response (55), 17 of the 20 patients receiving rTPA had a decrease in the degree of vascular obstruction compared with 4 of 16 patients receiving heparin (51). Pooled analysis of two studies (45,46) suggested a statistically significant improvement in the degree of pulmonary artery occlusion posttreatment in patients receiving streptokinase in comparison to those treated with heparin (61).

Recurrent pulmonary embolism and death

Data on the composite outcome of recurrent pulmonary embolism or death were available from all 11 trials and are shown in

Table 11.7 Recurrent PE or death.*

Trial year	Recurrent PE or death n/N (%)	
	Thrombolytic regime	UFH regime
Urokinase		
UPET trial 1973 (43)	10/82 (12)	14/78 (18)
Marini 1988 (44)	0/20 (0)	0/10 (0)
Streptokinase		
Tibbutt 1974 (45)	0/13 (0)	1/17 (6)
Ly 1978 (46)	1/14 (7)	2/11 (18)
Dotter 1979 (47)	1/15 (7)	3/16 (19)
Jerjes-Sanchez 1995 (48)	0/4 (0)	4/4 (100)
rTPA		
Levine 1990 (49)	1/33 (3)	0/25 (0)
PIOPED 1990 (50)	1/9 (11)	0/4 (0)
Dalla-Volta 1992 (51)	3/20 (15)	1/16 (6)
Goldhaber 1993 (52)	0/46 (0)	4/55 (7)
Konstantinides 2002 (53)	8/118 (7)	7/138 (5)

*PE, pulmonary embolism; rTPA, recombinant tissue plasminogen activator; UFH, unfractionated heparin.

Table 11.7. Seven of the 11 trials suggested a reduction in recurrent pulmonary embolism or death with thrombolysis compared with unfractionated heparin (43–47,51,53). The pooled estimate of data from all trials revealed a nonstatistically significant reduction in recurrent pulmonary embolism or death for thrombolysis compared with heparin (6.7% vs. 9.6%; RR 0.76, 95% CI 0.46–1.25). In a previous meta-analysis, similar estimates of treatment effect were obtained for the individuals outcomes of pulmonary embolism (2.7% vs. 4.3%; odds ratio (OR) 0.67, 95% CI 0.33–1.37) and death (4.3% vs. 5.9%; OR 0.70, 95% CI 0.37–1.30) (62).

Bleeding

Seven of the 11 trials reported an increase in risk of major bleeding in patients receiving thrombolysis in comparison to those treated with heparin. A pooled analysis of the 11 trials (Table 11.8) revealed a nonstatistically significant increase in major bleeding (9.1% vs. 6.1%; OR 1.42, 95% CI 0.81–2.46) and a statistically significant increase in nonmajor bleeding (22.7 vs. 10.0%; OR 2.63, 95% CI 1.53–4.54) (62). The incidence of intracranial bleeding was low in all patients.

Table 11.8 Major bleeding in patients with PE.*

Outcome	Thrombolysis n/N (%)	UFH n/N (%)	OR (95% CI)
Major bleeding	34/374 (9.1)	23/374 (6.1)	1.4 (0.8–2.4)
Nonmajor bleeding	53/233 (22.7)	22/221 (10.0)	2.6 (1.5–4.5)
Intracranial bleeding	2/374 (0.5)	1/374 (0.3)	1.0 (0.4–3.0)

*PE, pulmonary embolism; OR, odds ratio; UFH, unfractionated heparin.

B. Clinical question

What is the efficacy and safety of systemic thrombolysis compared with standard anticoagulant therapy in patients for the initial treatment of patients with hemodynamically unstable pulmonary embolism?

Eligible trials

Patients with PE who are hemodynamically unstable at presentation have a three-month mortality of 30%–50% and are therefore as a group most likely to benefit from thrombolytic therapy (63,64). Only one randomized trial was identified that restricted inclusion to patients who were hemodynamically unstable at presentation (48).

Outcomes

The one eligible trial was terminated prematurely after only eight patients has been randomized because the four patients allocated to heparin all died as a result of pulmonary embolism, whereas the four who received thrombolysis survived (48).

A subgroup analysis of the randomized trials comparing thrombolytic therapy with heparin for PE restricted to trials that also included hemodynamically unstable patients (five trials, 254 patients) demonstrated a significant reduction in recurrent pulmonary embolism or death (9.4% vs. 19.0%; OR 0.45; 95% CI 0.22–0.92) with a similar albeit nonsignificant reduction in death (OR 0.47, 95% CI 0.20–1.10) (62).

C. Clinical question

What is the efficacy and safety of systemic thrombolysis compared with standard anticoagulant therapy in patients for the initial treatment of patients with pulmonary embolism and right ventricular dysfunction at presentation?

Eligible trials

Registry data suggests that patients with PE and echocardiographic evidence of right ventricular dysfunction have a significantly increased risk of death in comparison to those patients who do not have this finding (63,64). As a result, it has been proposed that hemodynamically stable patients with acute pulmonary embolism and moderate or severe right ventricular dysfunction should be treated with thrombolytic therapy. The one study that directly addressed this question randomized 256 hemodynamically stable patients with acute pulmonary embolism and echocardiographic evidence of right ventricular dysfunction to receive either recombinant tissue plasminogen activator (rTPA) or heparin (52).

Outcomes

No difference in recurrent pulmonary embolism or death was observed (6.8% vs. 5.1%; OR 1.36; 95% CI 0.48–3.87) (62) although there was a significant reduction in the need for escalation of therapy among those treated with thrombolytic therapy (10.2% vs. 24.6%; $p = 0.004$).

D. Clinical question

What is the most effective route of administration of thrombolytic therapy for pulmonary embolism?

Eligible trials

Only a single trial was identified that directly comparing intrapulmonary and systemic intravenous administration of thrombolytic therapy (65).

Outcome

No difference was seen in the decrease in angiographically determined severity of embolism between those patients receiving intrapulmonary thrombolysis in comparison to those receiving intravenous systemic administration, either after an initial dose of 50 mg of rTPA of 50 given over two hours (12% vs. 15%) or following a further 50 mg of rTPA given over five hours (38% vs. 38%). The incidence of major bleeding was not reported by treatment group.

E. Authors' Conclusions

There is evidence that thrombolytic therapy compared with anticoagulation results in more rapid and complete thrombus lysis in patients with PE. However, there is no clear evidence that more rapid and complete thrombus resolution translates into a survival advantage, except perhaps in the subgroup of patients with PE who are hemodynamically unstable at presentation. Thrombolytic therapy increases the risk of bleeding, and in patients with acute coronary syndromes causes fatal intracranial bleeding. Therefore, thrombolysis should not be given to unselected patients with PE but be reserved for patients who are hemodynamically unstable at presentation or who become hemodynamically unstable during anticoagulant treatment.

F. Recommendations

1. In unselected patients with PE, we recommend against the routine use of thrombolytic therapy (Grade 1B).
2. In patients with PE that are hemodynamically unstable, we recommend that thrombolytic therapy be used as long as there are no clear contraindications (Grade 1B).
3. In patients with PE and echocardiographic evidence of right ventricular dysfunction, we suggest that thrombolytic not be used (Grade 2A).

Underlying values and preferences.
This recommendation ascribes a high value to the increased risk of bleeding with thrombolytic therapy.
4. In patients with PE treated with thrombolytic therapy, we recommend systemic administration (Grade 1B).

5. Future Directions

There is no evidence to support the routine use of thrombolysis in unselected patient with DVT or PE. Thrombolysis appears to have a role in patients with massive iliofemoral thrombosis and leg gangrene and in patients with PE who are hemodynamically unstable. Additional randomized comparisons are required to confirm the latter conclusions, and to clarify the risk-benefit ratio of thrombolysis in young patients with extensive iliofemoral DVT without limb ischemia at presentation and in patients with nonmajor PE who have RV dysfunction at presentation (66,67).

References

1 White RH. The epidemiology of venous thromboembolism. *Circulation.* 2003;**107**(23 Suppl 1):I4–8.
2 Büller HR, Agnelli G, Hull RD, et al. Antithrombotic therapy for venous thromboembolic disease: the Seventh ACCP Conference on Antithrombotic and Thrombolytic Therapy. *Chest.* 2004;**126**(3 Suppl): 401S–28S.
3 Barritt DW, Jordan SC. Anticoagulant drugs in the treatment of pulmonary embolism: a controlled trial. *Lancet.* 1960;**1**:1309–12.
4 Lagerstedt CI, Olsson CG, Fagher BO, et al. Need for long-term anticoagulant treatment in symptomatic calf-vein thrombosis. *Lancet.* 1985;**2**(8454):515–18.
5 Hull RD, Rascal GE, Hirsh J, et al. Continuous intravenous heparin compared with intermittent subcutaneous heparin in the initial treatment of proximal-vein thrombosis. *N Engle J Med.* 1986;**315**(18):1109–14.
6 Douketis JD, Kearon C, Bates S, et al. Risk of fatal pulmonary embolism in patients with treated venous thromboembolism. *JAMA.* 1998;**279**(6):458–62.
7 van Dongen CJ, van den Belt AG, Prins MH, et al. Fixed dose subcutaneous low molecular weight heparins versus adjusted dose unfractionated heparin for venous thromboembolism. *Cochrane Database Syst Rev.* 2004(4):CD001100.
8 Kahn SR. The post-thrombotic syndrome: progress and pitfalls. *Br J Haematol.* 2006;**134**(4):357–65.
9 Prandoni P, Cogo A, Bernardi E, et al. A simple ultrasound approach for detection of recurrent proximal-vein thrombosis. *Circulation.* 1993;**88**(4 Pt 1):1730–35.
10 Nijkeuter M, Hovens MM, Davidson BL, et al. Resolution of thromboemboli in patients with acute pulmonary embolism: a systematic review. *Chest.* 2006;**129**(1):192–97.
11 Wood KE. Major pulmonary embolism: review of a pathophysiologic approach to the golden hour of hemodynamically significant pulmonary embolism. *Chest.* 2002;**121**(3):877–905.
12 Atkins D, Best D, Briss PA, et al. Grading quality of evidence and strength of recommendations. *BMJ.* 2004;**328**(7454):1490.
13 Guyatt G, Gutterman D, Baumann MH, et al. Grading strength of recommendations and quality of evidence in clinical guidelines: report from an American College of Chest Physicians Task Force. *Chest.* 2006;**129**(1):174–81.
14 DerSimonian R, Laird N. Meta-analysis in clinical trials. *Control Clin Trials.* 1986;**7**(3):177–88.
15 Robertson B, Nilsson M, Nylander G. Value of streptokinase and heparin in treatment of acute deep vein thrombosis: a coded investigation. *Acta Chir Scand.* 1968;**134**:203–8.
16 Kakkar VV, Flanc C, Howe CT, et al. Treatment of deep vein thrombosis. A trial of heparin, streptokinase, and arvin. *Br Med J.* 1969;**1**(5647): 806–10.

17 Robertson BR, Nilsson IM, Nylander G. Thrombolytic effect of streptokinase as evaluated by phlebography of deep venous thrombi of the leg. *Acta Chir Scand.* 1970;**136**(3):173–80.

18 Tsapogas MJ, Peabody RA, Wu KT, et al. Controlled study of thrombolytic therapy in deep vein thrombosis. *Surgery.* 1973;**74**(6):973–84.

19 Porter JM, Seaman AJ, Common HH, et al. Comparison of heparin and streptokinase in the treatment of venous thrombosis. *Am Surg.* 1975;**41**(9):511–19.

20 Arnesen H, Heilo A, Jakobsen E, et al. A prospective study of streptokinase and heparin in the treatment of deep vein thrombosis. *Acta Med Scand.* 1978;**203**(6):457–63.

21 Elliot MS, Immelman EJ, Jeffery P, et al. A comparative randomized trial of heparin versus streptokinase in the treatment of acute proximal venous thrombosis: an interim report of a prospective trial. *Br J Surg.* 1979;**66**(12):838–43.

22 Schulman S, Granqvist S, Juhlin-Dannfelt A, et al. Long-term sequelae of calf vein thrombosis treated with heparin or low-dose streptokinase. *Acta Med Scand.* 1986;**219**(4):349–57.

23 Schweizer J, Kirch W, Koch R, et al. Short- and long-term results after thrombolytic treatment of deep venous thrombosis. *J Am Coll Cardiol.* 2000;**36**(4):1336–43.

24 Elsharawy M, Elzayat E. Early results of thrombolysis vs anticoagulation in iliofemoral venous thrombosis: a randomised clinical trial. *Eur J Vasc Endovasc Surg.* 2002;**24**(3):209–14.

25 Kiil J, Carvalho A, Sakso P, et al. Urokinase or heparin in the management of patients with deep vein thrombosis? *Acta Chir Scand.* 1981;**147**(7):529–32.

26 Goldhaber SZ, Hirsch DR, MacDougall RC, et al. Bolus recombinant urokinase versus heparin in deep venous thrombosis: a randomized controlled trial. *Am Heart J.* 1996;**132**(2 Pt 1):314–18.

27 Verhaeghe R, Besse P, Bounameaux H, et al. Multicenter pilot study of the efficacy and safety of systemic rt-PA administration in the treatment of deep vein thrombosis of the lower extremities and/or pelvis. *Thromb Res.* 1989;**55**(1):5–11.

28 Goldhaber SZ, Meyerovitz MF, Green D, et al. Randomized controlled trial of tissue plasminogen activator in proximal deep venous thrombosis. *Am J Med.* 1990;**88**(3):235–40.

29 Turpie AG, Levine MN, Hirsh J, et al. Tissue plasminogen activator (rt-PA) vs heparin in deep vein thrombosis. Results of a randomized trial. *Chest.* 1990;**97**(4 Suppl):172S–75S.

30 Common HH, Seaman AJ, Rosch J, et al. Deep vein thrombosis treated with streptokinase or heparin: follow-up of a randomized study. *Angiology.* 1976;**27**(11):645–54.

31 Johansson L, Nylander G, Hedner U, et al. Comparison of streptokinase with heparin: late results in the treatment of deep venous thrombosis. *Acta Med Scand.* 1979;**206**(1–2):93–8.

32 Arnesen H, Hoiseth A, Ly B. Streptokinase of heparin in the treatment of deep vein thrombosis: follow-up results of a prospective study. *Acta Med Scand.* 1982;**211**(1–2):65–8.

33 Bieger R, Boekhout-Mussert RJ, Hohmann F, et al. Is streptokinase useful in the treatment of deep vein thrombosis? *Acta Med Scand.* 1976;**199**(1–2):81–88.

34 Browse NL, Thomas ML, Pim HP. Streptokinase and deep vein thrombosis. *Br Med J.* 1968;**3**(5620):717–20.

35 Duckert F, Muller G, Nyman D, et al. Treatment of deep vein thrombosis with streptokinase. *Br Med J.* 1975;**1**(5956):479–81.

36 Watz R, Savidge GF. Rapid thrombolysis and preservation of valvular venous function in high deep vein thrombosis: a comparative study between streptokinase and heparin therapy. *Acta Med Scand.* 1979;**205**(4):293–98.

37 Silistreli E, Bekis R, Serbest O, et al. Platelet scintigraphy results of heparin versus streptokinase treatment in acute deep vein thrombosis. *Scand Cardiovasc J.* 2004;**38**(6):380–82.

38 Perkins JM, Magee TR, Galland RB. Phlegmasia caerulea dolens and venous gangrene. *Br J Surg.* 1996;**83**(1):19–23.

39 Tardy B, Moulin N, Mismetti P, et al. Intravenous thrombolytic therapy in patients with phlegmasia caerulea dolens. *Haematologica.* 2006;**91**(2):281–82.

40 Schwieder G, Grimm W, Siemens HJ, et al. Intermittent regional therapy with rt-PA is not superior to systemic thrombolysis in deep vein thrombosis (DVT)—a German multicenter trial. *Thromb Haemost.* 1995;**74**(5):1240–43.

41 Baldwin ZK, Comerota AJ, Schwartz LB. Catheter-directed thrombolysis for deep venous thrombosis. *Vasc Endovascular Surg.* 2004;**38**(1):1–9.

42 Janssen MC, Wollersheim H, Schultze-Kool LJ, et al. Local and systemic thrombolytic therapy for acute deep venous thrombosis. *Neth J Med.* 2005;**63**(3):81–90.

43 The urokinase pulmonary embolism trial: a national cooperative study. *Circulation.* 1973;**47**(2 Suppl):II1–108.

44 Marini C, Di Ricco G, Rossi G, et al. Fibrinolytic effects of urokinase and heparin in acute pulmonary embolism: a randomized clinical trial. *Respiration.* 1988;**54**(3):162–73.

45 Tibbutt DA, Davies JA, Anderson JA, et al. Comparison by controlled clinical trial of streptokinase and heparin in treatment of life-threatening pulmonary embolism. *Br Med J.* 1974;**1**(5904):343–47.

46 Ly B, Arnesen H, Eie H, Hol R. A controlled clinical trial of streptokinase and heparin in the treatment of major pulmonary embolism. *Acta Med Scand.* 1978;**203**(6):465–70.

47 Dotter CT, Seaman AJ, Rosch J, et al. Streptokinase and heparin in the treatment of major pulmonary embolism: a randomised comparison. *Vasc Surg.* 1979;**13**(1):42–52.

48 Jerjes-Sanchez C, Ramirez-Rivera A, de Lourdes Garcia M, et al. Streptokinase and heparin versus heparin alone in massive pulmonary embolism: a randomized controlled trial. *J Thromb Thrombolysis.* 1995;**2**(3):227–29.

49 Levine M, Hirsh J, Weitz J, et al. A randomized trial of a single bolus dosage regimen of recombinant tissue plasminogen activator in patients with acute pulmonary embolism. *Chest.* 1990;**98**(6):1473–79.

50 Anonymous. Tissue plasminogen activator for the treatment of acute pulmonary embolism: a collaborative study by the PIOPED Investigators. *Chest* 1990;**97**(3):528–33.

51 Dalla-Volta S, Palla A, Santolicandro A, et al. PAIMS 2: alteplase combined with heparin versus heparin in the treatment of acute pulmonary embolism. Plasminogen activator Italian multicenter study 2. *J Am Coll Cardiol.* 1992;**20**(3):520–26.

52 Konstantinides S, Geibel A, Heusel G, et al. Heparin plus alteplase compared with heparin alone in patients with submassive pulmonary embolism. *N Engle J Med.* 2002;**347**(15):1143–50.

53 Goldhaber SZ, Haire WD, Feldstein ML, et al. Alteplase versus heparin in acute pulmonary embolism: randomised trial assessing right-ventricular function and pulmonary perfusion. *Lancet.* 1993;**341**(8844):507–11.

54 Urokinase pulmonary embolism trial. Phase 1 results: a cooperative study. *JAMA.* 1970;**214**(12):2163–72.

55 Miller GA, Sutton GC, Kerr IH, Gibson RV, Honey M. Comparison of streptokinase and heparin in treatment of isolated acute massive pulmonary embolism. *Br Med J* 1971;**2**(5763):681–84.

56 Sharma GV, Folland ED, McIntyre KM, et al. Long-term benefit of thrombolytic therapy in patients with pulmonary embolism. *Vasc Med.* 2000;**5**(2):91–5.

57 Sharma GV, Burleson VA, Sasahara AA. Effect of thrombolytic therapy on pulmonary-capillary blood volume in patients with pulmonary embolism. *N Engle J Med.* 1980;**303**(15):842–45.

58 Giuntini C, Marini C, Di Ricco G, et al. A controlled clinical trial on the effect of heparin infusion and two regimens of urokinase in acute pulmonary embolism. *G Ital Cardiol.* 1984;14 Suppl 1:26–9.

59 Sasahara AA, Sharma GV, Parisi AF, et al. Pulmonary embolism, pulmonary microcirculation, and thrombolytic therapy. *Angiology.* 1982;**33**(6):368–74.

60 Faioni EM, Valsecchi C, Palla A, et al. Free protein S deficiency is a risk factor for venous thrombosis. *Thromb Haemost.* 1997;**78**(5): 1343–46.

61 Dong B, Jirong Y, Liu G, et al. Thrombolytic therapy for pulmonary embolism. *Cochrane Database Syst Rev.* 2006(2):CD004437.

62 Wan S, Quinlan DJ, Agnelli G, et al. Thrombolysis compared with heparin for the initial treatment of pulmonary embolism: a meta-analysis of the randomized controlled trials. *Circulation.* 2004;**110**(6): 744–49.

63 Kasper W, Konstantinides S, Geibel A, et al. Management strategies and determinants of outcome in acute major pulmonary embolism: results of a multicenter registry. *J Am Coll Cardiol.* 1997;**30**(5):1165–71.

64 Goldhaber SZ, Visani L, De Rosa M. Acute pulmonary embolism: clinical outcomes in the International Cooperative Pulmonary Embolism Registry (ICOPER). *Lancet.* 1999;**353**(9162):1386–89.

65 Verstraete M, Miller GA, Bounameaux H, et al. Intravenous and intrapulmonary recombinant tissue-type plasminogen activator in the treatment of acute massive pulmonary embolism. *Circulation.* 1988;**77**(2):353–60.

66 Dalen JE. Thrombolysis in submassive pulmonary embolism? No. *J Thromb Haemost.* 2003;**1**(6):1130–32.

67 Konstantinides S. Thrombolysis in submassive pulmonary embolism? Yes. *J Thromb Haemost.* 2003;**1**(6):1127–29.

12 Inferior Vena Cava Interruption

Michael B. Streiff, Christine L. Hann

This chapter will present an evidence-based overview of current "best practice" for the use of inferior vena cava interruption. Where possible, recommendations are based on published evidence; however, it is recognized that evidence is lacking in many areas within which vena caval interruption is widely practiced. Grading of the quality of evidence and strengths of recommendations in this chapter are based on the guidelines proposed by the international Grading of Recommendations Assessment, Development, and Evaluation Working Group (GRADE), adopting the modification used by the American College of Chest Physicians that merges the very low and low categories of quality of evidence (see chapter 1).

Do vena cava filters prevent pulmonary embolism?

The best evidence to support the efficacy of vena cava filters in the prevention of pulmonary embolism comes the PREPIC study, which randomized 400 patients with acute deep venous thrombosis (DVT) felt to be at high risk for pulmonary embolism (PE) to anticoagulation or anticoagulation and a vena cava filter. After 12 days of therapy, the incidence of PE (asymptomatic and symptomatic) was reduced by 78% in patients receiving filters compared with anticoagulation alone (2 PE 1.1% versus 9 PE 4.8%, odds ratio (OR) 0.22 [95% confidence interval (CI) 0.05–0.9] $p = 0.03$). At two years, the incidence of symptomatic PE tended to be lower in filter patients (6 PE 3.4% versus 12 PE 6.3% OR 0.5[95% CI 0.19–1.33], $p = 0.16$); a difference that became significant after eight years of follow-up (9 PE 6.2% versus 24 PE 15.1% hazard ratio (HR) 0.37 [95% CI 0.17–0.79] $p = 0.008$). Ninety-one percent of patients were discharged on vitamin K antagonists (VKA) and 94% were anticoagulated for three months (1). Thirty-eight percent were anticoagulated for two years, and 35% received VKA over the entire eight-year follow-up. Survival was equivalent at all time points between the groups (2). While this trial does not test the efficacy of filters in the population most likely to receive one (e.g., patients with acute venous thromboembolism [VTE] and a contraindication to anticoagulation), it does demonstrate that vena cava filters reduce the incidence of PE in DVT patients who received at least three months of anticoagulation.

Conclusion. Vena cava filters are effective in prevention of PE in patients with acute VTE receiving anticoagulation (Grade 2A).

What are the complications associated with vena cava filters?

The most clinically significant complications associated with the use of a vena cava filter are DVT, vena cava thrombosis, migration, vena cava penetration, and death. No fatal placement complications were reported in the PREPIC study (2). In observational cohort studies, periprocedural mortality was low, occurring in only 0.13% of patients (range, 0% to 0.34%, depending on filter model) (3). Deep venous thrombosis occurs more frequently 1.5-fold more commonly in filter recipients (57 DVT 35.7% versus 41 DVT 27.5%, HR 1.52 [95% CI 1.02–2.27], $p = 0.042$). Vena cava thrombosis occurred in 26 filter patients (13%) after eight years of follow-up. Thirty-five percent received anticoagulation throughout follow-up (2). In a prospective study of 142 patients receiving Vena Tech filters, Crochet et al., employing routine duplex and angiographic follow-up, documented vena cava occlusion radiographically in 33% of patients at nine years (4). These data may not be applicable to all filter models. In observational cohort studies, symptomatic migration and vena cava penetration were uncommon events, occurring in only 0.3% of patients (3). No episodes were reported in the PREPIC study. Although vena cava filters are associated with an increased risk of DVT, postthrombotic syndrome (PTS) was not more frequent in filter recipients in the PREPIC study (filter, 109, 70.3% versus no filter, 107, 69.7%

Evidence-based Hematology. Edited by Mark A. Crowther, Jeff Ginsberg, Holger J. Schünemann, Ralph M. Meyer, and Richard Lottenberg.

HR 0.87 [95% CI 0.66–1.13], $p = 0.3$), perhaps because of a significant prevalence of previous VTE (36%) and PTS (24%) among participants at enrollment (2).

Conclusion. Vena cava filters are associated with a 1.5-fold increase in DVT. Thirteen percent of patients develop vena cava thrombosis after eight years of follow-up (Grade 2A). Procedural mortality, symptomatic episodes of filter migration, or vena cava penetration are uncommon (Grade 2C).

Are clinical outcomes associated retrievable (optional) vena cava filters equivalent to those achieved with permanent vena cava filters?

Although permanent vena cava filters reduce the incidence of PE, permanent filters are associated with an increased incidence of unwanted adverse effects and their long-term safety remains unclear. In addition, many patients who receive a vena cava filter have transient contraindications to anticoagulation. Consequently, several retrievable filters have been tested and marketed in North America and Europe in recent years, including the Gunther Tulip filter (Cook, Inc., Bloomington, IN), the Nitinol OptEase filter (Cordis Endovascular, Miami Lakes, FL), the Recovery filter (Bard Peripheral Vascular, Tempe, AZ), and the ALN filter (ALN Implants Chirurgicaux, Ghisonaccia, France). No randomized clinical trials comparing different filter models exist. To estimate the comparative performance of different optional filters and permanent filters, the clinical outcomes derived from observational cohort studies of retrievable studies are displayed in Table 12.1. Of the four retrievable filters listed, the Recovery filter is no longer available because of episodes of filter migration. It has been replaced by the G2 Recovery filter that is not currently approved for retrieval by the U.S. Food and Drug Administration. A total of 1,754 patients have been enrolled in observational studies of optional filters (5–29). The mean retrieval percentage is less than 50%. Pulmonary embolism is infrequent (0.9%) among patients whose filters were successfully retrieved although the mean follow-up was short (10.8 months). Pulmonary embolism (1.7%), DVT (5.5%), and inferior vena cava (IVC) thrombosis (2.2%) occurred infrequently in patients whose optional filters remained in situ. These results are comparable to results among permanent filter recipients. In 110 published studies of 10,279 permanent filter recipients, 3.1% suffered a PE, 9.5% suffered a DVT, and 4.1% developed IVC thrombosis during a mean follow-up duration of 15.1 months (3). Focusing on the trauma patient population, permanent filters were placed in 2,119 patients, while retrievable filters were used in 792 patients. Symptomatic PE occurred in 0.71% of permanent filter recipients and 0.5% of retrievable filter patients (13,14,16,17,21,30–57).

Conclusion. The benefits and adverse effects of retrievable vena cava filters appear to quantitatively similar to permanent vena cava filters. Choice of a permanent or retrievable vena cava filter should be based on the predicted duration of filtration required (Grade 2C).

Is the presence of a vena cava filter an indication for indefinite anticoagulation?

Indefinite anticoagulation is commonly recommended for patients with a vena cava filter. This recommendation is based on the results of the PREPIC study and population-based observational studies that have noted an increased risk of venous thrombosis in vena cava filter recipients (2,58). No randomized clinical trials have been conducted directly examining this question. While anticoagulation with VKA is very effective in prevention of recurrent thromboembolism, it is associated with an incidence of major bleeding as high as 7%–8% per patient year of therapy (59). The morbidity and mortality of these bleeding events is substantial. The case fatality rate of major bleeding in patients receiving VKA for more than three months has been estimated to be 9.1%, and the incidence of anticoagulation associated intracranial bleeding is 0.65 per 100 patient-years (60). Concern regarding the adverse effects of a strict policy advocating indefinite anticoagulation for all patients with vena cava filters is supported by the results of the PREPIC study. Although only 35% of participants received anticoagulation throughout the eight-year follow-up period, major bleeding occurred in 57 subjects (14.3%) and was fatal in 17 (4.3%). In contrast, fatal thromboembolism only occurred in six patients (1.5%) (2). Clearly, a policy of routine anticoagulation among filter recipients undoubtedly would have resulted in a substantial increase in hemorrhagic morbidity and mortality among filter recipients. Therefore, clinicians caring for patients with permanent vena cava filters should carefully consider the risk of bleeding and thromboembolism in their filter patients when deciding on the duration of anticoagulation therapy.

Conclusion. There are insufficient data to support a recommendation that all filter patients should be treated with indefinite anticoagulation. Until further information is available, decisions on the duration of anticoagulation for patients with filter should be made on a case-by-case basis and incorporate an assessment of a patient's risk of thromboembolism and bleeding (Grade 2A).

Are vena caval filters effective for prevention of VTE in high-risk trauma patients?

VTE is a common complication of major trauma. In the absence of prophylaxis, 58% of trauma patients develop a DVT during the first few weeks of hospitalization. Eighteen percent of patients had a proximal DVT, and seven patients (1%) suffered a symptomatic PE, which was fatal in three patients (0.4%) (61). Routine contrast spiral CT scan surveillance has demonstrated that 24% (22/90) of trauma patients have evidence of PE (62). Although low-molecular-weight-heparin (LMWH) has been demonstrated

Table 12.1 Outcome for patients receiving optional (retrievable) vena cava filters.*

Filter Type	Study number	Patients (range, per study)	Mean implant time (range)	Retrieval attempted/ successful	Mean follow-up (months)	PE postretrieval	PE no retrieval	DVT no retrieval	IVC thrombosis no retrieval
Gunther Tulip MREye	15	945 (9–143)	17.9 days (8.2–43)	58%/90%	16.1	2/137 (1.5%)	5/383 (1.3%)	3/383 (0.8%)	10/383 (2.6%)
Nitinol OptEase	4	198 (27–94)	18 days (11–22)	65%/97%	2.3	2/124 (1.6%)	0/74	2/74 (2.7%)	1/74 (1.4%)
Bard Recovery	5	301 (13–106)	113 days (33–254)	28%/94%	3.5	0/79	5/222 (2.3%)	10/222 (4.5%)	0/222
ALN	4	328 (18–217)	83 days (51–179)	31%/92%	14.7	0/100	5/228 (2.2%)	35/228 (15.4%)	13/228 (5.7%)
Total Retrievable filters	28	1,754		49%/91%	10.8	4/440 (0.9%)	15/907 (1.7%)	50/907 (5.5%)	24/907 (2.6%)

*DVT, deep venous thrombosis; IVC, inferior vena cava; PE, pulmonary embolism.

Table 12.2 Outcome in cancer patients with VTE treated with vena cava filters or anticoagulation (AC).

Patient population	Study number	Patients (range, per study)	Mean follow up (months)	VTE (%)	DVT (%)	PE (%) fatal PE (%)	IVC thrombosis (%)	Major bleeding (%) fatal bleeding (%)
Cancer pts. with filters	18	1,287 (10–308)	9.5	102 (7.9%)	51 (4%)	27 (2.1%) NR	24 (1.9%)	NR
Cancer pts. with AC	4	1,216 (95–676)	4.6	129 (10.6%)	53 (6.9%)	32 (4.1%) 14 (1.8%)	NR	59 (4.9%) 1 (0.13%)

DVT, deep venous thrombosis; IVC, inferior vena cava; NR, not reported; PE, pulmonary embolism; VTE, venous thromboembolism.

to be effective in prevention of VTE in trauma patients, a substantial percentage of trauma patients have contraindications to pharmacologic prophylaxis on admission (63). While such contraindications may resolve with treatment or time, pulmonary embolism can occur early in the hospital course of trauma patients (6% within 24 hours); therefore, VTE prophylaxis should be initiated promptly on admission (64). Consequently, vena caval filters have been proposed as an alternative VTE prophylaxis strategy. Twenty-five single-center cohort studies encompassing 2,245 trauma patients with a mean weighted injury severity score (ISI) of 25.6 have examined the use of permanent vena caval filters in the prevention of VTE after trauma (30–45,48–55). Vena caval filters were placed in an average of 2.5% of the total trauma population (range, 0.4%–8.3%), an average of 6.3 days (3–11.4 days) after admission. PE occurred in 15 patients (0.71%) (range, 0.5–2.8%), three of which were fatal (0.14%) (range, 0%–1.6%). In comparison, 93 historical controls (2.1%, range, 1%–23%)) suffered PE, which was fatal in 43 patients (0.9%, range, 0.3%–10%). Symptomatic DVT occurred in 150 filter recipients (12.3%) (range, 2.4%–46.7%), while 24 suffered IVC thrombosis (2.5%) (range, 0.9%–22%).

The period during which pharmacologic VTE prophylaxis is contraindicated is transient; consequently, retrievable filters have become an increasingly popular option for mechanical VTE prophylaxis in trauma patients. Six single-center studies and one multicenter cohort study of retrievable filters, including 769 patients (range, 32–310 patients), have been published (13,14,16,17,21,56,57). Retrievable IVC filters were placed in 1.9% of patients (range, 1.3%–3.3%) with a weighted ISI of 26.5, a mean of 5.3 days after admission (range, 3–6 days). Filters were retrieved in 27.9% of patients, an average of 40.5 days after placement (10.2–94 days). Only one study documented follow-up after discharge in 51% of patients for a mean follow-up duration of 5.7 months (56). PE occurred in four patients (0.5%, range, 0%–3.2%), three of which occurred postfilter retrieval. None was fatal. DVT occurred in 19 patients (2.4%, range, 0%–19%), and IVC thrombosis was noted in seven (0.9%, range, 0%–1.3%). While these results suggest that retrievable filters are effective in PE prevention in trauma patients, one historically controlled study found no difference in the incidence of PE between periods of low and high prophylactic filter use (57).

Conclusion. The efficacy of retrievable and permanent IVC filters in PE prevention in trauma patients remains unclear. Randomized controlled trials are needed to establish the efficacy of IVC filters in the prevention of PE in trauma patients (Grade 2C).

Are vena cava filters effective for prevention of VTE in cancer patients? Are filters more effective than anticoagulation in cancer patients?

Cancer patients are four- to seven-fold more likely to develop VTE than patients without cancer (65,66). Anticoagulation is associated with a two- to three-fold higher risk of recurrent thromboembolism and two- to six-fold higher incidence of major bleeding in cancer patients compared with patients without cancer (67–69). Consequently, vena cava filters have been employed as an alternative treatment. Randomized controlled trials of cancer patients with venous thromboembolism treated with anticoagulation or vena cava filters have not been conducted. Therefore, only indirect comparisons can be made. Table 12.2 contains the results of studies using vena cava filters or anticoagulation in the treatment of VTE in cancer patients (70–86). Over 60% of patients in both treatment groups had extensive disease. In two vena cava filter studies providing data, anticoagulation was administered to 60% of patients in conjunction with caval filtration (85,86). The event rates noted in cancer patients treated with vena cava filters compare favorably to patients treated with anticoagulation and with data from all permanent IVC filter study participants who had a cumulative incidence of symptomatic PE, DVT, and IVCT of 3.1%, 9.5%, and 4.1%, respectively, over a mean follow-up of 15.1 months (3,67–69,87).

Conclusion. Vena cava filters appear to prevent PE in cancer patients with VTE with a low incidence of thrombotic complications. Available data are insufficient to accurately compare the outcome of cancer patients with VTE treated with vena cava filters versus anticoagulation. Additional prospective studies are warranted to assess the risks and benefits of vena cava filters in the cancer population. Until these data are available, filters should only be used in cancer patients who have contraindications to anticoagulation (Grade 2C).

Should patients with a free-floating thrombus be treated with a vena cava filter?

Several retrospective studies and one prospective study have identified proximal free-floating venous thrombus (FFT) as a risk factor for pulmonary embolism (88–93). Consequently, several authors have suggested that vena cava filters should placed in patients with FFT (88,91,92). In contrast, Pacouret et al. found no difference in the rate of subsequent PE between patients with (2/61, 3.3%) and without FFT (1/27, 3.7%) (94). A prospective case series of 22 patients with FFT suggested that these patients can be safely managed as outpatients with LMWH without recurrent VTE (95). The conflicting results of the aforementioned studies reflect the differences in diagnostic techniques (monoplanar versus biplanar venography, ventilation/perfusion scans versus pulmonary angiography) as well as relatively small subject populations. Although vena cava filters have been demonstrated to reduce the incidence of pulmonary embolism, their use has not been associated with a mortality benefit (2). Furthermore, they have not been formally evaluated in patients with known FFT. Therefore, it remains unknown whether their use will reduce the incidence of PE in this population. Routine use in this setting awaits additional information.

Conclusion. Insufficient data exist to support the routine use of vena cava filters for the treatment of patients with proximal FFT (Grade 2C).

Are vena caval filters effective for prevention of VTE in high-risk bariatric surgery patients?

The increasing prevalence in morbid obesity has driven a 7.7-fold increase in bariatric surgery procedures between 1998 and 2003 (96). PE is considered the leading cause of perioperative death in bariatric surgical patients with an estimated incidence of 1% in the immediate postoperative period (30 days) (97). In the Nationwide Inpatient Sample, 3.4 bariatric surgery patients per 1,000 suffered an episode of venous thromboembolism (98). Furthermore, nearly one-third of bariatric surgery patients who develop PE die (97).

Observational studies have identified a body mass index greater than 50 or 55 kg/m^{2}kg/M, a previous history of VTE, thrombophilia, venous stasis, and pulmonary hypertension as risk factors for VTE in the bariatric surgery population. The occurrence of postoperative VTE despite pharmacologic prophylaxis has stimulated the use of vena cava filters for PE prevention. Five cohort studies have examined the use of vena cava filters in the prevention of PE in 185 high-risk bariatric surgery patients (99–104). Pulmonary embolism occurred in one patient with a filter in place (0.5%) and in one patient after filter retrieval (0.5%). Seven patients (3.9%) developed a DVT, and two (1.1%) developed an IVC thrombosis. In one historically controlled study, PE occurred in four high-risk patients (13%) not receiving filters, while no PE developed in 33 high-risk patients during a subsequent period when all high-risk patients received IVC filters. All patients were treated with elastic stockings and sequential compression devices as well as 50 U/kg subcutaneous unfractionated heparin every 12 hours (99). However, several studies have shown that aggressive pharmacologic prophylaxis can also effectively prevent perioperative VTE in high-risk bariatric surgery patients (105,106). Since published studies of surgical VTE prophylaxis have enrolled subjects with an average body weight of 70–80 kg and body mass index of 25, weight-adjusted VTE pharmacologic prophylaxis regimens will need to be developed to optimize outcomes in bariatric surgery patients. Once optimal pharmacologic bariatric surgery VTE prophylaxis regimens are identified, rational investigation of the utility of vena cava filters in the prevention of PE in this population can be conducted.

Conclusion. The efficacy of vena cava filters in PE prevention in bariatric surgery patients remains unclear. Randomized controlled trials are needed to establish the efficacy of IVC filters in the prevention of PE in this patient population (Grade 2C).

Can patients with vena caval filters undergo magnetic resonance imaging?

Patients with vena caval filters are likely to require magnetic resonance (MR) imaging at some point during their medical care. No reports of filter migration as a result of MR imaging have been published thus far. Ferromagnetic alloys such as stainless steel, however, can produce "black-hole" artifacts on MR imaging (107). Several filters are composed of stainless steel, including the original stainless steel Greenfield filter, percutaneous Greenfield filter and the Bird's Nest filter; of these, the Bird's Nest Filter produced the greatest MR imaging artifact. Nonetheless, several small series have demonstrated that stainless steel filter components are stable in field strengths up to 1.5 T (108,109).

The majority of currently available vena cava filters are composed of low ferromagnetic alloys, which are stable at 1.5 T and do not produce significant MR image artifact (110). These include permanent filters such as the Simon Nitinol filter, Nitinol TrapEase, VenaTech filter, VenaTech LP filter, the Bard G2 filter, and the titanium Greenfield filter and retrievable filters such as the OptEase and Gunther Tulip (110–113). MR imaging as early as one week after placement was not associated with any consequences in a small series of patients with the Simon Nitinol filter (112). According to manufacturer's guidelines the Gunther Tulip, OptEase, and TrapEase filters, MR imaging can be performed safely immediately after placement. Although it is likely that other low ferromagnetic devices will behave similarly, data with other filter models would be useful for clinical decision making.

Conclusion. MR-imaging in patients with retrievable and permanent IVC filters appears to be safe. Small observational studies have not demonstrated filter migration during MR imaging. Larger studies are warranted to determine the safety of this practice (Grade 2C).

Are prophylactic vena cava filters indicated in patients undergoing pulmonary thromboembolectomy for chronic thromboembolic pulmonary hypertension?

A small subset (3.8%) of PE patients develop chronic thromboembolic pulmonary hypertension (CTEPH) due to the persistence of emboli despite treatment or multiple subclinical episodes of PE (114). Pulmonary endarterectomy has been demonstrated to be an effective treatment option for CTEPH patients (115,116). Despite the lack of randomized clinical trial data supporting this practice, vena caval filters are commonly placed preoperatively (117). Data on the utility of filters in this capacity are limited; however, given the severity and restricted treatment options for patients with CTEPH, indefinite anticoagulation and filters should be strongly considered in all patients undergoing pulmonary endarterectomy.

Conclusion. The efficacy of vena cava filters in PE prevention in pulmonary thromboembolectomy patients is unclear. Randomized controlled trials would be helpful to establish the efficacy of filters in this patient population. However, given the severity of illness in these patients and their limited treatment options, randomized controlled trials are unlikely to be performed (Grade 2C).

Are vena cava filters indicated for VTE prophylaxis in high-risk orthopedic patients?

In the absence of prophylaxis, patients undergoing orthopedic surgery such as total knee arthroplasty or total hip arthroplasty have a 10%–20% risk of developing proximal DVT and a 0.2%–5% of developing a fatal PE (118). The risk of thromboembolism persists for up to three months after surgery, thus patients may benefit from extended prophylaxis after discharge (119). While several observational case series attest to the efficacy of IVC filters in the prevention of PE in orthopedic patients (120–123), none of these studies incorporated random or masked treatment assignment or masked outcome assessment and follow-up was of limited intensity and duration. Furthermore, many advances in orthopedic VTE prophylaxis (LMWH, pentasaccharides, etc.) and anticoagulation monitoring (international normalized ratio) have occurred since the publication of these studies. Therefore, with the availability of modern methods of VTE prophylaxis, it is doubtful whether IVC filter placement represents a useful option for most orthopedic patients. Until well-designed studies demonstrate the utility of vena caval filters for this purpose, this indication for filter placement should be considered primarily of historical significance. As with any major surgical procedure, IVC filters, in particular, retrievable filters, remain a useful option for patients who develop VTE in the immediate perioperative period when full dose anticoagulation would be contraindicated (124).

Conclusion. The efficacy of vena cava filters in PE prevention in high-risk orthopedic surgery patients is unclear. Randomized controlled trials are needed to establish the efficacy of filters in this patient population (Grade 2C).

Should vena cava filters be used preferentially to treat VTE during pregnancy?

It is estimated that pregnant women have a fivefold increased risk of VTE compared with nonpregnant women of similar age. VTE has been reported to complicate 0.05%–3% of all pregnancies, and PE is considered a leading cause of maternal mortality in the United States (125). Several factors contribute to the increased VTE risk in this population, including pregnancy-related changes in coagulation factors (reductions in protein S activity, increases in factor VIII, fibrinogen, and von Willebrand factor activity), reduced activity, IVC compression, surgical mode of delivery, and age over 35 (126–128). Anticoagulation with heparin or LMWH is the recommended treatment for VTE in pregnancy. Major bleeding complications occur at a similar frequency among pregnant and nonpregnant women (129). Several observational case series have examined the use of vena caval filters during pregnancy for VTE (130–135). Randomized comparative studies are lacking.

Substantial evidence indicates that when appropriately monitored, anticoagulation is effective for the vast majority of pregnant patients (136). Therefore, the use of filters should be reserved for patients in whom anticoagulation is contraindicated. If a vena cava filter is necessary, an optional filter should be strongly considered, given the young age of potential recipients and the known long-term complications of IVC filters.

Conclusion. The efficacy of vena cava filters in PE prevention during pregnancy is unclear. Randomized controlled trials are needed to establish the efficacy of IVC filters in this patient population. (Grade 2C)

Should vena caval filters be used for PE prevention during thrombolysis of proximal deep venous thrombosis?

The principal complications of DVT are recurrent VTE and postthrombotic syndrome (PTS). Studies suggest that the use of systemic and catheter-directed thrombolysis may reduce the incidence of PTS (137–141). However, systemic thrombolysis of proximal DVT (particularly, iliofemoral or IVC thrombi) has resulted in several cases of fatal and nonfatal PE (142,143). Therefore, prophylactic placement of vena caval filters has been proposed as a strategy to prevent PE in patients undergoing thrombolysis.

Using a variety of temporary filters during systemic thrombolysis, however, a European multicenter registry noted four cases of fatal PE (2.1%) and three nonfatal PE (1.6%) despite filter protection (144). Conversely, only one fatal pulmonary embolus (0.3%) occurred during a multicenter registry of catheter-directed thrombolysis without routine filter use (141). In a retrospective single-institution study of 69 patients who received catheter-directed thrombolysis, 14 of whom received a vena caval filters, no PE was noted (145). Although far from conclusive, these data suggest that catheter-directed thrombolysis of most iliofemoral DVT is associated with a small risk of PE. In patients deemed at high risk for embolization (e.g., poorly adherent IVC or iliac thrombi) or mortality from PE (patients with concomitant PE or limited cardiopulmonary reserve), retrievable filters should be considered.

Conclusion. The data suggests that the risk of PE associated with catheter-directed thrombolysis of iliofemoral DVT is small. Use of a retrievable vena cava filter during thrombolysis may be considered in patients at high risk for embolization and should be based on the predicted competing risks of PE and adverse events associated with filter placement. Additional studies are warranted to assess the utility of retrievable filters in this patient population (Grade 2C).

What are appropriate indications for vena cava filter placement?

Vena cava filters reduce the incidence of PE in patients with DVT receiving anticoagulation at a cost of a higher incidence of DVT and vena cava thrombosis and an absence in mortality benefit. Although rare, fatal complications of insertion do occur in approximately one to two patients per thousand. Data supporting the utility of vena cava filters for other proposed indications are of low quality. Therefore, filters should be used primarily for patients with an acute episode of VTE who have contraindications to anticoagulation. Vena cava filters have also been proposed to be appropriate for patients with recurrent VTE despite adequate anticoagulation. Physicians caring for patients in this clinical situation should carefully weigh the risks and benefits of filters for these patients; several conditions associated with this presentation (Trousseau's syndrome, heparin-induced thrombocytopenia, antiphospholipid syndrome) are characterized by systematic activation of coagulation that cannot be managed by regional approaches to thromboembolism, and complications of filter placement tend to be greater in these patients. Additional data are required to justify filter use for other indications (3).

Conclusion. Vena cava filters are useful for treatment of acute VTE in patients with a contraindication to anticoagulation (Grade 2A). Vena cava filters are useful for patients with recurrent thromboembolism despite adequate anticoagulation (Grade 2C).

References

1 Decousus H, Leizorovicz A, Parent F, et al. A clinical trial of vena caval filters in the prevention of pulmonary embolism in patients with proximal deep-vein thrombosis. Prevention du Risque d'Embolie Pulmonaire par Interruption Cave Study Group [see comments]. *N Engl J Med.* 1998;**338**(7):409–15.

2 Decousus H, Barral FG, Buchmuller-Cordier A, et al. Eight-year follow-up of patients with permanent vena cava filters in the prevention of pulmonary embolism: the PREPIC (Prevention du Risque d'Embolie Pulmonaire par Interruption Cave) randomized study. *Circulation.* 2005;**112**(3):416–22.

3 Hann CL, Streiff MB. The role of vena caval filters in the management of venous thromboembolism. *Blood Rev.* 2005;**19**(4):179–202.

4 Crochet DP, Brunel P, Trogrlic S, et al. Long-term follow-up of Vena Tech-LGM filter: predictors and frequency of caval occlusion. *J Vasc Interv Radiol.* 1999;**10**(2 Pt 1):137–42.

5 Millward SF, Oliva VL, Bell SD, et al. Gunther Tulip Retrievable vena cava filter: results from the Registry of the Canadian Interventional Radiology Association. *J Vasc Interv Radiol.* 2001;**12**(9):1053–58.

6 de Gregorio MA, Gamboa P, Gimeno MJ, et al. The Gunther Tulip retrievable filter: prolonged temporary filtration by repositioning within the inferior vena cava. *J Vasc Interv Radiol.* 2003;**14**(10):1259–65.

7 Hoppe H, Nutting CW, Smouse HR, et al. Gunther Tulip filter retrievability multicenter study including CT follow-up: final report. *J Vasc Interv Radiol.* 2006;**17**(6):1017–23.

8 Looby S, Given MF, Geoghegan T, et al. Gunther Tulip retrievable inferior vena caval filters: indications, efficacy, retrieval, and complications. *Cardiovasc Intervent Radiol.* 2007;**30**(1):59–65.

9 Yamagami T, Kato T, Hirota T, et al. Evaluation of retrievability of the Gunther Tulip vena cava filter. *Cardiovasc Intervent Radiol.* 2007;**30**(2):226–31.

10 Wicky S, Doenz F, Meuwly JY, et al. Clinical experience with retrievable Gunther Tulip vena cava filters. *J Endovasc Ther.* 2003;**10**(5):994–1000.

11 Ponchon M, Gofette P, Hainaut P. Temporary vena caval filtration: preliminary clinical experience with removable vena caval filters. *Acta Clin Belg.* 1999;**54**(5):223–28.

12 Millward SF, Bhargava A, Aquino J Jr., et al. Gunther Tulip filter: preliminary clinical experience with retrieval. *J Vasc Interv Radiol.* 2000;**11**(1):75–82.

13 Allen TL, Carter JL, Morris BJ, et al. Retrievable vena cava filters in trauma patients for high-risk prophylaxis and prevention of pulmonary embolism. *Am J Surg.* 2005;**189**(6):656–61.

14 Morris CS, Rogers FB, Najarian KE, et al. Current trends in vena caval filtration with the introduction of a retrievable filter at a level I trauma center. *J Trauma.* 2004;**57**(1):32–6.

15 Terhaar OA, Lyon SM, Given MF, et al. Extended interval for retrieval of Gunther Tulip filters. *J Vasc Interv Radiol.* 2004;**15**(11):1257–62.

16 Hoff WS, Hoey BA, Wainwright GA, Reed JF, Ball DS, Ringold M, et al. Early experience with retrievable inferior vena cava filters in high-risk trauma patients. *J Am Coll Surg.* 2004;**199**(6):869–74.

17 Offner PJ, Hawkes A, Madayag R, et al. The role of temporary inferior vena cava filters in critically ill surgical patients. *Arch Surg.* 2003;**138**(6):591–94.

18 Ray CE Jr., Mitchell E, Zipser S, et al. Outcomes with retrievable inferior vena cava filters: a multicenter study. *J Vasc Interv Radiol.* 2006;**17**(10):1595–604.

19 Meier C, Keller IS, Pfiffner R, et al. Early experience with the retrievable OptEase vena cava filter in high-risk trauma patients. *Eur J Vasc Endovasc Surg.* 2006;**32**(5):589–95.
20 Oliva VL, Szatmari F, Giroux MF, et al. The Jonas study: evaluation of the retrievability of the Cordis OptEase inferior vena cava filter. *J Vasc Interv Radiol.* 2005;**16**(11):1439–45.
21 Rosenthal D, Wellons ED, Lai KM, et al. Retrievable inferior vena cava filters: early clinical experience. *J Cardiovasc Surg (Torino).* 2005;**46**(2):163–69.
22 Rosenthal D, Wellons ED, Lai KM, et al. Retrievable inferior vena cava filters: initial clinical results. *Ann Vasc Surg.* 2006;**20**(1):157–65.
23 Kalva SP, Athanasoulis CA, Fan CM, et al. "Recovery" vena cava filter: experience in 96 patients. *Cardiovasc Intervent Radiol.* 2006;**29**(4):559–64.
24 Grande WJ, Trerotola SO, Reilly PM, et al. Experience with the recovery filter as a retrievable inferior vena cava filter. *J Vasc Interv Radiol.* 2005;**16**(9):1189–93.
25 Binkert CA, Sasadeusz K, Stavropoulos SW. Retrievability of the recovery vena cava filter after dwell times longer than 180 days. *J Vasc Interv Radiol.* 2006;**17**(2 Pt 1):299–302.
26 Asch MR. Initial experience in humans with a new retrievable inferior vena cava filter. *Radiology.* 2002;**225**(3):835–44.
27 Mismetti P, Rivron-Guillot K, Quenet S, et al. A prospective long-term study of 220 patients with a retrievable vena cava filter for secondary prevention of venous thromboembolism. *Chest.* 2007;**131**(1):223–29.
28 Caronno R, Piffaretti G, Tozzi M, et al. Mid-term experience with the ALN retrievable inferior vena cava filter. *Eur J Vasc Endovasc Surg.* 2006;**32**(5):596–99.
29 Imberti D, Bianchi M, Farina A, et al. Clinical experience with retrievable vena cava filters: results of a prospective observational multicenter study. *J Thromb Haemost.* 2005;**3**(7):1370–75.
30 Rogers FB, Shackford SR, Wilson J, et al. Prophylactic vena cava filter insertion in severely injured trauma patients: indications and preliminary results. *J Trauma.* 1993;**35**(4):637–41.
31 Rogers FB, Shackford SR, Ricci MA, et al. Routine prophylactic vena cava filter insertion in severely injured trauma patients decreases the incidence of pulmonary embolism. *J Am Coll Surg.* 1995;**180**:641–47.
32 Rogers FB, Shackford SR, Ricci MA, et al. Prophylactic vena cava filter insertion in selected high-risk orthopaedic trauma patients. *J Orthop Trauma.* 1997;**11**(4):267–72.
33 Rogers FB, Strindberg G, Shackford SR, et al. Five-year follow-up of prophylactic vena cava filters in high-risk trauma patients. *Arch Surg.* 1998;**133**:406–11.
34 Sekharan J, Dennis JW, Miranda FE, et al. Long-term follow-up of prophylactic Greenfield filters in multisystem trauma patients. *J Trauma.* 2001;**51**(6):1087–90.
35 Wojcik R, Cipolle MD, Fearen I, et al. Long-term follow-up of trauma patients with a vena caval filter. *J Trauma.* 2000;**49**(5):839–43.
36 Van Natta TL, Morris JA Jr., Eddy VA, et al. Elective bedside surgery in critically injured patients is safe and cost-effective. *Ann Surg.* 1998;**227**(5):618–24.
37 McMurtry AL, Owings JT, Anderson JT, et al. Increased use of prophylactic vena cava filters in trauma patients failed to decrease overall incidence of pulmonary embolism. *J Am Coll Surg.* 1999;**189**(3):314–20.
38 Langan EM III, Miller RS, Casey WJ III, et al. Prophylactic inferior vena cava filters in trauma patients at high risk: follow-up examination and risk/benefit assessment. *J Vasc Surg.* 1999;**30**(3):484–48.
39 Leach TA, Pastena JA, Swan KG, et al. Surgical prophylaxis for pulmonary embolism. *Am Surg.* 1994;**60**(4):292–95.
40 Khansarinia S, Dennis JW, Veldenz HC, et al. Prophylactic Greenfield filter placement in selected high-risk trauma patients. *J Vasc Surg.* 1995;**22**(3):231–35.
41 Gosin JS, Graham AM, Ciocca RG, et al. Efficacy of prophylactic vena cava filters in high-risk trauma patients. *Ann Vasc Surg.* 1997;**11**(1):100–105.
42 Duperier T, Mosenthal A, Swan KG, et al. Acute complications associated with Greenfield filter insertion in high-risk trauma patients. *J Trauma.* 2003;**54**(3):545–49.
43 Zolfaghari D, Johnson B, Weireter LJ, et al. Expanded use of inferior vena cava filters in the trauma population. *Surg Annu.* 1995;**27**:99–105.
44 Patton JHJ, Fabian TC, Croce MA, et al. Prophylactic Greenfield filters: acute complications and long-term follow-up [see comments]. *J Trauma.* 1996;**41**(2):231–36.
45 Winchell RJ, Hoyt DB, Walsh JC, et al. Risk factors associated with pulmonary embolism despite routine prophylaxis: implications for improved protection. *J Trauma.* 1994;**37**(4):600–6.
46 Nunn CR, Neuzil D, Naslund T, et al. Cost-effective method for bedside insertion of vena caval filters in trauma patients [see comments]. *J Trauma.* 1997;**43**(5):752–58.
47 Tola JC, Holtzman R, Lottenberg L. Bedside placement of inferior vena cava filters in the intensive care unit. *Am Surg.* 1999;**65**(9):833–37.
48 Carlin AM, Tyburski JG, Wilson RF, et al. Prophylactic and therapeutic inferior vena cava filters to prevent pulmonary emboli in trauma patients. *Arch Surg.* 2002;**137**(5):521–25.
49 Sing RF, Camp SM, Heniford BT, et al. Timing of pulmonary emboli after trauma: implications for retrievable vena cava filters. *J Trauma.* 2006;**60**(4):732–34.
50 Rodriguez JL, Lopez JM, Proctor MC, et al. Early placement of prophylactic vena caval filters in injured patients at high risk for pulmonary embolism. *J Trauma.* 1996;**40**(5):797–802.
51 Rosenthal D, McKinsey JF, Levy AM, et al. Use of the Greenfield filter in patients with major trauma. *Cardiovasc Surg.* 1994;**2**(1):52–55.
52 Webb LX, Rush PT, Fuller SB, et al. Greenfield filter prophylaxis of pulmonary embolism in patients undergoing surgery for acetabular fracture. *J Orthop Trauma.* 1992;**6**(2):139–45.
53 Wilson JT, Rogers FB, Wald SL, et al. Prophylactic vena cava filter insertion in patients with traumatic spinal cord injury: preliminary results. *Neurosurgery.* 1994;**35**(2):234–39.
54 Benjamin ME, Sandager GP, Cohn EJ Jr., et al. Duplex ultrasound insertion of inferior vena cava filters in multitrauma patients. *Am J Surg.* 1999;**178**(2):92–97.
55 Greenfield LJ, Proctor MC, Michaels AJ, et al. Prophylactic vena caval filters in trauma: the rest of the story. *J Vasc Surg.* 2000;**32**(3):490–97.
56 Karmy-Jones R, Jurkovich GJ, Velmahos GC, et al. Practice patterns and outcomes of retrievable vena cava filters in trauma patients: an AAST multicenter study. *J Trauma.* 2007;**62**(1):17–24.
57 Antevil JL, Sise MJ, Sack DI, et al. Retrievable vena cava filters for preventing pulmonary embolism in trauma patients: a cautionary tale. *J Trauma.* 2006;**60**(1):35–40.
58 White RH, Zhou H, Kim J, Romano PS. A population-based study of the effectiveness of inferior vena cava filter use among patients with venous thromboembolism. *Arch Intern Med.* 2000;**160**(13):2033–41.
59 Ansell J, Hirsh J, Poller L, et al. The pharmacology and management of the vitamin K antagonists: the Seventh ACCP Conference on Antithrombotic and Thrombolytic Therapy. *Chest.* 2004;**126** (3 Suppl):204S–33S.

60 Linkins LA, Choi PT, Douketis JD. Clinical impact of bleeding in patients taking oral anticoagulant therapy for venous thromboembolism: a meta-analysis. *Ann Intern Med.* 2003;**139**(11):893–900.

61 Geerts WH, Code KI, Jay RM, et al. A prospective study of venous thromboembolism after major trauma. *N Engl J Med.* 1994;**331**:1601–6.

62 Schultz DJ, Brasel KJ, Washington L, et al. Incidence of asymptomatic pulmonary embolism in moderately to severely injured trauma patients. *J Trauma.* 2004;**56**(4):727–31.

63 Geerts WH, Jay RM, Code KI, et al. A comparison of low-dose heparin with low-molecular weight heparin as prophylaxis against venous thromboembolism after major trauma. *N Engl J Med.* 1996;**335**:701–7.

64 Owings JT, Kraut E, Battistella F, et al. Timing of the occurrence of pulmonary embolism in trauma patients. *Arch Surg.* 1997;**132**(8):862–66.

65 Heit JA, Silverstein MD, Mohr DN, et al. Risk factors for deep vein thrombosis and pulmonary embolism: a population-based case-control study. *Arch Intern Med.* 2000;**160**(6):809–15.

66 Blom JW, Doggen CJ, Osanto S, et al. Malignancies, prothrombotic mutations, and the risk of venous thrombosis. *JAMA.* 2005;**293**(6):715–22.

67 Prandoni P, Lensing AW, Piccioli A, et al. Recurrent venous thromboembolism and bleeding complications during anticoagulant treatment in patients with cancer and venous thrombosis. *Blood.* 2002;**100**(10):3484–88.

68 Hutten BA, Prins MH, Gent M, et al. Incidence of recurrent thromboembolic and bleeding complications among patients with venous thromboembolism in relation to both malignancy and achieved international normalized ratio: a retrospective analysis. *J Clin Oncol.* 2000;**18**(17):3078–83.

69 Palareti G, Legnani C, Lee A, et al. A comparison of the safety and efficacy of oral anticoagulation for the treatment of venous thromboembolic disease in patients with or without malignancy. *Thromb Haemost.* 2000;84(5):805–10.

70 Calligaro KD, Bergen WS, Haut MJ, et al. Thromboembolic complications in patients with advanced cancer: anticoagulation versus Greenfield filter placement. *Ann Vasc Surg.* 1991;**5**(2):186–89.

71 Cantelmo NL, Menzoian JO, Logerfo FW, et al. Clinical experience with vena caval filters in high-risk cancer patients. *Cancer.* 1982;**50**(2):341–44.

72 Lossef SV, Barth KH. Outcome of patients with advanced neoplastic disease receiving vena caval filters. *J Vasc Interv Radiol.* 19950;**6**(2):273–77.

73 Greenfield LJ, Proctor MC, Saluja A. Clinical results of Greenfield filter use in patients with cancer. *Cardiovasc Surg.* 1997;**5**(2):145–49.

74 Cohen JR, Tenenbaum N, Citron M. Greenfield filter as primary therapy for deep venous thrombosis and/or pulmonary embolism in patients with cancer. *Surgery.* 1991;**109**(1):12–15.

75 Hubbard KP, Roehm JOJ, Abbruzzese JL. The Bird's Nest filter: an alternative to long-term oral anticoagulation in patients with advanced malignancies. *Am J Clin Oncol.* 1994;**17**(2):115–17.

76 Muchmore JH, Dunlap JN, Culicchia F, et al. Deep vein thrombophlebitis and pulmonary embolism in patients with malignant gliomas. *South Med J.* 1989;**82**(11):1352–56.

77 Whitney BA, Kerstein MD. Thrombocytopenia and cancer: use of the Kim-Ray Greenfield filter to prevent thromboembolism. *South Med J.* 1987;**80**(10):1246–48.

78 Cohen JR, Grella L, Citron M. Greenfield filter instead of heparin as primary treatment for deep venous thrombosis or pulmonary embolism in patients with cancer. *Cancer.* 1992;**70**(7):1993–96.

79 Walsh DB, Downing S, Nauta R, et al. Metastatic cancer: a relative contraindication to vena caval filter placement. *Cancer.* 1987;**59**:161–63.

80 Rosen MP, Porter DH, Kim D. Reassessment of vena caval filter use in patients with cancer. *J Vasc Interv Radiol.* 1994;**5**(3):501–6.

81 Schwarz RE, Marrero AM, Conlon KC, et al. Inferior vena cava filters in cancer patients: indications and outcome. *J Clin Oncol.* 1996;**14**(2):652–57.

82 Ihnat DM, Mills JL, Hughes JD, et al. Treatment of patients with venous thromboembolism and malignant disease: should vena cava filter placement be routine? *J Vasc Surg.* 1998;**28**(5):800–7.

83 Jarrett BP, Dougherty MJ, Calligaro KD. Inferior vena cava filters in malignant disease.*J Vasc Surg.* 2002;**36**(4):704–7.

84 Wallace MJ, Jean JL, Gupta S, et al. Use of inferior vena caval filters and survival in patients with malignancy. *Cancer.* 2004;**101**(8):1902–7.

85 Zerati AE, Wolosker N, Yazbek G, et al. Vena cava filters in cancer patients: experience with 50 patients. *Clinics.* 2005;**60**(5):361–66.

86 Schunn C, Schunn GB, Hobbs G, et al. Inferior vena cava filter placement in late-stage cancer. *Vasc Endovascular Surg.* 2006;**40**(4):287–94.

87 Lee AY, Levine MN, Baker RI, et al. Low-molecular-weight heparin versus a coumarin for the prevention of recurrent venous thromboembolism in patients with cancer. *N Engl J Med.* 2003;**349**(2):146–53.

88 Norris CS, Greenfield LJ, Herrmann JB. Free-floating iliofemoral thrombus: a risk of pulmonary embolism. *Arch Surg.* 1985;120:806–8.

89 Voet D, Afschrift M. Floating thrombi: diagnosis and follow-up by duplex ultrasound. *Br J Radiol.* 1991;**64**:1010–14.

90 Baldridge ED, Martin MA, Welling RE. Clinical significance of free-floating venous thrombi. *J Vasc Surg.* 1990;**11**:62–9.

91 Radomski JS, Jarrell BE, Carabasi RA, et al. Risk of pulmonary embolus with inferior vena cava thrombosis. *Am Surg.* 1987;**53**:97–101.

92 Berry RE, George JE, Shaver WA. Free-floating thrombus: a retrospective analysis. *Ann Surg.* 1990;**211**:719–23.

93 Monreal M, Ruiz J, Salvador R, et al. Recurrent pulmonary embolism: a prospective study. *Chest.* 1989;**95**:976–79.

94 Pacouret G, Alison D, Pottier J-M, et al. Free-floating thrombus and embolic risk in patients with angiographically confirmed proximal deep venous thrombosis: a prospective study. *Arch Int Med.* 1997;**157**: 305–8.

95 Patel RK, Ramasamy K, Goss D, et al. Ambulatory therapy of patients with free-floating proximal deep vein thrombosis is safe. *Thromb Haemost.* 2005;**94**(6):1343–44.

96 Santry HP, Gillen DL, Lauderdale DS. Trends in bariatric surgical procedures. *JAMA.* 2005;**294**(15):1909–17.

97 Carmody BJ, Sugerman HJ, Kellum JM, et al. Pulmonary embolism complicating bariatric surgery: detailed analysis of a single institution's 24-year experience. *J Am Coll Surg.* 2006;**203**(6):831–37.

98 Poulose BK, Griffin MR, Zhu Y, et al. National analysis of adverse patient safety for events in bariatric surgery. *Am Surg.* 2005;**71**(5):406–13.

99 Gargiulo NJ III, Veith FJ, Lipsitz EC, et al. Experience with inferior vena cava filter placement in patients undergoing open gastric bypass procedures. *J Vasc Surg.* 2006;**44**(6):1301–5.

100 Schuster R, Hagedorn JC, Curet MJ, et al. Retrievable inferior vena cava filters may be safely applied in gastric bypass surgery. *Surg Endosc.* 2007;**21**:2277–9.

101 Ferrell A, Byrne TK, Robison JG. Placement of inferior vena cava filters in bariatric surgical patients—possible indications and technical considerations. *Obes Surg.* 2004;**14**(6):738–43.

102 Piano G, Ketteler ER, Prachand V, et al. Safety, feasibility, and outcome of retrievable vena cava filters in high-risk surgical patients. *J Vasc Surg.* 2007;**45**(4):784–88.
103 Keeling WB, Haines K, Stone PA, et al. Current indications for preoperative inferior vena cava filter insertion in patients undergoing surgery for morbid obesity. *Obes Surg.* 2005;**15**(7):1009–12.
104 Prystowsky JB, Morasch MD, Eskandari MK, et al. Prospective analysis of the incidence of deep venous thrombosis in bariatric surgery patients. *Surgery.* 2005;**138**(4):759–63.
105 Scholten DJ, Hoedema RM, Scholten SE. A comparison of two different prophylactic dose regimens of low molecular weight heparin in bariatric surgery. *Obes Surg.* 2002;**12**(1):19–24.
106 Hamad GG, Choban PS. Enoxaparin for thromboprophylaxis in morbidly obese patients undergoing bariatric surgery: findings of the prophylaxis against VTE outcomes in bariatric surgery patients receiving enoxaparin (PROBE) study. *Obes Surg.* 2005;**15**(10):1368–74.
107 Johnson SP, Raiken DP, Grebe PJ, et al. Single institution prospective evaluation of the over-the-wire Greenfield vena caval filter. *J Vasc Interv Radiol.* 1998;**9**(5):766–73.
108 Teitelbaum GP, Bradley WG Jr., Klein BD. MR imaging artifacts, ferromagnetism, and magnetic torque of intravascular filters, stents, and coils. *Radiology.* 1988;**166**(3):657–64.
109 Watanabe AT, Teitelbaum GP, Gomes AS, et al. MR imaging of the bird's nest filter. *Radiology.* 1990;**177**(2):578–79.
110 Teitelbaum GP, Ortega HV, Vinitski S, et al. Low-artifact intravascular devices: MR imaging evaluation. *Radiology.* 1988;**168**(3):713–19.
111 Grassi CJ, Matsumoto AH, Teitelbaum GP. Vena caval occlusion after Simon nitinol filter placement: identification with MR imaging in patients with malignancy. *J Vasc Interv Radiol.* 1992;**3**(3):535–39.
112 Kim D, Edelman RR, Margolin CJ, et al. The Simon nitinol filter: evaluation by MR and ultrasound. *Angiology.* 1992;**43**(7):541–48.
113 Kiproff PM, Deeb ZL, Contractor FM, et al. Magnetic resonance characteristics of the LGM vena cava filter: technical note. Cardiovasc Intervent Radiol. 1991;**14**(4):254–55.
114 Pengo V, Lensing AW, Prins MH, et al. Incidence of chronic thromboembolic pulmonary hypertension after pulmonary embolism. *N Engl J Med.* 2004;**350**(22):2257–64.
115 Jamieson SW, Nomura K. Indications for and the results of pulmonary thromboendarterectomy for thromboembolic pulmonary hypertension. *Semin Vasc Surg.* 2000;**13**(3):236–44.
116 Bonderman D, Skoro-Sajer N, Jakowitsch J, et al. Predictors of outcome in chronic thromboembolic pulmonary hypertension. *Circulation.* 2007;**115**(16):2153–58.
117 Mo M, Kapelanski DP, Mitruka SN, et al. Reoperative pulmonary thromboendarterectomy. *Ann Thorac Surg.* 1999;**68**(5):1770–76.
118 Geerts WH, Heit JA, Clagett GP, et al. Prevention of venous thromboembolism. *Chest.* 2001;**119**(1 Suppl):132S–75S.
119 White RH, Romano PS, Zhou H, et al. Incidence and time course of thromboembolic outcomes following total hip or knee arthroplasty. *Arch Intern Med.* 1998;**158**(14):1525–31.
120 Bicalho PS, Hozack WJ, Rothman RH, et al. Treatment of early symptomatic pulmonary embolism after total joint arthroplasty. *J Arthroplasty.* 1996;**11**(5):522–24.
121 Emerson RHJ, Cross R, Head WC. Prophylactic and early therapeutic use of the Greenfield filter in hip and knee joint arthroplasty. *J Arthroplasty.* 1991;**6**(2):129–35.
122 Vaughn BK, Knezevich S, Lombardi AVJ, et al. Use of the Greenfield filter to prevent fatal pulmonary embolism associated with total hip and knee arthroplasty. *J Bone Joint Surg Am.* 1989;**71**(10):1542–48.
123 Woolson ST, Harris WH. Greenfield vena caval filter for management of selected cases of venous thromboembolic disease following hip surgery. *Clin Orthoped Rel Res.* 1986;**204**:201–6.
124 Kearon C, Hirsh J. Management of anticoagulation before and after elective surgery. *N Engl J Med.* 1997;**336**(21):1506–11.
125 Heit JA, Kobbervig CE, James AH, et al. Trends in the incidence of venous thromboembolism during pregnancy or postpartum: a 30-year population-based study. *Ann Intern Med.* 2005;**143**(10):697–706.
126 Cerneca F, Ricci G, Simeone R. Coagulation and fibrinolysis changes in normal pregnancy: increased levels of procoagulants and reduced levels of inhibitors during pregnancy induce a hypercoagulable state, combined with a reactive fibrinolysis. *Eur J Obstet Gynecol Reprod Biol.* 1997;**73**(1):31–36.
127 Clark P, Brennand J, Conkie JA, et al. Activated protein C sensitivity, protein C, protein S and coagulation in normal pregnancy. *Thromb Haemost.* 1998;**79**(6):1166–70.
128 Gates S. Thromboembolic disease in pregnancy. *Curr Opin Obstet Gynecol.* 2000;**12**(2):117–22.
129 Bates SM, Ginsberg JS. How we manage venous thromboembolism during pregnancy. *Blood.* 2002;**100**(10):3470–78.
130 Aburahma AF, Boland JP. Management of deep vein thrombosis of the lower extremity in pregnancy: a challenging dilemma. *Am Surg.* 1999;**65**(2):164–67.
131 Aburahma AF, Mullins DA. Endovascular caval interruption in pregnant patients with deep vein thrombosis of the lower extremity. *J Vasc Surg.* 2001;**33**(2):375–78.
132 Banfield PJ, Pittam M, Marwood R. Recurrent pulmonary embolism in pregnancy managed with the Greenfield vena caval filter. *Int J Gynaecol Obstet.* 1990;**33**(3):275–78.
133 Narayan H, Cullimore J, Krarup K, et al. Experience with the cardial inferior vena cava filter as prophylaxis against pulmonary embolism in pregnant women with extensive deep venous thrombosis. *Br J Obstet Gynaecol.* 1992;**99**(8):637–40.
134 Neill AM, Appleton DS, Richards P. Retrievable inferior vena caval filter for thromboembolic disease in pregnancy [see comments]. *Br J Obstet Gynaecol.* 1997;**104**(12):1416–18.
135 Owen RJ, Krarup KC. Case report: the successful use and removal of the Gunther Tulip inferior vena caval filter in pregnancy. *Clin Radiol.* 1997;**52**(3):241–43.
136 Bates SM, Greer IA, Hirsh J, et al. Use of antithrombotic agents during pregnancy: the Seventh ACCP Conference on Antithrombotic and Thrombolytic Therapy. *Chest.* 2004;**126**(3 Suppl):627S–44S.
137 Arnesen H, Hoiseth A, Ly B. Streptokinase of heparin in the treatment of deep vein thrombosis: follow-up results of a prospective study. *Acta Med Scand.* 1982;**211**(1–2):65–8.
138 Elliot MS, Immelman EJ, Jeffery P, et al. A comparative randomized trial of heparin versus streptokinase in the treatment of acute proximal venous thrombosis: an interim report of a prospective trial. *Br J Surg.* 1979;**66**(12):838–43.
139 Elsharawy M, Elzayat E. Early results of thrombolysis vs anticoagulation in iliofemoral venous thrombosis. a randomised clinical trial. *Eur J Vasc Endovasc Surg.* 2002;**24**(3):209–14.

140 Grossman C, McPherson S. Safety and efficacy of catheter-directed thrombolysis for iliofemoral venous thrombosis. *AJR Am J Roentgenol.* 1999;**172**(3):667–72.

141 Mewissen MW, Seabrook GR, Meissner MH, et al. Catheter-directed thrombolysis for lower extremity deep venous thrombosis: report of a national multicenter registry. *Radiology.* 1999;**211**(1):39–49.

142 Grimm W, Schwieder G, Wagner T. Fatal pulmonary embolism in venous thrombosis of the leg and pelvis during lysis therapy. *Dtsch Med Wochenschr.* 1990;**115**(31–32):1183–87.

143 Martin M, Eickerling B. Todliche lungenembolie unter ultrahochdosierter Streptokinase-Behandlung. *Dtsch Med Wochenschr.* 1990;**115** (47):1812.

144 Lorch H, Welger D, Wagner V, et al. Current practice of temporary vena cava filter insertion: a multicenter registry. *J Vasc Interv Radiol.* 2000;**11**(1):83–8.

145 Protack CD, Bakken AM, Patel N, et al. Long-term outcomes of catheter directed thrombolysis for lower extremity deep venous thrombosis without prophylactic inferior vena cava filter placement. *J Vasc Surg.* 2007;**45**(5):992–97.

13 Management of Venous Thromboembolism in Pregnancy

Wee-Shian Chan

Questions

A. Diagnosis of venous thromboembolism (VTE) in pregnancy
   i. How do I diagnosis deep venous thrombosis (DVT) in pregnancy? Is there a role for D-dimer testing for DVT diagnosis in pregnancy?
   ii. How do I diagnosis pulmonary embolism (PE) in pregnancy? Do I use ventilation-perfusion scan or spiral computed tomography?

B. How do I treat VTE in pregnancy?
   i. Do I use unfractionated heparin (UH) or low-molecular-weight heparin (LMWH)?
   ii. How do I "weight-dose" my patient on LMWH?
   iii. How long should I treat for?
   iv. How do I manage anticoagulant in the peripartum period?

C. How do I manage thromboprophylaxis in pregnant patients?
   i. With prosthetic heart valves?
   ii. With one previous episode of DVT?
   iii. With previous adverse pregnancy outcome and thrombophilia?

Introduction

The risk of venous thromboembolism, or VTE (both DVT and PE) is increased tenfold during pregnancy (1–4), compared with age-matched non-pregnant women (3). The absolute risk of DVT or PE in pregnancy is nevertheless low, at 0.5 to 1 in 1,000 pregnancies (1–4). This risk, however, is increased in the postpartum period (1–4) and is dependent on the mode of delivery. Studies from four large population-based studies revealed that the risk of VTE is 0.9–7.5 per 10,000 patients for vaginal deliveries, compared with 7.8–59 per 10,000 patients for cesarean sections (1–4).

The increased risk of VTE during pregnancy might be a result of changes in the hemostatic and fibrinolytic systems (5,6), with increased levels of coagulation factors, such as fibrinogen and factor VIII (5) and decreased levels of coagulation inhibitors, such as protein S detected (6). In addition to changes in the coagulation system, physiological alterations during pregnancy cause venous stasis that could predispose to venous thrombosis (7–9). There is increased lower extremity venous diameter and decreased flow, likely because of hormonal influences on vascular tone and the compressive effects on the veins by the enlarging uterus (7,8). This latter physiological change, which is exaggerated for the left lower extremity venous system, could explain the resultant preponderance of left leg DVT observed during pregnancy (10).

The importance of VTE diagnosis and management during pregnancy cannot be overemphasized. In developed countries, VTE is still a major cause of maternal morbidity and mortality (11,12). Despite this, clinical studies of VTE management in pregnancy are few (13), and studies of VTE diagnosis are lacking.

In this chapter, data from studies in nonpregnant patients will be extrapolated to pregnant patients. Adopting results from those studies may be adequate for most clinical scenarios during pregnancy; however, as highlighted below, many questions remain unresolved. Grading of the quality of evidence and strengths of recommendations in this chapter are based on the guidelines proposed by the international Grading of Recommendations Assessment, Development, and Evaluation Working Group (GRADE), adopting the modification used by the American College of Chest Physicians that merges the very low and low categories of quality of evidence (see chapter 1).

Evidence-based Hematology. Edited by Mark A. Crowther, Jeff Ginsberg, Holger J. Schünemann, Ralph M. Meyer, and Richard Lottenberg.

A. Diagnosis of venous thromboembolism in pregnancy

i. Is there a role for D-dimer testing for DVT diagnosis in pregnancy?

Systematic search of the literature using PubMed and MeSH headings "DVT," Pregnancy, and "diagnosis" yielded four relevant studies in which the diagnosis of DVT was prospectively evaluated with objective testing (14–17). Two of these studies used impedance plethysmography (IPG) (14,15), and reported that pregnant women with suspected DVT can be managed safety following negative findings with IPG. This test is however, no longer used. The third study (16) was reported as an abstract and evaluated the use of D-dimer assay and compression leg ultrasound (CUS) in the diagnosis of DVT in pregnant women. This study reported that with negative D-dimer on initial presentation, a single CUS alone could be used to safely exclude DVT. The number of patients in this study is small ~50 patients, and the results need further validation. In a recently published study (also published as an abstract) (17), Chan et al. reported that D-dimer (whole-blood agglutination assay) was sensitive in excluding DVT in pregnant women (100%, 95% CI 77%–100%), and its specificity was 81/135 (60%, 95% CI 52 to 68%). In addition, the assay was specific enough to be used for at least two trimesters of pregnancy. Therefore, based on limited evidence from the literature with respect to DVT diagnosis in pregnant patients, our recommendations for diagnosis would be drawn from studies derived from non-pregnant patients.

Compression leg ultrasound (CUS) is studied extensively as the key diagnostic test for patients with symptomatic proximal DVTs (18), although it has never been evaluated prospectively in pregnant women. A pooled analysis of studies (18) investigating the test characteristics of CUS in the general population revealed that it is highly sensitive and specific for symptomatic proximal DVTs are 97% and 94%, respectively, when compared with the contrast venography (the gold standard). For DVTs isolated to the calf, this test is, however, less sensitive (18). Calf vein thromboses are significant because they make up about 20% of DVT in symptomatic patients, and 20% of them propagate proximally into the popliteal veins and have the potential to embolize (19). Although CUS is limited in its ability to diagnose calf DVT, the need for leg venography is safely obviated by performing serial testing with CUS over seven days (19), or with the use of other diagnostics tools like D-dimer testing or clinician's pretest probability (PTP). The use of clinician's PTP either based on "gestalt" or structured prediction rules and D-dimer testing in combination with CUS to aid in the diagnosis of DVT has been investigated prospectively in many studies (20–22). D-dimer testing, together with clinician's PTP (based on structured prediction rule) and CUS, can effectively exclude the presence of DVT on initial patient presentation, or identify patients who require further serial testing and other more invasive investigations (20–22). The use of both clinicians' PTP and D-dimer can therefore enhance the diagnostic sensitivity of a single CUS for DVT diagnosis in the general population. The use of Wells prediction rule (23) for assessing clinician's PTP has not been formally evaluated in pregnant women. Some of the presenting signs used to develop the prediction rule (e.g., leg edema) may be too poorly specific for use in pregnant women. Therefore, the generalizability of this prediction rule to pregnant women is uncertain.

D-dimer levels are known to increase with progressive trimesters of pregnancy, preterm labor, and hypertensive disorders during pregnancy (24–26). Studies investigating the utility of previously validated D-dimer assays for VTE diagnosis in nonpregnant patients (rapid ELISA-based, latex agglutination, and whole-blood agglutination assay) have reported mixed results for pregnant women (27–29). Expectedly, the more sensitive assays, at the current "cutoffs" (ELISA, latex agglutination) had poorer specificity in asymptomatic pregnant women; this was, however, not the case for the less sensitive whole-blood agglutination assay (27–29). Although this latter assay demonstrates promise for VTE diagnosis in pregnant women, the number of pregnant women managed prospectively using this assay to date is low (17); wide application of this assay for pregnant women should still be done with caution, as missing the diagnosis of DVT in pregnant carries serious consequences.

Currently, we recommend serial CUS in pregnant women with suspected DVT, at least over seven days (days 3 and 7) to ensure that significant disease does not go undiagnosed (Grade 1B) (Figure 13.1). However, in the case where DVT is highly

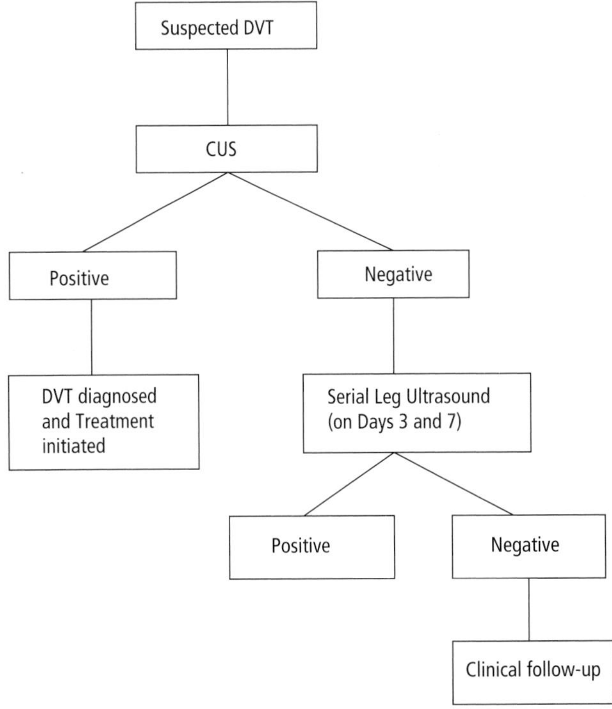

Figure 13.1 Diagnostic algorithm for the diagnosis of deep venous thrombosis (DVT) in pregnant patient.

suspicious (e.g., asymmetrically swollen and discolored leg), clinicians should consider further testing with magnetic resonance imaging, venography, or computed tomography (**Grade 1C**). D-dimer testing alone should not be used to dictate management (Grade 2B).

ii. How do I diagnosis pulmonary embolism (PE) in pregnancy? Do I use ventilation-perfusion scan or spiral computed tomography?

Systematic search of the literature using PubMed and MeSH headings "PE," "pregnancy," and "diagnosis" yielded one relevant study in which the diagnosis of PE was evaluated with objective testing (30).

In the retrospective study (30), Chan et al., reported on 120 pregnant women who had ventilation-perfusion (VQ) scanning during pregnancy. The prevalence of normal, nondiagnostic, and high-probability scans were strikingly different in 120 of these pregnant women compared with the nonpregnant population; pregnant women with suspected PE were more likely to have normal scans (74%) and less likely to have high-probability scans (2%) compared with 33% and 10%, respectively, in nonpregnant patients (31,32). This finding likely results from the fact that pregnant women are younger and tend to have less comorbid conditions that the general population. The subsequent follow-up conducted on 104 of these women with normal (n = 80) and nondiagnostic scans (n = 24) who did not receive anticoagulation, revealed that no VTE events were reported, and hence the likelihood of PE in these group of patients is low. Although these results from this retrospective review is reassuring with respect to the use of VQ scan in pregnant women, data surrounding the role of ancillary tests like CUS, clinician's prior impression, or D-dimer testing cannot be derived from this study. Therefore, data from studies in nonpregnant patients would be used to aid our recommendation (33–35).

The major concern surrounding the use of VQ scanning in pregnancy is, perhaps, fetal radiation. From epidemiological studies, the risk of radiation to the developing fetus is greatest when the fetal radiation dose exceeds 50–100 milliGray (mGy) (36); above this level, the risk of childhood malignancies may be increased. The risk of malformations or pregnancy losses with radiation doses of <50 mGy is likely low, although evidence is lacking (36). Regardless, the fetal radiation dose associated with VQ scanning is low (Table 13.1) (37), and does not exceed one-tenth of the threshold for childhood malignancies. From the study by Chan et al. (30), follow-up conducted on all live births revealed no increased risk of childhood malignancies or malformations in women exposed to VQ scanning while pregnant, and the rate of fetal losses did not differ significantly from those expected for the population (30).

Increasingly, spiral CT scan is becoming the primary diagnostic modality for PE (38,39). Spiral CT scanning is sensitive and specific for PE in the segmental arteries, but less sensitive for PE in the subsegmental arteries (39); in addition, many studies using spiral CT scan as the primary imaging modality have reported that this test can be safely used to diagnose and exclude PE as part of a management strategy (38,40). The additional advantage of the spiral CT scan over VQ scan is that other nonthrombotic causes can be diagnosed in a single test.

Table 13.1 Estimated fetal radiation exposure associated with diagnostic procedures for DVT and PE in pregnant women.

Test	Fetal radiation dose (milliGrays)
Perfusion lung scan with ^{99m}TcMAA	
3 mCi	0.18
1–2 mCi	0.06–0.12
Ventilation lung scan	
^{99m}TcDTPA	0.07–0.35
^{99m}TcSC	0.01–0.05
Contrast venography	
Pulmonary angiography via femoral route	4.05
Pulmonary angiography via brachial route	<0.50
Spiral computed tomography*	
First trimester	0.003–0.02
Second trimester	0.008–0.077
Third trimester	0.051–0.131
Chest X-ray	<0.01

* From Winer-Muram HT, Boone JM, Brown HL, Jennings SG, Mabie WC, Lombardo GT. Pulmonary embolism in pregnant patients: fetal radiation dose with helical CT. *Radiology.* 2002;224(**2**):487–92.

However, like VQ scanning, spiral CT scan has never been prospectively evaluated in pregnant women, and there is currently little data to support its use in pregnant women as the first-line test. Although the calculated radiation risk to the fetus is low (41) (Table 13.1) and below the threshold recommended for pregnancy (36, 37), there are three major concerns with adopting spiral CT as the diagnostic test of choice in pregnancy or as the central diagnostic test in our current study: (a) the iodinated contrast agent, administered as part of the study can result in neonatal hypothyroidism, the degree to which this is clinically significant has not been evaluated (42), (b) unlike VQ scanning (30), we do not yet have any short- or long-term data on fetal or pregnancy outcomes in pregnant women exposed to CT scanning, (c) the calculated minimum radiation dose to each breast of an average 60-kg woman is 20 mGy (43). This dose is equivalent to the dose received from seven mammograms, and is at least twice greater than the dose received from VQ scanning (<10 mGy). Increasingly, there is data linking an increased risk of breast cancer to diagnostic imaging procedures (44). Although the individual risk of breast cancer attributed to a single test cannot yet be defined from current studies, one must certainly be concerned with unnecessary breast radiation exposure especially when a clear alternative is still available. The use of spiral CT scan should be limited to specific situations in which information cannot be obtained from VQ scanning alone.

Our approach or PE diagnosis in pregnant women is shown in Figure 13.2 (Grade 1C). When PE is suspected, initial testing with CUS should be considered. Although the likelihood of asymptomatic DVT is likely low—if DVT is diagnosed, VQ scanning can

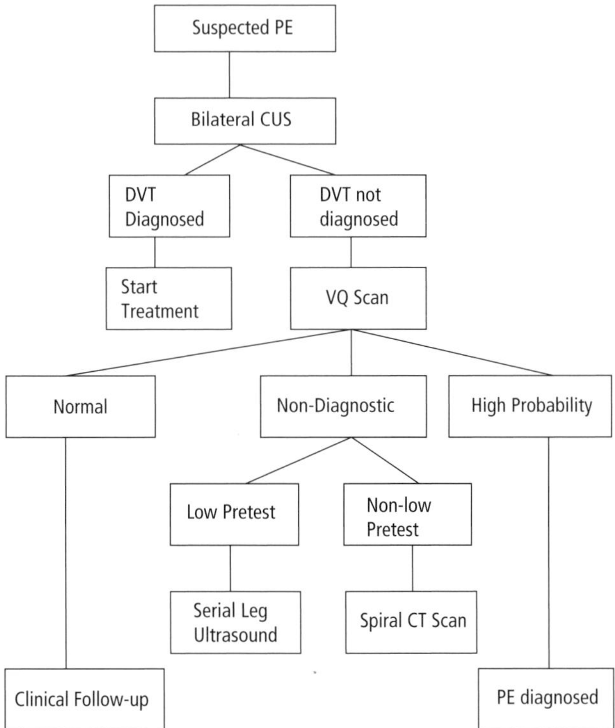

Figure 13.2 Diagnostic algorithm for the diagnosis of pulmonary embolism (PE) in pregnant patient.

be negated. If CUS is negative, a VQ scan or perfusion-only scan should be performed.

Based on the results of the VQ scan, no further testing is needed (if normal) or anticoagulation should be initiated (if high). In the situation when a scan is nondiagnostic, clinicians may elect to either proceed with spiral CT scan or with serial CUS testing alone (**Grade 1C**), based on clinical suspicion and presence of risk factors.

B. How do I treat VTE in pregnancy?

An initial search of the literature using PubMed and MeSH headings "pregnancy" and "unfractionated heparin" or "LMWH," applying the following limits: English, Clinical Trial, Meta-Analysis, Randomized Controlled Trial, Review, Case Reports, Female, Humans, yielded more than 600 articles; no clinical trials of LMWH or UH use for the treatment of venous thromboembolism in pregnancy were found. On closer scrutiny of the abstracts, there were three systematic reviews of the literature (45–47) involving LMWH use in pregnancy and one involving UH use in pregnancy (48). In addition, there was a large retrospective analysis, involving several hundred pregnant women exposed to LMWH (49). Several studies investigated the pharmacokinetics of LMWH in pregnant women (50–59), and other studies (mostly case reports and series) reported on the adverse effects of LMWH or UH in pregnant women (60–63).

i. Do I use UH or LMWH?

For many reasons, LMWH has supplanted UH as the anticoagulant of choice during pregnancy. LMWH, like UH, does not cross the placenta and hence is unlikely to cause teratogenicity in the developing fetus (64–66). Several large reviews of LMWH use in pregnant women have been published confirming the safety of LMWH exposure to the developing fetus (45–47,49). These reviews, however, do not confer superiority of one LMWH preparation over another. The advantage of LMWH over UH is clear: LMWHs are associated with a low risk of heparin-induced thrombocytopenia, 0% in over 2,000 pregnancies (47), low risk of osteoporosis—0.04% (95% confidence interval [CI] 0%–0.2%) (47), and low risk of bleeding—1.98% (95%CI 1.5%–2.5%) (47). However, like UH, LMWH use can result in erythematous cutaneous plaques at injection sites (1.8% 95% CI 1.3%–2.4%) (47). When these lesions appear, underlying heparin-induced thrombocytopenia (HIT) should be ruled out before a cautious switch to another preparation of LMWH (62) or danaparoid is made (67); even so, cross-reactivity to danaparoid and other LMWH have also been reported (68).

Although the efficacy of LMWH for pregnant women with acute VTE has not been evaluated in a clinical trial, based on clinical studies in nonpregnant patients, LMWH can be used to treat pregnant women with acute VTE (**Grade 1B**).

ii. How do I "weight-dose" my patient on LMWH, and do I need to monitor anti-Xa levels?

The LMWH dose administered is based on patient's weight (per manufacturer's recommendation). As the pregnancy progresses, it remains unclear if dose adjustment is needed based on changes in patient's weight, volume of distribution or renal excretion rate (68).

Several prospective cohort studies which followed anti-Xa levels three to four hours postinjection (therapeutic LMWH for acute VTE) have yielded mixed results (target peak 0.5–1.0 U/mL); Rodie et al. (58) reported (enoxaparin 1 mg/kg sc bid) that 3/33 women required dose reduction based on peak anti-Xa > 1.0 U/mL, Barbour et al. (57) (dalteparin 100 IU/kg bid) reported that 85% of pregnancies (11/13) required upward dose adjustment, and did Jacobsen et al. (56) (dalteparin 100 IU/kg bid who reported that 69% (9/13) of women required dose escalation. It is difficult to conclude from these small studies if dose-adjustment is needed or if anti-Xa monitoring is required at all (69). However, pharmacokinetic studies, on women on low-dose LMWH (51,53,54) do suggest that twice a day dosing may be superior to once daily dosing in pregnancy.

Therefore, we recommend that if LMWH is used to manage acute VTE in pregnancy, it should be administered as a once or twice daily dose based on weight (Grade 1C). With respect to ongoing dose-adjustment, one of three options can be adopted (Grade 1C): (a) no change be made once therapeutic dosing is initiated based on patient's weight, (b) perform monthly anti-Xa levels three to four hours postinjection, and adjust LMWH doses appropriately to target anti-Xa level 0.5–1.0 U/mL, or (c) adjust the LMWH doses as patient's weight increases.

iii. How do I manage anticoagulant around labor and delivery?

For patients receiving "therapeutic" doses of LMWH, induction of labor at term usually occurs to avoid the issues surrounding the use of neuraxial anagelsia (70). The last dose of LMWH is administered at least 24 hours prior to the planned induction (70) (Grade 1C). If spontaneous labor occurs within 12 hours after LMWH administration, or if emergent cesarean section is required within 12 hours after LMWH administration, neuraxial procedures should be avoided and alternate analgesia and anesthesia (i.e., general) be considered (70). It is often our practice to have these women be counseled by our anesthesia colleagues prior to term. In cases where excessive intrapatum bleeding results from the recent use of LMWH, protamine sulphate could be considered for partial reversibility of anticoagulant effects (71).

In certain high-risk situations whereby the risk of thromboembolic complications are high, such as acute VTE (less than four weeks), "bridging" anticoagulation with intravenous unfractionated heparin could be considered in the days prior to induction, and discontinued four to six hours after the onset of active labor to minimize "time-off" anticoagulation (Grade 1C). Alternately, a temporary filter could be considered (72) (Grade 2B).

For women in whom ongoing anticoagulant therapy is required in the postpartum period (i.e., those who develop active VTE in the antepartum), resumption of LMWH administration should only be considered six to eight hours after the removal of the catheter for neuraxial anagelsia (70) and if the risk of postpartum hemorrhage (in consultation with the obstetrical team) is minimal. In practice, LMWH is resumed 12 to 24 hours after delivery (Grade 1C).

The use of vitamin K antagonists (VKA), like coumadin, in the postpartum period is not contraindicated for breast-feeding (73).

iv. How long should I treat for?

The length of treatment with therapeutic LMWH during pregnancy for active VTE is unknown. Once VTE is diagnosed during pregnancy, therapeutic dosing with either adjusted-dose LMWH or UH should be initiated (74), followed by adjusted-dose UH or LMWH for at least three months or the duration of the pregnancy and for six weeks postpartum (74) (Grade 1C). From studies in nonpregnant patients with underlying malignancy (75) or with contraindications to anticoagulation (76), reducing intensity of anticoagulation after a period of therapeutic anticoagulation is safe (75,76). Although there are no clinical studies designed to address this specific issue in pregnancy, reducing the treatment doses after three months to prophylactic dosing, instead of maintaining therapeutic dosing till term, may be a reasonable option, particularly if the risk of bleeding (e.g., presence of placenta previa) is a concern (Grade 2C).

C. Thromboprophylaxis

i. How do I manage pregnant women with prosthetic heart valves?

A systematic search was made of PubMed for the past 10 years with respect to the management of prosthetic heart valves in pregnancy using MeSH headings "Prosthetic heart valves" and "pregnancy" from 1997 to March 2007. Our search yielded 10 relevant articles (77–86): case-reports, case-series, and cohorts of pregnant women with prosthetic heart valves managed during pregnancy. Although LMWH is more commonly used to manage these patients in the past decade instead of UH, there are now reported cases of valve thromboses in the pregnant women managed with LMWH; a recent review of the literature summarized this experience (87). There are still no published clinical trials on the efficacy of LMWH versus oral anticoagulants for the management of these patients during pregnancy.

The management of pregnant women remains problematic because of the need for therapeutic anticoagulation throughout pregnancy to prevent valve thrombosis and the lack of clinical trials to guide management for these women. The choices of anticoagulant therapy—UH, VKA, or LMWH—are all associated with risks to either the mother or the developing fetus.

In a pooled analysis of cohort and case-series studies (88), the use of warfarin (or VKA) is associated with fetal embryopathy (6.4%) and spontaneous losses (24.8%). Avoiding the use of warfarin between 6 and 12 weeks gestation age could negate the risk of warfarin embryopathy entirely (88); however, its use beyond the first trimester could still result in mild neurological impairment, as detected in school-age children exposed to in utero VKA (89). The use of both UH or LMWH during pregnancy is associated with minimal fetal risks (46,47,48); the major concern with the use of these two agents for prosthetic heart valve thromboprophylaxis during pregnancy is, however, their efficacy (87,88).

The use of UH for valve thromboprophylaxis is associated with valve thrombosis, even in adjusted doses (88). Although LMWH offers more predictable bioavailability and easier weight-based dosing, there are now increasing cases of valve thrombosis, associated with its use (87). Oran et al. (89) reported in a review that in 81 pregnancies managed with LMWH, the proportion of valve thrombosis was 8.84% (95% CI 2.52–14.76), the frequency of overall thromboembolic complications was 12.35% (95% CI 5.19%–19.51%). Among women who had factor Xa monitoring, only one patient had a thromboembolic event; among those women who had complications, 10 were on a fixed dose of LMWH, while one was on a low dose. The concern with LMWH use heightened further after a small randomized control trial was discontinued prematurely because two of the seven women treated with LMWH (versus warfarin therapy) developed valve thrombosis resulting in maternal deaths (74). This study also resulted in labeling changes and warnings against the use of LMWH for this cohort of patients.

Whether LMWH was efficacious in providing effective thromboprophylaxis to patients with prosthetic heart valves was examined by an expert panel recently (90). The panel reviewed studies on the use of LMWH for "bridging" anticoagulation in over 1,000 nonpregnant patients and reported that LMWH was effective for preventing valve thrombosis, at least during the short-term period of use. Pregnant women may be at higher risk of thrombosis because of "prothrombotic" tendencies and physiological changes altering the "bioavailability" of LMWH from changes in plasma volume and renal excretion (90). Currently, none of these theories can be adequately proved.

Based on the evidence from nonpregnant patients and the known risks associated with warfarin therapy during pregnancy, one of two approaches (74) could be considered in the management of thromboprophylaxis during pregnancy:

a. Adjusted-dose twice a day dosing with LMWH throughout pregnancy to keep a four-hour postinjection anti-Xa heparin level at 1.0–1.2 U/mL (Grade 1C).

b. LMWH (does adjusted) until 13 weeks gestational age, switch to warfarin until mid-third trimester, then resume LMWH till delivery (Grade 1C).

The addition of low-dose aspirin (75–162 mg/d) ((Grade 2C) should be considered if other high-risk features are present, for example, multiple prosthetic valves, atrial fibrillation, or history of previous thromboses.

For women who are on VKA, and who are considering pregnancy, a switch can be made to therapeutic dosing of LMWH and VKA discontinued prior to pregnancy. Alternatively, the patient can remain on VKA until pregnancy is achieved (detected on blood test), and a switch to LMWH can then be made (Grade 2C).

ii. My patient had a previous DVT and now wishes to get pregnant. Does she need thromboprophylaxis?

Women with a previous history of VTE are at an increased risk of recurrence during pregnancy. The risk of recurrent events have been reported to be between 0% and 13% (74). From a recent large retrospective cohort study of pregnant women (91), the risk of recurrent VTE was reported to be 6.2% (95% CI 1.6%–10.9%) in women who did not receive thromboprophylaxis during pregnancy compared with no women who did; the risk of VTE was also higher in this cohort of patients—5.2%, in the postpartum period. In an earlier prospective cohort study, Brill-Edwards et al. (92) reported that managing these women with no antepartum thromboprophlaxis therapy, but postpartum thromboprophylaxis for four to six weeks after, resulted in an overall recurrence rate of 2.4% (95% CI 0.2%–6.9%). Most of the recurrences occurred in women with thrombophilia or who had a previous unprovoked VTE (5.5%, 95 CI 1.2%–16%) compared with no women (95% CI 0%–8%) who did not have thrombophilia and had a previously provoked VTE.

With a lack of randomized controlled trials, these studies suggest that although the risk of VTE is increased in women with a previous history of VTE, antepartum thromboprophylaxis may not always be needed. For patients with a single event from transient risk factors (i.e., injury) and who does not have associated thrombophilia—antepartum thromboprophylaxis may not be necessary (Grade 2A). However, for all other patients—in the presence of thrombophilia, history of "unprovoked" or "estrogen-related" VTE events, antepartum thromboprophylaxis could be considered (Grade 1C).

The choice of thromboprophylactic therapy in the antepartum period would be low-dose LMWH or UH. For all women with a single unprovoked episode of VTE, postpartum thromboprophylaxis should be considered for four to six weeks after delivery.

iii. My patient was tested for inherited thrombophilia after one unsuccessful pregnancy. She does not have a previous venous thromboembolic event. Her obstetrician wants her to be on LMWH now that she is pregnant again. What do I do?

A search of PubMed for articles published in the past five years (March 2002–March 2007) using PubMed and MeSH headings "pregnancy" and "thrombophilia" yielded more than 700 articles. The abstracts of the articles were screened. There were at least 36 case-control studies investigating thrombophilias and adverse pregnancy outcomes. There were seven systematic reviews (93–99) in this area and three cohort studies (100–102) and one randomized trial (40 mg/d versus 80 mg/d of enoxaparin) (103) investigating the possible role of treatment in the secondary prevention of adverse pregnancy outcomes in patients with thrombophilia.

The findings from the seven systematic reviews (published between 2002 and 2006) of mostly case-control or cohort studies of the literature are consistent: the presence of thrombophilia is associated with adverse pregnancy events: early pregnancy losses (odds ratio [OR] 1.40–6.25), late pregnancy losses (ORs 1.31–20.09), pre-eclampsia (OR 1.37–3.49), intrauterine growth restriction (OR 1.24–2.92), and placental abruption (OR 1.42–7.71). The magnitude of association with various types of thrombophilic disorders however differs. The strength of association appears to be greatest with factor V Leiden (FVL) (97); it is associated with early recurrent fetal loss (2.01, 95% CI 1.13–3.58), late recurrent fetal loss, and stillbirths (3.26, 95% CI 1.82–5.83) and with the presence of prothrombin G20210A mutation (early recurrent 2.32 [95% CI 1.12–4.79] and stillbirths [2.30, 95% CI 1.09–4.87]). The evidence supporting the association of Protein S, Protein C, AT III deficiencies, and MTHFR 677 T genotype is weak (93–99). It is not known whether this association is nonexistent or that the number of patients with this defect is too small to provide any meaningful analysis. The presence of combined disorders (e.g., heterozygous FVL and MTHFR 677 CT) can enhance the risk of adverse outcomes such as stillbirth and pregnancy losses (105,106).

Several large, randomized-control studies are currently under way evaluating the effectiveness of thromboprophylaxis in preventing adverse pregnancy events in the presence of thrombophilia. The use of LMWH evaluated in the three small cohort studies of thrombophilic women with previous adverse pregnancy outcomes (100,101,102) was promising. In the Danish observational cohort study (100), the use of thromboprophylaxis in women with Protein C, S, or AT III deficiencies resulted in a reduced rate of fetal loss compared with deficient women who did not. From these studies, thromboprophylaxis may be beneficial for secondary prevention of adverse pregnancy outcomes. The magnitude of this prevention, however, is still unclear.

Women with inherited thrombophilia are also at increased risk of thrombosis in pregnancy (105–109); however, the absolute risks in most cases are small The estimated risk of VTE during pregnancy in patients with various thrombophilias (106): 1:500 for heterozygous FVL, 1:200 for heterozygous prothrombin G20210A mutation, 4.6:100 for double heterozygosity, 1:113 for protein C, 1:2.8 for Type I AT def, and 1:42 for Type II AT deficiency. The risk of VTE in homozygous FVL is reported to be 9%–16% (109). Double heterozygosity in FVL and prothrombin G20210A mutation is associated with an increased risk of VTE of 4% (95% CI 1.4–16.9).

The risk of VTE in pregnant women with homozygous MTHFR C677T is unknown, but hyperhomocysteinemia may be associated with VTE in the nonpregnant population (111). Homocysteine levels, however, are significantly lower in pregnancy because of physiological changes and with folate supplementation (112). Therefore, the need for thromboprophylactic measures with anticoagulant beyond folate supplementation may be unnecessary (112).

The decision to offer thromboprophylaxis based on the previous review would be

i. For women with previous pregnancy losses, who have inherited thrombophilia (FVL, prothrombin G20210A mutation, and Protein S, C, AT deficiencies), the use of low-dose LMWH may be appropriate throughout pregnancy for both the secondary prevention of pregnancy loss and VTE (Grade 2B).

ii. For women with MTHFR 677 TT, we suggest 5 mg of folate acid prior to conception or as soon as pregnancy is diagnosed (Grade 1C).

References

1 Lindqvist P, Dahlback B, Marsal K. Thrombotic risk during pregnancy: a population study. *Obstet Gynecol.* 1999;**94**:595–99.

2 Simpson EL, Lawrenson RA, Nightingale AL, et al. Venous thromboembolism in pregnancy and the puerperium: incidence and additional risk factors from a London perinatal database. *Br J Obstet Gynaecol.* 2001;**108**:56–60.

3 Macklon NS, Greer IA. Venous thromboembolic disease in obstetrics and gynaecology: the Scottish experience. *Scott Med J.* 1996;**41**:83–6.

4 Gherman RB, Goodwin TM, Leung B, et al. Incidence, clinical characteristics, and timing of objectively diagnosed venous thromboembolism during pregnancy. *Obstet Gynecol.* 1999;**94**:730–34.

5 Bonnar J. The blood coagulation and fibrinolytic system in the newborn and mother at birth. *Br L Obstet Gynecol.* 1971;**78**:355–60.

6 Comp PC, Thurnau GR, Welsh J, et al. Functional and immunologic protein S levels are decreased during pregnancy. *Blood.* 1986;**68**:881–85.

7 Cordts PR, Gawley TS. Anatomic and physiologic changes in lower extremity venous hemodynamics associated with pregnancy. *J Vasc Surg.* 1996;**24**:763–67.

8 Palmgren J, Kirkinen P. Venous circulation in the maternal lower limb: a Doppler study with the Valsalva maneuver. *Ultrasound Obstet Gynecol.* 1996;**8**:93–7.

9 Macklon NC, Greer IA, Bowman AW. An ultrasound study of gestational and postural changes in the deep venous system of the leg in pregnancy. *Br J Obstet Gynecol.* 1997;**104**:191–97.

10 Ray J, WS Chan. Deep vein thrombosis during pregnancy and puerperium: a meta-analysis of the period of risk and leg of presentation. *Obstet Gyn Surv.* 1999;**54**:265–71.

11 Sachs BP, Brown DA, Driscoll ST, et al. Maternal mortality in Massachusetts. Trends and prevention. *N Engl J Med.* 1987;**316**:607–72.

12 Report on confidential inquiries into maternal deaths for England and Wales 1979–1981. London: Her Majesty's Stationery Office, 1986.

13 Nijkeuter M, Ginsberg JS, Huisman MV. Diagnosis of deep vein thrombosis and pulmonary embolism in pregnancy: a systematic review. *J Thromb Haemost.* 2006;**4**(3):496–500. E-pub 2005 Dec 23.

14 Hull RD, Raskob GE, Carter CJ. Serial impedance plethysmography in pregnant patients with clinically suspected deep vein thrombosis. *Ann Intern Med.* 1990;**112**:663–67.

15 de Boer K, Buller HR, ten Cate JW, et al. Deep vein thrombosis in obstetric patients: diagnosis and risk factors. *Thromb Haemost.* 1992;**67**(1):4–7.

16 Chan WS, Chunilal S, Lee A, et al. A red blood cell agglutination D-dimer test to exclude deep venous thrombosis in pregnancy. *Ann Int Med.* 2007;**147**:165–70.

17 Chan WS, Chunilal SD, Lee AY, et al. Diagnosis of deep vein thrombosis during pregnancy: a pilot study evaluating the role of D-dimer and compression leg ultrasound during pregnancy. *Blood.* 2002;**100**: 275a.

18 Kearon C, Julian JA, Ginsberg JS, et al. Noninvasive diagnosis of deep venous thrombosis. *Ann Intern Med.* 1998;**128**:663–77.

19 Lohr JM, Kerr TM, Lutter KS, et al. Lower extremity calf thrombosis: to treat or not to treat? *J Vasc Surg.* 1991;**14**:618–23.

20 Bernardi E, Prandoni P, Lensing AW, et al. D-dimer testing as an adjunct to ultrasonography in patients with clinically suspected deep vein thrombosis: prospective cohort study. The Multicentre Italian D-dimer Ultrasound Study Investigators Group. *BMJ.* 1998;**317**(7165): 1037–40.

21 Perrier A, Desmaris S, Miron M-J, et al. Non-invasive diagnosis of venous thromboembolism in outpatients. *Lancet.* 1999;**353**:190–95.

22 Bates SM, Kearon C, Crowther M, et al. A diagnostic strategy involving a quantitative latex D-dimer assay reliably excludes deep venous thrombosis. *Ann Intern Med.* 2003;**138**(10):787–94.

23 Wells PS, Anderson DR, Bormanis J, et al. Value of assessment of pretest probability of deep-vein thrombosis in clinical management. *Lancet.* 1997;**350**:1795–98.

24 Nolan TE, Smith RP, Devoe LD. Maternal plasma D-dimer levels in normal and complicated pregnancies. *Obstet Gynecol.* 1993;**81**:235–38.

25 Proietti AB, Johnson MJ, Proietti FA, et al. Assessment of fibrin(nogen) dedradation products in preeclampsia using immunoblot enzyme-linked immunosorbent assay, and latex-bead agglutination. *Obstet Gynecol.* 1991;77:696–700.

26 Francalanci I, Comeglio P, Alessandrello A, et al. D-dimer concentrations during normal pregnancy, as measured by Elisa. *Thromb Res.* 1995;**78**:399–405.

27 Chan WS, SD Chunilal, Bates S, et al. The prevalence of positive soluble fibrin and D-dimer results in healthy asymptomatic pregnant women. *Blood.* 1999;**94**(10):20a.

28 Kline JA, Williams GW, Hernandez-Nino J. D-dimer concentrations in normal pregnancy: new diagnostic thresholds are needed. *Clin Chem.* 2005;**51**(5):825–29. E-pub 2005 Mar 11.

29 Morse M. Establishing a normal range for D-dimer levels through pregnancy to aid in the diagnosis of pulmonary embolism and deep vein thrombosis. *J Thromb Haemost.* 2004;**2**(7):1202–4.

30 Chan WS, Ray J, Coady G, et al. Clinical presentation of suspected pulmonary embolism during pregnancy, VQ lung scan: results, and subsequent maternal and pediatric outcomes. *Arch Intern Med.* 2002;**162**(10):1170–75.

31 Anonymous. Value of the ventilation/perfusion scan in acute pulmonary embolism: results of the prospective investigation of pulmonary embolism diagnosis (PIOPED). *JAMA.* 1990;**263**:2753–59.

32 Hull RD, Raskob GE, Coates G, et al. A new noninvasive management strategy for patients with suspected pulmonary embolism. *Arch Intern Med.* 1989;**149**:2549–55.

33 Wells PS, Ginsberg JS, Anderson DR, et al. Use of a clinical model for safe management of patients with suspected pulmonary embolism. *Ann Intern Med.* 1998;**129**:997–1005.

34 Kearon C, Ginsberg JS, Douketis J, et al. An evaluation of D-dimer in the diagnosis of pulmonary embolism: a randomized trial. *Ann Intern Med.* 2006;**144**(11):812–21.

35 Stein PD, Hull RD, Pineo G. Strategy that includes serial noninvasive leg tests for diagnosis of thromboembolic disease in patients with suspected acute pulmonary embolism based on data from PIOPED. Prospective Investigation of Pulmonary Embolism Diagnosis. *Arch Intern Med.* 1995;**155**(19):2101–4.

36 Doll R, Wakefield R. Risk of childhood cancer from fetal radiation. *Br J Radiol.* 1997;**70**:130–39.

37 Ginsberg JS, Hirsh J, Rainbow RJ. Risks to the fetus of radiologic procedures used in the diagnosis of maternal thromboembolic disease. *Thromb Haemost.* 1989;**61**:189–96.

38 Stein PD, Fowler SE, Goodman LR, et al. Multidetector computed tomography for acute pulmonary embolism. *N Engl J Med.* 2006;**354**(22):2317–27.

39 Mullins MD, Becker DM, Hagspiel KD, et al. The role of spiral volumetric computed computed tomography in the diagnosis of pulmonary embolism. *Arch Intern Med.* 2000;**160**:293–98.

40 Stein PD, Fowler SE, Goodman LR, et al. Multidetector computed tomography for acute pulmonary embolism. *N Engl J Med.* 2006;**354**(22):2317–27.

41 Hurwitz LM, Yoshizumi T, Reiman RE, et al. Radiation dose to the fetus from body MDCT during early gestation. *AJR Am J Roentgenol.* 2006;**186**(3):871–76.

42 Weber G, Vigone MC, Rapa A, et al. Neonatal transient hypothyroidism: aetiological study. Italian Collaborative Study on Transient Hypothyroidism. *Arch Dis Child Fetal Neonatal Ed.* 1998;**79**(1):F70–72.

43 Parker MS, Hui FK, Camacho MA, et al. Female breast radiation exposure during CT pulmonary angiography. *AJR Am J Roentgenol.* 2005;**185**:1228–33.

44 Berrington de Gonzalez A, Darby S. Risk of cancer from diagnostic X-rays: estimates for the UK and 14 other countries. *Lancet.* 2004;**363**:345–51.

45 WS Chan, Ray J. Low molecular weight heparin use in pregnancy: issues of safety and practicality. *Obstet Gynecol Surv.* 1999:**54**(10):649–54.

46 Sanson BJ, Lensing AWA, Prins MH, et al. Safety of low-molecular-weight heparin in pregnancy: a systematic review. *Thromb Haemost.* 1999;**81**:668–72.

47 Greer IA, Nelson-Piercy C. Low-molecular-weight heparins for thromboprophylaxis and treatment of venous thromboembolism in pregnancy: a systematic review of safety and efficacy. *Blood.* 2005;**106**(2):401–7. E-pub 2005 Apr 5. Review.

48 Ginsberg JS, Hirsh J. Anticoagulants during pregnancy. *Annu Rev Med.* 1989;**40**:79–86.

49 Lepercq J, Conard J, Borel-Derlon A, et al. Venous thromboembolism during pregnancy: a retrospective study of enoxaparin safety in 624 pregnancies. *Br J Obstet Gynaecol.* 2001;108(11):1134–40.

50 Blomback M, Bremme K, Hellgren M, et al. A pharmacokinetic study of dalteparin (Fragmin) during late pregnancy. *Blood Coagul Fibrinolysis.* 1998;**9**(4):343–50.

51 Casele HL, Laifer SA, Woelkers DA, et al. Changes in the pharmacokinetics of the low-molecular weight heparin enoxaparin sodium during pregnancy. *Am J Obstet Gynecol.* 1999;**181**:1113–17.

52 Crowther MA, Spitzer K, Julian J, et al. Pharmacokinetic profile of a low-molecular weight heparin (reviparin) in pregnant patients: a prospective cohort study. *Thromb Res.* 2000;**98**(2):133–38.

53 Norris LA, Bonnar J, Smith MP, et al. Low molecular weight heparin (tinzaparin) therapy for moderate risk thromboprophylaxis during pregnancy: a pharmacokinetic study. *Thromb Haemost.* 2004;**92**(4): 791–96.

54 Ensom MH, Stephenson MD. Pharmacokinetics of low molecular weight heparin and unfractionated heparin in pregnancy. *J Soc Gynecol Investig.* 2004;**11**(6):377–83.

55 Sephton V, Farquharson RG, Topping J, et al. A longitudinal study of maternal dose response to low molecular weight heparin in pregnancy. *Obstet Gynecol.* 2003;**101**(6):1307–11.

56 Jacobsen AF, Qvigstad E, Sandset PM. Low molecular weight heparin (dalteparin) for the treatment of venous thromboembolism in pregnancy. *Br J Obstet Gynaecol.* 2003;**110**(2):139–44.

57 Barbour LA, Oja JL, Schultz LK. A prospective trial that demonstrates that dalteparin requirements increase in pregnancy to maintain therapeutic levels of anticoagulation. *Am J Obstet Gynecol.* 2004;**191**(3):1024–29.

58 Rodie VA, Thomson AJ, Stewart FM, et al. Low molecular weight heparin for the treatment of venous thromboembolism in pregnancy: a case series. *Br J Obstet Gynaecol.* 2002;**109**(9):1020–24.

59 Blickstein D, Hod M, Bar J. Eczematous plaques related to unfractionated and low-molecular-weight heparin in pregnancy: cross-reaction with danaparoid sodium. *Blood Coagul Fibrinolysis.* 2003;**14**:765–8.

60 Pettila V, Kaaja R, Leinonen P, et al. Thromboprophylaxis with low molecular weight heparin (dalteparin) in pregnancy. *Thromb Res.* 1999;**96**(4):275–82.

61 Carlin AJ, Farquharson RG, Quenby SM, et al. Prospective observational study of bone mineral density during pregnancy: low molecular weight heparin versus control. *Hum Reprod.* 2004;**19**(5):1211–14.

62 Verdonkschot AE, Vasmel WL, Middeldorp S, et al. Skin reactions due to low molecular weight heparin in pregnancy: a strategic dilemma. *Arch Gynecol Obstet.* 2005;**271**(2):163–65.

63 Kim J, Smith KJ, Toner C, et al. Delayed cutaneous reactions to heparin in antiphospholipid syndrome during pregnancy. *Int J Dermatol.* 2004;**43**(4):252–60.

64 Forestier F, Daffos F, Capella-Pavlovsky M. Low molecular weight heparin (PK 10169) does not cross the placenta during the second trimester of pregnancy study by direct fetal blood sampling under ultrasound. *Thromb Res.* 1984;**34**(6):557–60.

65 Dimitrakakis C, Papageorgiou P, Papageorgiou I, et al. Absence of transplacental passage of the low molecular weight heparin enoxaparin. *Haemostasis.* 2000;**30**(5):243–48.

66 Omri A, Delaloye JF, Andersen H, et al. Low molecular weight heparin Novo (LHN-1) does not cross the placenta during the second trimester of pregnancy. *Thromb Haemost.* 1989;**61**(1):55–6.

67 Lindhoff-Last E, Kreutzenbeck HJ, Magnani HN. Treatment of 51 pregnancies with danaparoid because of heparin intolerance. *Thromb Haemost.* 2005;**93**(1):63–9.

68 Lindheimer MD, Katz AI. Renal physiology and disease in pregnancy. In: Sedin DW, Giebisch G, editors. *The kidney: physiology and pathophysiology.* New York: Raven Press, 1992. pp. 3371–3431.

69 Hunt BJ, Gattens M, Khamashta M, et al. Thromboprophylaxis with unmonitored intermediate-dose low molecular weight heparin in pregnancies with a previous arterial or venous thrombotic event. *Blood Coagul Fibrinolysis.* 2003;**14**(8):735–39.

70 Horlocker TT, Heit JA. Low molecular weight heparin: biochemistry, pharmacology, perioperative prophylaxis regimens, and guidelines for regional anesthetic management. *Anesth Analg.* 1997;**85**:874–85.

71 Wolzt M, Weltermann A, Nieszpaur-Los M, et al. Studies on the neutralizing effects of protamine on unfractionated and low molecular weight heparin (Fragmin) at the site of activation of the coagulation system in man. *Thromb Hemost.* 1995;**73**:439–43.

72 Kai R, Imamura H, Kumazaki S, et al. Temporary inferior vena cava filter for deep vein thrombosis and acute pulmonary thromboembolism: effectiveness and indication. *Heart Vessels.* 2006;**21**(4):221–25.

73 Clark SL, Porter TF, West FG. Coumarin derivatives and breast-feeding. *Obstet Gynecol.* 2000;**95**(6 Pt 1):938–40.

74 Bates SM, Greer IA, Hirsh J, et al. Use of antithrombotic agents during pregnancy: the Seventh ACCP Conference on Antithrombotic and Thrombolytic Therapy. *Chest.* 2004;**126**(3 Suppl):627S–644S. Review.

75 Lee AY, Levine MN, Baker RI, et al. Low-molecular-weight heparin versus a coumarin for the prevention of recurrent venous thromboembolism in patients with cancer. *N Engl J Med.* 2003;**349**(2): 146–53.

76 Monreal M, Lafoz E, Olive A, et al. Comparison of subcutaneous unfractionated heparin with a low molecular weight heparin (Fragmin) in patients with venous thromboembolism and contraindications to coumarin. *Thromb Haemost.* 1994;**71**(1):7–11.

77 Descarries LM, Leduc L, Khairy P, et al. Low-molecular-weight heparin in pregnant women with prosthetic heart valves. *J Heart Valve Dis.* 2006;**15**(5):679–85.

78 Plesinac SD, Darko PV, Pilic IZ, et al. Anticoagulation therapy during pregnancy of patients with artificial heart valves: fetomaternal outcome. *Arch Gynecol Obstet.* 2006;**274**(3):141–45.

79 Nassar AH, Hobeika EM, Abd Essamad HM, et al. Pregnancy outcome in women with prosthetic heart valves. *Am J Obstet Gynecol.* 2004;**191**(3):1009–13.

80 Hall DR, Oliver J, Rossouw GJ et al. Pregnancy outcome in women with prosthetic heart valves. *J Obstet Gynaecol.* 2001;**21**(2):149–53.

81 Mahesh B, Evans S, Bryan AJ. Failure of low molecular-weight heparin in the prevention of prosthetic mitral valve thrombosis during pregnancy: case report and a review of options for anticoagulation. *J Heart Valve Dis.* 2002;**11**(5):745–50. Review.

82 Leyh RG, Fischer S, Ruhparwar A, et al. Anticoagulation for prosthetic heart valves during pregnancy: is low-molecular-weight heparin an alternative? *Eur J Cardiothorac Surg.* 2002;**21**(3):577–79. Review.

83 Ayhan A, Yucel A, Bildirici I, et al. Feto-maternal morbidity and mortality after cardiac valve replacement. *Acta Obstet Gynecol Scand.* 2001;**80**(8):713–18.

84 Suri V, Sawhney H, Vasishta K, et al. Pregnancy following cardiac valve replacement surgery. *Int J Gynaecol Obstet.* 1999;**64**(3):239–46.

85 Lev-Ran O, Kramer A, Gurevitch J, et al. Low-molecular-weight heparin for prosthetic heart valves: treatment failure. *Ann Thorac Surg.* 2000;**69**(1):264–65.

86 Ashour ZA, Shawky HA, Hassan Hussein M. Outcome of pregnancy in women with mechanical valves. *Tex Heart Inst J.* 2000;**27**(3):240–45.

87 Oran B, Lee-Parritz A, Ansell J. Low molecular weight heparin for the prophylaxis of thromboembolism in women with prosthetic mechanical heart valves during pregnancy. *Thromb Haemost.* 2004;**92**(4):747–51.

88 WS Chan, Ginsberg, JS. Anticoagulation of pregnant women with mechanical heart valves: a systemic review of the literature. *Arch Int Med.* 2000;**160**(2):191–96.

89 Wesseling J, Van Driel D, Heymans HS, et al. Coumarins during pregnancy: long-term effects on growth and development of school-age children. *Thromb Haemost.* 2001;**85**(4):609–13.

90 Seshadri N, Goldhaber SZ, Elkayam U, et al. The clinical challenge of bridging anticoagulation with low-molecular-weight heparin in patients with mechanical prosthetic heart valves: an evidence-based comparative review focusing on anticoagulation options in pregnant and nonpregnant patients. *Am Heart J.* 2005;**150**(1):27–34.

91 Pabinger I, Grafenhofer H, Kaider A, et al. Risk of pregnancy-associated recurrent venous thromboembolism in women with a history of venous thrombosis. *J Thromb Haemost.* 2005;**3**(5):949–54.

92 Brill-Edwards P, Ginsberg JS, Gent M. Safety of withholding heparin in pregnant women with a history of venous thromboembolism. Recurrence of Clot in This Pregnancy Study Group. *N Engl J Med.* 2000;**343**(20):1439–44.

93 Howley HE, Walker M, Rodger MA. A systematic review of the association between factor V Leiden or prothrombin gene variant and intrauterine growth restriction. *Am J Obstet Gynecol.* 2005;**192**(3):694–708. Review.

94 Lin J, August P. Genetic thrombophilias and preeclampsia: a meta-analysis. *Obstet Gynecol.* 2005;**105**(1):182–92.

95 Kovalevsky G, Gracia CR, Berlin JA, et al. Evaluation of the association between hereditary thrombophilias and recurrent pregnancy loss: a meta-analysis. *Arch Intern Med.* 2004;**164**(5):558–63.

96 Krabbendam I, Franx A, Bots ML, et al. Thrombophilias and recurrent pregnancy loss: a critical appraisal of the literature. *Eur J Obstet Gynecol Reprod Biol.* 2005;**118**(2):143–53. Review.

97 Rey E, Kahn SR, David M, et al. Thrombophilic disorders and fetal loss: a meta-analysis. *Lancet.* 2003;**361**(9361):901–8.

98 Di Nisio M, Peters L, Middeldorp S. Anticoagulants for the treatment of recurrent pregnancy loss in women without antiphospholipid syndrome. *Cochrane Database Syst Rev.* 2005;**2**:CD004734. Review.

99 Robertson L, Wu O, Langhorne P, et al. Thrombophilia in pregnancy: a systematic review. *Br J Haematol.* 2006;**132**(2):171–96. Review.

100 Folkeringa N, Brouwer JL, Korteweg FJ, et al. Reduction of high fetal loss rate by anticoagulant treatment during pregnancy in antithrombin, protein C or protein S deficient women. *Br J Haematol.* 2007;**136**:656–61.

101 De Carolis S, Ferrazzani S, De Stefano V, et al. Inherited thrombophilia: treatment during pregnancy. *Fetal Diagn Ther.* 2006;**21**(3):281–86.

102 Kalk JJ, Huisjes AJ, de Groot CJ, et al. Recurrence rate of pre-eclampsia in women with thrombophilia influenced by low-molecular-weight heparin treatment? *Neth J Med.* 2004;**62**(3):83–7.

103 Brenner B, Hoffman R, Carp H, et al. Efficacy and safety of two doses of enoxaparin in women with thrombophilia and recurrent pregnancy loss: the LIVE-ENOX study. *J Thromb Haemost.* 2005;**3**(2): 227–29.

104 Nurk E, Tell GS, Refsum H, et al. Factor V Leiden, pregnancy complications and adverse outcomes: the Hordaland Homocysteine Study. *QJM.* 2006;**99**(5):289–98. E-pub 2006 Apr 13.

105 Coulam CB, Jeyendran RS, Fishel LA, et al. Multiple thrombophilic gene mutations rather than specific gene mutations are risk factors for recurrent miscarriage. *Am J Reprod Immunol.* 2006;**55**(5): 360–68.

106 Gerhardt A, Scharf RE, Beckmann MW, et al. Prothrombin and factor V mutations in women with a history of thrombosis during pregnancy and the puerperium. *N Engl J Med.* 2000;**342**(6):374–80.

107 McColl MD, Ramsay JE, Tait RC, et al. Risk factors for pregnancy associated venous thromboembolism. *Thromb Haemost.* 1997;**78**(4):1183–88.

108 Martinelli I, Mannucci PM, De Stefano V, et al. Different risks of thrombosis in four coagulation defects associated with inherited thrombophilia: a study of 150 families. *Blood.* 1998;**92**(7):2353–58.

109 Grandone E, Margaglione M, Colaizzo D, et al. Genetic susceptibility to pregnancy-related venous thromboembolism: roles of factor V Leiden, prothrombin G20210A, and methylenetetrahydrofolate reductase C677T mutations. *Am J Obstet Gynecol.* 1998;**179**(5):1324–28.

110 Friederich PW, Sanson BJ, Simioni P, et al. Frequency of pregnancy-related venous thromboembolism in anticoagulant factor-deficient women: implications for prophylaxis [erratum appears in *Ann Intern Med.* 1997;**127**(12):1138; *Ann Intern Med.* 1997;**126**(10):835]. *Ann Intern Med.* 1996;**125**(12):955–60.

111 den Heijer M, Koster T, Blom HJ, et al. Hyperhomocysteinemia as a risk factor for deep-vein thrombosis. *N Engl J Med.* 1996;**334**(12):759–62.

112 Walker MC, Smith GN, Perkins SL, et al. Changes in homocysteine levels during normal pregnancy. *Am J Obstet Gynecol.* 1999;**180**(3 Pt 1):660–64.

14 Pediatric Thrombosis

Anthony K. C. Chan, Paul Monagle

Introduction

Venous thromboembolism (VTE) is being diagnosed with increasing frequency in children. Unlike in adults, the majority of VTE in children is secondary. Central venous catheters (CVCs) are the most common cause of VTE in children (1). CVCs account for 90% of systemic VTE in neonates and renal vein thrombosis accounts for most of the non-CVC-related systemic VTE in the neonatal population (2). In older children, CVCs account for 60% of VTE, while malignancy and congenital heart diseases are the two most prominent disease categories associated with thrombosis (3). Approximately 0.7/100,000 children develop VTE (4). Given a conservative estimate that 1% of children with leukemia develop VTE, leukemia in children would therefore increase the risk of developing thrombosis by 1,400-fold. Most other underlying medical illnesses that predispose children to thrombosis are protein-losing conditions, such as nephrotic syndrome and inflammatory bowel disease (3,5–7). Accurately defining these risk factors will enable targeting of specific pediatric populations for thromboprophylaxis.

If one could prevent CVC-related thrombosis, most VTE in children would be prevented. In this chapter, we will review the evidence regarding whether to recommend thromboprophylaxis routinely in children with CVC and cancer. As neonatal renal vein thrombosis is the commonest VTE in neonates not caused by CVCs, we will also review the evidence for treatment of neonatal renal vein thrombosis.

This chapter will provide an "evidence-based" approach to "best management" of pediatric patients with venous thromboembolism. We acknowledge that evidence in many areas is sparse and may be extrapolated from contemporary management in adults. Grading of the quality of evidence and strengths of recommendations in this chapter are based on the guidelines proposed by the international Grading of Recommendations Assessment, Development, and Evaluation Working Group (GRADE), adopting the modification used by the American College of Chest Physicians that merges the very low and low categories of quality of evidence (see chapter 1).

Evidence-based Hematology. Edited by Mark A. Crowther, Jeff Ginsberg, Holger J. Schünemann, Ralph M. Meyer, and Richard Lottenberg.
 ISBN: 978-1-4051-5747-6.

Thromboprophylaxis in children with cancer

Background

Similar to adults, children with cancer are at a substantial risk of developing VTE. In the Canadian Pediatric Thrombophilia Registry, 20% of the patients with VTE had cancer (3). This figure is in contrast to only 2.3 cases of malignancy per 1,000 children and an estimated incidence of thrombosis of 0.7/100,000 in the general pediatric population. The reported prevalence of VTE in pediatric oncology ranges from less than 1% to as high as 44% (8). The reported prevalence depends on the study design (prospective versus retrospective), type of thrombosis being identified (symptomatic versus asymptomatic), and the type of cancer being studied.

Childhood acute lymphoblastic leukemia (ALL) is probably the most studied pediatric cancer with respect to VTE. In a randomized controlled trial, Mitchell et al. reported a prevalence of 5% symptomatic VTE and 31.7% asymptomatic VTE (9). This study illustrates that the prevalence depends on whether the reported VTE is symptomatic. The risk factors for VTE identified to date in this group of patients are the use of asparaginase and the type of corticosteroid given (10). The prevalence of VTE in pediatric ALL probably also depends on the type of chemotherapy protocol used. Three German studies showed that, despite studies done at similar times and on similar ethnic populations, there is a 10-fold difference on the incidence of VTE associated with different chemotherapeutic protocols (11–13).

Prevalence of thrombosis also varies dependent on the type of cancer. Brain tumors seem to carry little risk of thrombosis with a reported prevalence ranging from 0.6% to 3.2% in two large retrospective reviews (14,15). In contrast, pediatric sarcoma confers as much risk as leukemia, as demonstrated by a recent report that reported a prevalence of VTE of 14.3% (16). Although different types of cancer confer different risks of VTE, certain children with cancer have significantly higher risks of developing VTE and so can be a target population for thromboprophylaxis.

Two studies have reported potential treatments to address issues of primary thromboprophylaxis in children. The PARKAA trial studied use of antithrombin concentrate in pediatric ALL patients treated with L-asparaginase. In that study, there was a trend suggesting that the use of antithrombin may decrease the incidence of thrombosis (17). Unfortunately, the study was insufficiently powered to show efficacy. Ruud et al. studied the use of warfarin in the prevention of CVL-related thrombosis in children with cancer (18). Their study was terminated without full recruitment due to lack of efficacy. One limitation of the Ruud et al. study was that very few patients achieved the targeted international normalized ratio. Other case series have also addressed this issue. Elhasid et al. showed low-molecular-weight heparin (LMWH; mean dose 0.84 mg/kg once daily) to be safe, when compared with a historical control, in preventing thrombosis in ALL patients (19). Nowak-Gottl et al. gave LMWH (dose 1 mg/kg, once a day) as primary thromboprophylaxis to children and adolescents with Ewing's sarcoma (n = 36) and osteogenic sarcoma (n = 39). None of their patients developed any thromboembolic complications during the postoperative period (20). None of these series were adequate to address the efficacy problem because of sample size and study design.

Recommendation

In children with cancer, routine antithrombotic prophylaxis is not recommended because of the lack of evidence of efficacy and the potential for increased risk of bleeding (Grade 2C). This recommendation will be stronger in the types of cancer that have a low prevalence of VTE (e.g., brain tumor) because the numbers needed to treat will be significantly higher compared to cancer that has a higher prevalence (e.g., ALL).

Thromboprophylaxis in children with CVCs

Background

CVCs are the most important cause of thrombosis in children, as demonstrated by the national registries and some large case series (3,5,6,7,21,22). Prevalence of VTE in children with CVCs varies from 2% to 66.7%, depending on the type of study, specific patient population, and the diagnostic method used in each study (23–33). If patients with CVCs who are at high risk of thrombosis can be identified, thromboprophylaxis has great potential to safely reduce the risk of thrombotic complications in these children. There is only one randomized control trial to address thromboprophylaxis in the general pediatric population. The PROTEKT trial compared use of LMWH (Reviparin) to standard of practice in the prevention of CVC-related thrombosis (34). The study was concluded early because of lack of recruitment, which reduced the trial's power. The reported incidence of thrombosis is 14.1% in the LMWH group and 12.5% in the standard of practice group, a difference that was not statistically significant. Although no other studies have addressed primary prophylaxis, there are some studies on the use of secondary prophylaxis in specific disease groups. Studies related to cancer were described previously. In children with short-gut syndrome receiving long-term total parenteral nutrition, Newall et al. have demonstrated that warfarin increased the useful life span of CVCs (30).

Recommendations

1. Children with a CVC should not be given thromboprophylaxis (preferably with a LMWH for convenience) routinely (Grade 2C).
2. In children that require long-term CVCs as a means to sustain life (e.g., long-term total parenteral nutrition) and have developed CVC-related thrombosis, thromboprophylaxis is indicated (Grade 2C).

Treatment of neonatal renal vein thrombosis

Background

In one of the largest international neonatal thrombosis registries, the incidence of RVT was estimated to be 0.5/1,000 admissions to the neonatal intensive care unit (2), with only 21 cases being identified over 3.5 years. A registry from Germany estimated the incidence of symptomatic neonatal RVT to be 2.2/100,000 live births (35). Because the incidence of neonatal RVT is so low, performance of properly controlled studies either as single institution or even multi-institutional experience for therapy guidance will be difficult. No randomized control trial has been done to address the efficacy of antithrombotic therapy in neonatal RVT. There is a possibility that by the time RVT has been detected in a neonate, irreparable damage may have been done, and thus, antithrombotic therapy may not be beneficial.

To address the efficacy of antithrombotic therapy in neonatal RVT, a literature review was undertaken. Medical literature from 1992 to 2006 was identified through PubMed searches. Reports of less than two cases were excluded. As a result, 13 case series with 271 patients have been identified (2,36–47). Ten of the 13 case series had therapeutic information. Treatment modalities included supportive care (39.7%), unfractionated heparin (21.6%), LMWH (20.7%), and thrombolytic therapy (11.2%). Regardless of the treatment given, 70.6% of the affected kidneys were atrophic. Atrophic kidneys were identified in 75.3% of patients treated with UFH/LMWH and 72.5% of patients receiving supportive care. Four of the 173 neonates (2.3%) with unilateral RVT, in contrast to 4/73 neonates (5.5%) with bilateral RVT, developed chronic renal insufficiency. Therefore, although the benefit of anticoagulation as a treatment for unilateral RVT is unclear, bilateral renal vein thrombosis may require more aggressive therapy.

Recommendations

1. Neonates with unilateral renal vein thrombosis can be treated with LMWH or close monitoring of the size of the thrombi (Grade 2C).

2. In patients treated conservatively, if the size of the thrombus increases, the patient should be given anticoagulation therapy (Grade 2C).

3. In neonates with bilateral renal vein thrombosis or IVC involvement, the patient should be treated with anticoagulation therapy (Grade 2C).

4. Thrombolytic therapy can be considered in neonates with bilateral renal vein thrombosis (Grade 2C).

Future

Clinical management in pediatric thrombosis is largely based on low levels of evidence. More clinical studies are needed and only multinational investigations will provide enough statistical power to address most of the problems in pediatric thrombosis.

References

1 Andrew M, David M, Adams M, et al. Venous thromboembolic complications (VTE) in children: first analyses of the Canadian Registry of VTE. *Blood.* 1994;**83**(5):1251–57.

2 Schmidt B, Andrew M. Neonatal thrombosis: report of a prospective Canadian and international registry. *Pediatrics.* 1995;**96**(5 Pt 1):939–43.

3 Monagle P, Adams M, Mahoney M, et al. Outcome of pediatric thromboembolic disease: a report from the Canadian Childhood Thrombophilia Registry. *Pediatr Res.* 2000;**47**(6):763–66.

4 Chan AK, Deveber G, Monagle P, et al. Venous thrombosis in children. *J Thromb Haemost.* 2003;**1**(7):1443–55.

5 van Ommen CH, Heijboer H, Buller HR, et al. Venous thromboembolism in childhood: a prospective two-year registry in The Netherlands. *J Pediatr.* 2001;**139**(5):676–81.

6 Oren H, Devecioğlu O, Ertem M, et al. Analysis of pediatric thrombotic patients in Turkey. *Pediatr Hematol Oncol.* 2004;**21**(7):573–83.

7 Rask O, Berntorp E, Ljung R. Risk factors for venous thrombosis in Swedish children and adolescents. *Acta Paediatr.* 2005;**94**(6):717–22.

8 Wiernikowski JT, Athale UH. Thromboembolic complications in children with cancer. *Thromb Res.* 2006;**118**(1):137–52.

9 Mitchell LG, Andrew M, Hanna K, et al. A prospective cohort study determining the prevalence of thrombotic events in children with acute lymphoblastic leukemia and a central venous line who are treated with L-asparaginase: results of the Prophylactic Antithrombin Replacement in Kids with Acute Lymphoblastic Leukemia Treated with Asparaginase (PARKAA) Study. *Cancer.* 2003;**97**(2):508–16.

10 Athale UH, Chan AK. Thrombosis in children with acute lymphoblastic leukemia. Part II. Pathogenesis of thrombosis in children with acute lymphoblastic leukemia: effects of the disease and therapy. *Thromb Res.* 2003;**111**(4–5):199–212.

11 Mauz-Korholz C, Junker R, Gobel U, et al. Prothrombotic risk factors in children with acute lymphoblatic leukemia treated with delayed *E. coli* asparaginase (COALL-92 and 97 protocols). *Thromb Haemost.* 2000;**83**:840–43.

12 Nowak-Gottl U, Wermes C, Junker R, et al. Prospective evaluation of the thrombotic risk in children with acute lymphoblastic leukemia carrying the MTHFR TT 677 genotype, the prothrombin G20210A variant, and further prothrombotic risk factors. *Blood.* 1999;**93**:1595–99.

13 Nowak-Gottl U, Heinecke A, vonKries R, et al. Thrombotic events revisited in children with acute lym-phoblastic leukemia: impact of concomitant Escherichia coli asparaginase/prednisone administration. *Thromb Res.* 2001;**103**:165–72.

14 Tabori U, Beni-Adani L, Dvir R, et al. Risk of venous thromboembolism in pediatric patients with brain tumors. *Pediatr Blood Cancer.* 2004;**43**(6):633–36.

15 Deitcher SR, Gajjar A, Kun L, et al. Clinically evident venous thromboembolic events in children with brain tumors. *J Pediatr.* 2004;**145**(6): 848–50.

16 Athale U, Cox S, Siciliano S, et al. Thromboembolism in children with sarcoma. *Pediatr Blood Cancer.* 2006;**49**(2):171–76.

17 Mitchell L, Andrew M, Hanna K, et al. Trend to efficacy and safety using antithrombin concentrate in prevention of thrombosis in children receiving L-asparaginase for acute lymphoblastic leukemia. Results of the PAARKA study. *Thromb Haemost.* 2003;**90**(2):235–44.

18 Ruud E, Holmstrom H, De Lange C, et al. Low-dose warfarin for the prevention of central line-associated thromboses in children with malignancies—a randomized, controlled study. *Acta Paediatr.* 2006;**95**:1053–59.

19 Elhasid R, Lanir N, Sharon R, et al. Prophylactic therapy with enoxaparin during L-asparaginase treatment in children with acute lymphoblastic leukemia. *Blood Coagul Fibrinolysis.* 2001;**12**(5):367–70.

20 Nowak-Gottl U, Munchow N, Klippel U, et al. The course of fibrinolytic proteins in children with malignant bone tumors. *Eur J Pediatr.* 1999;**158**:S151–S53.

21 Chuansumrit A, Chiemchanya S, Khowsathit P, et al. Thromboembolic complications in Thai pediatric patients. *J Med Assoc Thai.* 2001;**84**(5):681–87.

22 Newall F, Wallace T, Crock C, et al. Venous thromboembolic disease: a single-centre case series study. *J Paediatr Child Health.* 2006;**42**(12):803–7.

23 Swaniker F, Fonkalsrud EW. Superior and inferior vena caval occlusion in infants receiving total parenteral nutrition. *Am Surg.* 1995;**61**(10):877–81.

24 Gauderer MW, Stellato TA. Subclavian broviac catheters in children—technical considerations in 146 consecutive placements. *J Pediatr Surg.* 1985;**20**(4):402–5.

25 Andrew M, Marzinotto V, Pencharz P, et al. A cross-sectional study of catheter-related thrombosis in children receiving total parenteral nutrition at home. *J Pediatr.* 1995;**126**(3):358–63.

26 Dollery CM, Sullivan ID, Bauraind O, et al. Thrombosis and embolism in long-term central venous access for parenteral nutrition. *Lancet.* 1994;**344**(8929):1043–45.

27 Marsh D, Wilkerson SA, Cook LN, et al. Right atrial thrombus formation screening using two-dimensional echocardiograms in neonates with central venous catheters. *Pediatrics.* 1988;**81**(2):284–86.

28 Pippus KG, Giacomantonio JM, Gillis DA, et al. Thrombotic complications of saphenous central venous lines. *J Pediatr Surg.* 1994;**29**(9):1218–19.

29 Sadiq HF, Devaskar S, Keenan WJ, et al. Broviac catheterization in low birth weight infants: incidence and treatment of associated complications. *Crit Care Med.* 1987;**15**(1):47–50.

30 Newall F, Barnes C, Savoia H, et al. Warfarin therapy in children who require long-term total parenteral nutrition. *Pediatrics.* 2003;**112**(5):e386.

31 Curnow A, Idowu J, Behrens E, et al. Urokinase therapy for silastic catheter-induced intravascular thrombi in infants and children. *Arch Surg.* 1985;**120**(11):1237–40.

32 Loeff DS, Matlak ME, Black RE, et al. Insertion of a small central venous catheter in neonates and young infants. *J Pediatr Surg.* 1982;**17**(6):944–49.

33 Schmidt-Sommerfeld E, Snyder G, Rossi TM, et al. Catheter-related complications in 35 children and adolescents with gastrointestinal disease on home parenteral nutrition. *JPEN J Parenter Enteral Nutr.* 1990;**14**(2):148–51.

34 Massicotte P, Julian JA, Gent M, et al. An open-label randomized controlled trial of low molecular weight heparin for the prevention of central venous line-related thrombotic complications in children: the PROTEKT trial. *Thromb Res.* 2003;**109**:101–8.

35 Nowak-Gottl U, von Kries R, Gobel U. Neonatal symptomatic thromboembolism in Germany: two-year survey. *Arch Dis Child Fetal Neonatal Ed.* 1997;**76**(3):F163–67.

36 Messinger Y, Sheaffer JW, Mrozek J, et al. Renal outcome of neonatal renal venous thrombosis: review of 28 patients and effectiveness of fibrinolytics and heparin in 10 patients. *Pediatrics.* 2006;**118**:e1478–84.

37 Winyard PJ, Bharucha T, De Bruyn R, et al. Perinatal renal venous thrombosis: presenting renal length predicts outcome. *Arch Dis Child Fetal Neonatal Ed.* 2006;**91**:F273–78.

38 Marks SD, Massicotte MP, Steele BT, et al. Neonatal renal venous thrombosis: clinical outcomes and prevalence of prothrombotic disorders. *J Pediatr.* 2005;**146**:811–16.

39 Proesmans W, van de Wijdeven P, Van Geet C. Thrombophilia in neonatal renal venous and arterial thrombosis. *Pediatr Nephrol.* 2005;**20**:241–42.

40 Kosch A, Kuwertz-Broking E, Heller C, et al. Renal venous thrombosis in neonates: prothrombotic risk factors and long-term follow-up. *Blood.* 2004;**104**:1356–60.

41 Heller C, Schobess R, Kurnik K, et al. Abdominal venous thrombosis in neonates and infants: role of prothrombotic risk factors—a multicentre case-control study. For the Childhood Thrombophilia Study Group. *Br J Haematol.* 2000;**111**:534–39.

42 Keidan I, Lotan D, Gazit G, et al. Early neonatal renal venous thrombosis: long-term outcome. *Acta Paediatr.* 1994;**83**:1225–27.

43 Nuss R, Hays T, Manco-Johnson M. Efficacy and safety of heparin anticoagulation for neonatal renal vein thrombosis. *Am J Pediatr Hematol Oncol.* 1994;**16**:127–31.

44 Laplante S, Patriquin HB, Robitaille P, et al. Renal vein thrombosis in children: evidence of early flow recovery with Doppler US. *Radiology.* 1993;**189**:37–42.

45 Orazi C, Fariello G, Malena S, et al. Renal vein thrombosis and adrenal hemorrhage in the newborn: ultrasound evaluation of 4 cases. *J Clin Ultrasound.* 1993;**21**:163–69.

46 Nowak-Gottl U, Schwabe D, Schneider W, et al. Thrombolysis with recombinant tissue-type plasminogen activator in renal venous thrombosis in infancy. *Lancet.* 1992;**340**:1105.

47 Bokenkamp A, von Kries R, Nowak-Gottl U, et al. Neonatal renal venous thrombosis in Germany between 1992 and 1994: epidemiology, treatment and outcome. *Eur J Pediatr.* 2000;**159**:44–8.

15 Bridging Anticoagulation in Patients Who Require Temporary Interruption of Warfarin for Surgery

James D. Douketis, Scott Kaatz

Introduction

The perioperative management of patients who require temporary interruption of warfarin because of surgery is a frequently encountered clinical scenario. There are 4 million people in North America and Europe with a mechanical heart valve, chronic atrial fibrillation, or venous thromboembolism who are receiving long-term warfarin to prevent arterial and venous thromboembolism, of whom approximately 400,000 are assessed each year for temporary interruption of warfarin and bridging anticoagulation (1).

Bridging anticoagulation refers to the administration of a short-acting heparin, typically therapeutic-dose (or full-dose) unfractionated heparin (UFH) or low-molecular-weight heparin (LWMH), for the 8–10 days before and after surgery, during which time warfarin therapy is interrupted and its anticoagulant effect is subtherapeutic (2). This management approach minimizes the time in the perioperative period that patients are not receiving therapeutic-dose anticoagulation and is intended to minimize the risk of potentially devastating thromboembolic events, such as a stroke, thrombosed mechanical heart valve, or recurrent venous thromboembolism (VTE) (2–6). Although the risk for thromboembolism during warfarin interruption is relatively low, the consequences can be devastating with a 15% mortality rate of a thrombosed mechanical heart valve, a 70% rate of major neurological deficit or death with an embolic stroke and an up to 25% case-fatality rate of recurrent VTE (7–9).

This chapter will address four common clinical questions: Which patients need bridging? Which procedures have a bleeding risk that is too high to use postprocedure bridging? How effective is bridging? How do we bridge? As randomized trials of bridging therapy are lacking, our proposed clinical formulations for bridging therapy in this chapter are based on data from observational studies, formulations from experts in this field and from our management of patients in large, multidisciplinary bridging anticoagulation clinics, and clinical practice guidelines. The data from observational studies were derived by searching the English-language MEDLINE database from 1990 to the present, using the following key words: *bridging anticoagulation, low-molecular-weight heparin, surgery, anticoagulation, warfarin interruption.* The database search was supplemented by a review of international conference abstract and by conferring with experts.

Which patients need bridging?

There are no randomized trials to help determine which patients need bridging and the risk of thromboembolic complications when warfarin is withheld for a procedure are estimated from observational cohort studies which makes it difficult to produce succinct guidelines. We have included the American College of Cardiology/American Heart Association/European Society of Cardiology (ACC/AHA/ESC) and American College of Chest Physicians (ACCP) grades of recommendation to our suggestion where appropriate (10,11). There is no consensus on a universal grading system for guidelines, though one is in development (12). The ACC/AHA/ESC and ACCP have different classifications for their recommendations: the ACC/AHA/ESC strongest to weakest are Class I, Class IIa, Class IIb, and Class III, with levels of evidence grades as A, B, and C; the ACCP classification, from strongest to weakest are 1A, 1C+, 1B, 1C, 2A, 2C+, 2B, and 2C.

Patients with a mechanical prosthetic heart valve. Bridging anticoagulant therapy should be considered in patients with a mechanical prosthetic heart valve who are at high or moderate risk for stroke or valve thrombosis. A suggested risk classification scheme is presented in (Table 15.1).

In patients with a mechanical heart valve, the risk of a thromboembolic event is determined by the type and position of the prosthetic valve and the presence of additional risk factors for stroke and intracardiac thrombosis. In patients who are probably at high

Evidence-based Hematology. Edited by Mark A. Crowther, Jeff Ginsberg, Holger J. Schünemann, Ralph M. Meyer, and Richard Lottenberg.
 ISBN: 978-1-4051-5747-6.

Table 15.1 Suggested risk stratification in patients with a mechanical heart valve.

Thromboembolism risk category	Patient characteristics	Suggested anticoagulant management
High risk	—Recent (within 3 months) stroke or transient ischemic attack —Any mechanical mitral valve —Caged-ball or tilting-disc aortic valve	—Bridging anticoagulation is recommended
Moderate risk	—Bileaflet aortic valve and 1 or more major stroke risk factor*	—Bridging anticoagulation should be considered
Low risk	—Bileaflet aortic valve and no major stroke risk factors*	—Bridging anticoagulation is optional

*Stroke risk factors include congestive heart failure or low ejection fraction; hypertension; age >75 years; diabetes; a history of stroke or transient ischemic attack; and atrial fibrillation.

risk for thromboembolism, such as those with a recent (within three months) stroke or transient ischemic attack, a mitral valve prosthesis, or an older-generation prosthesis (e.g., caged-ball, tilting disc), bridging anticoagulation is, in general, recommended by consensus groups (10,11) and experts (13–23). In patients at moderate risk for thromboembolism, such as those with a newer aortic valve prosthesis (e.g., bileaflet) and one or more stroke risk factors, bridging anticoagulant should be considered, although there are inconsistent clinical management guidelines from consensus groups (10,11). Finally, in patients who are probably at low risk for thromboembolism, such as those with a bileaflet aortic valve and no stroke risk factors, bridging anticoagulant therapy may not be required.

Patients with chronic atrial fibrillation. Bridging anticoagulation should be considered in selected patients with chronic atrial fibrillation who are at high or moderate risk for stroke. A suggested risk classification scheme is presented in Table 15.2.

High-risk patients include those with a recent (within three months) stroke or transient ischemic attack, and patients with rheumatic valvular heart disease (24,25). Recently, a scoring system ($CHADS_2$) was developed to assess risk for stroke in patients with nonvalvular atrial fibrillation. The score is calculated based on the presence or absence of one or more of the following major risk factors: a prior stroke or transient ischemic attack; congestive heart failure, hypertension, diabetes mellitus, and age >75 years, and a history of stroke or atrial fibrillation. (26). Bridging anticoagulation can be recommended in patients with a recent (within three months) stroke or transient ischemic attack or multiple (three or more risk factors), and it is optional in patients with one or two major stroke risk factors. In patients with atrial fibrillation and no stroke risk factors, bridging anticoagulation is not recommended because of the low risk for stroke (1%–2% per year), and these patients do not require warfarin treatment.

Venous thromboembolism. Bridging anticoagulant therapy should be considered in selected patients with venous thromboembolism, including those with deep vein thrombosis and pulmonary embolism, who are at high or moderate risk of disease recurrence. A suggested risk classification scheme is presented in Table 15.3.

High-risk patients in whom bridging anticoagulation is recommended are those who have had a recent (within one month)

Table 15.2 Suggested risk stratification in patients with chronic atrial fibrillation.

Thromboembolism risk category	Patient characteristics	Suggested anticoagulant management
High risk	—Recent (within 3 months) stroke or transient ischemic attack —Rheumatic valvular heart disease —3 or more major stroke risk factors*	—Bridging anticoagulation is recommended
Moderate risk	—1 or 2 major stroke risk factors*	—Bridging anticoagulation is optional
Low risk	—No major stroke risk factors*	—Bridging anticoagulation is not recommended

*Stroke risk factors include: congestive heart failure or low ejection fraction; hypertension; age >75 years; diabetes; and a history of stroke or transient ischemic attack.

Table 15.3 Suggested risk stratification in patients with venous thromboembolism.*

Thromboembolism risk category	Patient characteristics	Suggested anticoagulant management
High risk	—Prior VTE within last 3 months —Selected thrombophilia (deficiency of protein C, protein S or antithrombin, antiphospholipid antibodies, multiple thrombophilic abnormalities)	—Bridging anticoagulation is recommended
Moderate risk	—VTE within past 3–6 months —Active cancer (treated with post 6 months or palliative) —Recurrent VTE	—Bridging anticoagulation is optional
Low risk	—Prior VTE over 12 months ago	—Bridging anticoagulation is not recommended

episode of venous thromboembolism or have selected prothrombotic blood abnormalities, which consist of a deficiency of protein C, protein S, or antithrombin, antiphospholipid antibodies, homozygous factor V Leiden, or with multiple prothrombotic blood abnormalities (27–29). We do not consider isolated prothrombin gene mutation 20210a or heterozygous factor V Leiden as significant risk factors for a bridging decision. Moderate risk patients include those with prior venous thromboembolism during the last one to six months, in whom bridging anticoagulation should be considered. In patients with remote venous thromboembolism, occurring more than six months before the planned surgery, bridging anticoagulation is not recommended.

Which procedures is the bleeding risk too high to use postprocedure bridging?

Several bridging cohort studies have classified patients as high or low risk for postprocedure bleeding and have used different postprocedure protocols based on this stratification (30–33). However, this classification has been arbitrary and we were unable to find a validated model to classify surgical procedures as high or low risk for bleeding. If there is adequate postoperative hemostasis after surgery, the decision to resume anticoagulants will depend on the bleeding risk associated with the surgery. A suggested risk classification scheme for assessing risk for postoperative/postprocedural bleeding is presented in Table 15.4.

Patients at very high risk for postoperative bleeding include patients who have had excessive postoperative bleeding or have undergone a procedure associated with a very high risk for bleeding (e.g., intracranial neoplasm, coronary artery bypass surgery). It is always helpful to discuss such high-risk patients with the attending surgeon or proceduralist to better understand patient-specific issues relating to bleeding risk and to discuss the initiation of postoperative anticoagulation.

How effective is bridging?

There are no randomized trials to assess the efficacy of bridging therapy. However, cohort studies provide estimates of the expected thromboembolic and bleeding complication rates. The pooled incidence of arterial thromboembolism was approximately 1% and the pooled incidence of major bleeding was approximately 3% (13,18). These estimates should be help clinicians to weigh the risks and benefits of bridging therapy.

How do we bridge?

There are no standardized management guidelines regarding the use of bridging anticoagulation, mainly because of a lack of randomized controlled trials assessing different bridging anticoagulation management strategies. Most experts recommend that patients at high risk for thromboembolism should receive therapeutic-dose anticoagulation before and after surgery (13–22). The ACC/AHA/ESC and the ACCP recommend that patients at high risk for thromboembolism should receive therapeutic-dose anticoagulation during before and after surgery, while in patients at low-to-moderate risk, treatment recommendations vary. However, the distinction between “high-risk” and “low-to-moderate” risk for thromboembolism in these guidelines is not clear. In physicians surveys of bridging anticoagulation, over 90% of physicians administer bridging anticoagulation in patients at high risk for thromboembolism, whereas 20%–80% of physicians administer bridging to patients at lower risk (34–37).

Unfractionated Heparin

The traditional bridging anticoagulation method involves hospitalizing patients four to five days before surgery, stopping warfarin, and administering intravenous UFH while the anticoagulant effect

Table 15.4 Suggested risk stratification for bleeding associated with surgery or invasive procedure.*

		Postoperative resumption of anticoagulants	
Bleeding risk category	**Surgery or invasive procedure**	**Warfarin**	**Therapeutic-dose LMWH**
Very high risk	—Intracranial surgery —Spinal surgery —Coronary artery bypass surgery —Heart valve replacement	Evening of first or second day after surgery	No postoperative LMWH*
High risk	—Major vascular surgery —Permanent pacemaker insertion —Internal defibrillator placement —Prostatectomy —Bladder tumor resection —Lung resection surgery —Hip/knee joint replacement surgery —Intestinal anastomosis surgery —Bowel polypectomy —Kidney or prostate biopsy —Cervical cone biopsy	Evening of the day of surgery or the first day after surgery	48–72 hours after surgery
Moderate risk	—Other intra-abdominal surgery —Other intrathoracic surgery —Other orthopedic surgery —Bronchoscopy with anticipated biopsy	Evening of the day of surgery	24–48 hours after surgery
Low risk	—Laparoscopic cholecystectomy —Laparoscopic hernia repair —Dental surgery —Cutaneous surgery —Ophthalmologic surgery —Colonscopy with or without biopsy	Evening of the day of surgery	12–24 hours after surgery (i.e., day after surgery)
Very low risk	—Single tooth extraction or teeth cleaning —Selected skin biopsy —Selected cataract extraction	Warfarin interruption not needed	Bridging anticoagulation not needed

*Reproduced with permission from (46): Mannucci C, Douketis JD. The management of patients who require temporary reversal of vitamin K antagonists for surgery: a practical guide for clinicians. *Intern Emerg Med.* 2006;**1**:96–104. LMWH, low-molecular-weight heparin.

of warfarin recedes (2). UFH is stopped three to four hours before surgery and after surgery, UFH and warfarin are resumed, with UFH given for four or five days until therapeutic anticoagulation with warfarin is re-established. The administration of UFH requires laboratory monitoring with once- or twice-daily activated partial thromboplastin time (aPTT) testing (38). Bridging anticoagulation with UFH is not widely used, mainly because of limits on the cost and availability of hospital beds and the increasing number of surgical and other procedures that are being done without hospitalization.

Low-molecular-weight heparin

Bridging anticoagulation with LMWH is more convenient for perioperative patient management because it can be administered as a fixed, weight-adjusted subcutaneous injection, without the need for laboratory monitoring (38). LMWH as bridging anticoagulation obviates the need for hospitalization and can simplify patient care. Furthermore, the use of LMWH has the potential to reduce health care costs (39). These pragmatic issues make LMWH the preferred heparin for bridging.

Warfarin therapy interruption

Patients should be assessed at least five days before surgery to allow time for the anticoagulant effect of warfarin to be eliminated, after treatment is interrupted, and to instruct patients about LMWH self-injection if bridging anticoagulation is used (40). In patients who are receiving warfarin with an international normalized ratio (INR) range of 2.0–3.0, stopping treatment five days before surgery will, in most patients, ensure normal hemostasis at the time of surgery (40,41). However, the pharmacokinetic properties of warfarin differ between patients, especially the elderly who may require a longer time for the INR to normalize after VKA is stopped (41).

Monitoring the INR before surgery

Whenever feasible, INR testing should be done the day before surgery to ensure the INR <1.5, as patients with an INR ≥ 1.5 are at increased risk of postoperative bleeding (42). With an INR ≥1.5, giving 1 mg oral vitamin K will hasten the normalization of the INR in time for surgery (43,44). This small dose of vitamin K is unlikely to confer resistance to re-anticoagulation when warfarin is resumed after surgery (45). In patients who receive vitamin K, it is also reasonable to measure the INR on the morning of surgery to confirm that the INR is normal. If the INR is ≥1.5 on the day of surgery, additional vitamin K will not act rapidly enough and surgery will need to be rescheduled. Sometimes, fresh frozen plasma or prothrombin complex concentrate will be given to correct the INR so surgery is not delayed; however, we were unable to find any evidence to support this practice (46).

LMWH dosing before surgery

If once-daily LMWH is used as bridging anticoagulant therapy (e.g., tinzaparin, 175 IU/kg or dalteparin 200 IU/kg once daily), the dose should be administered in the mornings, and with the last preoperative dose administered on the morning of the day before surgery, and at least 24 hours before surgery. If twice-daily LMWH is used (e.g., dalteparin 100 IU/kg or enoxaparin, 1 mg/kg twice daily), the evening dose on the day before surgery should be omitted (47,48). With either regimen, the last dose of LMWH will be administered at least 24 hours before surgery to eliminate the likelihood of a residual anticoagulant effect at the time of the procedure.

The anticoagulant effect of LMWH is measured by the antifactor Xa level because the APTT does not reliably measure the anticoagulant effect of LMWH. Antifactor Xa level testing should not be routinely done in patients who are receiving LMWH because this testing is not available in many hospital or clinic laboratories, and the results may not be available for several hours, which is impractical in patients who are scheduled for surgery on the same day. Furthermore, since LMWHs have a predictable pharmacokinetic profile and elimination half-lives of three to four hours, there should not be a clinically important residual anticoagulant effect 24 hours after the preceding dose (38).

Resumption of bridging anticoagulation post procedure

The decision to resume bridging anticoagulation after surgery is based on whether there is adequate postoperative hemostasis and the bleeding risk associated with the surgery. If there is ongoing bleeding after surgery, the resumption of bridging anticoagulation should be deferred until the bleeding has subsided. In general, most postoperative bleeding will resolve within 24 hours after surgery.

If there is adequate postoperative hemostasis after surgery, the decision to resume anticoagulants will depend on the bleeding risk associated with the surgery. A suggested formulation for the resumption of bridging therapy with LMWH after surgery or an invasive procedure is presented in Table 15.4.

In patients undergoing surgery associated with a high risk of bleeding, such as prostatectomy or neurosurgery, the resumption of bridging anticoagulation should be deferred for at least 48–72 hours after surgery and, preferably, after consultation with the surgeon. In patients undergoing surgery that is associated with a moderate risk of bleeding, such as intra-abdominal or intrathoracic surgery, the resumption of bridging anticoagulation should be delayed until 24–48 hours after surgery, while in the case of a procedure with a low risk of bleeding, bridging anticoagulation can be resumed 12–24 hours after surgery.

In patients who develop major postoperative bleeding, all anticoagulants should be withheld until the bleeding source has been identified and treated. The need to prevent further bleeding supersedes the resumption of anticoagulants. If the cause of the bleeding is readily reversible, as with the repair of a blood vessel inadvertently severed during surgery, anticoagulants probably can be resumed within 24 hours after consultation with the surgeon.

Resumption of warfarin therapy

As with the resumption of bridging anticoagulation, the resumption of warfarin should be predicated on the patient's risk for postoperative bleeding. With most types of surgery or procedures that are associated with a low or moderate risk for bleeding, warfarin can be restarted on the evening of surgery since a clinically significant anticoagulant effect not occur for at least 48 hours after the initial dose of warfarin, and a full anticoagulant effect will not occur for four to five days (40,41). In patients who are undergoing a surgical or other procedure associated with a high or very high risk for postoperative bleeding, the initial dose of warfarin can be resumed on the evening of the first or second postoperative day. Overall, the graduated approach to resuming warfarin should parallel the resumption of bridging anticoagulation and should be individualized based on a postoperative assessment of the patient's risk for bleeding.

The starting dose of warfarin can be the patient's usual dose, according to their preprocedure dose regimen with adjustments for perioperative medications and dietary changes that can change the effects of warfarin. Consequently, the resumption of warfarin on the evening after surgery should not adversely affect postoperative hemostasis. If a patient has received high-dose vitamin K before surgery (i.e., 5–10 mg), this may result in resistance to re-anticoagulation when warfarin therapy is resumed. Because it is difficult to predict the warfarin dose requirements of such patients, it is reasonable to double their usual dose of warfarin for two consecutive days after surgery. If low-dose (1–2 mg) vitamin K has been given before surgery, it is reasonable to double the first dose of warfarin and to resume the usual dose on the following day.

Bridging anticoagulation should be stopped when a patient's INR level is within the therapeutic range. Preferably, INR testing should be done on day 3 and day 5 after surgery. The timing of postoperative INR testing may vary by one day earlier or later, depending on the day of the week that the surgery was done and patient availability for blood testing. In most patients, with a target

INR of 2.0–3.0, bridging anticoagulation will be required for three to four days after surgery, and in patients with a target INR of 2.5–3.5, approximately five days of bridging anticoagulation will be required.

Summary

The management of patients who require temporary interruption of warfarin requires an individual assessment of the patient's risk for thromboembolism during interruption of this treatment and their risk for bleeding associated with surgery. These considerations will determine whether patients receive bridging anticoagulation. In patients in whom bridging anticoagulation is considered appropriate, the risk for bleeding associated with the surgery or invasive procedure will determine when bridging anticoagulation is resumed after surgery. In recent years, much progress has been made in understanding the therapeutic benefits and risks of bridging anticoagulation through cohort studies and patient registries. However, several questions remain that, ultimately, are best addressed by randomized controlled trials. Most important, perhaps, is the need to address whether bridging anticoagulation is needed in patients who require temporary interruption of warfarin, especially in patients at low-to-moderate risk for thromboembolism in whom there is clinical equipoise about best practice and who constitute the vast majority of patients assessed. Additional unanswered questions relate to the timing of bridging anticoagulation before and after surgery and identifying types of surgery and procedures in which the risk for bleeding precludes postprocedure bridging anticoagulation.

References

1 American Heart Association. *Heart disease and stroke statistics update.* Dallas, Texas; 2001.

2 Douketis JD. Perioperative anticoagulation management in patients who are receiving oral anticoagulant therapy: a practical guide for clinicians. *Thromb Res.* 2002;**108**:3–13.

3 Spandorfer JM, Lynch S, Weitz HH, et al. Use of enoxaparin for the chronically anticoagulated patient before and after procedures. *Am J Cardiol.* 1999;**84**:478–80.

4 Carrel TP, Klingenmann W, Mohacsi PJ, et al. Perioperative bleeding and thromboembolic risk during non-cardiac surgery in patients with mechanical prosthetic heart valves: an institutional review. *J Heart Valve Dis.* 1999;**8**:392–98.

5 Vongpatanasin W, Hillis LD, Lange RA. Prosthetic heart valves. *N Engl J Med.* 1996;**335**:407–16.

6 Risk factors for stroke and efficacy of antithrombotic therapy in atrial fibrillation: analysis of pooled data from the five randomized controlled trials. *Arch Intern Med.* 1994;**154**:1449–57.

7 Douketis JD, Kearon C, Bates S, et al. Risk of fatal pulmonary embolism in patients with treated venous thromboembolism. *JAMA.* 1998;**279**:458–62.

8 Longstreth WT, Bernick C, Fitzpatrick A, et al. Frequency and predictors of stroke death in 5,888 participants in the Cardiovascular Health Study. *Neurology.* 2001;**56**:368–75.

9 Martinelli J, Jiminez A, Rabago G, et al. Mechanical cardiac valve thrombosis: is thrombectomy justified? *Circulation.* 1991;**84**(Suppl 3): 70–75.

10 Fuster V, Rydin LE, Cannon DS, et al. ACC/AHA/ESC 2006 guidelines for the management of patients with atrial fibrillation—an executive summary. A report of the American College of Cardiology/American Heart Association Task Force on Practice Guidelines with the European Society of Cardiology Task Force on Practice Guidelines. *Circulation.* 2006;**1114**:700–52.

11 Ansell J, Hirsh J, Poller L, et al. The pharmacology and management of the vitamin K antagonists: the Seventh ACCP Conference on Antithrombotic and Thrombolytic Therapy. *Chest.* 2004;**126**:204S–33S.

12 Grades of Recommendations, Assessment, Development, and Evaluation (GRADE) Working Group. Grading quality of evidence and strengths of recommendations. *BMJ.* 2004;**328**:1490–94.

13 Dunn AS, Turpie AG. Perioperative management of patients receiving oral anticoagulants: a systematic review. *Arch Intern Med.* 2003;**163**:901–8.

14 Jaffer AK, Brotman DJ, Chukaumerije N. When patients on warfarin need surgery. *Cleve Clin J Med.* 2003;**70**:973–84.

15 Spyropoulos AC, Jenkins P, Bornikova L. A disease management protocol for outpatient perioperative bridge therapy with enoxaparin in patients requiring temporary interruption of long-term oral anticoagulation. *Pharmacotherapy.* 2004;**24**:649–58.

16 Heit JA. Perioperative management of the chronically anticoagulated patient. *J Thromb Thrombolys.* 2001;**12**:81–87.

17 Hewitt RL, Chun KL, Flint LM. Current clinical concepts in perioperative anticoagulation. *Am Surg.* 1999;**65**:270–3.

18 Spyropoulos AC, Turpie AG. Perioperative bridging interruption with heparin for the patient receiving long-term anticoagulation. *Curr Opin Pulm Med.* 2005;**5**:373–80.

19 Jaffer A. Anticoagulation management strategies for patients on warfarin who need surgery. *Cleve Clin J Med.* 2006;73 Suppl 1:S100–105.

20 Jacobs LG, Nusbaum N. Perioperative management and reversal of antithrombotic therapy. *Clin Ger Med.* 2001;**17**:189–201.

21 Kearon C, Hirsh J. Management of anticoagulation before and after elective surgery. *N Engl J Med.* 1997;**336**:1506–11.

22 Shapira Y, Vaturi M, Sagie A. Anticoagulant management of patients with mechanical prosthetic valves undergoing non-cardiac surgery: indications and unresolved issues. *J Heart Valve Dis.* 2001;**10**:380–87.

23 Vongpatanasin W, Hillis LD, Lange RA. Prosthetic heart valves. *N Engl J Med.* 1996;**335**:407–16.

24 Risk factors for stroke and efficacy of antithrombotic therapy in atrial fibrillation: analysis of pooled data from the five randomized controlled trials. *Arch Intern Med.* 1994;**154**:1449–57.

25 Singer DE, Albers GW, Dalen JE, et al. Antithrombotic therapy in atrial fibrillation: the Seventh ACCP Conference on Antithrombotic and Thrombolytic Therapy. *Chest.* 2004;**126**:194S–206S.

26 Gage BF, Waterman AD, Shannon W, et al. Validation of clinical classification schemes for predicting stroke: results from the National Registry of Atrial Fibrillation. *JAMA.* 2001;**285**:2864–70.

27 Douketis JD, Foster GA, Crowther MA, et al. Clinical risk factors and timing of recurrent venous thromboembolism during the initial 3 months of anticoagulant therapy. *Arch Intern Med.* 2000;**160**:3431–36.

28 Kearon C, Gent M, Hirsh J, et al. A comparison of three months of anticoagulant therapy with extended anticoagulation for a first episode of idiopathic venous thromboembolism. *N Engl J Med.* 1999;**340**:901–7.

29 Schulman S, Svenungsson E, Granqvist S, et al. Anticardiolipin antibodies predict early recurrence of thromboembolism and death among patients with venous thromboembolism following anticoagulant therapy. *Am J Med.* 1998;**104**:332–38.

30 Douketis JD, Johnson JA, Turpie AG. Low-molecular-weight heparin as bridging anticoagulation during interruption of warfarin: assessment of a standardized peri-procedural anticoagulation regimen. *Arch Intern Med.* 2004;**164**:1319–26.

31 Kovacs MJ, Kearon C, Rodger M, et al. Single-arm study of bridging therapy with low-molecular-weight heparin for patients at risk of arterial embolism who require temporary interruption of warfarin. *Circulation.* 2004;**110**:1658–63.

32 Spyropoulos AC, Turpie AG, Dunn AS, et al. Clinical outcomes with unfractionated heparin or low-molecular-weight heparin as bridging therapy in patients on long-term oral anticoagulants: the REGIMEN registry. *J Thromb Haemost.* 2006;**4**:1246–52.

33 Dunn AS, Spyropoulos AC, Sirko SP, et al. Perioperative bridging therapy with enoxaparin in patients requiring interruption of long-term oral anticoagulant therapy: a multicenter cohort study. *Blood.* 2004;**104**:488a.

34 Douketis JD, Crowther MA, Cherian S, et al. Physician preferences for perioperative anticoagulation in patients with a mechanical heart valve who are undergoing elective non-cardiac surgery. *Chest.* 1999;**116**:1240–46.

35 Douketis JD, Crowther MA, Cherian SS. Perioperative anticoagulation in patients with chronic atrial fibrillation undergoing elective surgery: results of a physician survey. *Can J Cardiol.* 2000;**16**:326–30.

36 Garcia DA, Ageno W, Libby EN, et al. Perioperative anticoagulation for patients with mechanical heart valves: a survey of current practice. *J Thromb Thrombolys.* 2004;**18**:199–203.

37 Ageno W, Garcia D, Libby E, et al. Managing oral anticoagulant therapy in patients with mechanical heart valves undergoing elective surgery: results of a survey conducted among Italian physicians. *Blood Coagul Fibrinolys.* 2004;**15**:623–28.

38 Hirsh J, Raschke R. Heparin and low-molecular-weight heparin: the Seventh ACCP Conference on Antithrombotic and Thrombolytic Therapy. *Chest.* 2004; **126**:188S–203S.

39 Spyropoulos AC, Frost FJ, Hurley JS, et al. Costs and clinical outcomes associated with low-molecular-weight heparin vs unfractionated heparin for perioperative bridging in patients receiving long-term oral anticoagulant therapy. *Chest.* 2004;**125**:1642–50.

40 Palareti G, Legnani C. Warfarin withdrawal: pharmacokinetic-pharmacodynamic considerations. *Clin Pharmacokinet.* 1996;**30**:300–13.

41 White RH, McKitrick T, Hutchison R, et al. Temporary discontinuation of warfarin therapy: changes in the international normalized ratio. *Ann Intern Med.* 1995;**122**:400–402.

42 McKenna R. Abnormal coagulation in the postoperative period contributing to excessive bleeding. *Med Clin North Am.* 2001;**85**:1277–1310.

43 Crowther MA, Julian J, et al. Low dose oral vitamin K for the treatment of warfarin-associated coagulopathy. *Lancet.* 2000;**356**:1551–53.

44 Crowther MA, Donovan D, Harrison L, et al. Low-dose oral vitamin K reliably reverses over-anticoagulation due to warfarin. *Thromb Haemost.* 1998;**79**:1116–18.

45 Woods K, Douketis J, Kathirgamanathan K, et al. Low-dose oral vitamin K to normalize the international normalized ratio prior to surgery in patients who require temporary interruption of warfarin. *J Thromb Thrombolys.* 2007;**24**:93–7.

46 Mannucci C, Douketis JD. The management of patients who require temporary reversal of vitamin K antagonists for surgery: a practical guide for clinicians. *Intern Emerg Med.* 2006;**1**:96–104.

47 Douketis JD, Woods K, Foster GA, et al. Bridging anticoagulation with low-molecular-weight heparin after interruption of warfarin therapy is associated with a residual anticoagulant effect prior to surgery. *Thromb Haemost.* 2005;**94**:528–31.

48 O'Donnell MJ, Kearon C, Johnson J, et al. Preoperative anticoagulant activity after bridging low-molecular-weight heparin for temporary interruption of warfarin. *Ann Intern Med.* 2007;**146**:184–87.

16 Evidence-based Approach to the Diagnosis and Management of Thrombotic Thrombocytopenic Purpura

Brian Boulmay, Craig S. Kitchens

Thrombotic thrombocytopenic purpura (TTP) is a relatively rare disorder with an incidence of 3.7 per million (1). The classic clinical pentad, which included thrombocytopenia, hemolytic anemia, renal dysfunction, neurologic changes, and fever, was promulgated in 1966; TTP remains a clinical diagnosis (2). When this syndrome was initially described, outcomes were universally poor with greater than 90% mortality (2). Often the initial diagnosis of TTP was delayed because of confusion with other disorders such as disseminated intravascular coagulopathy (DIC). Other syndromes such as HELLP (hemolysis, elevated liver enzymes, and low platelets), eclampsia, and hemolytic uremic syndrome share similar clinical features implying an overlap in pathogenic mechanisms. Despite its labor intensity, the introduction of either plasma infusion (3) or plasma exchange (4) led to dramatic and effective improvements in outcomes. Thus, establishment of a firm diagnosis in a timely manner is imperative.

The hemolysis in TTP is related to red cell shearing from platelet thrombi formed in the microvasculature. Von Willebrand factor (VWF) is a glycoprotein produced by platelets and the endothelium; it is integral to platelet aggregation. VWF is initially produced as a large multimeric protein, the so-called ultra-large VWF multimer (ULVWF), which are the most reactive form of VWF in the activation of platelets. Normally ULVWF is cleaved by a protease specific for VWF termed ADAMTS13 (a disintegrin and metalloprotease with thrombospondin-1-like domains). In a majority of both congenital and idiopathic TTP syndromes, lack of ADAMTS13 results in accumulation of ULVWF, platelet thrombi formation, and obstruction of microcirculatory vessels. Idiopathic TTP likely results from autoantibodies directed against ADAMTS13 in most cases. However, congenital absence of ADAMTS13 accounts for a small but definite subgroup of TTP, particularly TTP recurring over decades.

This chapter provides an evidence-based overview of current "best practice" with regards to specific questions relevant to the management of patients with thrombotic thrombocytopenic purpura. Grading of the quality of evidence and strengths of recommendations in this chapter are based on the guidelines proposed by the international Grading of Recommendations Assessment, Development, and Evaluation Working Group (GRADE), adopting the modification used by the American College of Chest Physicians that merges the very low and low categories of quality of evidence (see chapter 1).

Evidence-based Hematology. Edited by Mark A. Crowther, Jeff Ginsberg, Holger J. Schünemann, Ralph M. Meyer, and Richard Lottenberg.

What are the Diagnostic Criteria for TTP?

A variety of signs, symptoms, and laboratory findings has been suggested as diagnostic criteria for TTP. These criteria are not universally agreed upon as diagnostic weight has yet to be fully established for any of these findings. The pentad of schistocytic hemolytic anemia, thrombocytopenia, renal abnormalities, fever, and mental alterations is descriptive yet rather nonspecific. Astute clinical judgment remains the key in prompt diagnosis of TTP.

Schistocytes result from pliable red blood cells (RBCs) being forced over and around microvascular endothelial surfaces roughened by the obstructive mass of ULVWF and its adherent platelets, often at considerable shear force. Whereas seemingly typical TTP has rarely been reported without any observable schistocytes on the peripheral blood smear (5), these cells are so frequently associated with TTP that their presence has assumed a near *sine quo non* status. However, other endothelial perturbations may be associated with observable schistocytes. Circulating blood from patients having undergone bone marrow transplantation may have up to 1% schistocytes in their peripheral blood (6) as can patients in whom various arterial stents have been inserted (7). Patients with pre-eclampsia may have up to 0.25% schistocytes, while those with mechanical heart valves may harbor 0.18%. Blood from perfectly normal subjects may display up to 0.05% schistocytes (8). Lesesve et al., determined that among patients considered possibly to have TTP, less than 1% schistocytes yielded a 98% negative predictive value for TTP while Burns et al. (8) described a mean schistocyte count of 8.4% (range 1%–18.4%) in patients with TTP.

Recently, a group of experts assembled to reach consensus regarding diagnostic criteria in TTP. They ranked a total of 27 putative clinical criteria and agreed that five criteria were optimal for the diagnosis and these included: (1) greater than 4% schistocytes on the peripheral blood smear; (2) de novo, prolonged, or progressive thrombocytopenia with platelet counts less than 50,000/mm^3 or at least a 50% reduction from previous platelet counts; (3) sudden and persistent increase in serum lactate dehydrogenase (LDH); (4) decrease in hemoglobin concentration or an increase in transfusion requirement; and (5) a decrease in serum haptoglobin levels. This group found that these readily available laboratory findings produced greater than 80% sensitivity and specificity for the diagnosis of transplant-associated microangiopathy (TAM) (9). Although these criteria were developed to be applied when one considers TAM-TTP, they represent the best-validated diagnostic criteria to date. Therefore, while these criteria have yet to be applied to acute idiopathic TTP, they should be considered useful when approaching a syndrome that appears to be acute TTP.

Immune-mediated idiopathic TTP is a result of inhibitory antibodies to ADAMTS13. Consequently, this has led some to propose that the ADAMTS13 activity assay be used as an aid in the diagnosis of the disorder (10). Assays for ADAMTS13 are neither routinely nor immediately available. In addition, ADAMTS13 activity can be reduced in a variety of conditions that are confused with TTP, such as systemic lupus erythematosus, immune thrombocytopenic purpura, and DIC (11). Both the sensitivity and specificity of this assay for idiopathic TTP is variously reported from 33% to 100% (12–16). Patients with idiopathic TTP often have ADAMTS13 activities of less than 5% of normal controls; other secondary forms of TTP, such as those associated with drugs, can have up to 100% ADAMTS13 activity (13). However, even in cases in which ADAMTS13 is normal but presentation is consistent with TTP, patients respond to conventional treatments such as plasma exchange. In the remission period, levels of ADAMTS13 less than 5% are indicative of the congenital absence-type ADAMTS13 deficiency, which may have prognostic or therapeutic implications.

Conclusion. Laboratory findings, including schistocytes, anemia, platelet counts of less that 50,000/mm^3, and renal failure in the absence of another alterative diagnosis, are strongly indicative of TTP (Grade 2C). Elevated LDH, decreased haptoglobin, and negative direct antiglobulin test will lend further weight to the diagnosis. A normal ADAMTS13 activity cannot be used to rule out a diagnosis of TTP. TTP remains a clinical diagnosis (Grade 1C).

Is therapeutic plasma exchange superior to plasma infusion for the treatment of TTP?

Plasma infusion benefits patients with idiopathic TTP secondary to replacement of the deficient VWF-cleaving protease ADAMTS-13. Therapeutic plasma exchange (TPE) allows both replacement of VWF-cleaving protease and removal of a presumed antibody to ADAMTS13. TPE involves the removal of the patient's plasma and replacing it with donor plasma, typically in the form of fresh frozen plasma (FFP). TPE should not be confused with simple plasmapheresis in which plasma is removed and replaced with, typically, albumin and saline. The efficacy of TPE has been established by 12 large uncontrolled case series with response rates of 60%–80% (17).

The Canadian Apheresis Study Group performed a randomized prospective trial, which enrolled 102 patients with the diagnosis of TTP to two treatment arms: (1) plasma infusion with 30 mL/kg of FFP on day 1 followed by 15 mL/kg per day, or (2) daily TPE using 1.0–1.5 times plasma volume exchange. Patients were treated daily with plasma infusion or TPE until the platelet count increased to 150,000/microliter with no neurologic dysfunction; patients then had five additional treatments administered over two weeks. Those who failed plasma infusion after nine days were allowed to crossover into the TPE arm. The patients in the TPE arm had an initial response rate of 47% as compared to 25% in the plasma infusion arm. Overall survival was statistically superior in the TPE arm: 78% versus 63%. In addition, the superiority of TPE persisted at six months with 78% of those remitted patients remaining in remission (18).

Although TPE has been shown to be superior to simple transfusion, it is unclear what the optimal exchange volume should be. The Canadian Apheresis Study Group used 1.5× exchange for D1-3 followed by 1× exchange (18). Observational data suggest the use of twice daily 1× plasma exchange may be employed if patients do not have an adequate response to initial exchange streategies (19).

A retrospective review evaluated thirty-seven patients treated with either high-dose plasma infusion (25–30 mL/kg per day) or TPE with single-volume plasma was performed (20). Sixteen of 19 patients treated with high-dose plasma infusion achieved remission with an average dose of 27.5 mL/kg/day. However, 8 of these 19 patients required a change of therapy due to fluid overload, unresponsiveness to initial therapy, or while plasma was being tapered. In the TPE group, 88% achieved a remission. These data suggest that high-dose plasma infusion is an appropriate initial therapy if TPE is unavailable.

Conclusion. TPE should be initiated as soon as the diagnosis of TTP has been established (Grade 1B). Initial 1.0–1.5 × TPE can be employed (Grade 2B) with a change to twice-daily single-volume exchanges if ineffective (Grade 2C). High-dose plasma infusion can be considered appropriate initial therapy if TPE is unavailable (Grade 2C).

Is cryoprecipitate-poor plasma preferred over FFP for treatment of TTP?

It is believed that large VWF multimers are central to the pathophysiology of TTP, and it has been postulated that cryoprecipitate-poor plasma (CPP) would be a superior exchange fluid because it has been rendered deficient in the donors' large VWF multimers. CPP has been reported as being efficacious as salvage therapy after failure with FFP in a few case series (21,22). The utility of CPP as upfront therapy was first evaluated in a nonrandomized retrospective series of 37 patients treated with FFP (19) or CPP (18) as exchange fluid (23). The groups were well matched for age, sex, race, and hematologic parameters. Patients in the CPP arm did receive more exchange therapies and were exposed to more blood product. However, a statistically significant survival advantage was noted in the CPP group: 72% versus 47% in the FFP group.

A retrospective Canadian series treated 40 newly diagnosed TTP patients with therapeutic plasma exchange, using CPP plasma as the exchange fluid (24). A 75% response rate was reported after seven exchanges and 95% were alive at one month. Although this study did not have an FFP arm, the study authors concluded that there was a significant difference compared with historical controls in which FFP was the primary exchange fluid ($p < 0.05$) in terms of response rates.

The North American TTP Group performed the only randomized prospective trial comparing FFP (13 patients) with CPP (14 patients) as initial therapy for idiopathic TTP (25). Patients treated in both arms had clinical parameters, including neurologic dysfunction, creatinine, platelet count, and hemoglobin measured at days +6 and +13 after initiation of therapy. There were no statistically significant differences in any of these measurements at both time points. Further, there was no difference in survival between the two treatment arms, with three deaths in each treatment arm.

Conclusion. Cryoprecipitate-poor TPE can be considered in patients refractory to initial therapy with FFP (Grade 2C). TPE using CPP is equivalent to FFP as initial therapy based on the only randomized data (Grade 2B).

Do antiplatelet agents have a role in the treatment of TTP?

Unbridled platelet adhesion onto VWF multimers is the putative underlying cause of the development of microvascular thrombosis in TTP. Although the mechanism of action of aspirin through the inhibition of thromboxane-dependent pathways would not be expected to specifically interfere with TTP pathophysiology, some have proposed blocking additional platelet aggregation with the use of aspirin and dipyridamole. Early studies suggested that antiplatelet therapy helped achieve disease remission (26); many protocols that use TPE as the backbone of therapy for TTP also include platelet inhibitors such as aspirin or dipyridamole (24,27).

An Italian prospective trial has directly addressed the efficacy of adding antiplatelet agents to TPE. Seventy-two patients with idiopathic TTP were randomized to receive TPE plus methylprednisolone with or without the use of aspirin/dipyridamole (10 mg/kg/day and 3 mg/kg/day, respectively). One volume TPE was employed daily for at least 7 of 10 days; if complete remission was achieved, two additional exchanges were done. At day 15, patient outcomes were assessed: 75% achieved a remission in the TPE/steroid arm and 91% in the TPE/steroid/antiplatelet arm; this difference was not statistically significant. There were a higher number of deaths in the arm treated with TPE and steroids alone; however, this difference also was not statistically significant (28).

An obvious potential complication of using antiplatelet therapy in thrombocytopenic patients is hemorrhage. One small retrospective series reported 35% of patients had serious bleeding complications when treated with antiplatelet agents as part of standard therapy (at relatively high doses of aspirin 900 mg–2,700 mg/day) (29). This observation was not borne out in the Italian Cooperative Group study, which used lower doses of antiplatelet agents. In the Italian study, 3 of 35 patients treated with aspirin/dipyridamole developed mucocutaneous bleeding and one developed a gastrointestinal hemorrhage, none of which were lethal or required a change in therapy (28).

Multiple clinical trials that have evaluated the use of plasma infusion/exchange strategies have variously employed antiplatelet therapies. All patients treated in the aforementioned Canadian Apheresis Study Group trial received aspirin (325 mg/day) and dipyridamole (400 mg/day) for a minimum of two weeks after entry into the study (24). A retrospective review evaluating plasma exchange/plasma infusion published reported 91% survival rates without the use of antiplatelet agents (27). Consensus guidelines published by the British Committee for Standards in Haematology have suggested the use of aspirin for patients when the platelet count rises above 50,000/mm^3 (30).

Conclusion. While use of aspirin and dipyridamole has not been definitively shown to be of clinical benefit in TTP management, they can be considered a reasonable part of therapy once the platelet count has improved to the point that life-threatening bleeding is of less concern (Grade 2C).

Do glucocorticosteroids have a role in the treatment of TTP?

Most cases of idiopathic TTP are thought to arise due to autoantibodies of the IgG subtype directed at ADAMTS13 (12). The addition of immunosuppressive agents such as glucocorticosteroids may result in a more durable remission if antibody production can be reduced. One case series has reported treating 54 patients with TTP but lacking neurologic abnormalities with only 200 mg/day of prednisone; 51% of these cases had a durable remission with neither TPE nor plasma infusion (27). The Canadian Apheresis Study Group, which evaluated TPE versus plasma infusion, did not employ steroid therapy as part of the treatment regimen (18). Outcomes data showed a 78% response rate in the TPE arm, which were similar to other exchange studies employing steroid treatment. No study has compared a steroid-containing arm to TPE alone.

Expert opinion and consensus statements suggest that steroid therapy can be added when response to initial therapy is poor (Grade 2C) (19). Alternatively, a short course of pulse-dose steroids (1 gram methylprednisolone daily for three days) could be considered as part of upfront treatment with TPE to achieve immunosuppression while minimizing long-term steroid exposure (Grade 2C) (30). Such therapy would also seem rationale when TPE is not readily available (Grade 2C).

In early remission should TPE be tapered or stopped?

No one laboratory or clinical endpoint is sufficient to direct clinicians in deciding when to stop therapy with plasma exchange. Instead, remission is typically defined as a resolution of the thrombocytopenia, a stable hemoglobin, resolved neurologic deficits, normal renal function, and normal (or normalizing) serum LDH. Once these initial parameters have been met, the decision to stop therapy can be entertained, but the decision in the final analysis is a *gestalt* based on the entire clinical and laboratory picture. Clearly, if a patient experiences disease exacerbation after the discontinuation of TPE, therapy will need to be resumed.

Consensus data and expert recommendations support that daily TPE should be continued two to three days after remission as a "consolidation" strategy, analogous to continuing chemotherapy after maximal response in malignant disorders (30). It is also a frequent practice to continue TPE but decrease treatments to every other day for a certain length of time before stopping completely. These strategies are not founded on any randomized trials but instead stem from our understanding of the underlying pathophysiology of TTP. The purely empiric decision to continue TPE despite achievement of remission needs to be weighed against the significant complication rate associated with an indwelling central venous catheter, exchange itself, and continued exposure to blood product. A review of 206 patients treated with TPE showed that 26% of patients developed blood-borne infections, hypotension, and deep vein thrombosis; most significantly, a 2% incidence of death was directly related to treatment (31).

Conclusion. Plasma exchange should be continued for two to three days postremission (Grade 2C). Tapering strategies for TPE are purely empiric.

Are there differing categories of TTP and does the differentiation guide therapy?

Idiopathic TTP is the most common presentation of the disease. However, several clinical scenarios, such as allogeneic stem cell transplant, systemic lupus erythematosus (SLE), and drug exposures, clearly lead to development of TTP or a TTP-like syndrome. Drugs most frequently associated with this disorder include mitomycin C (32), quinine (33), and ticlodipine (34). Whereas the clinical manifestations of many of these cases are consistent with microangiopathic hemolytic anemia, it is uncertain whether treatment with TPE is of benefit.

Patients who have undergone stem cell transplant (SCT) often develop what has been termed a "TTP-like" syndrome; that is, the presence of a microangiopathic anemia and thrombocytopenia without another obvious etiology (35). In addition, transplant patients often can have the "hallmark" signs of TTP such as fever, neurologic compromise, renal failure but not the actual disorder. The incidence of TTP associated with transplant has been variously reported from as low as 2% to as high as 76% (36). Unlike the majority of idiopathic TTP cases, patients with transplant-related TTP have a relatively normal level of ADAMTS13 (36). Instead, the underlying pathophysiologic mechanism is thought to be related to endothelial disruption from the preparative regimen. The implications for treatment is that conventional therapies applicable to idiopathic TTP that target ADAMTS13 deficiency do not have a basis in the transplant setting. One retrospective case series reviewed clinical outcomes in 17 patients who were given a "confident diagnosis" of TTP after allogeneic SCT. All of the patients received TPE, ranging from 2 to 30 exchanges; of these, 18% had a meaningful clinical response such as normalization of LDH and resolution of seizures. The patients diagnosed were more likely to have acute graft-versus-host disease (47% vs. 13%, $p < 0.01$), matched unrelated donor transplant (71% vs. 39%, $p = 0.02$), and systemic infection. Most significantly, however, is that only 1 of 17 patients was alive at 42 month follow-up. Clearly, patients who develop this TTP-like syndrome posttransplant do poorly compared with controls, and TPE may not be of benefit. Instead, more aggressive therapies directed to the underlying etiology of the microangiopathic process may be more appropriate (35).

The association of TTP with SLE has been reported extensively, with 56 case reports extant in the medical literature (37). The concurrent development of these two clinical entities could be explained by underlying and overlapping autoimmune processes. However, most case reports have either predated the recognition of, or not included data, on ADAMTS13 activity. Distinguishing TTP from SLE clinically can often prove difficult—in many ways analogous to the confusing picture seen with allogeneic transplantation. One extensive review of 40 case reports of SLE associated with TTP demonstrated that three distinct categories existed: TTP presenting after the diagnosis of SLE (73%), TTP presenting at the time the SLE diagnosis was given (12%), and a TTP diagnosis preceding SLE (15%) (38). While an active lupus "flair" may present with the classic pentad seen in active TTP, this series demonstrated that 43% of those with a known history of SLE do not have clinically active lupus at the time of the TTP diagnosis. The primary treatment strategy in the cases reviewed consisted of TPE (68%), plasma infusion (12%), steroids (10%), and no therapy (7%). Despite the use of TPE in a majority of cases, overall mortality was relatively high (34%); the mortality rate with TPE specifically was 32%. Based on these data, TTP in the setting of SLE carries with it a substantial mortality rate despite the use of standard therapies for idiopathic TTP.

Drug-associated TTP is an entity that has been described extensively in the literature: quinine, ticlopidine, and mitomycin-C are most commonly reported. The exact mechanism underlying the association is unclear. Although most idiopathic TTP cases have evidence for an ADAMTS13 inhibitor (13), many cases associated with drugs do not (14,39). In the case of ticlopidine-induced TTP, plasma from patients has been found to cause disruption of normal microvascular endothelium (40). With quinine exposure, IgG and IgM have been found that interact with both the glycoprotein Ib/IX or IIb/IIIa and likely play a role in the pathophysiology of the disease (41). Most literature describing mitomycin C-associated TTP report occurrence one to two months after the last dose of chemotherapy. Data suggest that there is a cumulative dose effect, with 60 mg most often reported as a threshold dose beyond which TTP becomes more common (42). The pathogenic mechanism is unclear, however. Data indicate that mitomycin-C increases platelet aggregation via inhibition of prostacyclin production (43), and there is clearly endovascular disruption similar to that seen in idiopathic TTP (44).

The mainstay of therapy in all cases of drug-associated TTP is withdrawal of the drug; most often standard therapies such as TPE are performed as an adjunctive therapy. One case series of 14 patients with quinine-associated TTP treated with plasma exchange showed a 21% mortality rate, in those that survived, there were no relapses (33). A retrospective case review in ticlopidine-associated TTP showed the overall mortality of those who did not receive TPE was 57.9%, while those receiving TPE had a mortality rate of 18.3% ($p < 0.001$) (34). Several types of therapies have been employed for the treatment of mitomycin-C–associated TTP, including TPE, plasma infusion, glucocorticosteroids, dialysis, and others. Despite these interventions, it carries a very poor prognosis with overall survival rates variously reported at 0%–25%. Most patients die by three months from the time of diagnosis no matter what treatments are used (42).

Conclusion. Several clinical situations (allogeneic transplantation, SLE) and drug exposures are associated with the development of TTP or a TTP-like syndrome. Despite less favorable outcomes as are seen in idiopathic TTP, clinicians can consider employing standard therapies such as TPE/plasma infusion or glucocorticosteroids in management of these patients (Grade 2C).

What is the role of rituximab in the treatment of TTP?

The underlying autoimmune nature of idiopathic TTP has resulted in the use of several adjunctive immunosuppressive strategies, such as glucocorticosteroids (described previously), chemotherapeutic agents, and splenectomy (see Table 16.1). Patients with idiopathic TTP and high titers of autoantibodies to ADAMTS13 appear to have a poor outcome (39); consequently, these cases may benefit from aggressive immunosuppression in addition to TPE. Rituximab is a chimeric anti-CD20 antibody with immunosuppressive properties currently used in the treatment of clonal B-cell lymphoproliferative disorders. Several off-label uses for this drug have been reported in autoimmune disorders. The only randomized clinical trial describing its use in such diseases has been in treatment of rheumatoid arthritis with positive outcomes (45).

Table 16.1 Immunosuppressive strategies in TTP.

Treatment strategy	Level of evidence
Vincristine (17,46)	Grade 2C
Cyclosporine (47)	Grade 2C
Azathiprine/Prednisone (48)	Grade 2C
Cyclophosphamide (49)	Grade 2C
Splenectomy (50–52)	Grade 2C

Published literature regarding the use of rituximab in TTP is in the form of case reports and small case series describing between one and five patients. Most were treated with four weekly rituximab doses at 375 mg/m^2. When summed together, all of the cases report a clinically significant response to rituximab, with relapses in only 4 of 29 patients; the median duration of response reported varies between 2 and 23 months. However, confounding these data is that there were no controls in any of the case series, and most of the patients received several other immunosuppressive agents in addition to rituximab (i.e., corticosteroids, vincristine). Laboratory correlates obtained in certain case series report marked increases in the ADAMTS13 activity and decrease in ADAMTS13 inhibitor after administration of rituximab (53).

Conclusion. Rituximab at a dose of 375 mg/m^2 weekly for four weeks can be considered for use in cases of refractory or recurrent episodes of TTP (Grade 2C).

References

1 Torok TJ, Holman RC, Chorba TL. Increasing mortality from thrombocytopenic purpura in the United States: analysis of national mortality data. *Am J Hematol.* 1995;**50**:84–90.

2 Amorosi EL, Ultmann JE. Thrombotic thrombocytopenic purpura: report of 16 cases and review of the literature. *Medicine.* 1966;**45**:139–59.

3 Byrnes JJ, Khurana M. Treatment of thrombocytopenic purpura with plasma. *N Eng J Med.* 1977;**297**:1386–89.

4 Bukowski RM, King JW, Hewlett JS. Plasmapheresis in the treatment of thrombotic thrombocytopenic purpura. *Blood.* 1977;**50**:413–17.

5 Daram SR, Philipneri M, Puri N, et al. Thrombotic thrombocytopenic purpura without schistocytes on the peripheral blood smear. *South Med J.* 2005;**98**(3):392–95.

6 Lesesve JF, Salignac S, Lecompte T, et al. Automated measurement of schistocytes after bone marrow transplantation. *Bone Marrow Transplant.* 2004;**34**(4):357–62.

7 Mansoor S, Roman A, Weinstein R. Intravascular stents do not cause microangiopathic hemolysis or thrombotic microangiopathy. *J Clin Apher.* 1999;**14**(3):130–34.

8 Burns ER, Lou Y, Pathak A. Morphologic diagnosis of thrombotic thrombocytopenic purpura. *Am J Hematol.* 2004;**75**(1):18–21.

9 Ruutu T, Barosi G, Benjamin RJ, et al. Diagnostic criteria for hematopoietic stem cell transplant-associated microangiopathy: results of a consensus process by an International Working Group. *Haematologica.* 2007;**92**(1):95–100.

10 Tsai HM. Is severe deficiency of ADAMTS-13 specific for thrombotic thrombocytopenic purpura? Yes. *J Thromb Haemost.* 2003;**1**(4): 625–31.

11 Mannucci PM, Canciani MT, Forza I, et al. Changes in health and disease of the metalloprotease that cleaves von Willebrand factor. *Blood.* 2001;**98**(9):2730–35.

12 Furlan M, Robles R, Galbusera M, et al. von Willebrand factor-cleaving protease in thrombotic thrombocytopenic purpura and the hemolytic-uremic syndrome. *N Engl J Med.* 1998;**339**(22):1578–84.

13 Vesely SK, George JN, Lammle B, et al. ADAMTS13 activity in thrombotic thrombocytopenic purpura-hemolytic uremic syndrome: relation to presenting features and clinical outcomes in a prospective cohort of 142 patients. *Blood.* 2003;**102**(1):60–8.

14 Vayrader A, Obert B, Houllier A, et al. Specific von Willebrand factor-cleaving protease in thrombotic microangiopathies: a study of 111 cases. *Blood.* 2001;**98**(6):1765–72.

15 Bianchi V, Robles R, Alberio L, et al. Von Willebrand factor-cleaving protease (ADAMTS13) in thrombocytopenic disorders: a severely deficient activity is specific for thrombotic thrombocytopenic purpura. *Blood.* 2002;**100**(2):710–13.

16 Remuzzi G, Galbusera M, Noris M, et al. von Willebrand factor cleaving protease (ADAMTS13) is deficient in recurrent and familial thrombotic thrombocytopenic purpura and hemolytic uremic syndrome. *Blood.* 2002;**100**(3):778–85.

17 Bobbio-Pallavincini E, Porta C, Centurioni R, et al. Vincristine sulfate for the treatment of thrombotic thrombocytopenic purpura refractory to plasma-exchange. The Italian Cooperative Group for TTP. *Eur J Haematol.* 1994;**52**:222–26.

18 Rock GA, Shumak KH, Buskard NA, et al. Comparison of plasma exchange with plasma infusion in the treatment of thrombotic thrombocytopenic purpura. Canadian Apheresis Study Group. *N Engl J Med.* 1991;**325**(6):393–97.

19 George JN. How I treat patients with thrombotic thrombocytopenic purpura-hemolytic uremic syndrome. *Blood.* 2000;**96**(4):1223–29.

20 Coppo P, Bussel A, Charrier S, et al. High-dose plasma infusion versus plasma exchange as early treatment of thrombotic thrombocytopenic purpura/hemolytic-uremic syndrome. *Medicine (Baltimore).* 2003;**82**(1):27–38.

21 Byrnes JJ, Moake JL, Klug P, et al. Effectiveness of the cryosupernatant fraction of plasma in the treatment of refractory thrombotic thrombocytopenic purpura. *Am J Hematol.* 1990;**34**(3):169–74.

22 Obrador GT, Zeigler ZR, Shadduck RK, et al. Effectiveness of cryosupernatant therapy in refractory and chronic relapsing thrombotic thrombocytopenic purpura. *Am J Hematol.* 1993;**42**(2):217–20.

23 Owens MR, Sweeney JD, Tahhan RH, et al. Influence of type of exchange fluid on survival in therapeutic apheresis for thrombotic thrombocytopenic purpura. *J Clin Apher.* 1995;**10**(4):178–82.

24 Rock G, Shumak KH, Sutton DM, et al. Cryosupernatant as replacement fluid for plasma exchange in thrombotic thrombocytopenic purpura. Members of the Canadian Apheresis Group. *Br J Haematol.* 1996;**94**(2):383–86.

25 Zeigler ZR, Shadduck RK, Gryn JF, et al. Cryoprecipitate poor plasma does not improve early response in primary adult thrombotic thrombocytopenic purpura (TTP). *J Clin Apher.* 2001;**16**(1):19–22.

26 Myers TJ, Wakem CJ, Ball ED, et al. Thrombotic thrombocytopenic purpura: combined treatment with plasmapheresis and antiplatelet agents. *Ann Intern Med.* 1980;**92**(2 Pt 1):149–55.

27 Bell WR, Braine HG, Ness PM, et al. Improved survival in thrombotic thrombocytopenic purpura-hemolytic uremic syndrome: clinical experience in 108 patients. *N Engl J Med.* 1991;**325**(6):398–403.

28 Bobbio-Pallavicini E, Gugliotta L, Centurioni R, et al. Antiplatelet agents in thrombotic thrombocytopenic purpura (TTP). Results of a randomized multicenter trial by the Italian Cooperative Group for TTP. *Haematologica.* 1997;**82**(4):429–35.

29 Rosove MH, Ho WG, Goldfinger D. Ineffectiveness of aspirin and dipyridamole in the treatment of thrombotic thrombocytopenic purpura. *Ann Intern Med.* 1982;**96**(1):27–33.

30 Allford SL, Hunt BJ, Rose P, et al. Guidelines on the diagnosis and management of the thrombotic microangiopathic haemolytic anaemias. *Br J Haematol.* 2003;**120**(4):556–73.

31 Howard MA, Williams LA, Terrell DR, et al. Complications of plasma exchange in patients treated for clinically suspected thrombotic thrombocytopenic purpura-hemolytic uremic syndrome. *Transfusion.* 2006;**46**(1):154–56.

32 Gordon LI, Kwaan HC. Thrombotic microangiopathy manifesting as thrombotic thrombocytopenic purpura/hemolytic uremic syndrome in the cancer patient. *Semin Thromb Hemost.* 1999;**25**(2):217–21.

33 Kojouri K, Vesely SK, George JN. Quinine-associated thrombotic thrombocytopenic purpura-hemolytic uremic syndrome: frequency, clinical features, and long-term outcomes. *Ann Intern Med.* 2001;**135**(12):1047–51.

34 Bennett CL, Davidson CJ, Raisch DW, et al. Thrombotic thrombocytopenic purpura associated with ticlopidine in the setting of coronary artery stents and stroke prevention. *Arch Intern Med.* 1999;**159**(21):2524–28.

35 Roy V, Rizvi MA, Vesely SK, et al. Thrombotic thrombocytopenic purpura-like syndromes following bone marrow transplantation: an analysis of associated conditions and clinical outcomes. *Bone Marrow Transplant.* 2001;**27**(6):641–46.

36 van der Plas RM, Schiphorst ME, Huizinga EG, et al. von Willebrand factor proteolysis is deficient in classic, but not in bone marrow transplantation-associated, thrombotic thrombocytopenic purpura. *Blood.* 1999;**93**(11):3798–802.

37 Guvenc B, Unsal C, Gurkan E, et al. Systemic lupus erythematosus and thrombotic thrombocytopenic purpura: a case report. *Transfus Apher Sci.* 2004;**31**(1):17–20.

38 Musio F, Bohen EM, Yuan CM, et al. Review of thrombotic thrombocytopenic purpura in the setting of systemic lupus erythematosus. *Semin Arthritis Rheum.* 1998;**28**(1):1–19.

39 Zheng XL, Kaufman RM, Goodnough LT, et al. Effect of plasma exchange on plasma ADAMTS13 metalloprotease activity, inhibitor level, and clinical outcome in patients with idiopathic and nonidiopathic thrombotic thrombocytopenic purpura. *Blood.* 2004;**103**(11):4043–49.

40 Mauro M, Zlatopolskiy A, Raife TJ, et al. Thienopyridine-linked thrombotic microangiopathy: association with endothelial cell apoptosis and activation of MAP kinase signalling cascades. *Br J Haematol.* 2004;**124**(2):200–10.

41 Gottschall JL, Neahring B, McFarland JG, et al. Quinine-induced immune thrombocytopenia with hemolytic uremic syndrome: clinical and serological findings in nine patients and review of literature. *Am J Hematol.* 1994;**47**(4):283–89.
42 Lesesne JB, Rothschild N, Erickson B, et al. Cancer-associated hemolytic-uremic syndrome: analysis of 85 cases from a national registry. *J Clin Oncol.* 1989;**7**(6):781–89.
43 Murgo AJ. Thrombotic microangiopathy in the cancer patient including those induced by chemotherapeutic agents. *Semin Hematol.* 1987;**24**(3):161–77.
44 Nagaya S, Wada H, Oka K, et al. Hemostatic abnormalities and increased vascular endothelial cell markers in patients with red cell fragmentation syndrome induced by mitomycin C. *Am J Hematol.* 1995;**50**(4): 237–43.
45 Cohen SB, Emery P, Greenwald MW, et al. Rituximab for rheumatoid arthritis refractory to anti-tumor necrosis factor therapy: results of a multicenter, randomized, double-blind, placebo-controlled, phase III trial evaluating primary efficacy and safety at twenty-four weeks. *Arthritis Rheum.* 2006;**54**(9):2793–806.
46 Gutterman LA, Stevenson TD. Treatment of thrombotic thrombocytopenic purpura with vincristine. *JAMA.* 1982;**247**:1433–36.
47 Kierdorf H, Maurin N, Heintz B. Cyclosporine for thrombotic thrombocytopenic purpura [Letter]. *Ann Intern Med.* 1993;**118**:987–88.
48 Moake JL, Rudy CK, Troll JH, et al. Therapy of chronic relapsing thrombocytopenic purpura with prednisone and azathioprine. *Am J Hematol.* 1985;**20**:73–79.
49 Zieschang M, Kohlhäufl M, Höffler D, et al. A case of thrombotic thrombocytopenic purpura successfully treated with cyclophosphamide [Letter]. *Nephron.* 1995;**69**:176.
50 Kappers-Klunne MC, Wijermans P, Fijnheer R, et al. Splenectomy for the treatment of thrombotic thrombocytopenic purpura. *Br J Haematol.* 2005;**130**:768–76.
51 Outschoorn UM, Ferber A. Outcomes in the treatment of thrombotic thrombocytopenic purpura with splenectomy: a retrospective cohort study. *Am J Hematol.* 2006;**81**:895–900.
52 Hovinga JA, Studt J, Biasiutti FD, et al. Splenectomy in relapsing and plasma-refractory acquired thrombotic thrombocytopenic purpura. *Haematologica.* 2004;**89**:320–24.
53 Hull MJ, Eichbaum QG. Efficacy of rituximab and concurrent plasma exchange in the treatment of thrombotic thrombocytopenic purpura. *Clin Adv Hematol Oncol.* 2006;**4**(3):210–14.

17 Diagnosis and Management of Disseminated Intravascular Coagulation

Julia A. M. Anderson

Disseminated intravascular coagulation (DIC) is a clinicopathologic syndrome characterized by the systemic activation of coagulation. The mainstay of the syndrome involves the dysregulation and excessive generation of thrombin and a reactive fibrinolytic response. This leads to the widespread deposition of fibrin in the circulation contributing to microvascular thrombosis and multiorgan failure, a recognized phenomenon from histological studies and animal experiments (1–3). Further activation of the coagulation system depletes platelets and coagulation factors and may precipitate bleeding manifestations. Clinical manifestations are diverse, forming a spectrum from asymptomatic lab abnormalities to hemorrhagic and thrombotic complications, with evidence for nonovert and overt clinical phases (4).

Until recently, DIC was poorly defined; its varied clinical presentation, heterogeneous causation (see Table 17.1; Figure 17.1) and lack of systematic randomized controlled trials have led to many recommendations based on expert opinion and consensus-driven guidelines with no secure evidence base. Increasing knowledge of important pathogenetic mechanisms has resulted in novel therapeutic approaches to patients with DIC. In an effort to facilitate basic and clinical research into DIC, the 2001 Scientific Subcommittee on DIC of the International Society on Thrombosis and Haemostasis (ISTH) proposed a practical working definition (5) and a diagnostic scoring system for "overt" DIC that now form a reference point for randomized controlled trials and a more evidence-based approach to the management of this syndrome.

A search of MEDLINE and PubMed for English language articles relating to humans published from 1966 to 2006 using the terms "disseminated intravascular coagulation" and related keywords, and a search of the American Society for Hematology and the ISTH meeting abstracts and ISTH abstracts for the years 1996 to 2005 yielded 11,682 publications, the majority of which are case reports, studies of pathophysiology, and reviews. There are three phase III randomized controlled trials evaluating the role of natural anticoagulants in the management of DIC.

This chapter highlights and grades the currently available evidence relevant to the diagnosis and management of DIC and poses the following questions:

1. How does the clinician make a diagnosis of DIC, and why is this a relevant clinical finding?
2. What is the role of specialized assays in the diagnosis of DIC?
3. What scoring systems are in use, and what are their limitations?
4. Why is an international working definition and scoring system important?
5. What are the primary management principles in the treatment of a patient in DIC?
6. Is there evidence to support the use of anticoagulants and fibrinolytic inhibitors?
7. Is there a role for the supplementation of natural anticoagulant pathways in the management of patients with DIC?

Grading of the quality of evidence and strengths of recommendations in this chapter are based on the guidelines proposed by the international Grading of Recommendations Assessment, Development, and Evaluation Working Group (GRADE), adopting the modification used by the American College of Chest Physicians that merges the very low and low categories of quality of evidence (see chapter 1).

How is the diagnosis of DIC made?

The presence of DIC increases the risk of mortality beyond that associated with the primary disease (4,6). No single test exists with sufficient diagnostic accuracy to confirm the diagnosis of DIC. Most importantly, the diagnosis of DIC rests on the correlation of clinical features, taking into account the relevant causative factor and laboratory findings. Monitoring the trend in serial tests is often more important than the absolute results.

Evidence-based Hematology. Edited by Mark A. Crowther, Jeff Ginsberg, Holger J. Schünemann, Ralph M. Meyer, and Richard Lottenberg.

Table 17.1 Clinical conditions associated with overt disseminated intravascular coagulation.

Diagnosis	Causes
Sepsis, severe infection	Gram negative and gram positive bacterial infections Viral infections Fungal infections Parasitic infections
Trauma	Shock, hypoxia, brain injury, burns, heat stroke
Malignancy	Solid tumors, including mucin-producing adenocarcinoma Hematological malignancies, especially acute promyelocytic leukemia
Obstetric emergencies	Amniotic fluid embolism, abruptio placentae, retained dead fetus, eclampsia
Vascular abnormalities	Large vessel aneurysms,* giant hemangioma, including Kasabach-Merrit syndrome
Toxic	Drugs (recreational) Venoms—snake and spider bites
Immunological	Drugs (therapeutic)—heparin-induced thrombocytopenia ABO incompatible transfusion
Advanced liver disease	LeVeen shunt

*See Figure 17.1.

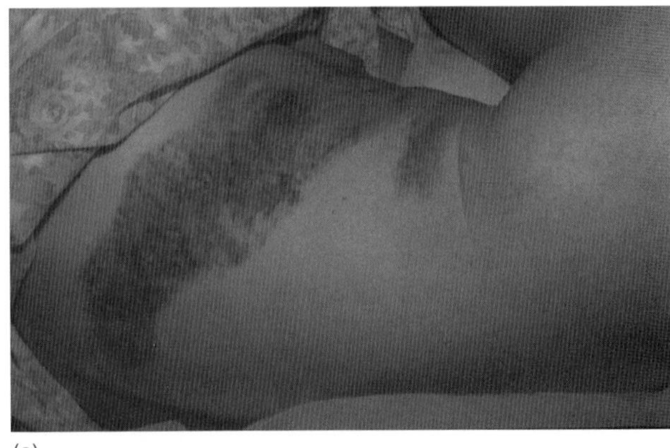

(a)

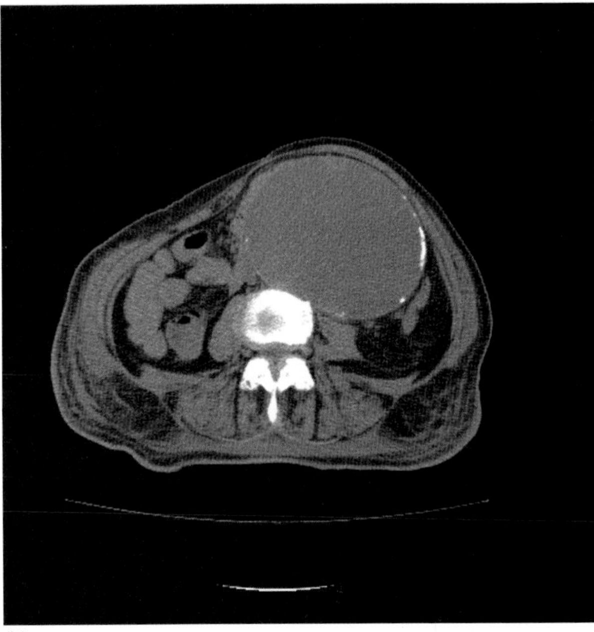

(b)

Figure 17.1 (a) Ecchymosis in a patient with chronic disseminated intravascular coagulation caused by (b) a massive thoracoabdominal aneurysm.

Screening for the presence of overt DIC can be made by a combination of simple, reliable, readily available laboratory tests, and forms the basis of two currently used scoring systems (5,6):

1. Complete blood count and examination of the blood film

A decreasing trend in the platelet count represents a sensitive, but nonspecific marker of DIC. Examination of the blood film may reveal red cell fragments but may also highlight the cause, for example, toxic granulation and Döhle bodies within neutrophils and blasts in acute leukemia (see Figure 17.2).

2. Global assays of hemostasis

The prothrombin time (PT), activated partial thromboplastin time (APTT), and thrombin clotting time (TCT) may show prolongation, a reflection of ongoing coagulation factor consumption, and impaired synthesis. These tests do not assess activation of coagulation. Measurement of coagulation factor activity, such as factor VII and factor V assays, and natural anticoagulants, such as antithrombin and protein C activities add to the laboratory picture.

3. Fibrinogen

Measurement of fibrinogen can be misleading as it acts as an acute phase reactant, and with increased turnover may remain within a normal range before falling due to consumption. Hypofibrinogenemia is detected in limited cases, including acute head injury, prostatic adenocarcinoma with hyperfibrinolysis, and obstetric emergencies (7). Low levels of fibrinogen otherwise reflect the late consumptive stage of DIC. The measurement of fibrinogen has recently been removed from the Japanese Association for Acute Medicine DIC scoring system (8), and it is postulated that the removal of fibrinogen levels from the calculation of ISTH DIC score will not affect the accuracy of its scoring system (9).

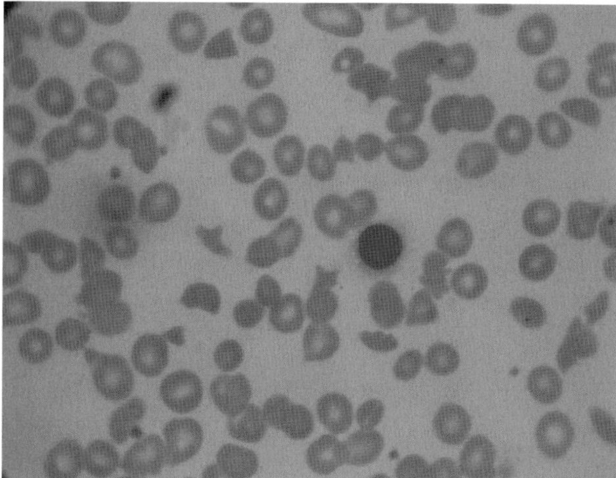

Figure 17.2 Importance of blood film examination in a patient with disseminated breast cancer: the blood film shows circulating tumor cells, thrombocytopenia and dramatic red cell fragmentation. Howell Jolly bodies are also evident, secondary to previous splenectomy.

4. Tests for fibrin(ogen) degradation products (FDPs)

A test for the presence of fibrin degradation products is considered a sine qua non for the diagnosis of DIC and should be elevated in almost all patients with DIC (10).

FDPs may be detected by:

i. A serum FDP assay that uses polyclonal antibodies to detect fibrin(ogen) degradation products D and E.

ii. A monoclonal antibody to detect the covalently linked D regions of FDPs (D-dimer) (11).

iii. By the addition of protamine sulfate or ethanol to cause precipitation in plasma of fibrin monomers and other fibrin-containing complexes.

What is the role of specialized assays in the diagnosis of DIC?

Nonovert DIC represents a more subtle form of hemostatic dysfunction, and its detection may provide better outcomes for the patient by facilitating earlier intervention (12). Specialized laboratory tests have been used in clinical trials and research settings to assess for the presence of nonovert DIC, and include:

- markers of soluble fibrin monomer: markers of soluble fibrin are highly sensitive but not specific. Quantification of soluble fibrin is also difficult with variation between available assays (13)
- markers of thrombin generation: prothrombin fragment 1+2 or thrombin-antithrombin complexes
- markers of endothelial activity (thrombomodulin)
- neutrophil (elastase) disturbance
- α_2-antiplasmin levels (often reduced in patients with hyperfibrinolysis, as in prostate disease or liver disease).

The analysis of a biphasic waveform displayed by an automated laboratory machine during the APTT assay is a relatively specific and sensitive marker for DIC at its early stage (14) but can only be performed on the MDA coagulation analyzer and is available in only a limited number of labs. Detection of a similar abnormal clotting pattern on other equipment may help diagnose nonovert DIC in the future (9).

What scoring systems are in use, and what are their limitations?

In 1983, the Japanese Research Committee on DIC sponsored by the Japanese Ministry of Health and Welfare (JMHW) proposed criteria for the diagnosis of DIC, and a scoring system was developed (6) but not widely adopted because of practical limitations (15,16). In 2001, a scoring system was reviewed by the Subcommittee on DIC of the ISTH (5) based on a retrospective analysis of studies in patients with DIC. The five-step diagnostic algorithm uses the aforementioned routinely used laboratory tests (platelet count, PT, decreased fibrinogen, plasma levels of fibrin[ogen] degradation products) and creates a scoring system (0–8 points). The overt scoring system has been prospectively validated in a cohort of intensive care patients confirming high sensitivity and specificity (9); a nonovert scoring system has been demonstrated to be workable and has prognostic relevance and uses additional coagulation assays of antithrombin and protein C (12).

Presently, the ISTH score fails to account for dynamic changes over a period of time. New clinical scores are being refined and validated (8,17) with the aim of improving the predictive power. Proposed modifications to the ISTH score include the removal of fibrinogen levels from the algorithm, and replacement of the PT by the international normalized ratio (INR), to further standardize the system. The optimal choice for a fibrin-related marker and the ideal cutoff value also need to be established. In most centers, measurement of D-dimers is used, but the measurement of soluble fibrin holds promise (18). A recent study has demonstrated that optimal cutoff points can be defined for the use of D-dimer results in the DIC score (19).

Why is an international working definition and scoring system important?

The ISTH Scoring system is not only a helpful bedside tool, but also an independent predictor of mortality when applied to large databases of patients with severe sepsis (7). The score may form the basis of patient selection for new therapies aimed at modulating the interface of coagulation and inflammatory cascades, such as recombinant human activated protein C (rhaPC). It also allows for more standardized patient stratification in clinical trials of critically ill patients treated with interventions aimed at the coagulation system (20). Intensivists may be able to combine the overt DIC score with other scores, such as the APACHE II score to better predict mortality in critically ill patients although a prospective study is required in this area (21).

What are the primary management principles in the treatment of a patient with DIC?

An individual approach is necessary with prompt recognition and removal of the precipitating cause. This may dramatically alleviate the coagulopathy as, for example, in obstetric cases with uterine evacuation for *abruptio placentae*. In other situations, for example, septicemia, the administration of antibiotics and other treatment measures may not alleviate the coagulopathy and DIC proceeds (4,22).

Supportive management includes the maintenance of adequate oxygenation, fluid, and electrolyte balance and the prevention of acidosis and hypothermia. Replacement folate to prevent cytopenias and vitamin K to prevent acquired coagulation deficiencies are important simple measures.

The efficacy of treatment with plasma, fibrinogen, cryoprecipitate, or platelets holds no evidence basis but is widely accepted as supportive and aimed at replacing depleted coagulation factors (23). Plasma and blood product therapies should not be administered on the basis of lab results alone. Administration of plasma and blood products may be appropriate in a patient with active bleeding, with a high bleeding risk, or if undergoing invasive procedures. Large volumes of plasma products may be necessary to correct a given defect.

In nonbleeding patients, prophylactic platelet transfusions should be considered to maintain a platelet count greater than $10–20 \times 10^9$/L. Higher target levels may be required in patients undergoing procedures, at risk for life-threatening bleeding (head injury or intracranial bleeding), or with significant blood loss. The threshold for platelet transfusion is based on randomized controlled trials in patients with thrombocytopenia following chemotherapy.

Cryoprecipitate administration should be considered in a symptomatic patient to maintain the plasma fibrinogen over 1.0g/L, and the administration of 10–15 mL/kg fresh frozen plasma is recommended to correct factor deficiencies in DIC-associated bleeding, with repeat PT and APTT tests to guide further therapy.

The use of coagulation factor concentrates, such as prothrombin complex concentrates, are not usually appropriate as they contain only single or a small combination of factors; minute traces of activated coagulation factors may precipitate thromboembolism or worsen the coagulopathy.

Is there evidence to support the use of anticoagulants and the use of fibrinolytic inhibitors in the management of DIC?

Anticoagulant therapy

Unfractionated heparin, low-molecular-weight heparin (LMWH), direct thrombin inhibitors, and other novel agents have been shown to be efficacious in experimental models of sepsis (24–26), but clinical studies are to date inconclusive (27).

The successful use of heparin and LMWH have been anecdotally reported in specific settings, such as chronic DIC associated with solid tumors (28), and in overt cases of thromboembolism or situations involving extensive fibrin deposition, such as purpura fulminans and acral necrosis. Case reports highlight the successful use of LMWH in managing chronic DIC in aortic aneurysms, but in a small clinical series of 15 patients with abdominal aortic aneurysm and markers of nonovert DIC, the preoperative administration of LMWH failed to improve intra-operative parameters such as operating time, blood loss, and transfusion demands, despite improvements preoperatively in platelet number and fibrinogen concentration (29).

The role of heparin in the treatment of the coagulopathy complicating acute promyelocytic leukaemia (APML) remains controversial (30). Before the introduction of all-trans retinoic acid therapy, although widely accepted as a standard of practice, no prospective, randomized controlled studies demonstrated the efficacy of heparin in this setting. Retrospective studies and small poorly controlled clinical trials attempted to address the issue, but results require cautious interpretation, and overall fail to demonstrate significant efficacy of early therapy with heparin in the reduction of early death in patients with APML (31–33). Because of advances in leukemia care, there is a need to re-evaluate prophylactic anticoagulant therapy, such as LMWH or fondaparinux, to reduce early hemorrhagic death from DIC in APML. Well-designed randomized controlled trials are required (34).

Novel anticoagulants may hold promise in the management of DIC, including recombinant nematode anticoagulant protein c2, a potent, specific inhibitor of the tissue factor/factor VIIa pathway (35). The favorable effects of recombinant hirudin on endotoxin-induced DIC have been demonstrated in animal studies (36) and also shown in human volunteers to blunt thrombin generation and the expression of tissue factor on monocytes (37). To date, there have been no controlled clinical trials of this drug in patients with DIC; the potential for bleeding (38) and lack of an antidote may prove limiting factors.

Conclusion. Heparin may play a role in selected cases of DIC involving thromboembolism, or fibrin deposition (Grade 2C). Its role in the management of DIC in APML remains controversial (Grade 2C).

Fibrinolytic inhibitors: (epsilon-aminocaproic acid [EACA] or tranexamic acid)

These agents act by blocking secondary fibrinogenolysis and in the setting of DIC may have adverse consequences such as the prevention of tissue perfusion. Consideration may be warranted in situations of intense fibrinogenolysis, such as the Kasabach–Merrit syndrome and other vascular malformations with anecdotal reports of the successful use of tranexamic acid in combination with danaparoid sodium in chronic DIC associated with abdominal aortic aneurysm (39).

Tranexamic acid has been used in the coagulopathies affecting metastatic prostate cancer and APML (40), although in a large retrospective study of 268 patients treated for APML with either heparin, antifibrinolytic agents (tranexamic acid, EACA, or aprotonin), and supportive therapy alone, no significant differences were demonstrated between the three groups (31).

Conclusion. Fibrinolytic inhibitors may have a limited role in the management of DIC associated with intense fibrinogenolysis (Grade 2C).

Is there a role for the supplementation of natural anticoagulant pathways?

Phase III clinical trials have been performed with three natural anticoagulants, antithrombin (AT) (41), activated protein C (aPC) (42), and tissue factor pathway inhibitor (TFPI) (43) in the setting of patients with severe sepsis (38).

TFPI

In 2001, a large (1,754 patients) phase III randomized, double-blind, placebo-controlled, multicenter trial of recombinant TFPI (rTFPI), the OPTIMIST trial, demonstrated rTFPI to be ineffective in patients with severe sepsis (43). There was a notable drug interaction with heparin and rTFPI with a trend to harm in the rTFPI arm when heparin was co-administered (rTFPI 34% vs. placebo 29.8%, $p = 0.12$). Disparate results in mortality rates were observed during the course of the trial and remain unexplained (44).

Antithrombin (AT)

The use of AT concentrates in patients with DIC has been studied extensively, mostly in patients with septicemia. As AT levels notably decrease in the presence of systemic infection, there is a clear rationale for its replacement in septic patients (45). All trials show a degree of beneficial effect in terms of improvement of lab parameters, shortening of the duration of DIC, or an improvement in organ function (38). A series of small trials has demonstrated a modest reduction in mortality in AT-treated patients, but no trial has demonstrated a statistically significant effect (46–48). In the KyberSept trial, a large multicenter phase III randomized placebo-controlled trial of patients with severe sepsis, there was no significant reduction in 28-day patient mortality in those with sepsis treated with AT concentrate (41) (38.9% AT group vs. 38.7% placebo group, $p = 0.94$). Questions relate to whether an optimal patient cohort was studied as the 90-day survival time analysis reached statistical significance with a mortality rate of 44.9% in the AT group and 52.5% in placebo group and whether the pre-specified target blood level of AT in the treated arm of >200% was achieved (44).

Recombinant activated protein C and protein C replacement therapies

Activated protein C concentrate has been demonstrated to have anti-inflammatory and anti-apoptotic properties in animal models of gram negative septicemia (49). Clinically, the beneficial effect of rhaPC has been demonstrated in two randomized controlled trials. Following a dose-ranging study (50), a large phase III multicenter randomized controlled trial in patients with severe sepsis demonstrated a dramatic statistically significant reduction in absolute risk of death of 6.1% and a relative risk reduction of 19.4% (prematurely stopped at second interim analysis because of a significant reduction in mortality in the aPC treated patients) (42). All-cause mortality at 28 days was 25% in the aPC group versus 31% in the control group, a 19.4% relative risk reduction. The administration of aPC was demonstrated to cause an amelioration of coagulation abnormalities, and aPC-treated patients had less organ failure (51).

Recombinant human aPC is now licensed for the treatment of patients with severe sepsis and two or more organ failures. It is administered as a 96-hour infusion, and caution is necessary in patients with thrombocytopenia ($<30 \times 10^9$/L) to avoid risk of intracranial hemorrhage.

The successful use of (unactivated) protein C replacement has been reported in meningococcal septicemia (52) and purpura fulminans (53). In situations in which protein C is not available, the strategy to replace protein C by plasma exchange has proven successful in a small case series (54).

Conclusion. Current evidence shows no role for the use of rTFPI (Grade 2B) or AT (Grade 2B) in the management of DIC associated with sepsis. There is a strong recommendation for the use of rhaPC in the management of DIC associated with severe sepsis (Grade 1A). Protein C may be replaced by factor concentrate or by plasma exchange and may hold a role in the setting of DIC in sepsis if rhaPC is unavailable (Grade 2C).

Summary points

- DIC is a syndrome characterized by enhanced thrombin generation leading to the intravascular deposition of fibrin within the microvasculature leading to organ dysfunction.
- The presence of DIC increases the risk of mortality beyond that associated with the primary disease state.
- Increased knowledge of the pathogenesis of DIC has enabled novel therapeutic strategies to be considered in clinical trials.
- The development of an internationally accepted working definition and scoring systems of overt and non-overt DIC may allow improved patient selection for future randomized clinical trials.

References

1 Shimamura K, Oka K, Nakazawa M, et al. Distribution patterns of microthrombi in disseminated intravascular coagulation. *Arch Pathol Lab Med.* 1983;**107**:543–47.

2 Kojima M, Shimamura K, Mori N, Oka K, et al. A histological study on microthrombin in autopsy cases of DIC. *Bibl Haematol.* 1983;**49**:95–106.

3 McHenry MC, Baggenstoss AH, Martin WJ. Bacteremia due to gram-negative bacilli: clinical and autopsy findings in 33 cases. *Am J Clin Pathol.* 1968;**50**:160–74.

4 Toh CH, Dennis M. Disseminated intravascular coagulation: old disease, new hope. *BMJ.* 2005;**327**:974–77.

5 Taylor FB, Toh CH, Hoots WK, et al. Towards definition, clinical and laboratory criteria and a scoring system for disseminated intravascular coagulation. *Thromb Haemost.* 2001;**86**:1327–30.

6 Kobayashi N, Maekawa T, Takada M, et al. Criteria for diagnosis of DIC based on the analysis of clinical and laboratory findings in 345 DIC patients collected by the Research Committee on DIC in Japan. *Bibl Haematol.* 1983;**49**:265–75.

7 Levi M. Settling the score for disseminated intravascular coagulation. *Crit Care Med.* 2005;**33**:2417–18.

8 Gando S, Iba T, Eguchi Y, et al. A multicenter, prospective validation of disseminated intravascular coagulation diagnostic criteria for critically ill patients: comparing current criteria. *Crit Care Med.* 2006;**34**:625–31.

9 Bakhtiari K, Meijers JC, de Jonge E, et al. Prospective validation of the International Society of Thrombosis and Haemostasis scoring system for disseminated intravascular coagulation. *Crit Care Med.* 2004;**32**:2416–21.

10 Levi M, de Jonge E, Meijers J. The diagnosis of disseminated intravascular coagulation. *Blood Rev.* 2002;**16**:217–23.

11 Carr JM, McKinney M, McDonagh J. Diagnosis of disseminated intravascular coagulation: role of D-dimer. *Am J Clin Pathol.* 1989;**91**:280–87.

12 Toh CH, Downey C. Performance and prognostic importance of a new clinical and laboratory scoring system for identifying non-overt disseminated intravascular coagulation. *Blood Coag Fibrinol.* 2005;**16**:69–74.

13 Dempfle CE. The use of soluble fibrin in evaluating the acute and chronic hypercoagulable state. *Thromb Haemost.* 1999;**82**:673–87.

14 Toh CH, Samis J, Downey C, et al. Biphasic transmittance waveform in the APTT coagulation assay is due to the formation of a Ca(++)-dependent complex of C-reactive protein with very-low-density lipoprotein and is a novel marker of impending disseminated intravascular coagulation. *Blood.* 2002;**100**:2522–29.

15 Wada H, Gabazza EC, Asakura H, et al. Comparison of diagnostic criteria for disseminated intravascular coagulation (DIC): diagnostic criteria of the International Society of Thrombosis and Hemostasis and of the Japanese Ministry of Health and Welfare for overt DIC. *Am J Hematol.* 2003;**74**:17–22.

16 Wada H, Wakita Y, Nakase T, et al. Outcome of disseminated intravascular coagulation in relation to the score when treatment was begun. *Thromb Haemost.* 1995;**74**:848–52.

17 Kinasewitz GT, Zein JG, Lee GL. Prognostic value of a simple evolving disseminated intravascular coagulation score in patients with severe sepsis. *Crit Care Med.* 2005;**33**:2214–21.

18 Dempfle CE, Wurst M, Smolinski M. Use of soluble fibrin antigen instead of D-dimer as fibrin-related marker may enhance the prognostic power of the ISTH overt DIC score. *Thromb Haemost.* 2004;**91**:812–18.

19 Lehman CM, Wilson LW, Rodgers GM. Analytic validation and clinical evaluation of the STA LIATEST immunoturbidimetric D-dimer assay for the diagnosis of disseminated intravascular coagulation. *Am J Clin Pathol.* 2004;**122**:178–84.

20 Dhainaut JF, Yan SB, Joyce DE, et al. Treatment effects of drotrecogin alfa (activated) in patients with severe sepsis with or without overt disseminated intravascular coagulation. *J Thromb Haemost.* 2004;**2**:1924–33.

21 Angstwurm MWA, Dempfle CE, Spannagl M. New disseminated intravascular coagulation score: a useful tool to predict mortality in comparison with Acute Physiology and Chronic Health Evaluation II and Logistic Organ Dysfunction scores. *Crit Care Med.* 2006;**34**:314–20.

22 Gando S, Kameue T, Nanzaki S, et al. Disseminated intravascular coagulation is a frequent complication of systemic inflammatory response syndrome. *Thromb Haemost.* 1996;**75**:224–28.

23 Levi M. Current understanding of disseminated intravascular coagulation. *Br J Haematol.* 2004;**124**:567–76.

24 du Toit H, Coetzee AR, Chalton DO. Heparin treatment in thrombin-induced disseminated intravascular coagulation in the baboon. *Crit Care Med.* 1991;**19**:1195–1200.

25 Slofstra SH, van't Veer C, Buurman WA, et al. Low molecular weight heparin attentuates multiple organ failure in a murine model of disseminated intravascular coagulation. *Crit Care Med.* 2005;**33**:1455–57.

26 Pernerstorfer T, Hollenstein U, Hansen J, et al. Heparin blunts endotoxin-induced coagulation activation. *Circulation.* 1999;**100**:2485–90.

27 Feinstein DI. Diagnosis and management of disseminated intravascular coagulation: the role of heparin therapy. *Blood.* 1982;**60**:284–87.

28 Sakuragawa N, Hasegawa H, Maki M, et al. Clinical evaluation of low-molecular weight heparin (FR-860) on disseminated intravascular coagulation (DIC)—a multicenter co-operative double blind trial in comparison with heparin. *Thromb Haemost.* 1993;**72**:475–500.

29 Jelenska MM, Szmidt J, Bojakowski K, et al. Compensated activation of coagulation in patients with abdominal aortic aneurysm: effects of heparin treatment prior to elective surgery. *Thromb Haemost.* 2004;**92**:997–1002.

30 Falanga A, Rickles FR. Pathogenesis and management of the bleeding diathesis in acute promyelocytic leukemia. *Best Pract Res Clin Haematol.* 2003;**16**:463–82.

31 Rodeghiero F, Avvisati G, Castaman G, et al. Early deaths and anti-hemorrhagic treatments in acute promyelocytic leukemia. a GIMEMA retrospective study in 268 consecutive patients. *Blood.* 1990;**75**: 2112–17.

32 Goldberg MA, Ginsburg D, Mayer RJ, et al. Is heparin administration necessary during induction chemotherapy for patients with acute promyelocytic leukemia? *Blood.* 1987;**69**:187–91.

33 Hoyle CF, Swirsky DM, Hayhoe FG. Beneficial effect of heparin in the management of patients with acute promyelocytic anemia. *Br J Haematol.* 1988;**68**:283–89.

34 Tallman MS, Brenner B, de la Serna J, et al. Meeting report. *Leuk Res.* 2005;**29**:347–51.

35 Moons AH, Peters RJ, Cate H, et al. Recombinant nematode anticoagulant protein c2, a novel inhibitor of tissue factor-factor VIIa activity, abrogates endotoxin-induced coagulation in chimpanzees. *Thromb Haemost.* 2002;**88**:627–31.

36 Hermida J, Montes R, Paramo JA, et al. Endotoxin-induced disseminated intravascular coagulation in rabbits: effect of recombinant hirudin on hemostatic parameters, fibrin deposits, and mortality. *J Lab Clin Med.* 1998;**131**:77–83.

37 Pernerstorfer T, Hollenstein U, Hansen JB, et al. Lepirudin blunts endotoxin-induced coagulation activation. *Blood.* 2000;**95**:1729–34.

38 Levi M, ten Cate H. Disseminated intravascular coagulation. *N Engl J Med.* 1999;**341**:586–92.

39 Ontachi Y, Asakura H, Arahata M, et al. Effect of combined therapy of danaparoid sodium and tranexamic acid on chronic disseminated intravascular coagulation associated with abdominal aortic aneurysm. *Circ J.* 2005;**69**:1150–53.

40 Avvisati G, Ten Cate JW, Büller HR, et al. Tranexamic acid for control of haemorrhage in acute promyelocytic leukaemia. *Lancet.* 1989:**2**;122–24.

41 Warren BL, Eid A, Singer P, et al. High-dose antithrombin III in severe sepsis: a randomised controlled trial. *JAMA.* 2001;**286**:1869–78.

42 Bernard GR, Vincent AL, Laterre PF, et al. Efficacy and safety of recombinant human activated protein C for severe sepsis. *N Engl J Med.* 2001;**344**:699–709.

43 Abraham E, Reinhart K, Opal S, et al. Efficacy and safety of tifacogin (recombinant tissue factor pathway inhibitor) in severe sepsis: a randomised controlled trial. *JAMA.* 2003;**290**:238–47.

44 LaRosa SP, Opal SM. Tissue factor pathway inhibitor and antithrombin trial results. *Crit Care Clin.* 2005;**21**:433–48.

45 Opal SM. Therapeutic rationale for antithrombin in sepsis. *Crit Care Med.* 2000;**28**:S34–S37.

46 Fourrier F, Chopin C, Huart JJ, et al. Double-blind, placebo-controlled trial of antithrombin III concentrates in septic shock with disseminated intravascular coagulation. *Chest.* 1993;**104**:882–88.

47 Baudo F, Caimi TM, Ravizza A, et al. Antithrombin III (ATIII) replacement therapy in patients with sepsis and/or postsurgical complications: a controlled double-blind, randomised, multicenter study. *Intensive Care Med.* 1998;**24**:336–42.

48 Eisele B, Lamy M, Thijs LG, et al. Antithrombin III in patients with severe sepsis. A randomized, placebo-controlled, double-blind multicenter trial plus a meta-analysis on all randomized, placebo-controlled, double-blind trials with antithrombin III in severe sepsis. *Intensive Care Med.* 1998;**24**:663–72.

49 Joyce DE, Gelbert L, Ciacca A, et al. Gene expression profile of antithrombotic protein C defines new mechanisms modulating inflammation and apoptosis. *J Biol Chem.* 2001;**276**:11199–203.

50 Bernard GR, Ely EW, Wright TJ. Safety and dose relationship of recombinant human activated protein C for coagulopathy in severe sepsis. *Crit Care Med.* 2001;**29**:2051–59.

51 Vincent JL, Angus DC, Artigas A, et al. Effects of drotrecogin alfa (activated) on organ dysfunction in the PROWESS trial. Recombinant Human Activated Protein C Worldwide Evaluation in Severe Sepsis (PROWESS) Study Group. *Crit Care Med.* 2003;**31**:834–40.

52 Smith OP, White B, Vaughan D, et al. Use of protein C concentrate, heparin and haemofiltration in meningococcus-induced purpura fulminans. *Lancet.* 1997;**359**:1590–93.

53 Schellongowski P, Bauer E, Holzinger U, et al. Treatment of adult patients with sepsis-induced coagulopathy and purpura fulminans using a plasma-derived protein C concentrate (Ceprotin). *Vox Sang.* 2006;**90**:294–301.

54 Baker PM, Keeling DM, Murphy M. Plasma exchange as a source of protein C for acute-onset protein C pathway failure. *Br J Haematol.* 2003;**120**:166–71.

18 Diagnosis and Management of Hereditary Bleeding Disorders

Including Congenital/Acquired Platelet Function Disorders

Nigel S. Key, Alice D. Ma

Introduction

The focus of this chapter is inherited disorders of hemostasis, including those entities that affect primary hemostasis (including von Willebrand disease (vWD) and inherited intrinsic platelet defects) and those that affect secondary hemostasis (specifically, hemophilia A and B). Since the introduction and widespread availability of clotting factor concentrates to treat hemophilia (and later vWD) beginning in the 1960s, there has been a vast improvement in the ability to prevent death and disability from hemorrhage and improve quality of life in these patients (1). Despite these advances, it has been pointed out that the quality of evidence supporting current recommendations on the optimal dose and duration of clotting factor replacement in various bleeding episodes is not supported by rigorous evidence from appropriately designed clinical trials (2). For example, early prospective randomized controlled trials (RCTs) demonstrated that when initiated within two hours, a single FVIII dose of 14 U/kg was superior to 7 U/kg, but no less effective than 28 U/kg (both doses were >95% effective at 48 hours) for all severities of hemarthrosis within this category (3). Yet, in the absence of supportive evidence, single doses of 30 U/kg are frequently recommended for the treatment of acute hemarthrosis in many recent texts (4). In other situations, such as following surgery, plasma FVIII activity levels are frequently used as a laboratory surrogate for hemostasis, and more recent comparisons of clotting factor concentrates have tended to focus on their pharmacokinetic rather than clinical bioequivalence (5), even though the precise hemostatic target level of FVIII or FIX in the postoperative setting remains uncertain (6). In fact, during the past 25 years, there have been very few RCTs addressing the minimal hemostatic level of FVIII or FIX in various bleeding scenarios.

The situation is even more complicated in hemophilic patients who have developed high titer FVIII inhibitors (>5 Bethesda units/mL), in whom bleeding events require treatment with one of the FVIII/IX bypassing agents, FEIBA (FEIBA-VH®, Baxter, Glendale, CA) or recombinant factor VIIa (rFVIIa; Novoseven®, Novo Nordisk, Inc, Bagsvaerd, Denmark). Not only are the mechanisms of action of both agents still debated, but there are no validated surrogate laboratory endpoints for hemostasis, and the dose response relationships remain incompletely defined (7). Furthermore, the economic impact of treating bleeding episodes in patients with FVIII inhibitors is considerable. Although the cost per patient has been shown to be similar to noninhibitor patients in some studies (8), others have demonstrated that individuals with an inhibitor may consume three times as many financial resources as those without inhibitors (9,10). All studies agree that a few refractory outlier patients can drive the average cost of treatment in this subgroup. Thus, in the developing world, where the resources available for the purchase of expensive clotting factor concentrates are limited, the answer to these short-term treatment questions becomes especially pertinent.

Against this background, several high-quality clinical studies have recently begun to address some of these important issues. In this chapter, we will address one diagnostic and two therapeutic questions in hereditary bleeding disorders for which high-quality studies do exist, as follows: (A) What is the role of the platelet function analyzer (PFA-100®) in the evaluation of disorders of primary hemostasis? (B) Is primary prophylaxis with factor VIII (FVIII) beneficial in preventing hemophilic arthropathy in children with hemophilia A? (C) What is the optimal agent to treat bleeding events in patients with congenital hemophilia A complicated by a high titer FVIII inhibitor?

We searched under "Platelet function analyzer" and "PFA-100" in MEDLINE for question A. We omitted articles dealing with acquired defects, including drug-induced thrombocytopathies. All other manuscripts were included. For question B, we included manuscripts found while searching under the combination of "hemophilia and prophylaxis" and "hemophilia and arthropathy prevention." For question C, we searched under "hemophilia

Evidence-based Hematology. Edited by Mark A. Crowther, Jeff Ginsberg, Holger J. Schünemann, Ralph M. Meyer, and Richard Lottenberg.
 ISBN: 978-1-4051-5747-6.

Table 18.1 PFA-100® closure times in congenital platelet disorders.*

	Total number of subjects reported	CADP CT	CEPI CT	References
Disorders with normal platelet counts				
Glanzmann thrombaesthenia	23	P	P	(13,22–24,29,54)
Aspirin-like defect	6	N	P	(29)
$P2Y_{12}$ deficiency	4	N or P	N or P	(20,22)
Dense granule deficiency	30	N or P	N or P	(13,22,23,29, 55)
Hermansky–Pudlak syndrome	44	N or P	N or P	(13,23,24,56)
Primary secretion defects	30	N	N or P	(21,23,55)
Platelet procoagulant defect	1	N	N	(22)
Disorders with normal or low platelet counts				
Bernard Soulier syndrome	8	P	P	(13,23)
Platelet-type von Willebrand syndrome	3	P	P	(29)
Grey platelet syndrome	3	P	P	(22,23)
Wiskott–Aldrich syndrome	5	N or P	N or P	(23)
Hereditary Macrothrombocytopenia associated with nonmuscle myosin heavy chain IIa syndromes	5	N	N or P	(22,57)
Macrothrombocytopenia of undefined cause	11	N or P	N or P	(23)
Undefined autosomal dominant thrombocytopenia	1	N	N	(22)

*Adapted with permission from Hayward, et al. (20, p. 313). CADP CT, collagen/ADP closure time; CEPI CT, collagen/epinephrine closure time; P, closure time prolonged; N, closure time normal.

A and inhibitors" and "Congenital hemophilia and inhibitors" and "Factor VIII inhibitors," excluding studies of acquired inhibitors.

Grading of the quality of evidence and strengths of recommendations in this chapter are based on the guidelines proposed by the international Grading of Recommendations Assessment, Development, and Evaluation Working Group (GRADE), adopting the modification used by the American College of Chest Physicians that merges the very low and low categories of quality of evidence (see chapter 1).

A. What is the role of the PFA-100 in the diagnostic evaluation of disorders of primary hemostasis?

The Platelet Function Analyzer (PFA-100) was designed to replace the bleeding time as a clinically useful measure of primary hemostasis (11). Citrated whole blood is aspirated through an aperture in a cartridge where it contacts a membrane impregnated with a mixture of either collagen and epinephrine (CEPI) or collagen and ADP (CADP). Contact with these agonists leads to platelet adhesion, aggregation, and activation, eventually resulting in occlusion of the aperture and cessation of blood flow. The time needed for this to occur is referred to as the closure time (CT) (11). If the flow is prolonged beyond 300 seconds, nonclosure is said to occur. The assay depends on von Willebrand factor (VWF) binding to platelet receptors (glycoprotein Ib/IX/V and IIb/IIIa) under high shear.

Several factors impact the results of the PFA-100 CT (12). It is recommended that each laboratory establish its own normal ranges, and coefficients of variation for CTs in normal samples have been reported to be between 6% and 13% (13,14). The test may be performed on blood anticoagulated with either 3.8% or 3.2% citrate. The higher concentration of citrate leads to longer CT values (15). Preanalytical variables, which may lead to spurious results, include running the assay more than four hours after sample collection (13) and transporting samples through a pneumatic tube (16). CT values are prolonged in the presence of anemia and thrombocytopenia (11), and neonates have shorter CTs, presumably due to higher hematocrits and higher levels of von Willebrand factor (VWF) (17). PFA-100 CTs are not affected by deficiencies of fibrinogen or factors VIII, IX, or XI (18,19).

A review on the use of the PFA-100 in the evaluation of platelet disorders and platelet function was recently summarized by the Platelet Physiology Subcommittee of the Scientific and Standardization Committee of the International Society of Thrombosis and Haemostasis. They concluded that "although the PFA-100® CT is abnormal in some forms of platelet disorders, the test does not have sufficient sensitivity or specificity to be used as a screening tool for platelet disorders. A role for the PFA-100® CT in therapeutic monitoring of platelet function remains to be established" (20). Table 18.1 is revised from this publication and lists the PFA-100 closure times in congenital and acquired platelet disorders.

Table 18.2 PFA-100® closure times in von Willebrand disease subtypes.*

vWD subtype	CADP CT	CEPI CT	References
1	N or P	N or P	(21,24,29,34,58–65)
2A	P	P	(24,29,34,58,59,61,62,64)
2B	P	P	(24,29,34,58,59,61,62,64)
2N	N	N	(29,58)
2M	P	P	(58,59,61)
3	P	P	(24,29,34,58–65)

*CADP CT, collagen/ADP closure time; CEPI CT, collagen/epinephrine closure time; P, closure time prolonged; N, closure time normal.

Congenital platelet disorders prolong the PFA-100 closure times in a manner proportional to their severity. Glanzmann thrombaesthenia, Bernard Soulier Syndrome, and pseudo von Willebrand disease all reliably prolong both the CEPI and CADP closure times, usually to nonclosure. Milder platelet abnormalities more commonly encountered in clinical practice, including storage pool disease and the macrothrombocytopenias, produce more heterogeneous results, with some only prolonging the CT in the CEPI cartridge.

Studies examining PFA-100 CTs in platelet disorders have generally studied small numbers of patients and have varied in clinical design and patient selection (Table 18.1). This has led to reports of sensitivities for the PFA-100 in platelet disorders, ranging from 24% to 80% (13,21–24). Undoubtedly, the heterogeneity of platelet disorders also contributes to this variable sensitivity.

There have been more studies evaluating the use of the PFA-100 in identifying patients with von Willebrand disease (vWD) (Table 18.2). This subject was reviewed by Favoloro in 2006 (18). Multiple reports document reliably prolonged CTs for both CEPI and CADP in severe vWD (Types 2A, 2B, 2M, and 3), with sensitivities for these disorders near 100% (19,25–27). By contrast, reports of sensitivities of CTs for detection of type 1 vWD are lower and more variable, ranging from 50% (21) to 100% (28–31). In general, the CT for CEPI is more likely to be prolonged, and the CT for CADP is more likely to be normal, similar to the pattern seen with aspirin ingestion. The variability in the sensitivity may lie with the different reference ranges for VWF measurements used in different laboratories and even the "slippery" criteria for defining patients with type 1 vWD (32). As a final consideration, the PFA-100 has been reported to have poor reproducibility, with variability between measurements as high as 20% (12,18).

Conclusions. The PFA-100 is a useful tool in the diagnosis of disorders of primary hemostasis. Closure times that are not prolonged will adequately exclude severe subtypes of vWD (2A, 2B, and 3) and severe platelet disorders (Bernard–Soulier syndrome, Glanzmann's thrombaesthenia, and platelet-type vWD) (Evidence Grade 1C). For milder disorders such as platelet storage pool disease, platelet secretion defects, and type 1 vWD, the PFA-100 CT lacks sufficient sensitivity but may be useful to follow the response to therapy (Evidence Grade 1C) (25,33,34). Like the APTT, the PFA-100 is only a screening tool. It is abnormal in a number of conditions and cannot identify specific defects in primary hemostasis. More specific testing such as measurements of VWF antigen and activity levels, platelet aggregation testing, and platelet flow cytometry are needed to make specific diagnoses.

B. Is primary prophylaxis with factor VIII (FVIII) of benefit in preventing hemophilic arthropathy in children with hemophilia A?

Recurrent joint hemorrhage in hemophilia predisposes to chronic synovitis and ultimately, end-stage destructive hemophilic arthropathy after an interval of years to decades. For at least 30 years, it has been proposed that periodic prophylactic administration of FVIII or FIX concentrate is superior to "on demand" therapy in preventing the later development of crippling arthropathy. The original rationale (and goal) of prophylactic therapy was to maintain circulating clotting factor levels above 1%–2% at all times in patients with baseline levels of FVIII or FIX below this level (i.e., severe hemophilia A or B, respectively). Prophylaxis may be administered before any—or at most after a minimal number—of hemarthroses in young boys with hemophilia, in which case it is usually referred to as "primary." "Secondary" prophylaxis, however, refers to the situation in which preventive therapy is initiated at some later time in life in an effort to prevent recurrent hemorrhage and thereby slow the progression of arthropathy.

Pioneering studies from Sweden demonstrated that long-term outcomes in patients receiving primary prophylaxis were superior to historical controls receiving on-demand therapy (35). At about the same time, the international Orthopaedic Outcome Study Group reported that after several years of follow-up, secondary prophylaxis decreased the rate of deterioration of hemophilic patients' joints even when they were already damaged by previous hemathroses (36). Despite favorable and consistent orthopedic results from these observational studies, prophylaxis was slow to be widely adopted in the 1980s and early 1990s, primarily because of concerns surrounding cost and blood-borne viral infections. In addition, many unresolved questions remained to be addressed, including the dose and frequency of administration of FVIII (or FIX), and how to monitor joint disease progression, for example, using clinical versus radiologic measures. Another critical issue was when to begin and when—if ever—to discontinue prophylaxis. In this regard, retrospective cohort studies from the Netherlands reported that the median age at first bleed in boys with severe hemophilia was 2.2 years (range 0.2–5.8). When prophylaxis was started shortly after the first bleed, arthropathy was minimal after two decades of follow-up; however, the risk of joint damage in adulthood increased in proportion to the delay in initiation of prophylaxis after the first hemarthrosis (37).

Despite the body of literature attesting to the value of prophylaxis in hemophilia, a Cochrane Collaboration review in 2005 concluded that there was "insufficient evidence from randomized controlled trials to determine whether prophylactic clotting factor concentrates decrease bleeding and bleeding-related complications in hemophilia A or B, compared to placebo, on-demand treatment, or prophylaxis based on pharmacokinetic data from individuals" (38, p. 2). This review identified four published small RCTs—the majority from the 1970s—involving 37 subjects, with inconclusive evidence of benefit, defined by the frequency of joint bleeds or circulating clotting factor levels. No RCTs that included long-term outcomes (clinical joint function, orthopedic joint score, radiologic joint score, or quality of life measurements) were identified. The review did however acknowledge 26 observational studies that included >1,600 patients with hemophilia on prophylaxis and almost 1,200 individuals treated on demand that were highly suggestive of a longer-term benefit of prophylaxis (38). Notably, the inherent difficulty that systematic reviews of RCTs have in addressing long-term outcomes in individuals with chronic lifelong diseases has been acknowledged elsewhere, leading some authors to emphasize that these reviews should also consider data from observational studies when addressing long-term outcomes (39).

Shortly after the publication of this controversial (40,41) review, the results of a North American RCT (the "Joint Outcome Study"), addressing the long-term outcomes of primary prophylactic therapy in severe hemophilia A, were reported (42). This open-label study, begun in 1996, randomized 65 boys with hemophilia A, aged <30 months, to prophylaxis (25 IU/kg of intravenous recombinant FVIII given every other day) or "enhanced episodic infusion," in which joint bleeds were treated with at least three doses of FVIII, totaling at least 80 IU/kg over three days, with extension of treatment duration to a maximum of four weeks, if needed. These children were eligible for randomization if they had experienced ≤2 bleeds into each of the six index joints (two knees, two elbows, two ankles). The primary outcome was preservation of joint structure by magnetic resonance imaging (MRI) in these six joints at six years of age, which was documented in 93% of children on prophylaxis and 55% in the episodic therapy cohort ($p = 0.002$). Interestingly, MRI findings correlated poorly with clinical evidence of hemarthroses, suggesting that frequent subclinical bleeding in patients on episodic therapy is as—or even more—important than clinically apparent hemarthrosis in determining the likelihood of chronic arthropathy. Therefore, this study provides additional evidence that short-term outcomes in RCTs, such as frequency of joint bleeding in hemophilia, may be a poor surrogate for the clinically important long-term outcome of greatest relevance (39).

Another 10-year RCT (the Evaluation Study on Prophylaxis: A Randomized Italian Trial, or ESPRIT) similar in design to the Joint Outcome Study, is currently nearing completion, and the results are awaited (43). In Canada, a nonrandomized study evaluating lower-intensity prophylactic regimens has been completed (44). In this five-year study, an inception cohort of 25 boys with severe hemophilia was treated initially with once weekly prophylaxis, with plans to escalate the dose for breakthrough bleeding. Children on this tailored regimen fared better than historical controls, with fewer bleeds per year, and a lower likelihood of developing "target joints" (chronic synovitis). This protocol may be an attractive alternative in circumstances in which financial resources or reluctance to self-administer frequent prophylactic concentrate may preclude the use of the more standard regimens.

Conclusion. Primary prophylaxis at a FVIII dose of 25 IU/kg every other day is superior to on-demand therapy in the prevention of hemophilic arthropathy for boys with severe hemophilia A, when begun at or shortly after the onset of hemarthroses. It is however unclear whether (if at all) continuous prophylaxis can be discontinued without risking the development of arthropathy (Grade 1A recommendation).

C. Treatment of hemarthrosis in hemophilia patients with high titer FVIII inhibitors

Clinical trials assessing the efficacy of hemostatic therapies in hemophilia complicated by high-titer inhibitors have generally focused on joint and muscle bleeds of mild to moderate severity, primarily because they represent the most common site of bleeding in hemophilia. Improvement in pain and restoration of range of motion in the affected joint at a predetermined time following the therapeutic intervention has been used as a convenient surrogate endpoint for hemostasis in these clinical trials.

Early RCTs of nonactivated prothrombin complex concentrates (PCCs; includes agents such as Proplex (T)®, Konyne (80)®, Bebulin®, Profilnine®, and Prothromblex®) established their therapeutic efficacy for the treatment of hemarthrosis in inhibitor patients (45–47). These agents were generally licensed for the treatment of hemophilia B uncomplicated by a FIX inhibitor but were prescribed "off-label" to treat acute bleeding episodes in FVIII- or FIX-deficient patients with inhibitors (Table 18.3). Importantly, one study demonstrated a 25% response (defined as improvement in joint mobility or pain) with the albumin placebo at six hours, compared with a 50%–60% response rate with PCCs (45). Shortly thereafter, activated PCCs (FEIBA (VH)® and Autoplex®) were introduced into clinical practice. In one prospective randomized study, FEIBA was shown to produce a statistically significant improvement in efficacy compared with Prothromblex, a nonactivated PCC (46), although in a second head-to-head comparison, Autoplex was not superior to Proplex (47) (Table 18.3). A limitation of these pioneering studies was the absence of information on the elapsed time between the onset of bleeding symptoms and administration of the first dose of clotting factor concentrate, and home therapy did not become widely adopted as the standard of care, as it did in hemophilia patients without inhibitors. Similarly, no prospective studies of PCCs/APCCs were performed in surgery, and in the absence of data on efficacy and safety, only surgery that could not be avoided was generally recommended for patients with inhibitors.

Recombinant factor VIIa (rFVIIa) was licensed by the U.S. Food and Drug Administration for the treatment of bleeding in hemophilia patients with inhibitors in 1999. Prelicensure

Table 18.3 Randomized control trials (RCTs) of FVIII/FIX bypassing agents (prothrombin complex concentrates [PCC], activated PCCs, and rFVIIa) in the treatment of mild to moderate bleeds in hemophilia complicated by an inhibitor.*

Study year (reference)	Study arms	Doses (n)	Total patients (n)	Response rate† (%)
1980 (45)	Konyne®	1	157	47
	Proplex®	1		53
	Placebo	1		25
1981 (46)	FEIBA®‡	1 or 2	150	64§
	Prothromblex®	1 or 2		52
1983 (47)	Autoplex®‡	1	82	52
	Proplex®	1		56
2007 (53)	FEIBA-VH®‡	1	48	76
	rFVIIa	2		65

*From (1) Key NS, Negrier C. Clotting factor concentrates; past, present and future. *Lancet.* 2007;**370**(9585):439–48. Copyright Elsevier (2007).

† Generally assessed by subjective judgment at 6 hours post infusion.

‡Activated PCC.

§$p < 0.05$.

randomized prospective dosing studies had demonstrated that when treated at a median of 8–10 hours following the onset of symptoms of bleeding (predominantly hemarthrosis), 35mcg/kg and 70mcg/kg of rFVIIa, administered by bolus every 2.5 ± 0.5 hours produced an equivalent efficacy of approximately 70% (48). Subsequently, several nonrandomized studies of rFVIIa demonstrated efficacy rates of about 90% for joint and muscle bleeds treated in the home setting with two or three doses of 90–120mcg/kg given every two to three hours (49,50). In these studies, the drug was administered less than 3 hours after the onset of bleeding, and in aggregate, the available literature suggests that early administration of rFVIIa is an important determinant in optimizing the clinical response.

A systematic literature review published in 2003 concluded that a paucity of high-quality studies precluded evidence-based recommendations on the management of bleeding in inhibitor patients (51). A subsequent Cochrane Collaboration review focused on the relative merits of rFVIIa versus plasma-derived concentrates (APCCs) in the treatment of acute bleeding episodes and concluded that the absence of any RCTs comparing the two strategies precluded the recommendation of one strategy over the other (52). However, since that time, the results of a multicenter RCT comparing rFVIIa (90–120mcg/kg body weight × 2 doses, administered 2 hours apart) to FEIBA (75–100 U/kg body weight, single dose) have been published (53). This prospective, open-label, so-called FEIBA Novoseven Comparative (FENOC) crossover study was designed to test clinical equivalence of these two agents in the treatment of large joint hemarthroses in inhibitor patients. Patients were instructed to initiate treatment within four hours of symptom onset and to crossover to the alternative option to treat the next qualifying hemarthrosis. The primary outcome was evaluation of the hemostatic effect at six hours after onset of treatment, at which time 81.3% of FEIBA-treated events were rated as "effective" or "'partially effective," compared with 78.1% of rFVIIa-treated events. However, the confidence intervals were such that the criteria for declaring the two products equivalent at this time point were not met ($p = 0.059$), although the two treatments were judged to be equivalent by the prespecified criteria at multiple later time points. Of interest, this trial demonstrated that almost one-third of patients rated the efficacy of the two agents differently, with some reporting a greater response to rFVIIa and others to FEIBA (53). This finding likely reflects the different mechanisms of action of these bypassing agents and the inability of any laboratory parameter to predict the response to either agent in a given patient.

Conclusion. In the treatment of acute hemarthrosis requiring bypassing therapy, rFVIIa and FEIBA are equivalent in their hemostatic effect. However, the strength of this recommendation is downgraded because a significant proportion of patients appear to respond discordantly to one or the other agent, and the FENOC study had insufficient power to gauge the relative thrombotic risks of the two therapies. In addition, the quality of the evidence is hampered by the failure to reach the primary predefined endpoint of equivalence (albeit a "near miss") in the FENOC study. Therefore, this is rated as a Grade 2B recommendation.

References

1 Key NS, Negrier C. Clotting factor concentrates; past, present and future. *Lancet.* 2007;**370**(9585):439–48.

2 Bolton-Maggs PH, Stobart K, Smyth RL. Evidence-based treatment of haemophilia. *Haemophilia.* 2004;**10** Suppl 4:20–24.

3 Aronstam A, Wassef M, Choudhury DP, et al. Double-blind controlled trial of three dosage regimens in treatment of haemarthroses in haemophilia A. *Lancet.* 1980;**1**(8161):169–71.

4 Manno C, PJ L. Transfusion therapy for coagulation factor deficiencies. In: Hoffman R, Benz E Jr, Shattil S, et al., editors. *Hematology basic principles and practice.* 4th ed. Philadelphia: Elsevier, Churchill, Livingstone; 2005. pp. 2469–79.

5 Kessler CM, Gill JC, White GC II, et al. B-domain deleted recombinant factor VIII preparations are bioequivalent to a monoclonal antibody purified plasma-derived factor VIII concentrate: a randomized, three-way crossover study. *Haemophilia.* 2005;**11**(2):84–91.

6 Srivastava A. Dose and response in haemophilia—optimization of factor replacement therapy. *Br J Haematol.* 2004;**127**(1):12–25.

7 Key NS. Inhibitors in congenital coagulation disorders. *Br J Haematol.* 2004;**127**(4):379–91.

8 Bohn RL, Aledort LM, Putnam KG, et al. The economic impact of factor VIII inhibitors in patients with haemophilia. *Haemophilia.* 2004;**10**(1):63–8.

9 Gringeri A, Mantovani LG, Scalone L, et al. Cost of care and quality of life for patients with hemophilia complicated by inhibitors: the COCIS Study Group. *Blood.* 2003;**102**(7):2358–63.

10 Goudemand J. Hemophilia. Treatment of patients with inhibitors: cost issues. *Haemophilia.* 1999;**5**(6):397–401.

11 Kundu SK, Heilmann EJ, Sio R, et al. Description of an in vitro platelet function analyzer—PFA-100. *Semin Thromb Hemost.* 1995;**21** Suppl 2:106–12.

12 Haubelt H, Anders C, Vogt A, et al. Variables influencing platelet function Analyzer-100 closure times in healthy individuals. *Br J Haematol.* 2005;**130**(5):759–67.

13 Harrison P, Robinson MS, Mackie IJ, et al. Performance of the platelet function analyser PFA-100 in testing abnormalities of primary haemostasis. *Blood Coagul Fibrinolysis.* 1999;**10**(1):25–31.

14 Ortel TL, James AH, Thames EH, et al. Assessment of primary hemostasis by PFA-100 analysis in a tertiary care center. *Thromb Haemost.* 2000;**84**(1):93–7.

15 Heilmann EJ, Kundu SK, Sio R, et al. Comparison of four commercial citrate blood collection systems for platelet function analysis by the PFA-100 system. *Thromb Res.* 1997;**87**(1):159–64.

16 Dyszkiewicz-Korpanty A, Quinton R, Yassine J, et al. The effect of a pneumatic tube transport system on PFA-100 trade mark closure time and whole blood platelet aggregation. *J Thromb Haemost.* 2004;**2**(2):354–56.

17 Israels SJ, Cheang T, McMillan-Ward EM, et al. Evaluation of primary hemostasis in neonates with a new in vitro platelet function analyzer. *J Pediatr.* 2001;**138**(1):116–19.

18 Favaloro EJ. The utility of the PFA-100 in the identification of von Willebrand disease: a concise review. *Semin Thromb Hemost.* 2006;**32**(5):537–45.

19 Jilma B. Platelet function analyzer (PFA-100): a tool to quantify congenital or acquired platelet dysfunction. *J Lab Clin Med.* 2001;**138**(3):152–63.

20 Hayward CP, Harrison P, Cattaneo M, Ortel TL, Rao AK. Platelet function analyzer (PFA)-100 closure time in the evaluation of platelet disorders and platelet function. *J Thromb Haemost.* 2006;**4**(2):312–19.

21 Quiroga T, Goycoolea M, Munoz B, et al. Template bleeding time and PFA-100 have low sensitivity to screen patients with hereditary mucocutaneous hemorrhages: comparative study in 148 patients. *J Thromb Haemost.* 2004;**2**(6):892–98.

22 Posan E, McBane RD, Grill DE, et al. Comparison of PFA-100 testing and bleeding time for detecting platelet hypofunction and von Willebrand disease in clinical practice. *Thromb Haemost.* 2003;**90**(3):483–90.

23 Harrison P, Robinson M, Liesner R, et al. The PFA-100: a potential rapid screening tool for the assessment of platelet dysfunction. *Clin Lab Haematol.* 2002;**24**(4):225–32.

24 Kerenyi A, Schlammadinger A, Ajzner E, et al. Comparison of PFA-100 closure time and template bleeding time of patients with inherited disorders causing defective platelet function. *Thromb Res.* 1999;**96**(6):487–92.

25 Favaloro EJ. Utility of the PFA-100 for assessing bleeding disorders and monitoring therapy: a review of analytical variables, benefits and limitations. *Haemophilia.* 2001;**7**(2):170–79.

26 Harrison P. The role of PFA-100 testing in the investigation and management of haemostatic defects in children and adults. *Br J Haematol.* 2005;**130**(1):3–10.

27 Favaloro EJ. Laboratory assessment as a critical component of the appropriate diagnosis and sub-classification of von Willebrand's disease. *Blood Rev.* 1999;**13**(4):185–204.

28 Lippi G, Franchini M, Brocco G, et al. Influence of the ABO blood type on the platelet function analyzer PFA-100. *Thromb Haemost.* 2001;**85**(2):369–70.

29 Fressinaud E, Veyradier A, Truchaud F, et al. Screening for von Willebrand disease with a new analyzer using high shear stress: a study of 60 cases. *Blood.* 1998;**91**(4):1325–31.

30 Fressinaud E, Veyradier A, Sigaud M, et al. Therapeutic monitoring of von Willebrand disease: interest and limits of a platelet function analyser at high shear rates. *Br J Haematol.* 1999;**106**(3):777–83.

31 Buyukasik Y, Karakus S, Goker H, et al. Rational use of the PFA-100 device for screening of platelet function disorders and von Willebrand disease. *Blood Coagul Fibrinolysis.* 2002;**13**(4):349–53.

32 Sadler JE. Slippery criteria for von Willebrand disease type 1. *J Thromb Haemost.* 2004;**2**(10):1720–23.

33 Favaloro EJ. Clinical application of the PFA-100. *Curr Opin Hematol.* 2002;**9**(5):407–15.

34 Favaloro EJ, Kershaw G, Bukuya M, et al. Laboratory diagnosis of von Willebrand disorder (vWD) and monitoring of DDAVP therapy: efficacy of the PFA-100 and vWF:CBA as combined diagnostic strategies. *Haemophilia.* 2001;7(2):180–89.

35 Nilsson IM, Berntorp E, Lofqvist T, et al. Twenty-five years' experience of prophylactic treatment in severe haemophilia A and B. *J Intern Med.* 1992;**232**(1):25–32.

36 Aledort LM, Haschmeyer RH, Pettersson H. A longitudinal study of orthopaedic outcomes for severe factor-VIII-deficient haemophiliacs. The Orthopaedic Outcome Study Group. *J Intern Med.* 1994;**236**(4):391–99.

37 Fischer K, van der Bom JG, Mauser-Bunschoten EP, et al. The effects of postponing prophylactic treatment on long-term outcome in patients with severe hemophilia. *Blood.* 2002;**99**(7):2337–41.

38 Stobart K, Iorio A, Wu JK. Clotting factor concentrates given to prevent bleeding and bleeding-related complications in people with hemophilia A or B. *Cochrane Database Syst Rev.* 2005(2):CD003429.

39 Elphick HE, Tan A, Ashby D, et al. Systematic reviews and lifelong diseases. *BMJ.* 2002;**325**(7360):381–84.

40 Aledort L, Ljung R, Blanchette V. Are randomized clinical trials the only truth? Not always. *J Thromb Haemost.* 2006;**4**(3):503–4.

41 More on: are randomized clinical trials the only truth? Not always. *J Thromb Haemost.* 2006;**4**(5):1167–68.

42 Manco-Johnson M, Abshire T, Shapiro AD. Prophylaxis versus episodic treatment to prevent joint disease in boys with severe hemophilia. *N Engl J Med.* 2007;**357**(6):535–44.

43 Gringeri A. Prospective controlled studies on prophylaxis: an Italian approach. *Haemophilia.* 2003;**9** Suppl 1:38–42; discussion 3.

44 Feldman BM, Pai M, Rivard GE, et al. Tailored prophylaxis in severe hemophilia A: interim results from the first 5 years of the Canadian Hemophilia Primary Prophylaxis Study. *J Thromb Haemost.* 2006;4(6):1228–36.

45 Lusher JM, Shapiro SS, Palascak JE, et al. Efficacy of prothrombin-complex concentrates in hemophiliacs with antibodies to factor VIII: a multicenter therapeutic trial. *N Engl J Med.* 1980;**303**(8):421–25.

46 Sjamsoedin LJ, Heijnen L, Mauser-Bunschoten EP, et al. The effect of activated prothrombin-complex concentrate (FEIBA) on joint and muscle bleeding in patients with hemophilia A and antibodies to factor VIII: a double-blind clinical trial. *N Engl J Med.* 1981;**305**(13):717–21.

47 Lusher JM, Blatt PM, Penner JA, et al. Autoplex versus proplex: a controlled, double-blind study of effectiveness in acute hemarthroses in hemophiliacs with inhibitors to factor VIII. *Blood.* 1983;**62**(5):1135–38.

48 Lusher JM, Roberts HR, Davignon G, et al. A randomized, double-blind comparison of two dosage levels of recombinant factor VIIa in the treatment of joint, muscle and mucocutaneous haemorrhages in persons with haemophilia A and B, with and without inhibitors. rFVIIa Study Group. *Haemophilia.* 1998;**4**(6):790–98.

49 Key NS, Aledort LM, Beardsley D, et al. Home treatment of mild to moderate bleeding episodes using recombinant factor VIIa (Novoseven) in haemophiliacs with inhibitors. *Thromb Haemost.* 1998;**80**(6): 912–18.

50 Santagostino E, Gringeri A, Mannucci PM. Home treatment with recombinant activated factor VII in patients with factor VIII inhibitors: the advantages of early intervention. *Br J Haematol.* 1999;**104**(1): 22–6.

51 Lloyd Jones M, Wight J, Paisley S, et al. Control of bleeding in patients with haemophilia A with inhibitors: a systematic review. *Haemophilia.* 2003;**9**(4):464–520.

52 Hind D, Lloyd-Jones M, Makris M, et al. Recombinant Factor VIIa concentrate versus plasma derived concentrates for the treatment of acute bleeding episodes in people with Haemophilia A and inhibitors. *Cochrane Database Syst Rev.* 2004(2):CD004449.

53 Astermark J, Donfield SM, DiMichele DM, et al. A randomized comparison of bypassing agents in hemophilia complicated by an inhibitor: the FEIBA NovoSeven Comparative (FENOC) study. *Blood.* 2007;**109**(2):546–51.

54 Mammen EF, Comp PC, Gosselin R, et al. PFA-100 system: a new method for assessment of platelet dysfunction. *Semin Thromb Hemost.* 1998;**24**(2):195–202.

55 Cattaneo M, Lecchi A, Agati B, et al. Evaluation of platelet function with the PFA-100 system in patients with congenital defects of platelet secretion. *Thromb Res.* 1999;**96**(3):213–17.

56 Harrison C, Khair K, Baxter B, et al. Hermansky-Pudlak syndrome: infrequent bleeding and first report of Turkish and Pakistani kindreds. *Arch Dis Child.* 2002;**86**(4):297–301.

57 Rodriguez V, Nichols WL, Charlesworth JE, et al. Sebastian platelet syndrome: a hereditary macrothrombocytopenia. *Mayo Clin Proc.* 2003;**78**(11):1416–21.

58 Cattaneo M, Federici AB, Lecchi A, Agati B, Lombardi R, Stabile F, et al. Evaluation of the PFA-100 system in the diagnosis and therapeutic monitoring of patients with von Willebrand disease. *Thromb Haemost.* 1999;**82**(1):35–9.

59 Nitu-Whalley IC, Lee CA, Brown SA, et al. The role of the platelet function analyser (PFA-100) in the characterization of patients with von Willebrand's disease and its relationships with von Willebrand factor and the ABO blood group. *Haemophilia.* 2003;**9**(3):298–302.

60 Carcao MD, Blanchette VS, Dean JA, et al. The Platelet Function Analyzer (PFA-100): a novel in-vitro system for evaluation of primary haemostasis in children. *Br J Haematol.* 1998;**101**(1):70–3.

61 Dean JA, Blanchette VS, Carcao MD, et al. von Willebrand disease in a pediatric-based population—comparison of type 1 diagnostic criteria and use of the PFA-100 and a von Willebrand factor/collagen-binding assay. *Thromb Haemost.* 2000;**84**(3):401–9.

62 Favaloro EJ, Facey D, Henniker A. Use of a novel platelet function analyzer (PFA-100) with high sensitivity to disturbances in von Willebrand factor to screen for von Willebrand's disease and other disorders. *Am J Hematol.* 1999;**62**(3):165–74.

63 Favaloro EJ. Template bleeding time and PFA-100 have low sensitivity to screen patients with hereditary mucocutaneous hemorrhages: comparative study of 148 patients—a rebuttal. *J Thromb Haemost.* 2004;**2**(12):2280–82; author reply, 3–5.

64 Schlammadinger A, Kerenyi A, Muszbek L, et al. Comparison of the O'Brien filter test and the PFA-100 platelet analyzer in the laboratory diagnosis of von Willebrand's disease. *Thromb Haemost.* 2000;**84**(1):88–92.

65 Wuillemin WA, Gasser KM, Zeerleder SS, et al. Evaluation of a platelet function Analyser (PFA-100) in patients with a bleeding tendency. *Swiss Med Wkly.* 2002;**132**(31–32):443–48.

19 Diagnosis and Management of Acquired Bleeding Disorders

Vitamin K Antagonists

Miguel A. Escobar

A review of the literature was done to identify all published trials using MEDLINE and PubMed databases from 1996 to December 2006 using the following terms: coumarin, anticoagulation, vitamin K, phytonadione, plasma, fresh frozen plasma (FFP), coagulation concentrate, prothrombin complex concentrate (PCC), recombinant factor VIIa, Novoseven. The results were limited to "human" and "English" language. Abstracts and conference proceedings were not generally included. Grading of the quality of evidence and strengths of recommendations in this chapter are based on the guidelines proposed by the international Grading of Recommendations Assessment, Development, and Evaluation Working Group (GRADE), adopting the modification used by the American College of Chest Physicians (ACCP) that merges the very low and low categories of quality of evidence (see chapter 1).

What is the risk of bleeding with the use of vitamin K antagonists?

Vitamin K antagonists (VKAs) are the mainstay of treatment for the primary and secondary prevention of venous thromboembolism, prevention of systemic embolism in patients with atrial fibrillation and prosthetic heart valves, prevention of stroke, recurrent myocardial infarction, or death in patients with acute myocardial infarction (1). VKAs exert their effect by interfering with the gamma-carboxylation of glutamate residues on the N-terminal domains of vitamin K–dependent proteins (2). They are metabolized in the liver through the cytochrome P450 system in particular involving the CYP2C9 isoenzyme. Acenocoumarol, warfarin, and phenprocoumon are the different VKAs with half-lives that vary between 10 hours, 40 hours, and 5 days, respectively. The clinical effectiveness of VKAs is dependent on maintaining a therapeutic level of anticoagulation based on the international normalized ratio (INR) of the prothrombin time (3). For most clinical indications, a target INR between 2.0 and 3.0 is recommended (1).

It is estimated that about 1% of the population in the United States and the United Kingdom receive long-term anticoagulation with VKAs (4,5). However, despite adequate monitoring, bleeding is the most common complication that can be seen in up to 7% per year of patients taking long-term anticoagulation (4). Genetic and environmental factors can alter the effect of VKAs. For example, mutations in the gene coding for the cytochrome P450 2C9 isoenzyme can account for the increased sensitivity of some individuals to VKAs. Intensity of anticoagulation, length of therapy, patient characteristics, and concomitant use of drugs that can interfere with hemostasis can also increase the risk of bleeding in some individuals (6). However, warfarin has a narrow therapeutic window that is associated with an unpredictable anticoagulation response, making it difficult to maintain the therapeutic target (7). Although there is no clear consensus with regards to contraindications to oral anticoagulation, clinicians can make their selection criteria using the exclusion criteria used in trials that evaluated the efficacy and tolerability of anticoagulation in patients with nonvalvular atrial fibrillation (see Table 19.1) (8). All contraindications to anticoagulation are relative, and the decision to start anticoagulation is usually individualized by assessing the risk-benefit of thromboembolism versus bleeding.

Intensity of anticoagulant effect

In randomized clinical trials, cohort studies, and case control studies the evidence supports a strong relationship between the intensity of anticoagulation and the risk of bleeding in patients treated for deep vein thrombosis, atrial fibrillation, ischemic stroke, or tissue and mechanical heart valves. In these studies, maintaining an INR between 2.0 and 3.0 decreases the frequency of bleeding by about half when compared with a target INR > 3.0 (9–12). Intensity of anticoagulation is also an independent risk factor for intracranial bleeding, especially when INR is above the 4.0 to 5.0 range (Grade 1C) (13,14).

Evidence-based Hematology. Edited by Mark A. Crowther, Jeff Ginsberg, Holger J. Schünemann, Ralph M. Meyer, and Richard Lottenberg.

Table 19.1 Exclusion criteria used in trials evaluating the efficacy and tolerability of anticoagulation (8).

Active bleeding
Active peptic ulcer disease
Known coagulation defects
Thrombocytopenia (<50,000) or platelet dysfunction
Recent hemorrhagic stroke
Noncompliant or unreliable patient
Patient is psychologically or socially unsuitable
Dementia or severe cognitive impairment
History of falls (>3 within the previous year or recurrent, injurious falls)
Excessive alcohol intake
Uncontrolled hypertension (>180/100 mm Hg)
Daily use of nonsteroidal anti-inflammatory agents
Planned invasive procedure or major surgery

Length of therapy

Higher frequencies of bleeding episodes early in the course of starting anticoagulation has been reported in four retrospective and one prospective study evaluating almost 5,000 patients (15–19). In one of these studies, the risk of bleeding decreased from 3.0% during the first month of outpatient treatment to 0.3% per month after the first year of therapy (17). Similar results were reported by the Italian Study on Complications of Oral Anticoagulant Treatment (ISCOAT) investigators who found that one-third of hemorrhagic events occurred during the first three months of treatment (18). The reason for the development of these early events in the aforementioned trials is somewhat unclear, but there are several possible explanations: (1) anticoagulation can predispose to bleeding from occult lesion; (2) fluctuation in laboratory values leading to supra-therapeutic levels that provoke hemorrhage; and (3) dose adjustments may be less well controlled at the beginning of treatment (17,18).

Patient Characteristics

It is debatable whether the risk of bleeding is higher in older individuals although prospective studies support age as an independent risk factor for major bleeding. In the ISCOAT (cohort of 2,745 individuals), bleeding was reported more frequently in those older than 70 years (10.5 per 100 patient-years of follow-up) when compared with patients younger than 70 years (6.0 per 100 patient-years of follow-up) (relative risk = 1.75) (18). In the SPAF-II trial (Stroke Prevention in Atrial Fibrillation Study), the impact of age was also evaluated in patients receiving long-term anticoagulation. The incidence of major hemorrhage was 1.7% per year in individuals younger than 75 years versus 4.2% per year in those aged greater than 75 years (20). Furthermore, among older patients (>75 years), the risk of intracranial hemorrhage was particularly increased when the INR was above therapeutic levels (14,21). Other comorbid conditions have also been associated with hemorrhage during warfarin therapy, including renal insufficiency, hypertension, cerebrovascular disease, ischemic stroke, serious heart disease, and malignancy (6).

Concomitant medications

The concomitant use of anticoagulants with medications like aspirin, acetaminophen, and nonsteroidal anti-inflammatory drugs (NSAIDs) may increase the likelihood of bleeding.

In three randomized trials that included more than 19,000 patients, warfarin (target INR between 1.5 and 2.5) plus low-dose aspirin (75 to 81 mg/day) was compared with aspirin alone (75–162 mg/day). In all trials, major bleeding was more common in the combination arm (22–24). Although medications like acetaminophen may potentially influence the metabolism of VKAs, two studies failed to show such an adverse effect (25,26).

Whether NSAIDs can increase the risk of bleeding in patients receiving VKAs is still unanswered given the lack of randomized trials. Only observational studies with a weak association have been published (27–30).

Can we calculate the actual risk of bleeding with the use of vitamin K antagonists?

In clinical practice, it is difficult to predict the risk of bleeding when an individual is placed in VKAs. Patient- and treatment-related risk factors have been developed and validated in two prediction models in outpatients treated with warfarin. Beyth et al. classified patients according to the risk of major bleeding based in four independent risk factors: age ≥65 years, history of gastrointestinal bleeding, history of stroke, and one or more of four specific comorbidities (recent MI, hematocrit <30%, serum creatinine >1.5mg/dL, or diabetes mellitus) (31). The risk of major bleeding at 48 months was 53% in the high-risk patients, 12% in the intermediate-risk patients, and 3% in the low-risk patients, with an overall rate of 5% per year (see Table 19.2). In both the derivation and validation cohorts, patients were considered appropriate candidates for outpatient anticoagulation, and there was no comment about patients who were not ineligible for enrollment.

Kuijer et al. validated a bleeding risk prediction score system based on age, gender, and the presence of malignancy in patients treated for venous thromboembolism (32). The frequency of major bleeding at three months was 7% in the high-risk group, 4% in the intermediate-risk group, and 1% in the low-risk group. These

Table 19.2 Cumulative incidence of major bleeding (31).

Time since start of outpatient treatment	Low risk* n = 80	Intermediate risk* n =166	High risk* n =18
1 month	0	2	0
6 months	3	8	16
12 months	3	8	30
48 months	3	12	53

*Low risk, no risk factors; intermediate risk, one or two risk factors; high risk, three or four risk factors.

"prediction" scores can assist physicians considering individuals for anticoagulation who have a diversity of risk factors.

The duration of therapy is a crucial determinant in the risk of bleeding; the risk of bleeding increases with duration of anticoagulants in each group (31). It is possible that for the high-risk individuals implementing measures like maintaining a lower target INR and closer laboratory monitoring can decrease the risk of bleeding complications (32).

What is the recommended management for bleeding due to vitamin K antagonists?

The frequent use of long-term VKAs for the management of a wide variety of thrombotic disorders has resulted in an increase in hemorrhagic complications as previously described in this chapter. Despite current improvements in the management of anticoagulation therapy, more than a third of the patients are unable to maintain a target INR range, putting them at risk for bleeding (33). Numerous guidelines on the management of patients with VKA-induced coagulopathy have been published; however, recommendations are based on very low levels of evidence (34). Currently, FFP, vitamin K, PCCs, and recombinant factor VIIa (rFVIIa) are available in most countries for the reversal of VKAs. There is a consensus that patients presenting with major bleeding secondary to excessive anticoagulation require rapid reversal of the coagulopathy. However, the management of patients with a high INR who are asymptomatic or who have minor bleeding is less defined. Dentali et al. (34) recently published a detailed review of the literature and proposed evidence-based treatment algorithms.

Management of the nonbleeding patient

Patients with supra-therapeutic INRs without evidence of bleeding is common. Theoretically, the decision to treat the coagulopathy can be based on balancing the risk that the patient will develop a bleeding complication by reducing the duration of INR prolongation versus enhancing the risk for thrombosis associated inadequate anticoagulation (34). However, in clinical practice the management of these patients varies widely among physicians as described in two different surveys performed in the United States and Canada, respectively (4,35).

Overall, the frequent treatment options available for this scenario are the following: (1) withhold the VKA until the INR slowly decreases to a therapeutic level or (2) withhold the VKA and administer vitamin K1. The administration of coagulation concentrates or FFP in this setting is not indicated based on a lack of evidence-based data.

Withholding anticoagulation is the most common practice; two retrospective studies support a conservative management of no intervention in patients with INRs greater than 6.0 (36,37). However, this strategy can be associated with a 9% overall risk of bleeding during the first 14 days while waiting for the INR to decrease to the target range as described in a prospective study of 114 patients (38). Limitations in this study include that most patients were elderly with a mean age of 71 years and 13% had INRs greater than 10 at entry of study; both of which are risk factors for bleeding.

Is there a role for subcutaneous vitamin K?

This route of administration is broadly used in the treatment of VKA-induced coagulopathy (4,35). Of three randomized controlled trials and one retrospective review involving 150 patients, the subcutaneous administration of vitamin K for rapid reversal of VKAs was suboptimal when compared with IV and oral routes (39–41). These studies support the unpredictable response of the subcutaneous administration of vitamin K for a rapid reversal of overanticoagulation with VKAs; for this reason, it is not recommended in this setting.

What is the recommended dose of oral Vitamin K?

Five randomized clinical trials compared oral vitamin K with placebo, subcutaneous, or intravenous administration of vitamin K (see Table 19.3) (42–46). Two double-blind, placebo-controlled RCTs confirmed that 1 and 2.5 mg of oral vitamin K, respectively, lowers the INR more promptly than does the withholding of warfarin alone (43,44). The only RCT comparing low-dose oral and subcutaneous vitamin K showed that the oral route was more effective in lowering the INR on the day following treatment ($p = 0.015$) (45). Lubetsky et al. randomly allocated 47 patients with INR values between 6.0 and 10.0 to receive 0.5 mg of intravenous (IV) or 2 mg of oral vitamin K (46). At six hours, 11 of the 24 patients that received IV vitamin K and 0 of 23 allocated to oral therapy had INR values between 2.0 and 4.0 ($p < 0.001$). At 24 hours, the INR values were similar between the two groups.

Whereas the effectiveness of vitamin K in reversing the coagulopathy of warfarin is well recognized, there is no clear consensus on the optimal dose for the treatment of the nonbleeding patient with a supra-therapeutic INR.

Management of the bleeding patient

The management of patients that present with hemorrhagic events due to anticoagulation with VKAs should be more individualized, depending on the severity of the symptoms. For minor bleeding episodes (i.e., wound bleeding, epistaxis) the use of local measures with or without decreasing or discontinuing the VKA may be sufficient. For major or life-threatening bleeding, the cessation of the VKA, administration of IV vitamin K, and replacement of deficient factors is essential (see Table 19.4).

Four RCT have compared different doses of IV vitamin K with oral and subcutaneous administration for the reversal of VKA coagulopathy in patients not requiring urgent reversal of anticoagulation (40,41,46,47). These studies concluded that IV administration of vitamin K caused a more rapid fall in the INR, and a dose

Table 19.3 Randomized clinical trials with the use of vitamin K*.

Reference	No. of patients	INR studied	Treatment	Outcome	Results
Pengo (42)	23	>5	A: Withhold warfarin × 1 day B:2 mg vit K PO	INR <5 at 24 and 48 hours	A: 7/12 (24h) 11/12 (48 h) B: 11/11 (24 h) 10/11 (48 h)
Crowther (43)	99	4.5–10.0	A: placebo B: 1 mg vit K PO	Mean INR values	A: 20% B: 56%
Patel (44)	30	6.0–10.0	A: placebo B: 2.5 mg vit K PO	INR < 4	Vit K superior to placebo
Crowther (45)	51	4.5–10.0	A: 1 mg vit K PO B: 1 mg vit K SC	INR between 1.8 and 3.2	A: 60% B: 24%
Lubetsky (46)	63	A, B: 6–10 C, D: >10	A: 2.5 mg vit K PO B: 0.5 mg vit K iv C: 5 mg vit K PO D: 1 mg vit K iv	INR at 24 and 48 hours	IV vit K caused a faster drop in the INR. At 24 h, there was no difference

*PO, oral administration; IV, intravenous administration; h, hour; vit, vitamin.

of 0.5 mg was more adequate in returning the INR to therapeutic range.

Allergic reactions, including anaphylaxis in patients receiving intravenously administered vitamin K, have been reported in the literature (48). In a retrospective study of 6,572 doses administered, the incidence of true anaphylaxis was 3 per 10,000 doses (49). The main factor responsible for the reaction seems to be the solubilizing vehicle, polyethoxylated castor oil. To diminish the risk of allergic reactions, vitamin K should be administered at an infusion rate of 1 mg/h or less using an infusion pump and mixed in a minimal volume of 50 mL of IV fluid (34,49).

FFP and PCCs are both plasma-derived products used for the urgent reversal of VKA coagulopathy. FFP can be administered at a dose of 15–20 mL/kg of body weight. This amount of volume if infused quickly can be associated with fluid overload, especially in elderly patients. In addition, thawing of FFP can delay treatment, and there is a small risk of a transfusion-transmitted disease given that lacks pathogen inactivation. Despite these observations, FFP remains the most common factor replacement product used in North America for the urgent reversal of coumarin overdose (34). For serious bleeding, the ACCP guidelines recommend FFP or PCC (Grade 1C) and the British Committee for Standards in Haematology recommends PCC in preference to FFP (Grade B level III) (1,50).

Table 19.4 Recommended guidelines for the treatment of VKA coagulopathy.*

INR	Symptoms	Other treatment	Grade
>1.3	Life-threatening bleeding	Withhold VKA PCC or plasma 5–10 mg IV vit K	1C
>1.3	Serious bleeding	Withhold VKA PCC or plasma 1–10 mg IV vit K	1C
4.5–10	No bleeding	Withhold VKA 1 mg oral vit K	2C
>10	No bleeding	Withhold VKA 2.5–5 mg oral vit K or 0.5–1.0 mg IV vit K	2C

*VKA, vitamin K antagonist; IV, intravenous administration; vit, vitamin.

PCCs contain coagulation factors II, VII, IX, and X, and their concentration is about 25 times higher than in plasma, hence requiring much less volume for infusion. In addition, they all undergo at least one step of viral inactivation. Given the heterogeneity of commercially available PCCs in their factor concentration and the lack of randomized trials, there is controversy regarding the optimal dose to reverse the coagulopathy of VKAs. Typical doses vary between 25 and 50 IU/kg of body weight or fixed doses (i.e., 500 IU). There are at least nine reports in the literature (~225 patients) on the use of PCCs for the reversal of warfarin overdose, most of which are in prospective cohorts, but no randomized clinical trials have been performed (34,51).

Makris et al. (52) and Cartmill et al. (53) published two prospective studies comparing the utility of PCCs compared with FFP in 53 patients using doses of 25–50 IU/kg. Patients receiving PCCs had a more rapid and complete reversal of the coagulopathy. More recently, Lankiewics and colleagues described a retrospective study in 58 patients using a PCC (25–50 IU/kg) to urgently reverse the effect of warfarin (median INR = 29). In addition, all patients received oral or parenteral vitamin K, and 50% also received FFP. Immediately after PCC administration 76% had INRs <1.5 and

96.5% had INRs <2.0. This effect persisted for over 24 hours. In this study, four patients experienced thrombotic events, although according to the authors none was attributable to the administration of the PCC (51).

More recently recombinant factor VIIa (rFVIIa) has been used as an alternative to FFP and PCC for the reversal of VKA coagulopathy. Its mechanism of action is based on activation of factor X on the surfaces of activated platelets with an immediate effect and a short half-life of approximately 2.5 hours. No RCT has been published in this setting, but in four case series (31 patients), rFVIIa was used to revert the coagulopathy of VKA with doses between 10 and 90 micrograms per kilogram of body weight. Most of the patients had intracerebral hemorrhage (54–57). In all cases, the INRs fully normalized and no thromboembolic complications were reported. Some of the patients also received FPP and vitamin K. For serious and life-threatening bleeding, the ACCP recommends the use of rFVIIa as an alternative to PCCs (Grade 1C). This recommendation is based in limited data.

Conclusions

Coagulopathy due to VKAs is a common problem encountered both in outpatient clinics, mostly with asymptomatic elevation of INRs, and in hospitalized patients when hemorrhagic complications occur. Treatment is based on guidelines that lack adequately powered, controlled trials. Recommendations given in this chapter and in other publications are based on studies that use the elevated INR as a surrogate marker for the risk of bleeding. Large randomized trials to establish the risk-benefit on the use of FFP, PCCs, and recombinant FVIIa are greatly needed.

References

1 Ansell J, Hirsh J, Poller L, et al. The pharmacology and management of the vitamin K antagonists: the Seventh ACCP Conference on Antithrombotic and Thrombolytic Therapy. *Chest.*2004;**126**(3 Suppl):204S–33S.
2 Whitlon DS, Sadowski JA, Suttie JW. Mechanism of coumarin action: significance of vitamin K epoxide reductase inhibition. *Biochemistry.* 1978;**17**(8):1371–77.
3 Standarization WECoB. Requirements for thromboplastins and plasma used to control oral anticoagulant therapy. Geneva; 1983.
4 Libby EN, Garcia DA. A survey of oral vitamin K use by anticoagulation clinics. *Arch Intern Med.* 2002;**162**(16):1893–96.
5 Sconce EA, Kamali F. Appraisal of current vitamin K dosing algorithms for the reversal of over-anticoagulation with warfarin: the need for a more tailored dosing regimen. *Eur J Haematol.* 2006;**77**(6):457–62.
6 Levine MN, Raskob G, Beyth RJ, et al. Hemorrhagic complications of anticoagulant treatment: the Seventh ACCP Conference on Antithrombotic and Thrombolytic Therapy. *Chest.* 2004;**126**(3 Suppl):287S–310S.
7 Baker RI, Coughlin PB, Gallus AS, et al. Warfarin reversal: consensus guidelines, on behalf of the Australasian Society of Thrombosis and Haemostasis. *Med J Aust.* 2004;**181**(9):492–97.
8 Sebastian JL, Tresch DD. Use of oral anticoagulants in older patients. *Drugs Aging.* 2000;**16**(6):409–35.
9 Hull R, Hirsh J, Jay R, et al. Different intensities of oral anticoagulant therapy in the treatment of proximal-vein thrombosis. *N Engl J Med.* 1982;**307**(27):1676–81.
10 Turpie AG, Gunstensen J, Hirsh J, et al. Randomised comparison of two intensities of oral anticoagulant therapy after tissue heart valve replacement. Lancet 1988;**1**(8597):1242–45.
11 Saour JN, Sieck JO, Mamo LA, et al. Trial of different intensities of anticoagulation in patients with prosthetic heart valves. *N Engl J Med.* 1990;**322**(7):428–32.
12 Altman R, Rouvier J, Gurfinkel E, et al. Comparison of two levels of anticoagulant therapy in patients with substitute heart valves. *J Thorac Cardiovasc Surg.* 1991;**101**(3):427–31.
13 Cannegieter SC, Rosendaal FR, Wintzen AR, et al. Optimal oral anticoagulant therapy in patients with mechanical heart valves. *N Engl J Med.* 1995;**333**(1):11–17.
14 Hylek EM, Singer DE. Risk factors for intracranial hemorrhage in outpatients taking warfarin. *Ann Intern Med.* 1994;**120**(11):897–902.
15 Fihn SD, McDonell M, Martin D, et al. Risk factors for complications of chronic anticoagulation: a multicenter study. Warfarin Optimized Outpatient Follow-up Study Group. *Ann Intern Med.* 1993;**118**(7):511–20.
16 Gurwitz JH, Goldberg RJ, Holden A, et al. Age-related risks of long-term oral anticoagulant therapy. *Arch Intern Med.* 1988;**148**(8):1733–36.
17 Landefeld CS, Goldman L. Major bleeding in outpatients treated with warfarin: incidence and prediction by factors known at the start of outpatient therapy. *Am J Med.* 1989;**87**(2):144–52.
18 Palareti G, Leali N, Coccheri S, et al. Bleeding complications of oral anticoagulant treatment: an inception-cohort, prospective collaborative study (ISCOAT). Italian Study on Complications of Oral Anticoagulant Therapy. *Lancet.* 1996;**348**(9025):423–28.
19 Petitti DB, Strom BL, Melmon KL. Duration of warfarin anticoagulant therapy and the probabilities of recurrent thromboembolism and hemorrhage. *Am J Med.* 1986;**81**(2):255–59.
20 Warfarin versus aspirin for prevention of thromboembolism in atrial fibrillation: Stroke Prevention in Atrial Fibrillation II Study. *Lancet.* 1994;**343**(8899):687–91.
21 Risk factors for stroke and efficacy of antithrombotic therapy in atrial fibrillation: analysis of pooled data from five randomized controlled trials. *Arch Intern Med.* 1994;**154**(13):1449–57.
22 Randomised double-blind trial of fixed low-dose warfarin with aspirin after myocardial infarction. Coumadin Aspirin Reinfarction Study (CARS) Investigators. *Lancet.* 1997;**350**(9075):389–96.
23 Thrombosis prevention trial: randomised trial of low-intensity oral anticoagulation with warfarin and low-dose aspirin in the primary prevention of ischaemic heart disease in men at increased risk. The Medical Research Council's General Practice Research Framework. *Lancet.* 1998;**351**(9098):233–41.
24 Fiore LD, Ezekowitz MD, Brophy MT, et al. Department of Veterans Affairs Cooperative Studies Program Clinical Trial comparing combined warfarin and aspirin with aspirin alone in survivors of acute myocardial infarction: primary results of the CHAMP study. *Circulation.* 2002;**105**(5):557–63.
25 Hylek EM, Heiman H, Skates SJ, et al. Acetaminophen and other risk factors for excessive warfarin anticoagulation. *JAMA.* 1998;**279**(9):657–62.
26 Gadisseur AP, Van Der Meer FJ, Rosendaal FR. Sustained intake of paracetamol (acetaminophen) during oral anticoagulant therapy with

coumarins does not cause clinically important INR changes: a randomized double-blind clinical trial. *J Thromb Haemost.* 2003;**1**(4):714–17.

27 Michot F, Ajdacic K, Glaus L. A double-blind clinical trial to determine if an interaction exists between diclofenac sodium and the oral anticoagulant acenocoumarol (nicoumalone). *J Int Med Res.* 1975;**3**(3):153–57.

28 Shorr RI, Ray WA, Daugherty JR, et al. Concurrent use of nonsteroidal anti-inflammatory drugs and oral anticoagulants places elderly persons at high risk for hemorrhagic peptic ulcer disease. *Arch Intern Med.* 1993;**153**(14):1665–70.

29 Mieszczak C, Winther K. Lack of interaction of ketoprofen with warfarin. *Eur J Clin Pharmacol.* 1993;**44**(2):205–6.

30 Knijff-Dutmer EA, Schut GA, van de Laar MA. Concomitant coumarin-NSAID therapy and risk for bleeding. *Ann Pharmacother.* 2003;**37**(1):12–16.

31 Beyth RJ, Quinn LM, Landefeld CS. Prospective evaluation of an index for predicting the risk of major bleeding in outpatients treated with warfarin. *Am J Med.* 1998;**105**(2):91–9.

32 Kuijer PM, Hutten BA, Prins MH, et al. Prediction of the risk of bleeding during anticoagulant treatment for venous thromboembolism. *Arch Intern Med.* 1999;**159**(5):457–60.

33 Veeger NJ, Piersma-Wichers M, Tijssen JG, et al. Individual time within target range in patients treated with vitamin K antagonists: main determinant of quality of anticoagulation and predictor of clinical outcome. A retrospective study of 2300 consecutive patients with venous thromboembolism. *Br J Haematol.* 2005;**128**(4):513–19.

34 Dentali F, Ageno W, Crowther M. Treatment of coumarin-associated coagulopathy: a systematic review and proposed treatment algorithms. *J Thromb Haemost.* 2006;**4**(9):1853–63.

35 Wilson SE, Douketis JD, Crowther MA. Treatment of warfarin-associated coagulopathy: a physician survey. *Chest.* 2001;**120**(6):1972–76.

36 Glover JJ, Morrill GB. Conservative treatment of overanticoagulated patients. *Chest.* 1995;**108**(4):987–90.

37 Lousberg TR, Witt DM, Beall DG, et al. Evaluation of excessive anticoagulation in a group model health maintenance organization. *Arch Intern Med.* 1998;**158**(5):528–34.

38 Hylek EM, Chang YC, Skates SJ, Hughes RA, Singer DE. Prospective study of the outcomes of ambulatory patients with excessive warfarin anticoagulation. *Arch Intern Med.* 2000;160(11):1612–17.

39 Whitling AM, Bussey HI, Lyons RM. Comparing different routes and doses of phytonadione for reversing excessive anticoagulation. *Arch Intern Med.* 1998;**158**(19):2136–40.

40 Nee R, Doppenschmidt D, Donovan DJ, et al. Intravenous versus subcutaneous vitamin K1 in reversing excessive oral anticoagulation. *Am J Cardiol.* 1999;**83**(2):286–88, A6–7.

41 Raj G, Kumar R, McKinney WP. Time course of reversal of anticoagulant effect of warfarin by intravenous and subcutaneous phytonadione. *Arch Intern Med.* 1999;**159**(22):2721–24.

42 Pengo V, Banzato A, Garelli E, et al. Reversal of excessive effect of regular anticoagulation: low oral dose of phytonadione (vitamin K1) compared with warfarin discontinuation. *Blood Coagul Fibrinolysis.* 1993;**4**(5): 739–41.

43 Crowther MA, Julian J, McCarty D, et al. Treatment of warfarin-associated coagulopathy with oral vitamin K: a randomised controlled trial. *Lancet* 2000;**356**(9241):1551–53.

44 Patel RJ, Witt DM, Saseen JJ, et al. Randomized, placebo-controlled trial of oral phytonadione for excessive anticoagulation. *Pharmacotherapy.* 2000;**20**(10):1159–66.

45 Crowther MA, Douketis JD, Schnurr T, et al. Oral vitamin K lowers the international normalized ratio more rapidly than subcutaneous vitamin K in the treatment of warfarin-associated coagulopathy: a randomized, controlled trial. *Ann Intern Med.* 2002;**137**(4):251–54.

46 Lubetsky A, Yonath H, Olchovsky D, et al. Comparison of oral vs intravenous phytonadione (vitamin K1) in patients with excessive anticoagulation: a prospective randomized controlled study. *Arch Intern Med.* 2003;**163**(20):2469–73.

47 Hung A, Singh S, Tait RC. A prospective randomized study to determine the optimal dose of intravenous vitamin K in reversal of over-warfarinization. *Br J Haematol.* 2000;**109**(3):537–39.

48 Fiore LD, Scola MA, Cantillon CE, et al. Anaphylactoid reactions to vitamin K. *J Thromb Thrombolysis.* 2001;**11**(2):175–83.

49 Riegert-Johnson DL, Volcheck GW. The incidence of anaphylaxis following intravenous phytonadione (vitamin K1): a 5-year retrospective review. *Ann Allergy Asthma Immunol.* 2002;**89**(4):400–406.

50 Baglin TP, Keeling DM, Watson HG. Guidelines on oral anticoagulation (warfarin): third edition—2005 update. *Br J Haematol.* 2006;**132**(3):277–85.

51 Lankiewicz MW, Hays J, Friedman KD, et al. Urgent reversal of warfarin with prothrombin complex concentrate. *J Thromb Haemost.* 2006;**4**(5):967–70.

52 Makris M, Greaves M, Phillips WS, et al. Emergency oral anticoagulant reversal: the relative efficacy of infusions of fresh frozen plasma and clotting factor concentrate on correction of the coagulopathy. *Thromb Haemost.* 1997;**77**(3):477–80.

53 Cartmill M, Dolan G, Byrne JL, et al. Prothrombin complex concentrate for oral anticoagulant reversal in neurosurgical emergencies. *Br J Neurosurg.* 2000;**14**(5):458–61.

54 Deveras RA, Kessler CM. Reversal of warfarin-induced excessive anticoagulation with recombinant human factor VIIa concentrate. *Ann Intern Med.* 2002;**137**(11):884–88.

55 Freeman WD, Brott TG, Barrett KM, et al. Recombinant factor VIIa for rapid reversal of warfarin anticoagulation in acute intracranial hemorrhage. *Mayo Clin Proc.* 2004;**79**(12):1495–500.

56 Lin J, Hanigan WC, Tarantino M, et al. The use of recombinant activated factor VII to reverse warfarin-induced anticoagulation in patients with hemorrhages in the central nervous system: preliminary findings. *J Neurosurg.* 2003;**98**(4):737–40.

57 Sorensen B, Johansen P, Nielsen GL, et al. Reversal of the international normalized ratio with recombinant activated factor VII in central nervous system bleeding during warfarin thromboprophylaxis: clinical and biochemical aspects. *Blood Coagul Fibrinolysis.* 2003;**14**(5): 469–77.

20 Diagnosis and Management of Heparin-Induced Thrombocytopenia

Theodore E. Warkentin, Andreas Greinacher

Introduction

Heparin-induced thrombocytopenia (HIT) is an acquired, transient, prothrombotic disorder that paradoxically is triggered by the anticoagulant, heparin (1). HIT is caused by platelet-activating antibodies of IgG class (HIT antibodies) that recognize complexes of (cationic) platelet factor 4 (PF4) and (anionic) heparin (2–4). Detectability of platelet-activating heparin-dependent antibodies is a sine qua non for diagnosis; hence, HIT is a "clinicopathologic" syndrome in which one or more clinical events (most often, thrombocytopenia with or without thrombosis) occur together with HIT antibodies (5).

HIT is strongly associated with thrombosis (odds ratio, 20 to 40) (6–8), both venous and arterial, with hypercoagulability (increased in vivo thrombin generation) (9) secondary to platelet activation, formation of procoagulant, platelet-derived microparticles, and, possibly, activation of endothelium and monocytes (Figure 20.1) (10).

What are the clinical features that suggest a diagnosis of HIT?

HIT should be suspected in a patient who develops an otherwise unexplained fall in the platelet count (thrombocytopenia) or thrombosis that begins 5 to 14 days after starting heparin (typical onset), or within 24 hours (rapid onset) after initiating heparin in a patient with a recent exposure to heparin (especially within the past month) (11). Sometimes, HIT begins several days after all heparin has been stopped (delayed onset) (12).

Thrombocytopenia is best defined by a proportional (relative) platelet count fall (using as "baseline" the highest platelet count preceding the HIT-associated platelet count fall), rather than an absolute platelet count threshold (8). This clinical picture can be summarized by the 4T's clinical scoring system (13): *T*hrombocytopenia plus *T*hrombosis plus *T*iming (of thrombocytopenia or thrombosis in relation to heparin use) in the absence of o*T*her explanation(s) (Table 20.1).

Table 20.2 lists the clinical sequelae of HIT (14–17). As many as 50% to 75% of symptomatic thrombi that begin during or shortly after a course of heparin are associated with HIT (18,19). Often, thrombosis is the first manifestation of HIT, with the platelet count fall becoming apparent within the next few days (17,20).

Recommendation. The potential diagnosis of HIT is suggested by any of the following: onset of thrombocytopenia that begins 5 to 10 days after initiating a course of heparin and/or onset of thrombosis or other characteristic sequelae (e.g., adrenal hemorrhage, necrotizing or erythematous skin lesions, post-bolus anaphylactoid reaction), that begin 5 to 14 days after initiating a course of heparin, or within 1 day if there has been recent heparin exposure, especially within the past month).

What laboratory tests are clinically useful for detecting HIT antibodies?

Two types of laboratory assay are available to detect HIT antibodies: platelet activation assays and PF4-dependent immunoassays (21). Platelet activation assays that utilize "washed" platelets, such as the platelet serotonin-release assay (SRA) and heparin-induced platelet activation (HIPA) assay, have the highest combination of sensitivity and specificity (22). This reflects their detection of antibodies based on their key biologic feature (strong platelet agonists). Two PF4-dependent enzyme(-linked) immuno(sorbent) assays—EIAs (or ELISAs)—are commercially available. Both detect the major immunoglobulin classes (IgG, IgA, IgM) (21), even though only IgG antibodies are potentially platelet-activating through the platelet FcγIIa receptors (2,22). The EIAs are very sensitive for HIT antibodies but have lower diagnostic specificity, since they detect both platelet-activating and non-platelet-activating

Evidence-based Hematology. Edited by Mark A. Crowther, Jeff Ginsberg, Holger J. Schünemann, Ralph M. Meyer, and Richard Lottenberg.
© 2008 Blackwell Publishing, ISBN: 978-1-4051-5747-6.

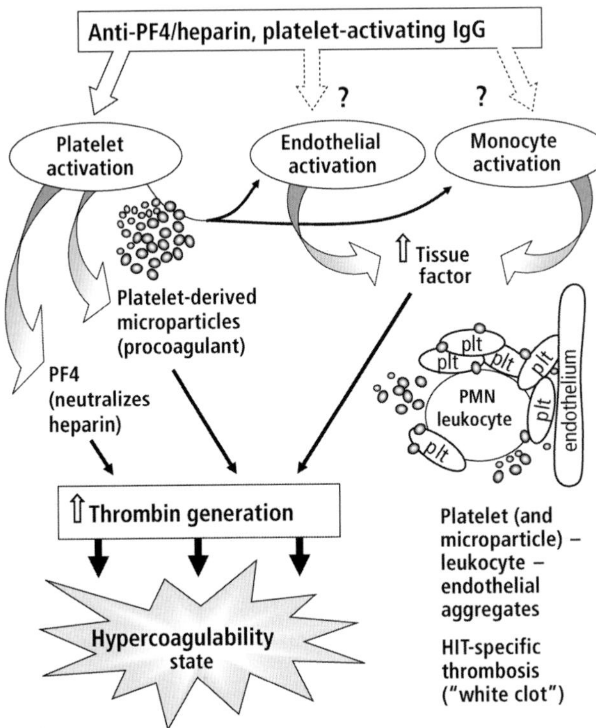

Figure 20.1 Pathogenesis of HIT: a central role for thrombin generation. The figure illustrates two explanations for thrombosis in HIT. (1) Activation of platelets (Plt) by anti-PF4/heparin IgG antibodies (HIT antibodies), leading to formation of procoagulant, platelet-derived microparticles and neutralization of heparin by PF4 released from activated platelets, leads to marked increase in thrombin ("hypercoagulability state"), characterized by an increased risk of venous and arterial thrombosis, as well as increased risk for coumarin-induced venous limb gangrene. (2) However, it is also possible that unique pathogenetic mechanisms operative in HIT explain unusual thromboses, such as arterial "white clots." For example, HIT antibodies have been shown to activate endothelium and monocytes (leading to cell surface tissue factor expression), although this stimulation may be largely "indirect" through poorly-defined mechanisms involving platelet activation and, possibly, formation of platelet-derived microparticles. Further, aggregates of platelets and polymorphonuclear (PMN) leukocytes have been described in HIT. To what extent these cooperative interactions between platelets, platelet-derived microparticles, PMN leukocytes, monocytes, and endothelium lead to arterial (or venous) thrombotic events in HIT, either in large or small vessels, remains unclear. (From Warkentin TE. An overview of the heparin-induced thrombocytopenia syndrome. *Semin Thromb Hemost.* 2004;**30**:273–83 (10), with permission.)

antibodies (21,22) (Figure 20.2). Routine use of EIAs for "confirming" HIT will result in about half of patients being inappropriately labeled as having HIT, if it is assumed that HIT requires the presence of platelet-activating antibodies detected by a platelet activation assay (23). The likelihood of HIT increases with the magnitude of the positive test result (i.e., positive EIA >1.0 optical density (OD) units is more likely to indicate HIT than a weak positive result (23,24). HIT antibodies are transient (11) and thus acute serum should be tested. In practice, EIAs represent a standardized approach to screen for HIT antibodies and when used in conjunction with clinical scoring, are satisfactory for resolving a putative diagnosis of HIT in about 80%–90% of cases; the remainder require a platelet activation assay for resolution (23).

Recommendation. Tests for HIT antibodies should only be ordered when HIT is clinically suspected. The PF4-dependent EIAs are highly sensitive for screening. However, if the EIA yields a "weak" positive result (<1.0 units) or the clinical profile suggests a plausible alternative diagnosis, referral for a washed platelet activation assay (SRA, HIPA) is appropriate.

What alternative anticoagulants are efficacious for treatment of thrombosis complicating HIT?

Three non-heparin anticoagulants—danaparoid, lepirudin, and argatroban—have been shown to be efficacious for treatment of HIT (25–35). Two other agents—bivalirudin and fondaparinux—are rational therapies for HIT (36), although controlled studies are lacking.

The strong association between HIT and thrombosis, and the tendency for thrombotic events to occur early in the course of HIT, means that many—perhaps most—patients will have symptomatic thrombosis at the time that HIT is recognized (7,8,14,17,18,20). Three alternative non-heparin anticoagulants—danaparoid, lepirudin, argatroban (in order of market entry)—are approved for treatment of HIT (although approvals vary among countries) (Table 20.3). Only one agent (danaparoid) was evaluated in a randomized controlled trial (against dextran-70) (25). The other two agents, lepirudin, and argatroban, which are direct thrombin inhibitors (DTIs), were assessed in prospective cohort studies with historical controls (28–35). Tables 20.4a to 20.4c list studies supporting their efficacy for treatment or prevention of thrombosis complicating HIT. Consensus conference guidelines regarding therapy of HIT also have been published (36,37) Table 20.5 summarizes the key treatment principles for managing HIT (17). Current trends and expert opinion support using DTI dosing that is substantially less than that indicated in the manufacturers' package inserts (see also Table 20.3).

Recommendation. For patients with strongly suspected (or confirmed) acute HIT complicated by thrombosis, treatment with an alternative non-heparin anticoagulant in therapeutic doses, such as danaparoid, lepirudin, or argatroban, is recommended. [This recommendation is based on a literature review using the OVID database searched between 1966 and 2006 using the text words "heparin induced thrombocytopenia" (text words were used since HIT does not have a MESH heading) and identifying controlled (either randomized prospective, historical retrospective, or retrospective contemporaneous) studies of HIT (with or without thrombosis) reporting twenty-five or more subjects. This search revealed 11 studies (25–35).]

Table 20.1 Estimating the pretest probability of HIT: The "4 T's" scoring system.

	Points (0, 1, or 2 for each of 4 categories: maximum possible score = 8)		
Date: 20___-m____-d____	**2**	**1**	**0**
Thrombocytopenia Score = _____	>50% platelet fall to nadir ≥20	30–50% platelet count fall (or >50% directly resulting from surgery); or nadir 10–19	<30% platelet fall; or nadir <10
*Timing** of platelet count fall, thrombosis, or other sequelae (first day of heparin course = day 0) Score = ______	Day 5–10 onset*; or ≤1 day (with recent heparin exposure within past 5–30 days)	Consistent with day 5–10 fall, but not clear (e.g., missing platelet counts); or, ≤1 day (heparin exposure within past 31–100 days); or, platelet fall after day 10	Platelet count fall ≤4 days without recent heparin exposure
Thrombosis (incl. adrenal infarction) or other sequelae (e.g., skin lesions, ASR) Score = ______	Proven new thrombosis; or skin necrosis (at injection site); or post-i.v. heparin bolus ASR	Progressive or recurrent thrombosis; or erythematous skin lesions; or suspected thrombosis (not proven)	None
Other cause for thrombocytopenia Score = ______	No explanation for platelet count fall is evident	Possible other cause is evident	Definite other cause is present

TOTAL SCORE = ______ **Pretest probability score**: **6–8 = HIGH; 4–5 = INTERMEDIATE; 0–3 = LOW**
Changes to score based upon new information, e.g., further fall in platelets, new thrombosis, other cause for thrombocytopenia proven, etc.
Date: 20___–___–___ Describe change ____

*First day of immunizing heparin exposure considered day 0; the day the platelet count begins to fall is considered the day of onset of thrombocytopenia (it generally takes 1 to 3 more days until an arbitrary threshold that defines thrombocytopenia is passed. Usually, heparin administered at or near surgery is the most immunizing situation).
The scoring system shown has undergone minor modifications from previously publications.
ASR, acute systemic reaction; i.v., intravenous.

Table 20.2 Clinical sequelae of HIT.

Sequela(e)	**Comment**
Venous thromboembolism	Deep-vein thrombosis (~50%) and pulmonary embolism (~25%) are the two most common sequelae of HIT, especially in postoperative patients
Arterial thrombosis	Order of frequency is: limb artery thrombosis (10–15%) > thrombotic stroke (5–10%) > myocardial infarction (3–5%) > other (<5%); platelet-rich "white clots" are characteristic
Thrombotic stroke	Besides cerebral artery thrombosis, venous infarction can be caused by thrombosis of dural sinuses and/or cerebral veins
Overt DIC	About 10–20% of HIT patients have overt (decompensated) disseminated intravascular coagulation (DIC), as shown by reduced fibrinogen levels, increased prothrombin time/international normalized ratio, positive protamine sulfate paracoagulation assay, microangiopathic hemolysis, or circulating normoblasts (nucleated red cells)
Coumarin necrosis	Two syndromes: venous limb gangrene (acral necrosis in limb with deep-vein thrombosis) > "classic" skin necrosis (subdermal and dermal necrosis, usually in a non-acral location, such as breast, abdomen, thigh, and calf); characterized by microvascular thrombosis
Adrenal hemorrhage	Associated with thrombosis of adrenal veins; unilateral adrenal hemorrhage presents as abdominal or flank pain; when adrenal hemorrhage is bilateral, there is high risk of adrenal crisis
Skin lesions at heparin injection site(s)	Necrotizing skin lesions at heparin injection sites are specific for HIT; erythematous plaques at heparin injection sites can also indicate HIT; some patients with dramatic skin lesions do not evince thrombocytopenia
Acute systemic reaction	One or more signs or symptoms that begin 5–30 min. after i.v. heparin injection (or s.c. LMWH injection): cardiac (tachycardia, chest pain, hypertension, cardiac arrest), respiratory (dyspnea, tachypnea, chest pain, respiratory arrest), inflammatory (fever, chills, rigors, flushing), neurologic (pounding headache, transient global amnesia syndrome), gastrointestinal (diarrhea); these features are *not* that of anaphylaxis

Table 20.3 Comparison of three alternative anticoagulants used to treat HIT.

	Danaparoid	Lepirudin	Argatroban
Drug type (molecular mass)	Heterogeneous, polydispersed mix of anticoagulant GAGs: heparan sulfate (84%), dermatan sulfate (12%), chondroitin sulfate (4%) (6,000 Da [mean])	65–amino acid polypeptide made using recombinant biotechnology (6,980 Da); derivative of hirudin (leech anticoagulant)	Small-molecule arginine derivative (527 Da) invented in a Japanese laboratory
Anticoagulant action	Indirect (antithrombin-dependent) inhibition of factor Xa and thrombin (anti-Xa:anti-thrombin ratio, ~22)	High affinity (Ki = 0.0001 nmol/L) binding to two sites on thrombin, the fibrinogen-binding site and the active site pocket (*bi*valent DTI)	Moderate affinity (Ki = 40 nmol/L) binding to active site of thrombin (*uni*valent DTI)
Immunologic features	In vitro XR for HIT Abs in 15–40% of patients (usually not clinically significant); in high therapeutic concentrations, inhibits PF4-containing immune complexes	Neither promotes nor inhibits HIT Ab binding to PF4/polyanion complexes; lepirudin is immunogenic (allergic/anaphylactic reactions are reported)	Neither promotes nor inhibits HIT Ab binding to PF4/polyanion complexes; argatroban is not immunogenic
Half-life	25 h (anti-Xa action) (assumes normal renal function)	80 min (assumes normal renal function)	40–50 min (assumes normal hepatobiliary function)
Dosing regimen	Bolus: 2250 U (1500 U for b.w. <60 kg; 3000 U for b.w. 75–90 kg; 3750 U for b.w. >90 kg); followed by 400 U/h x 4 h, then 300 U/h x 4 h, then 150–200 U/h thereafter	Bolus (optional): 0.2–0.4 mg/kg; infusion, start at 0.05–0.10 mg/kg/h (adjusted according to APTT)*,**; marked dose reduction if renal dysfunction**	No bolus; 1 to 2 mcg/kg/min (adjusted according to APTT)***; marked dose reduction if hepatobiliary dysfunction****
Drug accumulation	Renal dysfunction (minor danaparoid accumulation)	Renal dysfunction (major lepirudin accumulation)	Hepatobiliary dysfunction (major argatroban accumulation)
Laboratory monitoring	Anti-factor Xa levels (target therapeutic range: 0.5 to 0.8 anti-Xa U/mL)	APTT (estimate of drug level*****)	APTT (estimate of drug level*****)

* Note that this dosing regimen differs considerably from that contained in the manufacturer's package insert.

** The initial lepirudin infusion rate should be no higher than 0.10 mg/kg/h (serum creatinine <90 umol/L), with lower infusion rates for patients with higher serum creatinine levels (90 to 140 umol/L, start at 0.05 mg/kg/h; 140 to 400, start at 0.01 mg/kg/h; >400, start at 0.005 mg/kg/h). APTT monitoring be performed at 4-h intervals until it is apparent that steady state within the therapeutic range (1.5 to 2.5-times patient baseline [or mean laboratory] APTT) has been achieved.

*** Although manufacturer's package insert recommends that dosing start at 2 mcg/kg/min, many clinicians start at lower doses, e.g. 1 mcg/kg/min, especially in patients who are critically ill or who have cardiac failure.

**** For patients with moderate or greater liver dysfunction, the starting dose is 0.5 mcg/kg/min.

***** The APTT is not reliable for anticoagulant monitoring in patients with preexisting congenital or acquired coagulopathies, overt DIC, prolonged APTT due to "lupus anticoagulant," or effects of warfarin

Ab, antibody; APTT, activated partial thromboplastin time; b.w., body weight; Da, Daltons; DIC, disseminated intravascular coagulation; GAGs, glycosaminoglycans; PF4, platelet factor 4; U, units; XR, cross-reactivity.

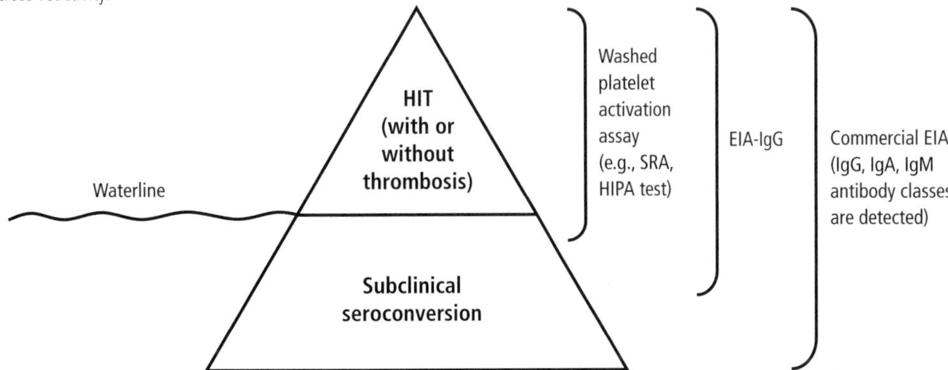

Figure 20.2 Iceberg model of HIT: implications for differing diagnostic specificities of tests for HIT. Clinical HIT (with or without thrombosis) is represented by the portion of the iceberg above the waterline. Three different types of assays for HIT antibodies are shown: washed platelet activation assays, PF4/heparin EIAs that detects only IgG class antibodies (EIA-IgG), and a commercially available PF4/polyanion EIA that detects anti-PF4/heparin antibodies of all three major immunoglobulin classes (EIA-IgG/IgA/IgM). The model indicates that the three assays have different specificity for clinical HIT (in the rank order, washed platelet activation assay > EIA-IgG > EIA-IgG/IgA/IgM), but that all three assays have similar high diagnostic sensitivity for HIT. EIA, enzyme-immunoassay; HIPA, heparin-induced platelet activation; SRA, serotonin release assay.

Table 20.4a Summary of studies describing efficacy of danaparoid as treatment for thrombosis complicating HIT.

Study type RCT	Intervention/Dosing	Complete clinical resolution of existing thrombi	Overall clinical effectiveness*	Major bleeds	Comment
Chong et al. (25)	Danaparoid (Dan) bolus 2,400 U, then 200 U/h x 5 d** Dextran 70 (Dex) 1,000 mL day 1, then 500 mL x 4 d	Dan: 24/43*** (56%) Dex: 5/36*** (14%) $p = 0.02$	Dan: 22/25 (88%) Dex: 8/17 (47%) $p = 0.01$	Dan: 0/25 (0) Dex: 0/17 (0)	Open-label trial (stratified for thrombosis severity); 83% tested positive for HIT Abs; no prior XR testing; no anticoagulant monitoring
Non-RCT studies		**New thrombosis**	**Composite end-point*****		
Farner et al. (26)	Dan: Bolus 2500 U, then 200 U/h x 5 d Lep: Bolus 0.4 mg/kg, then 0.15 mg/kg/h****	Dan: 5/53 (9%) Lep: 9/114 (8%) $p = 0.74$	Dan: ~20%****** Lep: ~20%****** $p = 0.91$	Dan: 3/122 (2%)******* Lep: 18/173 (8%)******* $p = 0.009$	Dan patients served as contemporaneous control group for prospective lep studies
Lubenow et al. (27)	Dan (± warfarin): various doses Anc (ancrod and/or coumarin)	Dan: 11/62 (18%) Anc: 24/56 (43%) $p = 0.0044$	Dan: 15/62 (24%) Anc: 28/56 (50%) $p = 0.0043$	Dan: 8/62 (13%) Anc: 19/56 (34%) $p = 0.0084$	Data shown are day 35; superior efficacy and bleeding end points with Dan were also seen at day 7 (primary study endpoint)

* subjective clinical judgment of investigators.
** After initial 2,400 U bolus, patients received 400 U/h x 2 h, then 300 U/h x 2 h, then 200 U/h x 5 d.
*** Denominator is number of thrombi, rather than number of patients.
**** APTT adjusted to 1.5-2.5 times baseline APTT.
***** Composite end point: all-cause mortality, all-cause limb amputation, and new thrombosis (each patient counted only once).
****** Estimated cumulative event-rate at 42 days, as read from fig. 2 in Farner et al. [26].
******* Includes all patients (with or without thrombosis at baseline) who received danaparoid in either prophylactic or therapeutic doses.
Abs, antibodies; APTT, activated partial thromboplastin time; RCT, randomized controlled trial; XR, cross-reactivity.

Table 20.4b Summary of studies describing efficacy of the DTIs (lepirudin, argatroban) as treatment for thrombosis complicating HIT.

Study	Intervention/Dosing	New thrombosis	Composite end-point*	Major bleeds	Comment
Lubenow et al. 2005 (31)	Lep: Bolus 0.4 mg/kg; 0.15 mg/kg/ h** Con: variable	Lep (HAT-1): 3/51 (6%) Lep (HAT-2): 7/65 (11%) Lep (HAT-3): 5/98 (5%) Con: 30/120 (25%) $p < 0.0001$	Lep (HAT-1): 7/51 (14%) Lep (HAT-2): 16/65 (25%) Lep (HAT-3): 18/98 (18%) Con: 52/120 (47%) $p < 0.0001$	Lep (HAT-1): 7/51 (14%) Lep (HAT-2): 6/65 (9%) Lep (HAT-3): 20/98 (20%) Con: 7/120 (6%) $p = 0.0015$	All patients tested positive for HIT antibodies (HIPA test); *p* values are for combined HAT-1/2/3 studies vs controls (outcomes from start of treatment)
Lewis et al. (33,34)	Arg: 2 mcg/kg/min (no bolus)*** Con: variable	Arg-911: 28/144 (19%) Arg-915: 30/229 (13%) Con: 16/46 (35%) $p = 0.0032$	Arg-911: 63/144 (44%) Lep-915: 95/229 (41%) Con: 26/46 (57%) $p = 0.083$	Arg-911: 16/144 (3%) Arg-915: 14/229 (6%) Con: 1/46 (2%) p = 0.23	Patients did not require positive test for HIT Abs****; *p* values are for combined Arg-911 and -915 studies vs controls

* Composite end point: all-cause mortality, all-cause limb amputation, and new thrombosis (each patient counted only once).
** APTT adjusted to 1.5–2.5-times baseline APTT; also, average lepirudin treatment duration was 16.4 days in the HAT-1, -2, and -3 trials.
*** APTT adjusted to 1.5–3.0-times baseline APTT; also, average argatroban treatment duration was 5.9 and 7.1 days in the Arg-911 and -915 trials, respectively.
**** 65% of argatroban-treated patients with thrombosis tested positive for HIT Abs in the Arg-911 study (data not available for Arg-915 study).
Abs, antibodies; APTT, activated partial thromboplastin time; Con, control group; HIPA, heparin-induced platelet activation; RCT, randomized controlled trial; XR, cross-reactivity.

Table 20.4c Summary of studies describing efficacy of the DTIs (lepirudin, argatroban) as treatment for isolated HIT.

Study	Intervention/Dosing	New thrombosis	Composite end-point*	Major bleeds	Comment
Lubenow et al. 2004 (32)	Lep: No bolus; 0.10 mg/kg/h** Con: variable	Lep: 4/91 (4%) Con: 7/47 (15%) $p = 0.02$ (log-rank test)	Lep: 18/91 (20%) Con: 14/47 (30%) $p = 0.0281$ (log-rank test)	Lep: 13/91 (14%) Con: 4/47 (9%) $p = 0.42$	All patients tested positive for HIT antibodies (HIPA test)
Lewis et al. (33,34)	Arg: 2 mcg/kg/min (no bolus)*** Con: variable	Arg-911: 13/160 (8%) Arg-915: 11/189 (6%) Con: 33/147 (22%) $p < 0.001$	Arg-911: 41/160 (26%) Arg-915: 53/189 (28%) Con: 57/147 (39%) $p = 0.010$	Arg-911: 5/160 (3%) Arg-915: 10/189 (5%) Con: 12/147 (8%) $p = 0.088$	Patients did not require positive test for HIT Abs****; *p* values are for combined Arg-911 and -915 studies vs controls

* Composite end point: all-cause mortality, all-cause limb amputation, and new thrombosis (each patient counted only once).
** APTT adjusted to 1.5–2.5-times baseline APTT; also, average lepirudin treatment duration was 13.9 days in the HAT-1, -2, and -3 trials (data combined).
*** APTT adjusted to 1.5–3.0-times baseline APTT; also, average argatroban treatment duration was 5.9 and 7.1 days in the Arg-911 and -915 trials, respectively.
**** 50% of argatroban-treated patients tested positive for HIT Abs in the Arg-911 study (data not available for Arg-915 study).
Abs, antibodies; APTT, activated partial thromboplastin time; RCT, randomized controlled trial; XR, cross-reactivity.

Table 20.5 Six treatment principles of HIT

Two Do's	Stop heparin Start alternative, non-heparin anticoagulant, usually in therapeutic doses
Two Don'ts	Avoid or postpone coumarin pending substantial platelet count recovery (give intravenous vitamin K if coumarin already given when HIT is recognized Avoid platelet transfusions
Two Diagnostics	Test for HIT antibodies Investigate for lower-limb DVT (duplex ultrasonography)

Why is warfarin (coumarin) anticoagulation contraindicated during acute HIT?

Acute HIT is a major risk factor for warfarin (coumarin) necrosis, which manifests either as venous limb gangrene or "classic" skin necrosis (9,38–40). The pathogenesis is microthrombosis due to depletion of the vitamin K-dependent natural anticoagulant, protein C, in the setting of increased thrombin generation from HIT (i.e., disturbed procoagulant-anticoagulant balance) (9).

Venous limb gangrene is characterized by (a) an underlying hypercoagulability disorder such as HIT; (b) acral (distal extremity) necrosis in a limb affected by DVT; and (c) a supratherapeutic international normalized ratio (INR) that is usually >3.5 (surrogate marker for severe depletion in protein C). Classic skin necrosis is characterized by necrosis of skin and subcutaneous tissues at central (non-acral) sites (e.g., breast, abdomen, thigh, calf).

Besides its failure to inhibit thrombin, and its risk for producing severe protein C depletion, coumarins also prolong the activated partial thromboplastin time (APTT), thus predisposing to underdosing of DTI therapy (as DTIs are usually monitored by the APTT) (40). The risk of coumarin necrosis in HIT has been estimated at 5% to 10%, which is much greater than the risk in non-HIT populations (~0.01%). For these reasons, vitamin K therapy is recommended if a diagnosis of HIT is made when warfarin has already been started (36,40) (Figure 20.3).

Recommendation. For patients with strongly suspected (or confirmed) HIT, warfarin (coumarin) therapy is contraindicated, at least until after the platelet count has substantially recovered (preferably, $>150 \times 10^9$/L), and only then during overlapping alternative anticoagulation (e.g., danaparoid, lepirudin, argatroban), with a minimum five-day overlap, beginning warfarin in low, maintenance doses (maximum, 5 mg), and stopping the alternative anticoagulant when the platelet count has reached a stable plateau and with at least the last two days the INR within the target therapeutic range. For patients already receiving coumarin at the time of diagnosis of HIT, vitamin K (e.g., 10 mg IV) is recommended.

What is the natural history of isolated HIT?

"Isolated HIT," which denotes absence of clinically evident thrombosis at the time of HIT diagnosis, is associated with a high subsequent risk of symptomatic thrombosis (35%–50%; sudden thrombotic death, 4%–5%) irrespective of whether the heparin is stopped promptly or not (15,24,30,41,42) (Table 20.6). The high risk of thrombosis in part reflects the high frequency (~50%) of HIT-associated subclinical lower-limb DVT (42). Treatment of isolated HIT prevents some thrombotic events (Table 20.4c).

Recommendation. For patients with strongly suspected (or confirmed) isolated HIT, treatment with an alternative non-heparin anticoagulant, such as danaparoid, lepirudin, or argatroban, is recommended, until the platelet count recovers to a stable plateau. Systematic investigation of the lower limbs for subclinical thrombosis by duplex ultrasonography should be performed.

Can HIT be prevented?

The risk of HIT can be reduced in some clinical situations by choosing low-molecular-weight heparin (LMWH) or fondaparinux over unfractionated heparin (UFH). There are four risk factors for HIT: (a) duration of heparin therapy beyond four days; (b) type of heparin (UFH > LMWH >? fondaparinux); (c) type of patient (surgery > medical > obstetric/pediatric); and (d) patient sex (female > male) (7,8,43–47). In the setting of postsurgery thromboprophylaxis, UFH is more likely than LMWH both to cause formation of anti-PF4/heparin antibodies and to cause HIT (7,8,19,22,44,45). One meta-analysis (45) estimated the risk of HIT to be 10-fold greater with UFH compared with LMWH. Although the risk of forming antibodies is also greater in medical patients receiving UFH compared with LMWH, a difference in risk of HIT between the two heparin types has not been proven, perhaps because the lower risk among medical patients makes such studies more difficult.

The synthetic pentasaccharide anticoagulant, fondaparinux, which is modeled after the heparin-binding region of antithrombin, interacts with PF4 in such a way as to cause some approximation of PF4 tetramers to one another (4); however, unlike the situation with heparin, anti-PF4/heparin antibodies do not react well against PF4/fondaparinux complexes in vitro or in vivo (48). Although formation of anti-PF4/heparin antibodies has been reported with fondaparinux postorthopedic surgery thromboprophylaxis (48), the risk of HIT with this agent appears to be negligible.

Despite the increased risk of HIT among women, it is noteworthy that HIT is rare during pregnancy (46), and has not been reported with LMWH therapy during pregnancy (49).

Table 20.6 Natural history of isolated HIT.

Study	Test for HIT antibodies	Thrombosis frequency (%)	Comment
Retrospective cohort (15)	SRA	32/62 (52%)	Sudden death in 3/62 (4.8%) patients
Retrospective cohort (41)	PAT	43/113 (38%)	Trend to higher rate of thrombosis when heparin was stopped "early" (<48 hr) after recognition of HIT
Retrospective cohort (42)	PAT	8/16 (50%)	Asymptomatic thrombi of lower limbs detected by routine duplex ultrasound
Prospective cohort (30)	HIPA	6.1% per patient day	Thrombotic event-rate (per day) during mean 1.7-day period awaiting HIT Ab test results prior to trial entry
Retrospective cohort (34)	PAT	32/139 (23%)	Thrombotic death reported in 6/139 (4.3%) patients
Retrospective cohort (24)	EIA-IgG/A/M (>1.00 OD units)	5/14 (36%)	Lower thrombosis rate (3/34 = 9%; p = 0.07) observed in "isolated HIT" patients with weak positive EIA (<1.00 units)

EIA-IgG/A/M, enzyme-immunoassay that detects anti-PF4/polyanion antibodies of IgG, IgA, and IgM classes; HIPA, heparin-induced platelet activation test; OD, optical density; PAT, platelet aggregation test (using platelet-rich plasma); SRA, serotonin-release assay (using washed platelets).

Recommendation. For postoperative orthopedic patients, use of LMWH or fondaparinux is recommended over UFH. Preferential use of LMWH or fondaparinux instead of UFH in other postoperative patients should be considered as a possible HIT reduction strategy.

Should routine platelet count monitoring for HIT be performed in some circumstances?

Routine platelet count monitoring is appropriate in situations at relatively high risk for HIT, since identification of isolated HIT and early recognition of HIT-associated thrombosis may improve clinical outcomes. The rationale for platelet count monitoring every two to three days includes the following considerations: (a) HIT is relatively common in some clinical settings (1%–5% for one to two weeks of postsurgical UFH thromboprophylaxis) (7,8,19,47); (b) HIT has a narrow temporal onset (day 5–10) (11,14), allowing for a focused period of monitoring; (c) there is a relatively specific definition of thrombocytopenia apropos for surgical patients (>50% platelet count fall from the postoperative peak) (8); (d) platelet count declines in HIT occur over a median of two to three days (14); and (e) treatment of isolated HIT—which by definition can only be detected by platelet count monitoring—reduces the risk of subsequent thrombosis (32–35; Table 20.4c). (f) As most postoperative patients develop a reactive thrombocytosis characterized by rising platelet counts between postoperative days 4 to 14 that reach levels 50 to 100% above the presurgery baseline, in the case of postoperative HIT-induced thrombosis, the diagnostically relevant platelet count decrease might only be apparent if the preceding postoperative platelet count values are available. Accordingly, it is suggested (36) that in high-risk situations for HIT at least every-other-day platelet count monitoring be performed from day 4 to day 14, or until heparin is stopped (whichever occurs first).

At the other extreme, HIT has not been reported with LMHW during pregnancy (49). In this and other low-risk situations, routine platelet count monitoring may not be warranted. For patients at intermediate risks of HIT (e.g., UFH for medical patients; LMWH for surgical patients), platelet count monitoring every two or three days between days 4 to 14 (while receiving heparin) is suggested.

Recommendation. For patients considered at high risk for HIT (e.g., postoperative prophylactic-dose UFH), at least every-other-day platelet count monitoring from day 4 until day 14 (or until UFH is stopped, whichever occurs first), is suggested. For patients considered at intermediate risk for HIT (e.g., therapeutic-dose UFH; postoperative patients receiving LMWH prophylaxis; medical patients receiving UFH prophylaxis), platelet count monitoring every two or three days from day 4 until day 14 (or until UFH is stopped, whichever occurs first), is suggested. For patients considered at low risk for HIT (e.g., medical/obstetric patients receiving LMWH), routine platelet count monitoring is not recommended.

Is deliberate reexposure to heparin ever warranted in a patient with previous HIT?

Intraoperative Figure 20.3 anticoagulation with UFH for cardiac or vascular surgery is appropriate in a patient with previous HIT (11,36,50), provided that heparin-dependent platelet-activating antibodies are no longer detectable at the time of planned surgery. Heparin is safe in this situation because: (a) HIT-IgG antibodies are remarkably transient (median time to nondetectability, 50 to 80 days, depending on the assay performed) (11); (b) tests for HIT antibodies are sensitive (high confidence that clinically relevant antibodies have been excluded) (21,22); (c) there is no anamnestic (immune memory) response to heparin reexposure (antibodies

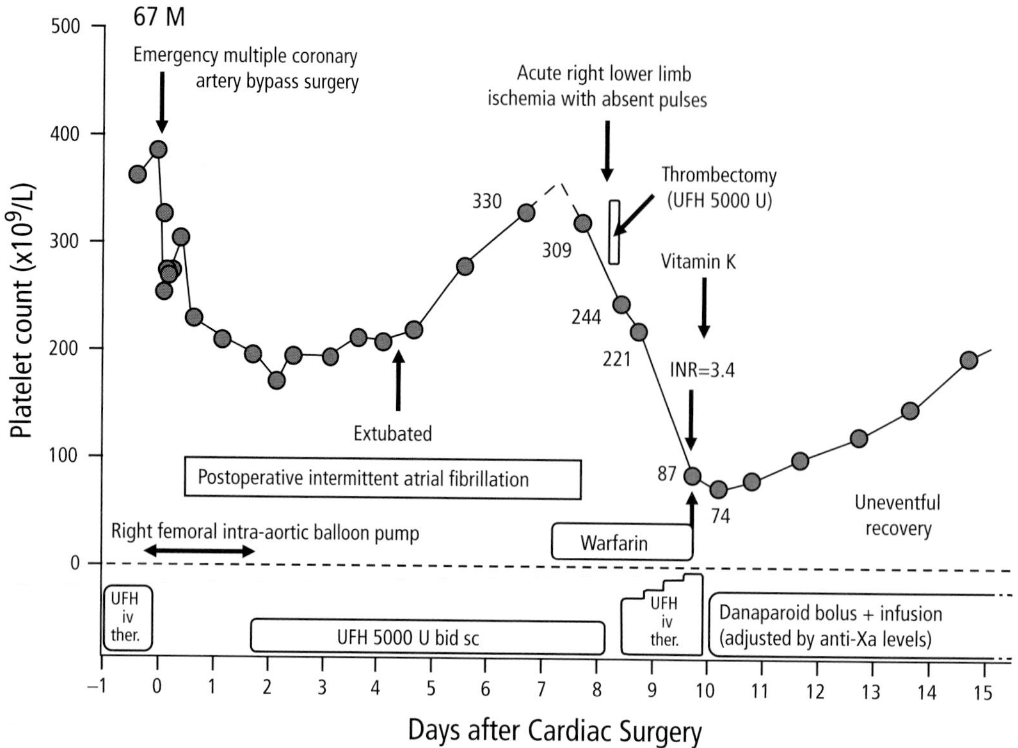

Figure 20.3 A 67-year-old male developed acute right lower limb ischemia with absent pulses 8 days after emergency cardiac surgery. The platelet count had fallen only minimally (from 330 to 309 $\times$ 10^9/L) and the limb ischemia was attributed to either cardiac embolism (secondary to postoperative atrial fibrillation) or local right femoral artery injury (secondary to recent use of an intra-aortic balloon pump). After limb-salvaging thrombectomy (with intraoperative use of UFH), the patient received postoperative therapeutic-dose UFH monitored by the APTT. Progressive decline in the platelet count by 78% to 74 $\times$ 10^9/L prompted the diagnosis of HIT, at which time the UFH was switched to danaparoid, and vitamin K was given to reverse warfarin anticoagulation. Interestingly, a cool and painful left foot improved rapidly following treatment with vitamin K and danaparoid. Reproduced, with permission (17).
bid, twice-daily; iv ther., intravenous therapeutic-dose; sc, subcutaneous; U, units; UFH, unfractionated heparin.

are not regenerated for at least five days after surgery, if at all) (11,50); and (d) there are significant risks with alternative non-heparin anticoagulants (lack of antidotes, minimal experience during surgery utilizing cardiopulmonary bypass). However, in most other situations in which anticoagulation is required for a patient with previous HIT (e.g., postoperative antithrombotic prophylaxis), use of nonheparin anticoagulants (e.g., warfarin) or agents with negligible risk of HIT (e.g., danaparoid, fondaparinux) are recommended over heparin use.

Recommendation UFH is the drug-of-choice for management of cardiac and vascular surgery among patients with previous HIT whose antibodies are no longer detectable. Postoperative anticoagulation is usually performed with non-heparin anticoagulants.

References

1 Arepally GM, Ortel TL. Clinical practice: heparin-induced thrombocytopenia. *N Engl J Med.* 2006;**355**:809–17.

2 Kelton JG, Sheridan D, Santos A, et al. Heparin-induced thrombocytopenia: laboratory studies. *Blood.* 1988;**72**:925–30.

3 Amiral J, Bridey F, Dreyfus M, et al. Platelet factor 4 complexed to heparin is the target for antibodies generated in heparin-induced thrombocytopenia [letter]. *Thromb Haemost.* 1992;**68**:95–6.

4 Greinacher A, Gopinadhan M, Günther JU, et al. Close approximation of two platelet factor 4 tetramers by charge neutralization forms the antigens recognized by HIT antibodies. *Arterioscler Thromb Vasc Biol.* 2006;**26**:2386–93.

5 Warkentin TE, Chong BH, Greinacher A. Heparin-induced thrombocytopenia: towards consensus. *Thromb Haemost.* 1998;**79**:1–7.

6 Warkentin TE. Management of heparin-induced thrombocytopenia: a critical comparison of lepirudin and argatroban. *Thromb Res.* 2003;**110**:73–82.

7 Warkentin TE, Levine MN, Hirsh J, et al. Heparin-induced thrombocytopenia in patients treated with low-molecular-weight heparin or unfractionated heparin. *N Engl J Med.* 1995;**332**:1330–35.

8 Warkentin TE, Roberts RS, Hirsh J, et al. An improved definition of immune heparin-induced thrombocytopenia in postoperative orthopedic patients. *Arch Intern Med.* 2003;**163**:2518–24.

9 Warkentin TE, Elavathil LJ, Hayward CPM, et al. The pathogenesis of venous limb gangrene associated with heparin-induced thrombocytopenia. *Ann Intern Med.* 1997;**127**:804–12.

10 Warkentin TE. An overview of the heparin-induced thrombocytopenia syndrome. *Semin Thromb Hemost.* 2004;**30**:273–83.

11 Warkentin TE, Kelton JG. Temporal aspects of heparin-induced thrombocytopenia. *N Engl J Med.* 2001;**344**:1286–92.

12 Warkentin TE, Kelton JG. Delayed-onset heparin-induced thrombocytopenia and thrombosis. *Ann Intern Med.* 2001;**135**:502–6.

13 Lo GK, Juhl D, Warkentin TE, et al. Evaluation of pretest clinical score (4 T's) for the diagnosis of heparin-induced thrombocytopenia in two clinical settings. *J Thromb Haemost.* 2006;**4**:759–65.

14 Warkentin TE. Clinical picture of heparin-induced thrombocytopenia. In: Warkentin TE, Greinacher A, editors. *Heparin-induced thrombocytopenia.* 4th ed. New York: Informa Healthcare USA 2007; pp. 21–66.

15 Warkentin TE, Kelton JG. A 14-year study of heparin-induced thrombocytopenia. *Am J Med.* 1996;**101**:502–7.

16 Warkentin TE. Heparin-induced skin lesions. *Br J Haematol.* 1996;**92**:494–97.

17 Warkentin TE. Think of HIT. *Hematology: Am Soc Hematol Educ Program.* 2006;408–14.

18 Warkentin TE. Think of HIT when thrombosis follows heparin. *Chest.* 2006;**130**:631–32.

19 Greinacher A, Eichler P, Lietz T, et al. Replacement of unfractionated heparin by low-molecular-weight heparin for postorthopedic surgery antithrombotic prophylaxis lowers the overall risk of symptomatic thrombosis because of a lower frequency of heparin-induced thrombocytopenia [letter]. *Blood.* 2005;**106**:2921–22.

20 Greinacher A, Farner B, Kroll H, et al. Clinical features of heparin-induced thrombocytopenia including risk factors for thrombosis: aretrospective analysis of 408 patients. *Thromb Haemost.* 2005;**94**:132–35.

21 Warkentin TE, Sheppard JI. Testing for heparin-induced thrombocytopenia antibodies. *Transfus Med Rev.* 2006;**20**:259–72.

22 Warkentin TE, Sheppard JI, Moore JC, et al. Laboratory testing for the antibodies that cause heparin-induced thrombocytopenia: how much class do we need? *J Lab Clin Med.* 2005;**146**:341–46.

23 Lo GK, Sigouin CS, Warkentin TE. What is the potential for overdiagnosis of heparin-induced thrombocytopenia? *Am J Hematol.* 2007;**82**:1037–43.

24 Zwicker JI, Uhl L, Huang WY, et al. Thrombosis and ELISA optical density values in hospitalized patients with heparin-induced thrombocytopenia. *J Thromb Haemost.* 2004;**2**:2133–37.

25 Chong BH, Gallus AS, Cade JF, et al. Prospective randomized open-label comparison of danaparoid with dextran 70 in the treatment of heparin-induced thrombocytopenia with thrombosis: a clinical outcome study. *Thromb Haemost.* 2001;**86**:1170–75.

26 Farner B, Eichler P, Kroll H, et al. A comparison of danaparoid and lepirudin in heparin-induced thrombocytopenia. *Thromb Haemost.* 2001;**85**:950–957.

27 Lubenow N, Warkentin TE, Greinacher A, et al. Results of a systematic evaluation of treatment outcomes for heparin-induced thrombocytopenia in patients receiving danaparoid, ancrod, and/or coumarin explain the rapid shift in clinical practice during the 1990s. *Thromb Res.* 2006;**117**:507–15.

28 Greinacher A, Völpel H, Janssens U, et al. Recombinant hirudin (lepirudin) provides safe and effective anticoagulation in patients with the immunologic type of heparin-induced thrombocytopenia: a prospective study. *Circulation.* 1999;**99**:73–80.

29 Greinacher A, Janssens U, Berg G, et al. Lepirudin (recombinant hirudin) for parenteral anticoagulation in patients with heparin-induced thrombocytopenia. *Circulation.* 1999;**100**:587–93.

30 Greinacher A, Eichler P, Lubenow N, et al. Heparin-induced thrombocytopenia with thromboembolic complications: meta-analysis of two prospective trials to assess the value of parenteral treatment with lepirudin and its therapeutic aPTT range. *Blood.* 2000;**96**:846–51.

31 Lubenow N, Eichler P, Lietz T, et al. Lepirudin in patients with heparin-induced thrombocytopenia—results of the third prospective study (HAT-3) and a combined analysis of HAT-1, HAT-2, and HAT-3. *J Thromb Haemost.* 2005;**3**:2428–36.

32 Lubenow N, Eichler P, Lietz T, et al. Lepirudin for prophylaxis of thrombosis in patients with acute isolated heparin-induced thrombocytopenia: an analysis of 3 prospective studies. *Blood.* 2004;**104**:3072–77.

33 Lewis BE, Wallis DE, Berkowitz SD, et al. Argatroban anticoagulant therapy in patients with heparin-induced thrombocytopenia. *Circulation.* 2001;**103**:1838–43.

34 Lewis BE, Wallis DE, Leya F, et al. Argatroban anticoagulation in patients with heparin-induced thrombocytopenia. *Arch Intern Med.* 2003;**163**:1849–56.

35 Lewis BE, Wallis DE, Hursting MJ, et al. Effects of argatroban therapy, demographic variables, and platelet count on thrombotic risks in heparin-induced thrombocytopenia. *Chest.* 2006;**129**:1407–16.

36 Warkentin TE, Greinacher A. Heparin-induced thrombocytopenia: recognition, treatment, and prevention: the Seventh ACCP Conference on Antithrombotic and Thrombolytic Therapy. *Chest.* 2004;**126**(3 Suppl):311S–37S.

37 Keeling D, Davidson S, Watson H, et al. The management of heparin-induced thrombocytopenia. *Br J Haematol.* 2006;**133**:259–69.

38 Smythe MA, Warkentin TE, Stephens JL, et al. Venous limb gangrene during overlapping therapy with warfarin and a direct thrombin inhibitor for immune heparin-induced thrombocytopenia. *Am J Hematol.* 2002;**71**:50–52.

39 Srinivasan AF, Rice L, Bartholomew JR, et al. Warfarin-induced skin necrosis and venous limb gangrene in the setting of heparin-induced thrombocytopenia. *Arch Intern Med.* 2004;**164**:66–70.

40 Warkentin TE. Should vitamin K be administered when HIT is diagnosed after administration of coumarin? [letter]. *J Thromb Haemost* 2006;**4**:894–96.

41 Wallis DE, Workman DL, Lewis BE, et al. Failure of early heparin cessation as treatment for heparin-induced thrombocytopenia. *Am J Med.* 1999;**106**:629–35.

42 Tardy B, Tardy-Poncet B, Fournel P, et al. Lower limb veins should be systematically explored in patients with isolated heparin-induced thrombocytopenia. *Thromb Haemost.* 1999;**82**:1199–1200.

43 Smythe MA, Koerber JM, Mattson JC. The incidence of recognized heparin-induced thrombocytopenia in a large tertiary care teaching center. *Chest.* 2007;**131**:1644–9.

44 Warkentin TE, Sheppard JI, Sigouin CS, et al. Gender imbalance and risk factor interactions in heparin-induced thrombocytopenia. *Blood.* 2006;**108**:2937–41.

45 Martel N, Lee J, Wells PS. Risk for heparin-induced thrombocytopenia with unfractionated and low-molecular-weight heparin thromboprophylaxis: a meta-analysis. *Blood.* 2005;**106**:2710–15.

46 Fausett MB, Vogtlander M, Lee RM, et al. Heparin-induced thrombocytopenia is rare in pregnancy. *Am J Obstet Gynecol.* 2001;**185**:148–152.

47 Lee DH, Warkentin TE. Frequency of heparin-induced thrombocytopenia. In: Warkentin TE, Greinacher A, editors. *Heparin-induced thrombocytopenia.* 4th ed. New York: Informa Healthcare USA 2007; pp. 67–116.

48 Warkentin TE, Cook RJ, Marder VJ, et al. Anti-platelet factor 4/heparin antibodies in orthopedic surgery patients receiving antithrombotic prophylaxis with fondaparinux or enoxaparin. *Blood.* 2005;**106**:3791–96.

49 Greer IA, Nelson-Piercy C. Low-molecular-weight heparins for thromboprophylaxis and treatment of venous thromboembolism in pregnancy: a systematic review of safety and efficacy. *Blood.* 2005;**106**:401–7.

50 Pötzsch B, Klövekorn WP, Madlener K. Use of heparin during cardiopulmonary bypass in patients with a history of heparin-induced thrombocytopenia [letter]. *N Engl J Med.* 2000;**343**:515.

21 Management of Antiphospholipid Antibody Syndrome

Wendy Lim, Mark A. Crowther

Introduction

Antiphospholipid antibodies (aPL) were first described in 1906 by Wassermann and colleagues among patients with positive serologic tests for syphilis (1). These autoantibodies were subsequently found to target phospholipid-binding proteins, with a subgroup of aPL causing prolongation of phospholipid-dependent coagulation assays including the activated partial thromboplastin time (APTT). Despite this laboratory finding, patients with aPL more commonly develop thrombotic rather than bleeding complications, and the presence of aPL in patients with arterial or venous thromboembolism or recurrent pregnancy morbidity comprises the antiphospholipid antibody syndrome (APS).

The aPL measured in the laboratory for the diagnosis of APS include (1) lupus anticoagulants (LA); (2) anticardiolipin (aCL) antibodies; and (3) anti-β_2-glycoprotein I (anti-β_2-GPI) antibodies.

The mainstay of treatment of patients with APS is antithrombotic therapy given the high risk of recurrent thromboembolism that characterizes this condition. Immunosuppressive therapy and plasmapheresis are rarely used in the treatment of patients with APS and are generally reserved for patients with the catastrophic variant of APS. The antithrombotic management of patients with APS is challenging because of a lack of standardized laboratory tests to confirm the diagnosis, limited data on its natural history, and a paucity of randomized treatment trials. In this chapter, we review the laboratory testing and diagnostic criteria for APS and summarize the level of evidence supporting the optimal antithrombotic management of patients with APS. Grading of the quality of evidence and strengths of recommendations in this chapter are based on the guidelines proposed by the international Grading of Recommendations Assessment, Development, and Evaluation Working Group (GRADE), adopting the modification used by the American College of Chest Physicians that merges the very low and low categories of quality of evidence (see chapter 1).

Evidence-based Hematology. Edited by Mark A. Crowther, Jeff Ginsberg, Holger J. Schünemann, Ralph M. Meyer, and Richard Lottenberg.

The clinical questions

1. How are aPL measured in the laboratory?
2. How is APS diagnosed?
3. What is the value of LA, aCL, and anti-β_2-GPI assays in the evaluation of patients with suspected APS?
4. What is the optimal management of patients with aPL without thrombosis?
5. What is the optimal management of patients with aPL and venous thromboembolism?
6. What is the optimal management of patients with aPL and arterial thromboembolism?
7. What is the optimal management of patients with aPL and recurrent thrombosis?
8. What is the optimal management of women with aPL and pregnancy morbidity?

How are aPL measured in the laboratory?

The laboratory testing for aPL is complicated because of uncertainty regarding their antigenic target. However, there is increasing evidence that many aPL, including LA and aCL bind β_2-glycoprotein I, a phospholipid-binding plasma protein (2–5). Other antigenic targets have been identified (6–8) but are not currently included in the laboratory diagnostic criteria for APS. Consensus guidelines describing the optimal laboratory techniques for measuring aCL and LA have been published (9,10), and recommended procedures for measuring anti-β_2-GPI antibodies have been proposed (11).

Lupus anticoagulants

Lupus anticoagulants, also known as nonspecific inhibitors, are antibodies that block phospholipid surfaces important for coagulation. They reduce the coagulant potential of plasma and prolong the clotting time in APTT-based coagulation tests (12). Failure of the prolonged clotting time to correct after a 1:1 mix with normal platelet-free plasma and correction of the clotting time after addition of excess phospholipids confirms the presence of a LA (13). Consensus guidelines recommend screening for LA with two or more phospholipid-dependent coagulation tests, including the APTT, dilute Russell Viper Venom Time, kaolin clotting time, dilute prothrombin time, Textarin Time, or Taipan Time (13). The detection of LA in patients receiving anticoagulant therapy can be problematic because the clotting times are prolonged; however, this is usually overcome by mixing patient and normal plasma prior to LA measurement (14).

Anticardiolipin antibodies

Anticardiolipin antibodies bind cardiolipin, a bovine protein. They are detected using an enzyme-linked immunosorbent assay (ELISA) and consist of IgG, IgM, and IgA isotypes. The IgG isotype is thought to have the strongest association with thrombosis (15). The ELISA tests for aCL are not well standardized, and aCL testing has shown poor concordance among laboratories (12). ACL are reported as a titer specific to the isotype (GPL, MPL, or APL units), but because the accuracy and reliability of assays are limited, consensus guidelines recommend semiquantitative reporting of results as low, medium, or high titer (16).

Anti-β_2-glycoprotein I antibodies

Anti-β_2-glycoprotein I antibodies are one of the aPL subtypes (17). Binding of β_2-glycoprotein I by anti-β_2-GPI antibodies results in dimerization of β_2-glycoprotein I and increases the binding affinity of β_2-glycoprotein I for cell-surface phospholipids, resulting in endothelial, monocyte, platelet, and complement activation, which is a postulated mechanism for aPL-associated thrombosis (18–20). Like aCL, the immunoglobulin isotypes may be IgG, IgM, or IgA and are detected using an ELISA. Laboratory testing for these antibodies is currently poorly standardized (21).

How is APS diagnosed?

Preliminary criteria for definite APS were first proposed in 1999 (known as the Sapporo criteria) (22) and updated in 2005 (17). APS is present in patients with at least one clinical and one laboratory criterion. Clinical criteria include objectively confirmed arterial, venous, or small vessel thrombosis, or pregnancy morbidity consisting of recurrent fetal loss before the 10th week of gestation, one of more unexplained fetal deaths at or beyond the 10th week of gestation, or premature birth due to placental insufficiency, eclampsia, or pre-eclampsia. Laboratory criteria include the presence of LA, medium or high-titer IgG, or IgM aCL (>40 GPL or MPL or >99th percentile), or IgG or IgM anti-β_2-GPI at titers >99th percentile; all aPL must be present on two or more occasions at least 12 weeks apart (17). The consensus recommendations suggest classifying patients with APS as to whether these antibodies occur alone or in combination (17).

Although these consensus-derived diagnostic criteria require repeated measurement to establish a diagnosis of APS, there is no evidence that transient aPL are less important than persistent antibodies. Thus, although useful for research purposes, these criteria have limited utility when making treatment decisions about individual patients.

What is the value of LA, aCL, and anti-β_2-GPI assays in the evaluation of patients with suspected APS?

Cross-sectional studies measuring aPL among healthy blood donors report a prevalence of 10% (23,24), and aPL are present in 30% to 50% of patients with systemic lupus erythematosis (SLE) (25,26). Among patients with thrombosis the prevalence of aPL ranges from 4% to 21% (27,28).

Although there is an association between aPL and thrombosis, it is unknown whether these antibodies directly cause thrombosis. Increasing aCL titers are associated with increasing risks of thrombosis, suggesting a causal association, although it is notable that low titer aCL is likely of little clinical relevance. The association between aPL and thrombosis is stronger with LA than with aCL; the mean odds ratio (OR) for thrombosis is 1.6 for aCL and 11.0 for LA (29). However, it is notable that meta-analyses assessing this association have been limited by the quality of the included studies since there are no large prospective studies of unselected patients whose aPL status was determined prior to objective documentation of thrombotic complications.

Thrombosis is presumed to cause many of the pregnancy complications associated with APS. In women without SLE, a retrospective review of more than 13,000 patients found a prevalence of aPL of 20% among women with recurrent fetal loss, compared with 5% in healthy women (30). The association between aPL and fetal loss is strongest for loss occurring after 10 weeks (31), and data for eclampsia, pre-eclampsia, and intrauterine growth restriction remains controversial. Further, the toxicity of treatments evaluated in these studies may contribute to pregnancy complications and may confound the association between aPL and adverse pregnancy outcomes (32).

What is the optimal management of patients with aPL?

The optimal antithrombotic management in patients with APS requires assessments of the risk of thrombosis, the effectiveness of antithrombotic therapies for preventing thrombosis, and the risk of bleeding. In the following section, we outline the bleeding risk and the risk of thrombosis in patients with aPL based on their clinical presentation and describe the studies supporting the optimal antithrombotic management. The antithrombotic recommendations are based on the following grading system: Grade 1, strong recommendation, Grade 2, less certain recommendation; this is followed by an assessment of the quality of the data, where consistent results from randomized clinical trials receive a Grade A, inconsistent results from randomized trials receive a Grade B, and observational studies receive a Grade C.

Bleeding risk

Estimates of bleeding risk are derived from studies evaluating the efficacy of warfarin in patients with APS. Major bleeding occurs at a frequency of 2%–3% per year, which is comparable to the bleeding rates observed in anticoagulated patients without APS (33,34). Patients with aPL directed against prothrombin can manifest an acquired hemophilia and may present with a bleeding diathesis — the term *lupus anticoagulant* was actually coined based on the presentation of two patients with this form of acquired hemophilia (35).

What is the optimal management of patients with aPL without thrombosis?

Risk of thrombosis in patients with aPL without prior thromboembolism

In a prospective cohort of 551 patients with SLE of whom 49% had either LA or aCL, the incidence of thrombosis was 2 per 100 person-years (36). The OR of thrombosis was 3.20 (95% confidence interval [CI] 1.43–7.14) for LA and 6.80 (95% CI 1.53–30.20) for high-titer aCL when compared with patients who did not have an aPL. However, patients with SLE have a high prevalence of thrombosis even in the absence of aPL (25), and there are only limited data describing the risk of thrombosis in patients with an isolated aPL who do not have SLE. Among 552 randomly selected blood donors, no thrombotic events were observed after 12 months of follow-up among patients found to have aCL (24). Consequently, the risk of thrombosis among patients with incidentally detected aPL is uncertain but is likely to be low.

The risk of thrombosis among women with aPL and fetal loss only may be increased compared with those without fetal loss, based on the results of a retrospective study comparing aspirin to no prophylaxis in 65 nonpregnant women with aPL and a history of pregnancy loss (37). During a mean of 8.1 years, 20 of 34 (59%) nontreated patients experienced venous or arterial thrombosis (7.4/100 patient-years) compared with a baseline risk of thrombosis of 1 per 10,000 per year in unselected premenopausal women (38).

Antithrombotic recommendations

The management of patients who are incidentally found to have aPL and have no prior thrombosis has not been adequately studied, except in patients with SLE. Prospective studies in patients with aPL and no prior thrombosis evaluating aspirin compared with placebo and aspirin compared with warfarin plus aspirin are ongoing. Until the results of these trials are completed, treatment recommendations are based on consensus opinion, which suggest no treatment or low-dose aspirin (81 mg/d) for asymptomatic, nonpregnant patients (39) (Grade 2C).

What is the optimal management of patients with aPL and venous thromboembolism?

Risk of thrombosis in patients with aPL and venous thromboembolism

Deep vein thrombosis of the lower extremities and pulmonary embolism are the most common initial manifestation among patients with APS, occurring in 32% of patients who meet consensus criteria for the diagnosis (40).

The risk of recurrent venous thromboembolism among patients with aPL is based on retrospective studies of untreated patients or studies of patients followed prospectively after their anticoagulants have been discontinued (41). Three prospective studies suggest there is an increased risk of recurrence, ranging from 10% to 67% per year (42–44). In the largest prospective study, 412 patients with a first episode of venous thromboembolism who completed six months of anticoagulation were tested for aCL and followed prospectively after anticoagulants were discontinued. Over four years, 20 of 68 (29%) patients with elevated aCL had recurrent thrombosis, compared with 47 of 334 (14%) patients without aCL (relative risk [RR] 2.1, 95% CI 1.3–3.3) (42). Most patients included in these studies did not conform to the current consensus definition for APS since aPL testing was performed only once, and testing was often performed after recurrence. In patients who received no antithrombotic treatment, retrospective studies report recurrence rates of 0.19 events (45) to 0.29 events per year of follow-up (46); recurrence is reported to occur in 52% to 69% of patients during five to six years of follow-up regardless of the type of antithrombotic therapy (45,46). The incidence of thrombosis is highest during the first six months following discontinuation of warfarin therapy, with an event rate of 1.30 events per year of follow-up (46). Recurrent thrombosis tends to occur in the same vascular distribution as the original event; patients with venous thrombosis generally recur with venous events, and patients with arterial thrombosis have recurrent arterial events (45,47).

Antithrombotic recommendations

Initial treatment. Treatment of venous thromboembolism in patients with APS consists of initial therapy with heparin (unfractionated or low-molecular-weight heparin) for at least four to five days, followed by warfarin therapy (48).

Long-term treatment. Retrospective case series suggested that high-intensity warfarin (INR greater than 3.0) was more effective than either aspirin or warfarin administered with a target INR less than 3.0 (45,46). However, two randomized trials have shown that high-intensity warfarin is not superior to moderate

Table 21.1 Optimal antithrombotic therapy in patients with antiphospholipid antibodies.*

Clinical Scenario	Recommendation	Grade
Transient aPL—no prior thrombosis, with or without SLE	No treatment	Grade 2C
Persistent aPL—no prior thrombosis, with or without SLE	No treatment or low-dose aspirin	Grade 2C
Persistent aPL and venous thrombosis—first presentation or recurrent disease off therapeutic dose warfarin	Long-term warfarin, target INR 2.0 to 3.0	Grade 1A (intensity); Grade 1C (duration)
Persistent aPL and cerebral arterial thrombosis—first presentation or recurrent disease off therapeutic antithrombotic therapy	Long-term warfarin, target INR 1.4 to 2.8 or aspirin	Grade 1A
Persistent aPL and noncerebral arterial thrombosis—first presentation or recurrent disease off therapeutic antithrombotic therapy	Long-term warfarin, target INR 2.0 to 3.0	Grade 2C
Persistent aPL and recurrent thrombosis on therapeutic dose warfarin	Long-term therapeutic dose low-molecular-weight heparin, higher dose warfarin or warfarin target INR 2.0 to 3.0 and aspirin	Grade 2C
Prevention of pregnancy morbidity		
Persistent aPL and no prior thrombosis or recurrent fetal loss	No treatment, or low-dose aspirin, or prophylactic heparin or low-molecular-weight heparin	Grade 2B (no treatment); Grade 2C (aspirin, heparin, low-molecular-weight heparin)
Persistent aPL and no prior thrombosis, but presence of late fetal loss	Low-dose aspirin (81 mg/d), plus heparin, or low-molecular-weight heparin added viable intrauterine pregnancy is documented	Grade 2B
Persistent aPL and prior thrombosis	Most already on long-term warfarin (see above); replace warfarin with heparin during pregnancy	Grade 1C

*aPL, antiphospholipid antibody; INR, international normalized ratio; SLE, systematic lupus erythematosis.

intensity warfarin (international normalized ratio [INR] 2.0–3.0) in preventing recurrent thrombosis (33,34). In the first trial, among 114 APS patients randomized (74% with previous venous thrombosis) and followed for a mean of 2.7 years, the incidence of recurrent thrombosis was 10.7% among patients who received high-intensity warfarin and 3.4% among those who received moderate-intensity warfarin (hazard ratio [HR] 3.1, 95% CI 0.6–15.0) (33). Major bleeding rates were comparable, occurring in 5.4% of patients treated with high-intensity and 6.9% of patients receiving moderate-intensity warfarin (HR 1.0, 95% CI 0.2–4.8).

In the second trial of 109 APS patients followed for a median of 3.6 years, the incidence of recurrent thrombosis was 11.1% among patients who received high-intensity warfarin and 5.5% among those who received moderate-intensity warfarin (HR 1.97, 95% CI 0.49–7.89). Bleeding rates were not significantly different (27.8% versus 14.6%; HR 2.18, 95% CI 0.92–5.15) (34).

Both of these studies were designed to demonstrate that high-intensity warfarin was superior to warfarin administered to achieve an INR of 2.0 to 3.0 for prevention of recurrent thrombosis. Neither study was powered to demonstrate equivalence of the two interventions. When the results of the two studies were combined in a meta-analysis, a significant excess of minor bleeding was evident in patients allocated to high-intensity warfarin (OR 2.3, 95% CI 1.16–4.58, $p = 0.02$) (34). The pooled data did not demonstrate a significant difference in recurrent thrombosis (OR 2.49, 95% CI 0.93–6.67), total bleeding (OR 1.73, 95% CI 0.93–3.31) or major bleeding (OR 0.73, 95% CI 0.23–2.31).

Duration of treatment. The optimal duration of anticoagulation to prevent recurrent venous thrombosis in patients with aPL is unknown. The risk of recurrence appears to be highest in the six-month period immediately following discontinuation of anticoagulants. In one prospective study, patients with a single positive test for aCL, who were randomly assigned to stop warfarin after six months, experienced 23 recurrent events among 105 patients, compared with 3 recurrences in 106 patients receiving indefinite anticoagulation (HR 7.7, 95% CI 2.4–25.0) (42). All patients who experienced recurrent events in the indefinite treatment arm had discontinued warfarin prior to developing recurrent thrombosis. In a second prospective observational study, which measured both LA and aCL after presentation with a first episode venous thromboembolism, the HR for recurrence at three months was 4.0 (95% CI 1.2–13) for aPL-positive patients compared with aPL-negative patients (43). Consequently, the general consensus is to treat patients with APS and venous thrombosis with indefinite duration anticoagulation (48).

In summary, patients with aPL and a first episode venous thrombosis should be treated with warfarin administered to achieve an INR of 2.0 to 3.0 (Grade 1A). The optimal duration of anticoagulation is uncertain but based on prospective data suggesting a high rate of recurrence after warfarin discontinuation, indefinite anticoagulation is recommended (Grade 1C).

What is the optimal management of patients with aPL and arterial thromboembolism?

Risk of thrombosis in patients with aPL and arterial thromboembolism

The most common presentation of arterial disease in APS is ischemic stroke, which is the initial presentation in 13% and transient ischemic attack in 7% of patients with APS (40). The association between APS and other arterial thrombosis, including myocardial infarction, is less certain (49,50).

The risk of arterial thrombosis in patients with aPL is not well defined. Prospective studies have shown the presence of aPL is associated with increased stroke (51,52) although more recent studies suggest no association with aCL (53,54), or this risk may only be significant in women (55).

Antithrombotic recommendations

Antithrombotic recommendations are based on the results of the APL and Stroke Study (APASS) (56), a prospective cohort study within the Warfarin Aspirin Recurrent Stroke Study (WARSS) (57), a randomized double-blind trial comparing warfarin (INR 1.4–2.8) and aspirin 325 mg/d for preventing recurrent stroke or death. In this study, 1,770 patients with a first ischemic stroke were classified into two groups based on the presence or absence of aPL. There was no difference in the risk of thrombotic events in patients treated with warfarin (relative risk [RR] 0.99, 95% CI 0.75–1.31) compared with aspirin (RR 0.94, 95% CI 0.70–1.28). The presence of either LA or aCL was not predictive of recurrent thrombotic events, with 24.2% of patients with aPL and 24.0% of patients without aPL having recurrent events at two years (adjusted RR 0.98, 95% CI 0.80–1.20).

There are no prospective studies evaluating optimal treatment of patients with aPL-associated noncentral nervous system arterial thrombosis. Many patients with myocardial infarction and aPL are treated empirically with long-term warfarin therapy administered to achieve an INR of 2.0 to 3.0 (data extrapolated from venous thromboembolism studies).

In summary, patients with first ischemic stroke and a single positive aPL test who do not have another indication for anticoagulation should be treated with aspirin 325 mg/d or moderate-intensity warfarin (INR 1.4–2.8) (58) (Grade 1A). Aspirin is likely to be preferred because of its ease of use and lack of need for anticoagulant monitoring. Since there are no studies evaluating aPL and noncerebral arterial thrombosis, treatment recommendations are based on consensus opinion, which suggest moderate-intensity warfarin may be appropriate (Grade 2C).

What is the optimal management of patients with aPL and recurrent thrombosis?

Management of patients with APS who have recurrent thrombotic events has not been studied in prospective or randomized studies (59). Patients not receiving anticoagulants should be anticoagulated with heparin followed by warfarin. Patients with recurrent thrombotic events while receiving warfarin should have their INR examined carefully; a subtherapeutic INR at the time of, or immediately prior to, thrombosis represents inadequate anticoagulation as opposed to warfarin failure. These patients may be managed in the same manner as a patient presenting with new thrombosis off warfarin. Possible treatment options for recurrent thrombosis despite therapeutic anticoagulation with warfarin include: (1) increasing the intensity of warfarin; (2) switching to therapeutic doses of unfractionated heparin or low-molecular-weight heparin; or (3) adding an antiplatelet agent to warfarin. Plasma exchange or intravenous immune globulin, particularly in patients with catastrophic APS, has also been recommended (60).

In summary, antithrombotic recommendations for recurrent thrombosis in APS are based on consensus opinion. Patients who are not anticoagulated at the time of recurrence are started on anticoagulation with heparins overlapping with long-term warfarin. Patients who are already therapeutically anticoagulated with warfarin may be treated with high-intensity warfarin, heparins, or addition of aspirin (Grade 2C).

What is the optimal management of women with aPL and pregnancy morbidity?

Risk of pregnancy complications in women with aPL without prior thromboembolism

The risk of fetal loss and premature birth among asymptomatic women who have aPL appears to be increased, based on studies comparing the rates of these outcomes in women with and without aPL (61–64). Comparison of these studies is complicated by differences in the definition of pregnancy loss and the timing of testing for aPL. Nevertheless, each of the studies demonstrated a lower live-birth rate in women with aPL, ranging from 62% to 84%, compared with 90% to 98% in women without these antibodies (65).

Risk of pregnancy complications in women with aPL with prior pregnancy loss with and without prior thromboembolism

Pregnancy complications are likely increased among women with aPL who have a prior history of pregnancy loss and also likely increased among women with aPL who have a prior history of thrombosis (meeting criteria for APS), compared with women with aPL and no prior pregnancy loss or thrombosis, respectively, but the magnitude of risk is uncertain and has not been formally studied.

Antithrombotic recommendations

Although asymptomatic pregnant women with aPL have an increase in the risk of pregnancy complications, the absolute risk remains small. In one small randomized study of 19 women, there was no difference in pregnancy outcome among women who received low-dose aspirin (81 mg daily) compared with usual care (66). The small number of events in this trial precludes definitive conclusions, and since many experts believe these patients have an increased risk of thrombosis during pregnancy, aspirin (75–162 mg daily) or prophylactic dose heparin or low-molecular-weight heparin is recommended (67).

The optimal treatment of pregnant women with aPL and one or more fetal losses after 10 weeks gestation without thrombosis is controversial. Randomized trials and prospective observational studies have shown varying results, likely related to the lack of standardization of the aPL assays (65). A systematic review of 13 randomized trials involving 849 pregnant women with a history of pregnancy loss and aPL found that combination therapy with unfractionated heparin (5,000 units subcutaneously twice daily) and aspirin (75–81 mg daily) significantly reduced pregnancy loss compared with aspirin alone (RR 0.46, 95% CI 0.29–0.71) (68), although the analysis was based on only two trials of 140 patients (69,70). In one study of 98 patients, the combination of low-molecular-weight heparin (5,000 units subcutaneously daily) and aspirin (75 mg/d) compared with aspirin alone did not significantly reduce pregnancy loss (RR 0.78, 95% CI 0.39–1.57) (71). Aspirin 50–81 mg daily compared with placebo or usual care did not reduce the rate of pregnancy loss in three trials (RR 1.05, 95% CI 0.66–1.68) (66, 72, 73). Low doses of subcutaneous unfractionated heparin (5,000 units twice daily) appear to be as effective as high-dose heparin (10,000 units twice daily) (RR 0.83, 95% CI 0.29, 2.38) (69).

Consensus recommendations suggest that women with aPL and a history of two or more early pregnancy losses or one or more late pregnancy losses (who have no prior history of thrombosis) receive treatment with combination aspirin and heparin during pregnancy (67). Aspirin 81 mg/d is started with attempted conception and heparin (5,000–10,000 units every 12 hours) or low-molecular-weight heparin in prophylactic doses is started when a viable intrauterine pregnancy is documented and continued until late in the third trimester (74).

Pregnant women with aPL and prior thrombosis are generally receiving long-term anticoagulation with warfarin prior to pregnancy. The optimal management of these patients has not been formally evaluated. Warfarin is teratogenic between the 6th and 12th weeks of gestation and has been reported to cause nasal hypoplasia and stippled epiphysis (75). Consequently, warfarin is routinely replaced with low-molecular-weight heparin or unfractionated heparin prior to planned conception or during early gestation. The dose of low-molecular-weight heparin or unfractionated heparin requires monitoring and adjustment as pregnancy progesses (based on weight or peak anti-Xa levels for low-molecular-weight heparin and mid-interval APTT for unfractionated heparin). Resumption of long-term oral anticoagulation with warfarin is initiated postpartum.

In summary, pregnant women with aPL without prior pregnancy complications or thrombosis are at low risk and no treatment is recommended (Grade 2B) or low-dose aspirin or prophylactic heparin or low-molecular-weight heparin (Grade 2C). The management of pregnant women with aPL and prior pregnancy complications without thrombosis ranges is variable; most available data support use of prophylactic heparin or low-molecular-weight heparin and aspirin (Grade 2B). Pregnant women with aPL and prior thrombosis (meeting criteria for APS) should receive prepregnancy counseling, and the risks and benefits of management throughout pregnancy should be discussed (Grade 2C). During pregnancy, adjusted-dose low-molecular-weight heparin or unfractionated heparin is recommended, with resumption of long-term oral anticoagulation postpartum (Grade 1C).

References

1 Wassermann A, Neisser A, Bruck C. Eine serodiagnostische Reaction bei Syphilis. *Dtsch Med Wochensehr.* 1906;**32**:745–746.

2 McNeil HP, Simpson RJ, Chesterman CN, et al. Anti-phospholipid antibodies are directed against a complex antigen that includes a lipid-binding inhibitor of coagulation: beta 2-glycoprotein I (apolipoprotein H). *Proc Natl Acad Sci USA.* 1990;**87**(11):4120–24.

3 Galli M, Luciani D, Bertolini G, et al. Anti-beta 2-glycoprotein I, antiprothrombin antibodies, and the risk of thrombosis in the antiphospholipid syndrome. *Blood.* 2003;**102**(8):2717–23.

4 de Groot PG, Derksen RHWM. Pathophysiology of the antiphospholipid syndrome. *J Thromb Haemost.* 2005;**3**:1854–60.

5 de Laat HB, Derksen RH, Urbanus RT, et al. beta2-glycoprotein I-dependent lupus anticoagulant highly correlates with thrombosis in the antiphospholipid syndrome. *Blood.* 2004;**104**(12):3598–602.

6 de Groot PG, Horbach DA, Simmelink MJ, et al. Anti-prothrombin antibodies and their relation with thrombosis and lupus anticoagulant. *Lupus.* 1998;**7**(Suppl 2):S32–S36.

7 Cesarman-Maus G, Rios-Luna NP, Deora AB, et al. Autoantibodies against the fibrinolytic receptor, annexin 2, in antiphospholipid syndrome. *Blood.* 2006;**107**(11):4375–82.

8 Satoh A, Suzuki K, Takayama E, et al. Detection of anti-annexin IV and V antibodies in patients with antiphospholipid syndrome and systemic lupus erythematosus. *J Rheumatol.* 1999;**26**(8):1715–20.

9 Tincani A, Allegri F, Sanmarco M, et al. Anticardiolipin antibody assay: a methodological analysis for a better consensus in routine determinations—a cooperative project of the European Antiphospholipid Forum. *Thromb Haemost.* 2001;**86**(2):575–83.

10 Brandt JT, Barna LK, Triplett DA. Laboratory identification of lupus anticoagulants: results of the Second International Workshop for Identification of Lupus Anticoagulants. On behalf of the Subcommittee on Lupus Anticoagulants/Antiphospholipid Antibodies of the ISTH. *Thromb Haemost.* 1995;**74**(6):1597–1603.

11 Reber G, Tincani A, Sanmarco M, et al. Proposals for the measurement of anti-beta2-glycoprotein I antibodies: Standardization Group of the European Forum on Antiphospholipid Antibodies. *J Thromb Haemost.* 2004;**2**(10):1860–62.

12 Triplett DA. Antiphospholipid antibodies. *Arch Pathol Lab Med.* 2002;**126**:1424–29.

13 Brandt JT, Triplett DA, Alving B, et al. Criteria for the diagnosis of lupus anticoagulants: an update. On behalf of the Subcommittee on Lupus Anticoagulant/Antiphospholipid Antibody of the Scientific and Standardisation Committee of the ISTH. *Thromb Haemost.* 1995;**74**(4): 1185–90.

14 Tripodi A, Chantarangkul V, Clerici M, et al. Laboratory diagnosis of lupus anticoagulants for patients on oral anticoagulant treatment: performance of dilute Russell viper venom test and silica clotting time in comparison with Staclot LA. *Thromb Haemost.* 2002;**88**(4):583–86.

15 Harris EN, Pierangeli SS. Revisiting the anticardiolipin test and its standardization. *Lupus.* 2002;**11**(5):269–75.

16 Harris EN. Special report: the Second International Anti-cardiolipin Standardization Workshop/the Kingston Anti-Phospholipid Antibody Study (KAPS) group. *Am J Clin Pathol.* 1990;**94**(4):476–84.

17 Miyakis S, Lockshin MD, Atsumi T, et al. International consensus statement on an update of the classification criteria for definite antiphospholipid syndrome (APS). *J Thromb Haemost.* 2006;**4**(2):295–306.

18 Roubey RA, Eisenberg RA, Harper MF, et al. "Anticardiolipin" autoantibodies recognize beta 2-glycoprotein I in the absence of phospholipid: importance of Ag density and bivalent binding. *J Immunol.* 1995;**154**(2):954–60.

19 Willems GM, Janssen MP, Pelsers MM, et al. Role of divalency in the high-affinity binding of anticardiolipin antibody-beta 2-glycoprotein I complexes to lipid membranes. *Biochemistry.* 1996;**35**(43):13833–42.

20 Kuwana M, Matsuura E, Kobayashi K, et al. Binding of beta 2-glycoprotein I to anionic phospholipids facilitates processing and presentation of a cryptic epitope that activates pathogenic autoreactive T cells. *Blood.* 2005;**105**(4):1552–57.

21 Reber G, Tincani A, Sanmarco M, et al. Variability of anti-beta2 glycoprotein I antibodies measurement by commercial assays. *Thromb Haemost.* 2005;**94**(3):665–72.

22 Wilson WA, Gharavi AE, Koike T, et al. International consensus statement on preliminary classification criteria for definite antiphospholipid syndrome: report of an international workshop. *Arthritis Rheum.* 1999;**42**(7):1309–11.

23 Shi W, Krilis SA, Chong BH, et al. Prevalence of lupus anticoagulant and anticardiolipin antibodies in a healthy population. *Aust N Z J Med.* 1990;**20**(3):231–36.

24 Vila P, Hernandez MC, Lopez-Fernandez MF, et al. Prevalence, follow-up and clinical significance of the anticardiolipin antibodies in normal subjects. *Thromb Haemost.* 1994;**72**(2):209–13.

25 Long AA, Ginsberg JS, Brill-Edwards P, et al. The relationship of antiphospholipid antibodies to thromboembolic disease in systemic lupus erythematosus: a cross-sectional study. *Thromb Haemost.* 1991;**66**(5): 520–24.

26 Bruce IN, Clark-Soloninka CA, Spitzer KA, et al. Prevalence of antibodies to beta2-glycoprotein I in systemic lupus erythematosus and their association with antiphospholipid antibody syndrome criteria: a single center study and literature review. *J Rheumatol.* 2000;**27**(12):2833–37.

27 Ginsberg JS, Wells PS, Brill-Edwards P, et al. Antiphospholipid antibodies and venous thromboembolism. *Blood.* 1995;**86**(10):3685–91.

28 Mateo J, Oliver A, Borrell M, et al. Laboratory evaluation and clinical characteristics of 2,132 consecutive unselected patients with venous thromboembolism—results of the Spanish Multicentric Study on Thrombophilia (EMET-Study). *Thromb Haemost.* 1997;**77**(3): 444–51.

29 Galli M, Luciani D, Bertolini G, et al. Lupus anticoagulants are stronger risk factors for thrombosis than anticardiolipin antibodies in the antiphospholipid syndrome: a systematic review of the literature. *Blood.* 2003;**101**:1827–32.

30 Oshiro BT, Silver RM, Scott JR, et al. Antiphospholipid antibodies and fetal death. *Obstet Gynecol.* 1996;**87**(4):489–93.

31 Rai RS, Clifford K, Cohen H, et al. High prospective fetal loss rate in untreated pregnancies of women with recurrent miscarriage and antiphospholipid antibodies. *Hum Reprod.* 1995;**10**(12):3301–4.

32 Laskin CA, Bombardier C, Hannah ME, et al. Prednisone and aspirin in women with autoantibodies and unexplained recurrent fetal loss. *N Engl J Med.* 1997;**337**(3):148–53.

33 Crowther MA, Ginsberg JS, Julian J, et al. A comparison of two intensities of warfarin for the prevention of recurrent thrombosis in patients with the antiphospholipid antibody syndrome. *N Engl J Med.* 2003;**349**(12):1133–38.

34 Finazzi G, Marchioli R, Brancaccio V, et al. A randomized clinical trial of high-intensity warfarin vs. conventional antithrombotic therapy for the prevention of recurrent thrombosis in patients with the antiphospholipid syndrome (WAPS). *J Thromb Haemost.* 2005;**3**(5): 848–53.

35 Erkan D, Bateman H, Lockshin MD. Lupus anticoagulant-hypoprothrombinemia syndrome associated with systemic lupus erythematosus: report of 2 cases and review of literature. *Lupus.* 1999;**8**(7):560–64.

36 Petri M. Thrombosis and systemic lupus erythematosus: the Hopkins Lupus Cohort perspective. *Scand J Rheumatol.* 1996;**25**:191–93.

37 Erkan D, Merrill JT, Yazici Y, et al. High thrombosis rate after fetal loss in antiphospholipid syndrome: effective prophylaxis with aspirin. *Arthritis Rheum.* 2001;**44**(6):1466–67.

38 Anderson FA Jr, Wheeler HB, Goldberg RJ, et al. A population-based perspective of the hospital incidence and case-fatality rates of deep vein thrombosis and pulmonary embolism. The Worcester DVT Study. *Arch Intern Med.* 1991;**151**(5):933–38.

39 Alarcon-Segovia D, Boffa MC, Branch W, et al. Prophylaxis of the antiphospholipid syndrome: a consensus report. *Lupus.* 2003;**12**(7):499–503.

40 Cervera R, Piette JC, Font J, et al. Antiphospholipid syndrome: clinical and immunologic manifestations and patterns of disease expression in a cohort of 1,000 patients. *Arthritis Rheum.* 2002;**46**(4):1019–27.

41 Crowther MA, Wisloff F. Evidence based treatment of the antiphospholipid syndrome II. Optimal anticoagulant therapy for thrombosis. *Thromb Res.* 2005;**115**(1–2):3–8.

42 Schulman S, Svenungsson E, Granqvist S, et al. Anticardiolipin antibodies predict early recurrence of thromboembolism and death among patients with venous thromboembolism following anticoagulant therapy. *Am J Med.* 1998;**104**:332–38.

43 Kearon C, Gent M, Hirsh J, et al. A comparison of three months of anticoagulation with extended anticoagulation for a first episode of idiopathic venous thromboembolism. *N Engl J Med.* 1999;**340**:901–7.

44 Kearon C, Ginsberg JS, Kovacs MJ, et al. Comparison of low-intensity warfarin therapy with conventional-intensity warfarin therapy for long-term prevention of recurrent venous thromboembolism. *N Engl J Med.* 2003;**349**(7):631–39.

45 Rosove MH, Brewer PMC. Antiphospholipid thrombosis: clinical course after the first thrombotic event in 70 patients. *Ann Intern Med.* 1992;**117**(4):303–8.

46 Khamashta MA, Cuadrado MJ, Mujic F, et al. The management of thrombosis in the antiphospholipid-antibody syndrome. *N Engl J Med.* 1995;**332**:993–97.

47 Finazzi G, Brancaccio V, Moia M, et al. Natural history and risk factors for thrombosis in 360 patients with antiphospholipid antibodies: a four-year prospective study from the Italian registry. *Am J Med.* 1995;**100**: 530–36.

48 Büller HR, Agnelli G, Hull RD, et al. Antithrombotic therapy for venous thromboembolic disease: the Seventh ACCP Conference on Antithrombotic and Thrombolytic Therapy. *Chest.* 2004;**126**(3 Suppl): 401S–28S.

49 Tenedios F, Erkan D, Lockshin MD. Cardiac involvement in the antiphospholipid syndrome. *Lupus.* 2005;**14**(9):691–96.

50 Veres K, Lakos G, Kerenyi A, et al. Antiphospholipid antibodies in acute coronary syndrome. *Lupus.* 2004;**13**(6):423–27.

51 Brey RL, Abbott RD, Curb JD, et al. beta(2)-Glycoprotein 1-dependent anticardiolipin antibodies and risk of ischemic stroke and myocardial infarction: the Honolulu Heart Program. *Stroke.* 2001;**32**(8):1701–6.

52 Brey RL, Stallworth CL, McGlasson DL, et al. Antiphospholipid antibodies and stroke in young women. *Stroke.* 2002;**33**(10):2396–400.

53 Ginsburg KS, Liang MH, Newcomer L, et al. Anticardiolipin antibodies and the risk for ischemic stroke and venous thrombosis. *Ann Intern Med.* 1992;**117**(12):997–1002.

54 Ahmed E, Stegmayr B, Trifunovic J, et al. Anticardiolipin antibodies are not an independent risk factor for stroke: an incident case-referent study nested within the MONICA and Vasterbotten cohort project. *Stroke.* 2000;**31**(6):1289–93.

55 Janardhan V, Wolf PA, Kase CS, et al. Anticardiolipin antibodies and risk of ischemic stroke and transient ischemic attack: the Framingham cohort and offspring study. *Stroke.* 2004;**35**(3):736–41.

56 The APASS Writing Committee. Antiphospholipid antibodies and subsequent thrombo-occlusive events in patients with ischemic stroke. *JAMA.* 2004;**291**:576–84.

57 Mohr JP, Thompson JL, Lazar RM, et al. A comparison of warfarin and aspirin for the prevention of recurrent ischemic stroke. *N Engl J Med.* 2001;**345**(20):1444–51.

58 Brey RL, Chapman J, Levine SR, et al. Stroke and the antiphospholipid syndrome: consensus meeting Taormina 2002. *Lupus.* 2003;**12**(7):508–13.

59 Dentali F, Manfredi E, Crowther M, et al. Long-duration therapy with low molecular weight heparin in patients with antiphospholipid antibody syndrome resistant to warfarin therapy. *J Thromb Haemost.* 2005;**3**(9):2121–3.

60 Asherson RA, Cervera R, de Groot PG, et al. Catastrophic antiphospholipid syndrome: international consensus statement on classification criteria and treatment guidelines. *Lupus.* 2003;**12**(7):530–34.

61 Pattison NS, Chamley LW, McKay EJ, et al. Antiphospholipid antibodies in pregnancy: prevalence and clinical associations. *Br J Obstet Gynaecol.* 1993;**100**(10):909–13.

62 Lynch A, Marlar R, Murphy J, et al. Antiphospholipid antibodies in predicting adverse pregnancy outcome: a prospective study. *Ann Intern Med.* 1994;**120**(6):470–75.

63 Lockwood CJ, Romero R, Feinberg RF, et al. The prevalence and biologic significance of lupus anticoagulant and anticardiolipin antibodies in a general obstetric population. *Am J Obstet Gynecol.* 1989;**161**(2):369–73.

64 Yasuda M, Takakuwa K, Tokunaga A, et al. Prospective studies of the association between anticardiolipin antibody and outcome of pregnancy. *Obstet Gynecol.* 1995;**86**:555–59.

65 Derksen RH, Khamashta MA, Branch DW. Management of the obstetric antiphospholipid syndrome. *Arthritis Rheum.* 2004;**50**(4):1028–39.

66 Cowchock S, Reece EA. Do low-risk pregnant women with antiphospholipid antibodies need to be treated? Organizing Group of the Antiphospholipid Antibody Treatment Trial. *Am J Obstet Gynecol.* 1997;**176**(5):1099–100.

67 Bates SM, Greer IA, Hirsh J, et al. Use of antithrombotic agents during pregnancy: the Seventh ACCP Conference on Antithrombotic and Thrombolytic Therapy. *Chest.* 2004;**126**(3 Suppl):627S–44S.

68 Empson M, Lassere M, Craig J, et al. Prevention of recurrent miscarriage for women with antiphospholipid antibody or lupus anticoagulant. *Cochrane Database Syst Rev.* 2005;(2):CD002859.

69 Kutteh WH. Antiphospholipid antibody-associated recurrent pregnancy loss: treatment with heparin and low-dose aspirin is superior to low-dose aspirin alone. *Am J Obstet Gynecol.* 1996;**174**(5):1584–89.

70 Rai R, Cohen H, Dave M, et al. Randomised controlled trial of aspirin and aspirin plus heparin in pregnant women with recurrent miscarriage associated with phospholipid antibodies (or antiphospholipid antibodies). *BMJ.* 1997;**314**(253):257.

71 Farquharson RG, Quenby S, Greaves M. Antiphospholipid syndrome in pregnancy: a randomized, controlled trial of treatment. *Obstet Gynecol.* 2002;**100**(3):408–13.

72 Pattison NS, Chamley LW, Birdsall M, et al. Does aspirin have a role in improving pregnancy outcome for women with the antiphospholipid syndrome? A randomized controlled trial. *Am J Obstet Gynecol.* 2000;**183**(4):1008–12.

73 Tulppala M, Marttunen M, Soderstrom-Anttila V, et al. Low-dose aspirin in prevention of miscarriage in women with unexplained or autoimmune related recurrent miscarriage: effect on prostacyclin and thromboxane A2 production. *Hum Reprod.* 1997;**12**(7):1567–72.

74 Tincani A, Branch W, Levy RA, et al. Treatment of pregnant patients with antiphospholipid syndrome. *Lupus.* 2003;**12**(7):524–29.

75 Hall JG, Pauli RM, Wilson KM. Maternal and fetal sequelae of anticoagulation during pregnancy. *Am J Med.* 1980;**68**(1):122–40.

3 Benign Hematologic Disorders

Richard Lottenberg

22 Clinical Questions in Iron Overload

Antonello Pietrangelo, Nicola Magrini

Although iron is essential for many vital functions, there is no regulated means by which excess iron can be disposed in humans. Therefore, whenever body iron exceeds its needs and storage capabilities are saturated, toxicity due to iron overload may arise. There exist many causes of iron overload in humans, both genetics and acquired (Table 22.1) (1). Among all, hereditary hemochromatosis (HC) and transfusion-dependent iron overload in hereditary anemias, particularly thalassemia, are central when considering epidemiological impact, extent of iron burden, and risk for iron-related morbidity and mortality.

We have focused this chapter on HC and transfusion-dependent iron overload and developed four clinically relevant explicit questions with supporting definitions. Each question has guided a systematic literature review in the MEDLINE (PubMed version), EMBASE (Dialog version), Cinahl (Dialog version), the Cochrane Library databases from 1966 through November 2006, and the quality of reported evidence has been graded according to Grading of Recommendations Assessment, Development, and Evaluation Working Group (GRADE) definitions (2,3).

Study selection was based on specific inclusion and exclusion criteria (see Appendix 22.1, website http://www.blackwellpublishing.com/medicine/bmj/hematology). Two recent high-quality systematic reviews (4,5) were updated following the specified criteria through November 2006.

What is the best noninvasive method to diagnose tissue iron overload?

Assessment of tissue iron content is an important aspect for diagnosis and management of patients with suspected or ascertained iron loading conditions. The liver is the main iron storage depot in mammals and is the most easily accessible tissue for accurately assessing iron stores. Quantitative assay of hepatic iron concentration (HIC; synonymous for liver iron concentration, or LIC) by liver biopsy has been historically considered the gold standard for ascertaining tissue iron overload (6,7) and used widely in the literature. An alternative reference method for quality assessment of the extent of body iron overload has been the measure of total number of phlebotomies required to obtain a normal serum iron and ferritin (7–9).

The "gold standard" not only entails a liver biopsy, with potential morbidity and mortality risks, but also presents limitations and source of inaccuracy, such as insufficient liver biopsy tissue, presence of cirrhosis and uneven deposition of iron within the liver, difference of in vitro biopsy processing methods (e.g., wet- vs. dry-weight biopsies), and lack of standardized reference values (10–12) (Table 22.2). Finally, while early studies proposed LIC assay for prediction of iron loading in other organs (13), a number of subsequent studies have clearly indicated that LIC in thalassemia is a poor predictor of the extent of iron accumulated in the heart (14–17) or development of cardiomyopathy (14,15,18,19).

The most widely used biochemical surrogate for iron overload is serum ferritin. According to validation studies where body iron stores were assessed by phlebotomy, serum ferritin is a highly sensitive test for iron overload in hemochromatosis (20), thalassemia (21), and dialysis patients (22). Thus, normal levels essentially "rule out" iron overload. However, ferritin has low specificity as elevated values can be the result of a range of inflammatory and neoplastic states or mask other conditions, such as diabetes and metabolic syndrome, alcohol abuse, and viral hepatitis. In prognostic settings, serum ferritin above 1,000 ng/mL may indicate underlying cirrhosis in hemochromatosis patients (23–25). Monitoring serum ferritin during phlebotomy is standard practice in hemochromatosis (26,27). In thalassemic patients undergoing chelation, serum ferritin seems to be a poor predictor of iron accumulation in the heart as assessed by MRI (15,17,28). In general, while single measures are clearly inadequate for assessment of current iron chelation status, average ferritin values over several months seem reliable for trends.

Iron content of serum ferritin had been proposed as a new test that measures human body iron stores unconfounded by

Evidence-based Hematology. Edited by Mark A. Crowther, Jeff Ginsberg, Holger J. Schünemann, Ralph M. Meyer, and Richard Lottenberg.

Table 22.1 Human iron overload disorders.

Hereditary	Acquired	Miscellaneous
• Hereditary hemochromatosis (HC) (HFE-, TfR2-, HJV, HAMP-related) • Ferroportin disease • Aceruloplasminemia • Atransferrinemia • H-ferritin related iron overload • Hereditary iron loading anemias	• Dietary • Parental • Acquired hemolytic anemias • Long-term hemodialysis • Chronic liver disease ○ Hepatitis C and B ○ Alcoholic cirrhosis ○ Nonalcoholic fatty liver • Porphyria cutanea tarda • Alloimmune neonatal hemochromatosis	• African siderosis

inflammation (29). This has been challenged by subsequent studies in which, however, the reference standard has been liver iron assessed by imaging methods and not by biopsy (30,31). The serum iron, transferrin, transferrin saturation, and transferrin receptor concentration do not quantitatively reflect body iron stores and should then not be used as surrogate for tissue iron overload.

In recent years, noninvasive imaging methods to measure hepatic iron content have been extensively investigated (Table 22.2). Superquantum magnetic susceptibility determinations (SQUID) are capable of measuring hepatic iron concentrations over a wide range and are sensitive and specific (12,22,32). However, there is limited availability of devices and expertise, while the use of incorrect conversion factors to translate in vivo wet-weight LICs to dry-weight values has negatively affected the conduct of clinical trials or their use in clinical practice, as recently pointed out by Fisher et al. (33).

The recent advent of high Tesla magnetic resonance imaging instruments has shown some promise as a noninvasive way to estimate tissue iron content. An increased tissue iron content decreases, due to the paramagnetic properties of iron, the T2 relaxation time and the organ signal's intensity. Gradient-recalled-echo techniques have been recently shown to be accurate in quantifying

Table 22.2 Features of available methods to detect iron overload.*

Methods	Advantages	Disadvantages	References
Liver biopsy	Accurately reflects total body iron status; useful to assess liver pathology	Invasive; inaccurate if insufficient liver biopsy tissue, presence of cirrhosis and uneven deposition of iron; variability depending on in vitro biopsy processing methods; lack of standardization; imperfect surrogate for cardiac iron	(6,7,10–12,14–19)
Serum ferritin	Highly sensitive; noninvasive; inexpensive and widely available; average value over 6 months reliable during iron-chelation in thalassemia; reliable for monitoring iron depletion during phlebotomy	Highly variable; acute-phase reactant and affected by liver diseases and metabolic disorders; single measures inadequate for assessment of current status in thalassemics undergoing iron-chelation therapy; imperfect surrogate for cardiac iron	(20–24 15,17,25–27,28)
Superquantum magnetic susceptibility determinations (SQUID)	Validated in clinical studies in comparison to liver biopsy; hepatic iron assessment less prone to error due to uneven iron distribution	Expensive instruments; available in a few centers; calibration variability	(12,22,32,33)
Hepatic MRI	Noninvasive; less prone to error due to uneven iron distribution; validated in clinical studies in comparison to liver biopsy	Imperfect surrogate for cardiac iron; needs calibration and standardization between machines in different centers	(34–38)
Cardiac MRI	Surrogate for risk of heart failure due to iron; noninvasive measure of cardiac iron status; potentially useful for patient assessment and follow-up	Not widely available; not yet proven that improved T2* by chelation improves cardiac disease or death from iron overload; not yet calibrated in humans for quantitative assessment	(14,15,40–46, 47–50.)

* Modified from reference (50a).

both mild and more severe iron overload states as validated by paired assessment of LIC by biopsy (34–38). Myocardial iron accumulation is the main cause for cardiac complications in thalassemia (39). At variance with the assay of serum ferritin or hepatic iron deposition (see above), cardiac MRI measurement seems in agreement with cardiac iron as assessed by heart biopsy (40). A further development in assessing iron accumulation in the heart is based on multiecho T2* MR technique. This method has been validated in early studies (14,41), and it is seems reproducible on different machines (42–44). Patients with myocardial siderosis have been shown to be at increased risk of left ventricular systolic and diastolic dysfunction, arrhythmias, and heart failure (14,15,41,45). T2* can be used to monitor relative changes in human myocardial iron (46) and improvement of cardiac function under chelation (47,48), but it has not been calibrated for absolute values of cardiac iron in humans. Recent proposed improvements of cardiac MRI are spin-spin relaxation rate, R2, measurements (49) or multislice multiecho T2* MRI, which is supposed to overcome the heterogeneous distribution of myocardial iron (50).

Recommendations

- All patients with suspected iron overload should be offered a serum ferritin assay (Grade 1C).
- All patients with ascertained iron overload undergoing iron depletion therapy should be monitored by serum ferritin (Grade 1C).
- In selected patients with suspected iron overload and disorders potentially associated with increased serum ferritin levels (inflammatory disorders, metabolic syndrome, fatty liver, alcohol abuse, etc.), hepatic MRI could be offered (Grade 1C).
- Cardiac MRI should be offered to all patients with thalassemia major (Grade 1C).

What is the disease burden of hereditary hemochromatosis?

Hereditary hemochromatosis results from a genetically determined failure to stop iron from entering the circulatory iron pool when is not needed (51). Without therapeutic intervention, there is a distinct risk that tissue iron overload will occur, with the potential for damage and disease. The prototype, and by far the most common form of HC, is the classic disorder related to the C282Y homozygote mutation of HFE (52). We will therefore focus on HFE hemochromatosis, while rarer forms recently attributed to loss of TfR2, HAMP, or HJV or to a subtype of FPN mutations (1), on which limited and more sparse clinical and epidemiologic data are available, will not be discussed (Table 22.1). While two common HFE mutations exist, C282Y and H63D, only C282Y homozygosity is potentially associated with clinical manifestations. Apart for the C282Y/H63D compound heterozygosity, which has been claimed to be associated with some clinical expressivity, nor the H63D homozygosity or compound heterozygosity for other rarer HFE mutations, such as H65C, seem to convey a risk for organ disease in the absence of comorbidity (53–55).

There exist two main obstacles in HC to define burden of disease. Case definition in the literature varies greatly, from late stages of liver disease to iron overload or even elevated serum iron measures. Another problem is that very few longitudinal studies are available, and only a few studies have used age-, gender-, and race-matched comparison groups (Table 22.3).

The estimated prevalence of the C282Y mutation in Caucasians is high (1:200–300), while it is much lower in Hispanics, Asian Americans, Pacific Islanders, and African Americans (56). Elevated transferrin saturation has been reported in 71% to 86% men and 40% to 100% women homozygotes and elevated serum ferritin in 34% to 100% men and 9% to 63% women (57– 62). Both parameters are affected by race, gender, and age (60). However, studies involving unselected population (that is, not selected a priori for presence of symptoms or elevated iron levels), have shown that clinical penetrance is much lower. In a recent meta-analysis by Waalen et al. (54) prevalence of general symptoms, such as fatigue and joint pain, good health, diabetes, joint involvement, and skin pigmentation associated with iron overload in C282Y homozygotes was not significantly greater than in age- and sex-matched controls. Moreover, HFE homozygotes seem not to be lost from the population with age and no evidence of a decrease in life expectancy was found (54). As to the hepatic dysfunction, elevated aminotransferase have been reported in most controlled cross-sectional studies in unselected populations, while the rate of increased fibrosis and cirrhosis vary (54). A systematic review using strict case HC definition criteria (that is, documented hepatic iron overload) (63), found that about 1 in 357 persons to 1 in 625 persons in the general population to rates almost as high as 1 in 135 persons among Norwegian men, have HC (9). However, no prospective cohort studies comparing survival or complications in patients with or without HC defined by either biochemical or tissue iron levels are available (9). In particular, the available longitudinal studies did not consistently identify increasing serum ferritin levels over time and did not demonstrate an overt progression to clinical HC (60,64). Only 5% of patients identified by primary care screening had cirrhosis; yet, six studies demonstrated that the presence of cirrhosis at the time of diagnosis carry poor prognosis (9). Another systematic review was undertaken for the U.S. Preventive Services Task Force (4): HC here was defined as the presence of clinical signs and symptoms. They concluded that disease penetrance and burden was low as previously reported by Schmitt et al. (9). Pooled cross-sectional data obtained from health clinics, blood donor settings, mass screening, and family screening provided information on 67,771 individuals identified from general screening and 200 family members of probands. Of those individuals identified as C282Y homozygotes as a result of non-family-based genetic screening, 38% demonstrated iron overload, 25% liver fibrosis, and 6% cirrhosis upon further evaluation. A larger proportion of family members of probands had iron overload (49% to 86%) and cirrhosis (8%). Similar conclusions have

Table 22.3 Burden of disease in HFE hemochromatosis.*

Study, year (reference)	Prevalence of C282Y homozygotes	Elevated transferrin saturation in homozygotes	Elevated serum ferritin level in homozygotes	Patients with iron overload due to hereditary hemochromatosis	Patients with diabetes	Patients with other diseases/elevated LFT results	Fibrosis or cirrhosis
Longitudinal: general population (2 studies)							
Andersen et al., 2004 (60)	2.5/1000	Men: 5 of 7 (71%) Women: 9 of 16 (56%) (both tests elevated)		Selected C282YY: ND All C282YY: ND	All C282YY: 1 of 23 (4.4%)	Liver disease: 0 of 23 Hypogonadism: 0 of 23 Cardiomyopathy: 0 of 23 Arthralgia: 2 of 23 Subclinical hemochromatosis: 1 of 23	ND
Olynyk et al., 2004 (64)	4/1000	Men: 4 of 4 (100%) Women: 2 of 6 (33%) (both tests elevated)		Selected C282YY: 5 of 6 (83%) All C282YY: 5 of 10 (50%)	1 of 10	Arthralgia: 4 of 10	Selected C282YY: 3 of 6 (1 also consumed alcohol) All C282YY: 3 of 10 (30%)
Cross-sectional studies—General population (7 studies)							
Total population: n = 67,771 (57,59,62,102–105) Total patients with C282YY studied: n = 282	4.2/1000	Men: 75%–94% Women: 40%–94%	Men: 58%–76% Women: 54%–58%	Selected C282Y: 26 of 69 (38%) All C282Y: 30 of 127 (24%)	All C282YY: 0%–5.6%	All C282YY: LFT, ND	Cirrhosis or fibrosis: Selected C282YY: 5 of 16 (31%) All C282YY: 5 of 72 (6.9%) Fibrosis: Selected C282YY: 4 of 16 (25%) All C282YY: 4 of 72 (6%) Cirrhosis: Selected C282YY: 1 of 16 (6%) All C282YY: 1 of 72 (1.4%)

*Updated from reference 4. C282YY = C282Y/C282Y; LFT = liver function tests; ND = no data reported or not acceptable.
Selected C282YY refers to percentage positive only in those tested; all C282YY refers to percentage positive in all patients with C282YY.

been reached by studies in asymptomatic family members identified through screening (65–68) (Table 22.3). More recently, in the Hemochromatosis and Iron Overload Screening (HEIRS) study, self-reported diabetes was not significantly associated with HFE mutations (69), whereas liver fibrosis was present in up to 18.2% of C282Y homozygotes (70). In another recent study in an Australian community general population, HFE mutations were not associated with an increased prevalence of arthritis (71). It is likely that for development of organ disease, concurrent factors are necessary, both genetics and environmental (51). Coinheritance of mutations in hepcidin (72) or hemojuvelin (73) aggravates the phenotype of C282Y homozygotes. Among acquired factors, evidence for a strong association of alcohol and development of liver cirrhosis has been presented (74) while the cofactorial role steatosis-fat and high BMI are still under scrutiny (75,76).

Recommendation

• C282Y homozygosity does not indicate hemochromatosis unless iron overload is present (Grade lB).

What is the best diagnostic strategy to identify hereditary hemochromatosis?

We analyzed this question under two different clinical scenarios: symptomatic or asymptomatic individuals.

Based on the previous discussion on HFE-HC epidemiology and penetrance, it can be stated that diagnosis of HC in symptomatic untreated patients, that is, in patients with signs and symptoms or organ disease suggestive of HC, requires the presence of circulatory and tissue iron overload and C282Y homozygosity. In other words, untreated C282Y homozygotes with a related organ disease, such as cirrhosis, diabetes, or cardiomiopathy, invariably present with abnormal transferrin saturation and serum ferritin levels. Liver biopsy, the gold standard for diagnosis in the pre-HFE era, is no longer required for diagnosis, once HFE homozygosity has been detected in a subject with high transferrin saturation and serum ferritin (51). Liver biopsy is still important in prognostic settings in C282Y homozygotes: a serum ferritin above 1,000 ng/L, increased transaminases, and hepatomegaly may indicate the presence of underlying fibrosis or cirrhosis and represent indications for liver biopsy, particularly in subjects older than 40 years (23–25). Symptomatic subjects with clear signs of circulatory and tissue iron overload, but no diagnostic HFE test may carry pathogenic mutations in other rarer HC genes.

A systematic review by Schmitt et al. (9) has addressed the diagnostic value of biochemical tests in asymptomatic primary care patients. None of the reviewed studies compared the screening tests for iron overload (transferrin saturation and serum ferritin) with the gold standard (i.e., LIC by liver biopsy or the amount of iron removed by phlebotomy) (9). The diagnostic cutoff levels for transferrin saturation and serum ferritin have varied across studies as well: the higher cutoff levels (transferrin saturation 62% and serum ferritin levels >500 μg/L) identified a subgroup in which all patients had HC (77,78); the least stringent criteria (transferrin saturation >45% and serum ferritin levels >200 g/L) identified a group in which only 11.5% had HC (76).

A more recent systematic review has investigated the evidence for targeted genetic screening of special groups of patients with signs or symptoms consistent with undiagnosed, early-stage hemochromatosis (4). Seven cross-sectional studies showed that a slightly higher proportion of C282Y homozygotes could be identified by conducting genotyping only in patients from a liver clinic or diabetic patients hospitalized for poor control or complications or patients referred to specialists for chronic fatigue and arthralgias, particularly if prescreened for transferrin saturation >40% and serum ferritin >300 ng/mL (4).

Recommendations

• Liver biopsy is not necessary to diagnose hemochromatosis in the presence of C282Y homozygosity (Grade 1C).

• Liver biopsy should be offered for prognostic reasons in the presence of C282Y homozygosity and serum ferritin above 1000 ng/L (Grade 1B).

• If testing is performed for primary care patients with HC associated symptom(s) or disease(s), the cutoff values for serum ferritin level of more than 200 g/L in women or more than 300 g/L in men and transferrin saturation greater than 55% may be used as criteria for case-finding (Grade 2C).

• Patients with liver dysfunction, decompensated diabetes, or are referred for chronic fatigue and arthralgias should be screened with transferrin saturation and serum ferritin (Grade 1C), and could be offered genetic HFE testing (Grade 2C).

• Family members of individuals with HFE-HC should be screened with transferrin saturation and serum ferritin (Grade 1B), and should be offered genetic HFE testing (Grade 2C).

What are the best treatment strategies for iron overload?

Hereditary hemochromatosis

Therapeutic phlebotomy is the mainstay of treatment for HC. Phlebotomy is generally thought to have few side effects and effective in removing iron from tissues. No randomized, controlled trial was performed that compared phlebotomy to no treatment or early as opposed to delayed treatment. The systematic review by Whitlock et al. (4) selected only case series that provided data on 447 individuals (only 85 with genotypically confirmed hemochromatosis) (79–81): the 10-year survival of individuals recently diagnosed with HC or treated prior to the development of cirrhosis did not differ from that in age- and sex-matched population controls. In an additional retrospective study selected by the systematic review of Schmitt et al. (9), 158 Danish patients were followed for a median period of 8.5 years: survival of patients who were adequately phlebotomized was much higher than survival of those who were not adequately phlebotomized (estimated Kaplan–Meier survival:

Table 22.4 Marketed Iron chelators.

Active substance	Brand name	Route of administration	EMEA currently approved therapeutic indication *(approval date)*	FDA currently approved therapeutic indication *(approval date)*
Desferrioxamine	Desferal®	Intramuscular, subcutaneous, intravenous	Licensed for treatment of iron overload according to national approvals.	Treatment of acute iron intoxication and of chronic iron overload due to transfusion-dependent anemias (April 1, 1968) (generic drug authorized on March 17, 2004, and on March 31, 2006).
Deferiprone	Ferriprox®	Oral	Treatment of iron overload in patients with thalassemia major when deferoxamine therapy is contraindicated or inadequate (centralized authorization on August 25, 1999).	Marketing authorization not approved (October 12, 2005). Included in the orphan drug list from December 12, 2001, for the treatment of iron overload in patients with hematologic disorders requiring chronic transfusion therapy.
Deferasirox	Exjade®	Oral	Treatment of chronic iron overload due to frequent blood transfusions ($\geq$ 7 ml/kg/mo of packed red blood cells) in patients with beta thalassemia major aged 6 years and older. Also indicated for the treatment of chronic iron overload due to blood transfusions when deferoxamine therapy is contraindicated or inadequate in the following patient groups: —in patients with other anemias, —in patients aged 2 to 5 years, —in patients with beta thalassemia major with iron overload due to infrequent blood transfusions ($<$7 ml/kg/mo of packed red blood cells). (centralized authorization released on August 28, 2006). N.B.: This substance was prior designated as orphan drug (for the treatment of chronic iron overload requiring chelation therapy).	Treatment of iron overload in patients with iron overload due to multiple transfusions (November 9, 2005).

93% versus 48% at 5 years and 78% versus 32% at 10 years). Furthermore, adequately treated patients with cirrhosis or diabetes had better survival than those who were not adequately treated (82). Regarding the effect of phlebotomy on disease progression in individuals with biopsy-proven liver fibrosis, phlebotomy was associated with an improvement of 13% to 50%, with the greatest improvement among individuals with the least degree of liver fibrosis (66,79). Similar results have been reported in a recent study by Falize et al. (83) in 36 HC patients undergoing paired liver biopsy: a significant fibrosis stage regression was detected in 69% of patients with severe fibrosis and 35% with cirrhosis. Several observational studies support that some, though not all, other disease processes and symptoms respond to phlebotomy, such as reduced daily insulin dosage in type 1 diabetes mellitus, aminotransferase, weakness, lethargy, or abdominal pain (4).

Transfusion iron loading anemias

Three chelators are currently available in the market for treatment of transfusion-dependent iron overload (Table 22.4).

Desferrioxamine (DFO; Desferal), is the first-line, iron-chelating drug for treating transfusional iron overload since the 1970s: it is relatively safe, although hypersensitivity or toxic side effects have been reported and extends life (39). Yet, the mandatory subcutaneous infusion 10–12 hours a day is unacceptable to many patients and at least a third of them do not adhere to it (84). High-dose continuous DFO, administered via central catheter, can reverse cardiac toxicity of iron overload (85). Based on a recent *Cochrane Database of Systematic Review* (86), we evaluated according to GRADE guidelines the available evidence for both benefits and arms of desferrioxamine (see Table 22.5 on website: http://www.blackwellpublishing.com/medicine/bmj/hematology).

Although the drug represents the standard of care for transfusion-dependent iron overload, the available evidence is based on few studies of moderate quality and small sample size.

Deferiprone (L1, Ferriprox) has been the first orally active iron chelator to enter human trials, as alternative to DFO, and has been increasingly used for DFO "failures" or intolerance (87). Typical dosage for deferiprone is 75 mg/kg/d in three divided doses, up to 100 mg/kg daily. Idiosyncratic side effects include arthritis (from 5% to 20%) and neutropenia (up to 5%–8% of patients), including severe agranulocytosis (less than 1% of patients) (88,89). Two prospective studies have shown that deferiprone reduces or maintains iron stores in the majority of patients receiving regular red cell transfusions (see Table 22.6 on website: http://www.blackwellpublishing.com/medicine/bmj/hematology). Similar effects have been reported in patients with low rates of transfusional iron loading due to other hereditary anemias (90–93). In difficult-to-treat patient, raising the dose of deferiprone to 100 mg/kg/d or combining therapy with deferoxamine has usually proven very effective in reducing iron stores (94–98), although only in a few published studies direct comparison to desferrioxamine has been made (99–101). Retrospective studies first suggested that deferiprone might be more effective than deferoxamine in chelating cardiac iron (47) (see Table 22.6 website), the cause of most of the mortality (39) and negative prognostic factor in transfusional iron overload (102). A retrospective study of cardiac-related morbidity and mortality (see Table 22.6 website) and a randomized, prospective trial of cardiac iron (using as surrogate the MRI T2* value) and function (48), seem to indicate a preferential effect of deferiprone on removal of cardiac iron.

Deferasirox (ICL670, Exjade) belongs to a new class of oral iron chelators. Once-daily dosing permits the drug to circulate at all times, and deferasirox-iron complexes are excreted in the stool. Deferasirox has undergone clinical trials, including a phase III study designed to test noninferiority to deferoxamine (see Table 22.6, website). The study in 586 patients with thalassemia in 65 sites failed to meet its overall primary endpoint (i.e., at low doses of deferasirox, 5–10 mg/kg/d, increased HIC was observed), while at doses of 20 to 30 mg/kg/d, noninferiority of deferasirox compared with DFO was established, with 60% versus 59% achieving a successful outcome, respectively. Adverse drug reactions in deferasirox trials have included modest rise in creatinine level, rarely clinically relevant, occasional increase in transaminases, transient gastrointestinal symptoms, and rash (see Table 22.6, website).

Recommendations

- Therapeutic phlebotomy is recommended as the standard treatment for all patients with HFE-HC and documented iron overload (Grade 1B).
- Desferrioxamine is recommended as the standard treatment for patients with transfusion iron overload (Grade 1C).
- For patients intolerant to desferrioxamine, not adequately controlled, or poorly compliant, the recommended drug should be deferasirox (Grade 1B). Or, where available, deferiprone (Grade 1C).
- Deferiprone should be offered to patients with transfusion iron overload and cardiac iron excess documented by recent MRI techniques (e.g., T2*) (Grade 2C).

References

1 Pietrangelo A. Hereditary hemochromatosis. *Annu Rev Nutr.* 2006;**26**:251–70.

2 Atkins D, Best D, Briss PA, et al. Grading quality of evidence and strength of recommendations. *Br Med J.* 2004;**328**:1490.

3 Guyatt G, Gutterman D, Baumann MH, et al. Grading strength of recommendations and quality of evidence in clinical guidelines: report from an American College of Chest Physicians task force. *Chest.* 2006;**129**:174–81.

4 Whitlock EP, Garlitz BA, Harris EL, et al. Screening for hereditary hemochromatosis: a systematic review for the U.S. Preventive Services Task Force. *Ann Intern Med.* 2006;**145**:209–23.

5 Qaseem A, Aronson M, Fitterman N, et al. Screening for hereditary hemochromatosis: a clinical practice guideline from the American College of Physicians. *Ann Intern Med.* 2005;**143**:517–21.

6 Olynyk JK, Luxon BA, Britton RS, et al. Hepatic iron concentration in hereditary hemochromatosis does not saturate or accurately predict phlebotomy requirements. *Am J Gastroenterol.* 1998;**93**:346–50.

7 Angelucci E, Brittenham GM, McLaren CE, et al. Hepatic iron concentration and total body iron stores in thalassemia major. *N Engl J Med.* 2000;**343**:327–31.

8 Phatak PD, Barton JC. Phlebotomy-mobilized iron as a surrogate for liver iron content in hemochromatosis patients. *Hematology.* 2003;**8**:429–32.

9 Schmitt B, Golub RM, Green R. Screening primary care patients for hereditary hemochromatosis with transferrin saturation and serum ferritin level: systematic review for the American College of Physicians. *Ann Intern Med.* 2005;**143**:522–36.

10 Villeneuve JP, Bilodeau M, Lepage R, et al. Variability in hepatic iron concentration measurement from needle-biopsy specimens. *J Hepatol.* 1996;**25**:172–77.

11 Butensky E, Fischer R, Hudes M, et al. Variability in hepatic iron concentration in percutaneous needle biopsy specimens from patients with transfusional hemosiderosis. *Am J Clin Pathol.* 2005;**123**:146–52.

12 Fischer R, Piga A, Harmatz P, et al. Monitoring long-term efficacy of iron chelation treatment with biomagnetic liver susceptometry. *Ann N Y Acad Sci.* 2005;**1054**:350–57.

13 Olivieri NF, Brittenham GM. Iron chelating therapy and the treatment of thalassemia. *Blood.* 1997;**89**(3):739–61.

14 Anderson LJ, Holden S, Davis B, et al. Cardiovascular T2-star (T2*) magnetic resonance for the early diagnosis of myocardial iron overload. *Eur Heart J.* 2001;**22**:2171–79.

15 Tanner MA, Galanello R, Dessi C, et al. Myocardial iron loading in patients with thalassemia major on deferoxamine chelation. *J Cardiovasc Magn Reson.* 2006;**8**:543–47.

16 Christoforidis A, Haritandi A, Tsitouridis I, et al. Correlative study of iron accumulation in liver, myocardium, and pituitary assessed

with MRI in young thalassemic patients. *J Pediatr Hematol Oncol.* 2006;**28**:311–15.

17 Christoforidis A, Haritandi A, Tsatra I, et al. Four-year evaluation of myocardial and liver iron assessed prospectively with serial MRI scans in young patients with beta-thalassaemia major: comparison between different chelation regimens. *Eur J Haematol.* 2006;**78**(1):52–7.

18 Berdoukas V, Dakin C, Freema A, et al. Lack of correlation between iron overload cardiac dysfunction and needle liver biopsy iron concentration. *Haematologica.* 2005;**90**:685–86.

19 Anderson LJ, Westwood MA, Prescott E, et al. Development of thalassaemic iron overload cardiomyopathy despite low liver iron levels and meticulous compliance to desferrioxamine. *Acta Haematol.* 2006;**115**:106–8.

20 Beutler E, Felitti V, Ho NJ, et al. Relationship of body iron stores to levels of serum ferritin, serum iron, unsaturated iron binding capacity and transferrin saturation in patients with iron storage disease. *Acta Haematol.* 2002;**107**:145–49.

21 Olivieri NF, Brittenham GM. Iron-chelating therapy and the treatment of thalassemia [see comments] [erratum appears in *Blood.* 1997;**89**(7):2621]. *Blood.* 1997;**89**:739–61.

22 Canavese C, Bergamo D, Ciccone G, et al. Validation of serum ferritin values by magnetic susceptometry in predicting iron overload in dialysis patients. *Kidney Int.* 2004;**65**:1091–98.

23 Guyader D, Jacquelinet C, Moirand R, et al. Noninvasive prediction of fibrosis in C282Y homozygous hemochromatosis. *Gastroenterology.* 1998;**115**:929–36.

24 Beaton M, Guyader D, Deugnier Y, et al. Noninvasive prediction of cirrhosis in C282Y-linked hemochromatosis. *Hepatology.* 2002;**36**:673–78.

25 Morrison ED, Brandhagen DJ, Phatak PD, et al. Serum ferritin level predicts advanced hepatic fibrosis among U.S. patients with phenotypic hemochromatosis. *Ann Intern Med.* 2003;**138**:627–33.

26 van Oost BA, van den Beld B, van Asbeck BS, et al. Monitoring of intensive phlebotomy therapy in iron overload by serum ferritin assay. *Am J Hematol.* 1985;**18**:7–12.

27 Tavill AS. Diagnosis and management of hemochromatosis. *Hepatology.* 2001;**33**:1321–28.

28 Kolnagou A, Economides C, Eracleous E, et al. Low serum ferritin levels are misleading for detecting cardiac iron overload and increase the risk of cardiomyopathy in thalassemia patients: the importance of cardiac iron overload monitoring using magnetic resonance imaging T2 and T2*. *Hemoglobin.* 2006;**30**:219–27.

29 Herbert V, Jayatilleke E, Shaw S, et al. Serum ferritin iron, a new test, measures human body iron stores unconfounded by inflammation. *Stem Cells.* 1997;**15**(4):291–96.

30 Nielsen P, Gunther U, Durken M, et al. Serum ferritin iron in iron overload and liver damage: correlation to body iron stores and diagnostic relevance. *J Lab Clin Med.* 2000;**135**:413–18.

31 Nielsen P, Engelhardt R, Dullmann J, et al. Non-invasive liver iron quantification by SQUID-biosusceptometry and serum ferritin iron as new diagnostic parameters in hereditary hemochromatosis. *Blood Cells Mol Dis.* 2002;**29**:451–58.

32 Fischer R, Longo F, Nielsen P, et al. Monitoring long-term efficacy of iron chelation therapy by deferiprone and desferrioxamine in patients with beta-thalassaemia major: application of SQUID biomagnetic liver susceptometry. *Br J Haematol.* 2003;**121**:938–48.

33 Fischer R, Harmatz P, Nielsen P. Does liver biopsy overestimate liver iron concentration? *Blood.* 2006;**108**:1775–76.

34 St Pierre TG, Clark PR, Chua-Anusorn W, et al. Non-invasive measurement and imaging of liver iron concentrations using proton magnetic resonance. *Blood.* 2004;**105**:855–61.

35 Gandon Y, Olivie D, Guyader D, et al. Non-invasive assessment of hepatic iron stores by MRI. *Lancet.* 2004;**363**:357–62.

36 Wood JC, Enriquez C, Ghugre N, et al. MRI R2 and R2* mapping accurately estimates hepatic iron concentration in transfusion-dependent thalassemia and sickle cell disease patients. Blood. 2005;**106**: 1460–65.

37 St Pierre TG, Clark PR, Chua-Anusorn W. Measurement and mapping of liver iron concentrations using magnetic resonance imaging. *Ann N Y Acad Sci.* 2005;**1054**:379–85.

38 Rose C, Vandevenne P, Bourgeois E, et al. Liver iron content assessment by routine and simple magnetic resonance imaging procedure in highly transfused patients. *Eur J Haematol.* 2006;**77**:145–49.

39 Borgna-Pignatti C, Rugolotto S, De Stefano P, et al. Survival and complications in patients with thalassemia major treated with transfusion and deferoxamine. *Haematologica.* 2004;**89**:1187–93.

40 Mavrogeni SI, Markussis V, Kaklamanis L, et al. A comparison of magnetic resonance imaging and cardiac biopsy in the evaluation of heart iron overload in patients with beta-thalassemia major. *Eur J Haematol.* 2005;**75**:241–47.

41 Wood JC, Tyszka JM, Carson S, et al. Myocardial iron loading in transfusion-dependent thalassemia and sickle cell disease. *Blood.* 2004;**103**:1934–36.

42 Westwood M, Anderson LJ, Firmin DN, et al. A single breath-hold multiecho T2* cardiovascular magnetic resonance technique for diagnosis of myocardial iron overload. *J Magn Reson Imaging.* 2003;**18**: 33–9.

43 Westwood MA, Firmin DN, Gildo M, et al. Intercentre reproducibility of magnetic resonance T2* measurements of myocardial iron in thalassaemia. *Int J Cardiovasc Imaging.* 2005;**21**:531–38.

44 Tanner MA, He T, Westwood MA, et al. Multi-center validation of the transferability of the magnetic resonance T2* technique for the quantification of tissue iron. *Haematologica.* 2006;**91**:1388–91.

45 Westwood MA, Sheppard MN, Awogbade M, et al. Myocardial biopsy and T2* magnetic resonance in heart failure due to thalassaemia. *Br J Haematol.* 2005;**128**:2.

46 Anderson LJ, Westwood MA, Holden S, et al. Myocardial iron clearance during reversal of siderotic cardiomyopathy with intravenous desferrioxamine: a prospective study using T2* cardiovascular magnetic resonance. *Br J Haematol.* 2004;**127**:348–55.

47 Anderson LJ, Wonke B, Prescott E, et al. Comparison of effects of oral deferiprone and subcutaneous desferrioxamine on myocardial iron concentrations and ventricular function in beta-thalassaemia. *Lancet.* 2002;**360**:516–20.

48 Pennell DJ, Berdoukas V, Karagiorga M, et al. Randomized controlled trial of deferiprone or deferoxamine in beta-thalassemia major patients with asymptomatic myocardial siderosis. *Blood.* 2006;**107**:3738–44.

49 Alexopoulou E, Stripeli F, Baras P, et al. R2 relaxometry with MRI for the quantification of tissue iron overload in beta-thalassemic patients. *J Magn Reson Imaging.* 2006;**23**:163–70.

50 Pepe A, Lombardi M, Positano V, et al. Evaluation of the efficacy of oral deferiprone in beta-thalassemia major by multislice multiecho T2*. *Eur J Haematol.* 2006;**76**:183–92.

50a Neufeld EJ. Oral chelators deferasirox and deferiprone for transfusional iron overload in thalassemia major: new data, new questions. *Blood.* 2006;**107**:3436–441.

51 Pietrangelo A. Hereditary hemochromatosis—a new look at an old disease. *N Engl J Med.* 2004;**350**:2383–97.

52 Feder JN, Gnirke A, Thomas W, et al. A novel MHC class I-like gene is mutated in patients with hereditary haemochromatosis. *Nat Genet.* 1996;**13**:399–408.

53 Gochee PA, Powell LW, Cullen DJ, et al. A population-based study of the biochemical and clinical expression of the H63D hemochromatosis mutation. *Gastroenterology.* 2002;**122**:646–51.

54 Waalen J, Nordestgaard BG, Beutler E. The penetrance of hereditary hemochromatosis. *Best Pract Res Clin Haematol.* 2005;**18**:203–20.

55 Samarasena J, Winsor W, Lush R, et al. Individuals homozygous for the H63D mutation have significantly elevated iron indexes. *Dig Dis Sci.* 2006;**51**:803–7.

56 Adams PC, Reboussin DM, Barton JC, et al. Hemochromatosis and iron-overload screening in a racially diverse population. *N Engl J Med.* 2005;**352**:1769–78.

57 Beutler E, Felitti VJ, Koziol JA, et al. Penetrance of 845G–> A (C282Y) HFE hereditary haemochromatosis mutation in the USA. *Lancet.* 2002;**359**:211–18.

58 Jackson HA, Carter K, Darke C, et al. HFE mutations, iron deficiency and overload in 10,500 blood donors. *Br J Haematol.* 2001;**114**: 474–84.

59 Deugnier Y, Jouanolle AM, Chaperon J, et al. Gender-specific phenotypic expression and screening strategies in C282Y-linked haemochromatosis: a study of 9396 French people. *Br J Haematol.* 2002;**118**:1170–78.

60 Andersen RV, Tybjaerg-Hansen A, Appleyard M, et al. Hemochromatosis mutations in the general population: iron overload progression rate. *Blood.* 2004;**103**:2914–19.

61 Chambers V, Sutherland L, Palmer K, et al. Haemochromatosis-associated HFE genotypes in English blood donors: age-related frequency and biochemical expression. *J Hepatol.* 2003;**39**:925–31.

62 Olynyk JK, Cullen DJ, Aquilia S, et al. A population-based study of the clinical expression of the hemochromatosis gene [see comments]. *N Engl J Med.* 1999;**341**:718–24.

63 McLaren CE, Barton JC, Adams PC, et al. Hemochromatosis and iron overload screening (HEIRS) study design for an evaluation of 100,000 primary care-based adults. *Am J Med Sci.* 2003;**325**:53–62.

64 Olynyk JK, Hagan SE, Cullen DJ, et al. Evolution of untreated hereditary hemochromatosis in the Busselton population: a 17-year study. *Mayo Clin Proc.* 2004;**79**:309–13.

65 Barton JC, Rothenberg BE, Bertoli LF, et al. Diagnosis of hemochromatosis in family members of probands: a comparison of phenotyping and HFE genotyping. *Genet Med.* 1999;**1**:89–93.

66 Powell LW, Dixon JL, Ramm GA, et al. Screening for hemochromatosis in asymptomatic subjects with or without a family history. *Arch Intern Med.* 2006;**166**:294–301.

67 Gleeson F, Ryan E, Barrett S, et al. Clinical expression of haemochromatosis in Irish C282Y homozygotes identified through family screening. *Eur J Gastroenterol Hepatol.* 2004;**16**:859–63.

68 McCune CA, Ravine D, Carter K, et al. Iron loading and morbidity among relatives of HFE C282Y homozygotes identified either by population genetic testing or presenting as patients. *Gut.* 2006;**55**: 554–62.

69 Acton RT, Barton JC, Passmore LV, et al. Relationships of serum ferritin, transferrin saturation, and HFE mutations and self-reported diabetes in the hemochromatosis and iron overload Screening (HEIRS) study. *Diabetes Care.* 2006;**29**:2084–89.

70 Adams PC, Passmore L, Chakrabarti S, et al. Liver diseases in the hemochromatosis and iron overload screening study. *Clin Gastroenterol Hepatol.* 2006;**4**:918–23.

71 Sherrington CA, Knuiman MW, Divitini ML, et al. Population-based study of the relationship between mutations in the hemochromatosis (HFE) gene and arthritis. *J Gastroenterol Hepatol.* 2006;**21**:595–98.

72 Jacolot S, Le Gac G, Scotet V, et al. HAMP as a modifier gene that increases the phenotypic expression of the HFE pC282Y homozygous genotype. *Blood.* 2004;**103**:2835–40.

73 Le Gac G, Scotet V, Ka C, et al. The recently identified type 2A juvenile haemochromatosis gene (HJV), a second candidate modifier of the C282Y homozygous phenotype. *Hum Mol Genet.* 2004;**13**: 1913–18.

74 Fletcher LM, Dixon JL, Purdie DM, et al. Excess alcohol greatly increases the prevalence of cirrhosis in hereditary hemochromatosis. *Gastroenterology.* 2002;**122**:281–89.

75 Powell EE, Ali A, Clouston AD, et al. Steatosis is a cofactor in liver injury in hemochromatosis. *Gastroenterology.* 2005;**129**:1937–43.

76 Adams LA, Angulo P, Abraham SC, et al. The effect of the metabolic syndrome, hepatic steatosis and steatohepatitis on liver fibrosis in hereditary hemochromatosis. *Liver Int.* 2006;**26**:298–304.

77 Baer DM, Simons JL, Staples RL, et al. Hemochromatosis screening in asymptomatic ambulatory men 30 years of age and older. *Am J Med.* 1995;**98**:464–68.

78 Phatak PD, Sham RL, Raubertas RF, et al. Prevalence of hereditary hemochromatosis in 16031 primary care patients. *Ann Int Med.* 1998;**129**(11):954-61.

79 Niederau C, Fischer R, Purschel A, et al. Long-term survival in patients with hereditary hemochromatosis [see comments]. *Gastroenterology.* 1996;**110**:1107–19.

80 Adams PC, Speechley M, Kertesz AE. Long-term survival analysis in hereditary hemochromatosis. *Gastroenterology.* 1991;**101**:368–72.

81 Bomford A, Williams R. Long term results of venesection therapy in idiopathic haemochromatosis. *Q J Med.* 1976;**45**:611–23.

82 Milman N, Pedersen P, Steig T, et al. Clinically overt hereditary hemochromatosis in Denmark 1948–1985: epidemiology, factors of significance for long-term survival, and causes of death in 179 patients. *Ann Hematol.* 2001;**80**:737–44.

83 Falize L, Guillygomarc'h A, Perrin M, et al. Reversibility of hepatic fibrosis in treated genetic hemochromatosis: a study of 36 cases. *Hepatology.* 2006;**44**:472–77.

84 Gabutti V, Piga A. Results of long perm iron chelating therapy. *Acta Haematologica.* 1996;**95**(1):26–36.

85 Davis BA, Porter JB. Long-term outcome of continuous 24-hour deferoxamine infusion via indwelling intravenous catheters in high-risk beta-thalassemia. *Blood.* 2000;**95**:1229–36.

86 Roberts DJ, Rees D, Howard J, et al. Desferrioxamine mesylate for managing transfusional iron overload in people with transfusion-dependent thalassaemia. *Cochrane Database Syst Rev.* 2005(4): Article No. CD004450.

87 Hoffbrand AV, Cohen A, Hershko C. Role of deferiprone in chelation therapy for transfusional iron overload. *Blood.* 2003;**102**:17–24.

88 al-Refaie FN, Hershko C, Hoffbrand AV, et al. Results of long-term deferiprone (L1) therapy: a report by the International Study Group on Oral Iron Chelators. *Br J Haematol.* 1995;**91**:224–29.

89 Taher A, Chamoun FM, Koussa S, et al. Efficacy and side effects of deferiprone (L1) in thalassemia patients not compliant with desferrioxamine. *Acta Haematol.* 1999;**101**:173–77.

90 Olivieri NF, Koren G, Matsui D, et al. Reduction of tissue iron stores and normalization of serum ferritin during treatment with the oral iron chelator L1 in thalassemia intermedia. *Blood.* 1992;**79**: 2741–48.

91 Pootrakul P, Sirankapracha P, Sankote J, et al. Clinical trial of deferiprone iron chelation therapy in beta-thalassaemia/haemoglobin E patients in Thailand. *Br J Haematol.* 2003;**122**:305–10.

92 Chan JC, Chim CS, Ooi CG, et al. Use of the oral chelator deferiprone in the treatment of iron overload in patients with Hb H disease. *Br J Haematol.* 2006;**133**:198–205.

93 Voskaridou E, Douskou M, Terpos E, et al. Deferiprone as an oral iron chelator in sickle cell disease. *Ann Hematol.* 2005;**84**:434–40.

94 Wonke B, Wright C, Hoffbrand AV. Combined therapy with deferiprone and desferrioxamine. *Br J Haematol.* 1998;**103**:361–64.

95 Kattamis A, Ladis V, Berdousi H, et al. Iron chelation treatment with combined therapy with deferiprone and deferioxamine: a 12-month trial. *Blood Cells Mol Dis.* 2006;**36**:21–5.

96 Kolnagou A, Kontoghiorghes GJ. Effective combination therapy of deferiprone and deferoxamine for the rapid clearance of excess cardiac IRON and the prevention of heart disease in thalassemia. The Protocol of the International Committee on Oral Chelators. *Hemoglobin.* 2006;**30**:239–49.

97 Farmaki K, Angelopoulos N, Anagnostopoulos G, et al. Effect of enhanced iron chelation therapy on glucose metabolism in patients with beta-thalassaemia major. *Br J Haematol.* 2006;**134**:438–44.

98 Origa R, Bina P, Agus A, et al. Combined therapy with deferiprone and desferrioxamine in thalassemia major. *Haematologica.* 2005;**90**:1309–14.

99 Daar S, Pathare AV. Combined therapy with desferrioxamine and deferiprone in beta thalassemia major patients with transfusional iron overload. *Ann Hematol.* 2006;**85**:315–19.

100 Mourad FH, Hoffbrand AV, Sheikh-Taha M, et al. Comparison between desferrioxamine and combined therapy with desferrioxamine and deferiprone in iron overloaded thalassaemia patients. *Br J Haematol.* 2003;**121**:187–89.

101 Gomber S, Saxena R, Madan N. Comparative efficacy of desferrioxamine, deferiprone and in combination on iron chelation in thalassemic children. *Indian Pediatr.* 2004;**41**:21–7.

102 Davis BA, O'Sullivan C, Jarritt PH, et al. Value of sequential monitoring of left ventricular ejection fraction in the management of thalassemia major. *Blood.* 2004;**104**:263–69.

23 Aplastic Anemia, Paroxysmal Nocturnal Hemoglobinuria, and Pure Red Cell Aplasia

Shivani Srivastava, Richard W. Childs

Literature search

Each question has guided a systematic literature review in MEDLINE (PubMed version) from 1950 through January 2007. Grading of the quality of evidence and strengths of recommendations in this chapter are based on the guidelines proposed by the international Grading of Recommendations Assessment, Development, and Evaluation Working Group (GRADE) adopting the modification used by the ACCP that merges the very low and low categories of quality of evidence (see chapter 1).

Exclusion criteria

1. Non-human study
2. Non-English-language
3. Design: Case series with less than five patients, editorial, review.

Inclusion criteria

1. Age: no age limit
2. Design: Questions on therapeutics: RCTs and observational studies.

Aplastic anemia

Introduction

Acquired aplastic anemia (AA) is characterized by peripheral blood pancytopenia with a hypocellular, often "empty" bone marrow and absence of other causes of marrow failure (Table 23.1).

Evidence-based Hematology. Edited by Mark A. Crowther, Jeff Ginsberg, Holger J. Schünemann, Ralph M. Meyer, and Richard Lottenberg.
 ISBN: 978-1-4051-5747-6.

Clinical diagnosis and features

The clinical presentation includes symptoms related to thrombocytopenia, anemia, and neutropenia. The criteria for severe aplastic anemia (SAA) are a marrow biopsy showing less than 25% of normal cellularity or a bone marrow biopsy showing less than 50% normal cellularity in which fewer than 30% of the cells are hematopoietic and at least two of the following are present: absolute reticulocyte count <40,000/μL, absolute neutrophil count (ANC) <500/μL, or a platelet count <20,000/μL. Patients with SAA can be further categorized as having very severe aplastic anemia (vSAA) if the ANC is <200/μL. Patients with pancytopenia who do not fulfill the criteria of severe disease are characterized as having moderate aplastic anemia (1–3). In children and young adults, acquired AA should be distinguished from the inherited forms of bone marrow failure such as Fanconi's anemia as the differentiation has therapeutic implications. Patients with Fanconi's anemia often have physical anomalies, but the distinction depends on the laboratory finding of abnormal chromosome fragility seen readily in metaphase preparations of peripheral blood lymphocytes cultured with phytohemagglutinin. Chromosomal breakage is strikingly enhanced compared with controls if clastogenic agents, such as diepoxybutane, are added to the culture. However, in most older patients, the major differential diagnosis is between aplastic anemia and myelodysplasia. Bone marrow cytogenetics can help in establishing the proper diagnosis.

Pathophysiology

In about 70% of cases, aplastic anemia is thought to be caused by autoimmune-mediated suppression of the bone marrow by T cells releasing tumor necrosis factor (TNF) and interferon (IFN)-gamma causing apoptosis of CD34+ progenitor cells (4,5). The inciting event that triggers this autoimmune process has yet to be identified. Although it is important to identify potential agents inducing marrow suppression, drugs are only rarely identified as the cause of aplastic anemia.

Table 23.1 Differential diagnosis of pancytopenia.

Pancytopenia associated with hypocellular bone marrow
- Acquired aplastic anemia
- Inherited aplastic anemia (i.e., Fanconi anemia and others)
- Hypocellular myelodysplastic syndrome
- Aleukemic leukemia (acute myelogenous leukemia)
- Acute lymphoblastic leukemia
- Lymphoma involving of the bone marrow
- Drug-mediated marrow suppression
- Paroxysmal nocturnal hemoglobinuria

Hypocellular bone marrow with or without cytopenias
- Q fever
- Legionnaires' disease
- Mycobacteria
- Tuberculosis
- Anorexia nervosa, starvation
- Hypothyroidism

What is the treatment approach for a newly diagnosed patient with severe aplastic anemia?

Treatment includes withdrawal of offending agents in the rare patient in which such an agent is identified. Blood and platelet transfusions should be used selectively in patients who are potential candidates for hematopoietic cell transplantation to avoid alloimmunization. Irradiated and preferably cytomegalovirus (CMV)-negative blood products should be used with strict avoidance of blood products obtained from family members. Allogeneic hematopoietic stem cell transplantation (HSCT) offers a high probability of cure, particularly for younger patients (i.e., age ≤30 years). For SAA patients who lack an HLA matched sibling stem cell donor, those who lack the considerable financial resources necessary for a transplant or for patients who are older (i.e., age >40 years) who have a higher risk of transplant-related morbidity/mortality, treatment with immunosuppressive therapy (usually antithymocyte globulin [ATG] + cyclosporine A [CSA]) is usually pursued as first-line therapy (Figure 23.1) (6).

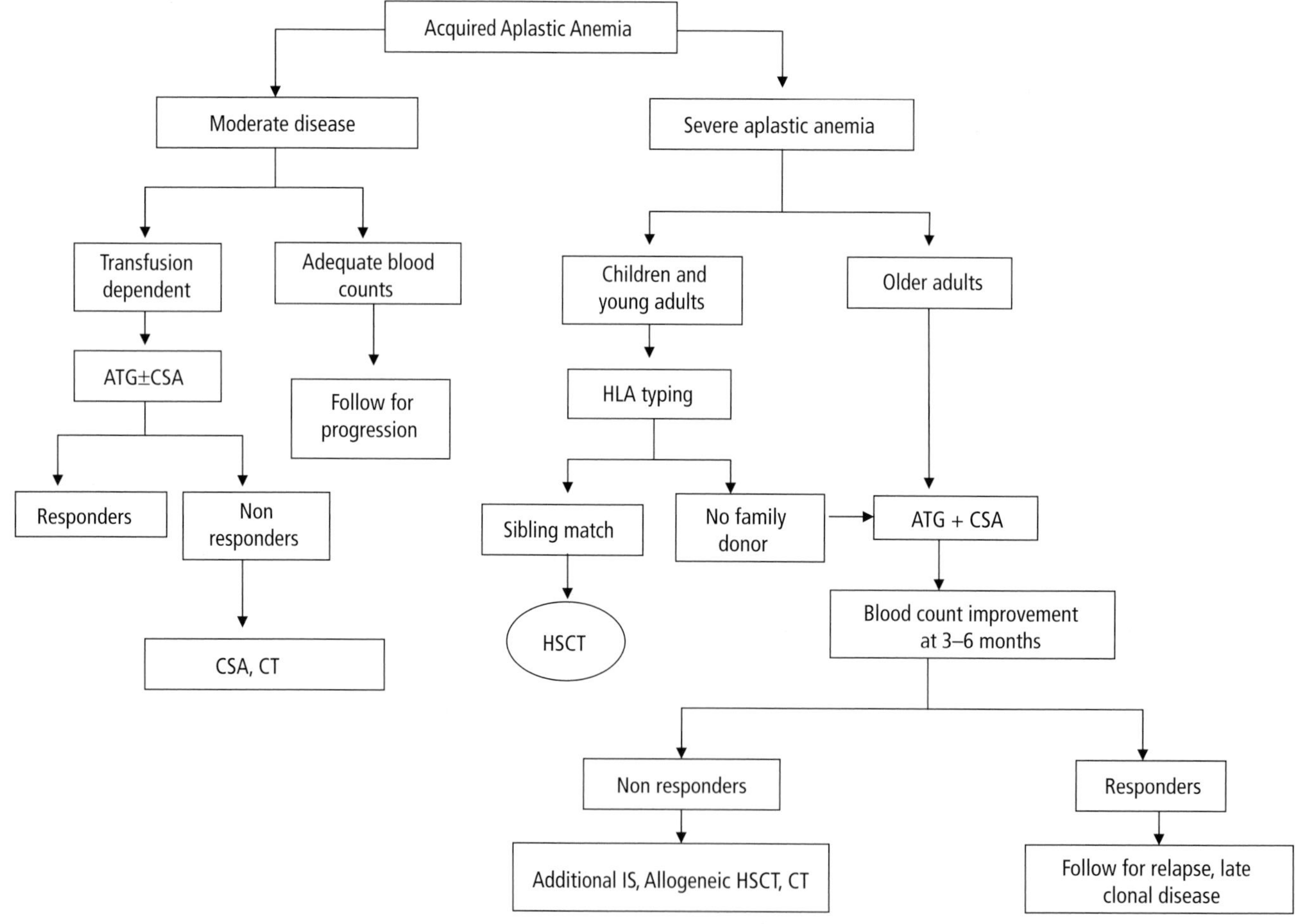

Figure 23.1 Algorithm-based treatment for patients with aplastic anemia. ATG, antithymocyte globulin; HSCT, hematopoietic stem cell transplantation; CSA, cyclosporine A; HLA, human leukocyte antigen; IS, immunosuppression; CT, clinical trial.

Does the combination of ATG and CSA as first-line treatment have long-term benefit?

In a single-arm interventional research protocol of 122 patients with SAA treated with immunosuppressive therapy (ATG 40mg/kg for four days; CSA 10–12 mg/kg for six months and 1mg/kg of methylprednisolone for about 2 weeks), 61% had a response associated with transfusion independence at 6 months with overall actuarial survival being 55% at 7 years (7). Relapse defined as a requirement for additional immunosuppression occurred in 30%–40% of responding patients but was usually not associated with severe pancytopenia. Importantly, relapse did not confer a poor prognosis and could be remedied in most cases with the reinstitution of CSA or a second round of ATG (7).

Recommendation. Patients with SAA who are appropriate candidates for immunosuppressive treatment should be treated with the combination of ATG and CSA (Grade 1B).

Is repeating immunosuppression useful in relapsed or refractory SAA?

Response rates to a second cycle of ATG in patients failing to respond to a first course of ATG have ranged from 22% to 64% (8). The use of rabbit ATG in SAA patients who have failed to respond to equine ATG can be effective in approximately 50% of patients (9). Retreatment with ATG and CSA is particularly advantageous for relapsed patients who have previously responded to immunosuppressive therapy. A response to retreatment has been associated with better survival compared with patients established to have treatment-refractory SAA.

Recommendation. In refractory or relapsed SAA, treatment with another cycle of ATG and CSA should be considered (Grade 1C).

What are the therapeutic options for patients with SAA refractory to treatment with ATG and CSA?

Because of its profoundly immunosuppressive effects, cyclophosphamide is used to treat a number of autoimmune disorders. A randomized phase III trial in patients with SAA comparing cyclophosphamide (50 mg/kg intravenously [IV] per day for 4 days) plus cyclosporine versus ATG and cyclosporine was initiated in the late 1990s but was terminated after accrual of only 31 patients because of an increase in invasive fungal infections and excess deaths as a consequence of protracted neutropenia in the cohort receiving cyclophosphamide (10). However, one study reported 9 of 17 patients with SAA who had failed other forms of immunosuppressive therapy had durable complete or partial responses following treatment with cyclophosphamide as a single agent (11).

Recommendation. We recommend retreatment with ATG and CSA as above (Grade 1C). Cyclophosphamide (50 mg/kg/d for four consecutive days) has been administered in this setting with a reported response rate of about 50% (12) (Grade 2C). For patients lacking an HLA matched sibling, transplantation from an alternative donor is most often offered to children who have failed a single course of immunosuppression or to older adults failing two rounds of ATG-based therapy (Grade 2C). Such transplants include T-cell depleted allografts obtained from haploidentical family donors, bone marrow or peripheral blood stem cell transplants from HLA matched unrelated donors, and more recently partially matched umbilical cord blood transplants.

What is the treatment approach for patients with moderate aplastic anemia?

Very few clinical trials have addressed treatment for patients defined as having moderate aplastic anemia. However, a multicenter prospective randomized controlled trial comparing CSA alone or the combination of equine ATG and CSA in nonsevere aplastic anemia showed the combination was superior and could reverse moderate pancytopenia and alleviate transfusion requirements (13). Treatment with daclizumab, a humanized monoclonal antibody to the interleukin-2 receptor, was shown in a pilot trial to improve blood counts and relieved transfusion requirements in 6 of 16 patients with moderate aplastic anemia (14).

Recommendations. In addition to observation, the use of ATG and CSA is recommended for patients that become transfusion dependent (Grade1B). Daclizumab might be considered in selected transfusion-dependent patients with moderate aplastic anemia who have not responded to ATG and CSA (Grade 2C).

What is the prognosis on long-term follow-up of patients following treatment for SAA?

There is an appreciable risk of progression to clonal hematopoietic stem cell disorder (e.g., myelodysplastic syndrome, acute myeloid leukemia, paroxysmal nocturnal hemoglobinuria) following immunosuppression-based therapy for SAA. A report from the European Bone Marrow Transplantation–Severe Aplastic Anemia Working Party (EBMT-SAA) estimated a 10-year incidence of malignancy of 19% (mostly MDS or AML), based on a retrospective multi-insititutional study of 860 patients treated with immunosuppression versus 748 patients who have received bone marrow transplants (an overall relative risk of cancer was 5.2 after immunosuppressive therapy as compared with an age-matched general population). In contrast, the risk of a hematological malignancy following allogeneic transplantation was not increased compared with age-matched controls (15).

Hematopoietic stem cell transplantation for severe aplastic anemia

Nearly 90% of patients under age 30 who undergo HSCT using an HLA matched sibling donor and conventional cyclophosphamide-based transplant conditioning can be expected to achieve long-term disease-free survival (16–18). Graft failure is more likely to occur in patients who delay transplantation, wherein a long lag period between diagnosis and transplantation exists. Multiple transfusions before transplantation increase the risk of alloimmunization, which is associated with a higher risk of allograft rejection.

Transplants from HLA-identical related donors

What is the optimal conditioning regimen to prevent graft rejection in SAA patients undergoing an allogeneic HSCT from an HLA matched sibling donor?

Cyclophosphamide as a single agent can be used to condition patients undergoing HSCT. The addition of ATG to cyclophosphamide conditioning appears to reduce the risk of graft rejection significantly. A report of 39 consecutive patients who received cyclophosphamide (total 200 mg/kg in four daily doses) and ATG (total 90 mg/kg in three doses using an HLA matched sibling donor) conditioning for a first transplant from an HLA matched sibling donor reported a graft rejection rate of only 5%. The three-year survival rate was 92% compared with the 72% in matched historical controls receiving cyclophosphamide alone (19). A more recent series of 81 patients with SAA at Fred Hutchinson Cancer Research Center undergoing this transplant approach reported 96% of the patients had sustained engraftment with 88% of patients being long-term survivors at a median follow-up of 9.2 years (17).

Recommendation. For patients with SAA undergoing allogeneic HSCT who are not at increased risk for rejection, the conditioning should include cyclophosphamide and ATG (Grade 1B).

What is the optimal method to minimize the risk of graft rejection in SAA patients undergoing allogeneic HSCT?

Patients with SAA who are older (i.e., >40 years of age), have failed prior immunosuppressive therapy, or who are heavily transfused have a higher risk of graft failure after HSCT. One approach to reduce graft rejection is the incorporation of radiation into the conditioning regimen (20,21). The introduction of fludarabine in combination with cyclophosphamide with or without ATG allows for the elimination of irradiation from the conditioning regimen (22–24). Recently, a single institution study of 26 patients with SAA, paroxysmal nocturnal hemoglobinuria (PNH), or pure red cell aplasia (PRCA) undergoing allogeneic HLA matched sibling transplant with cyclophosphamide, fludarabine, and with and without ATG showed that 24 of 26 patients were alive at a median of 21 months. The cumulative incidence of acute (65%) and chronic (56%) GVHD was high; only one patient died of treatment-related causes (22).

Recommendation. The addition of fludarabine to cyclophosphamide and ATG may improve transplant outcome and obviate the need for irradiation in patients with SAA who are at high risk for graft rejection (Grade 2B).

What are the transplant options and outcomes for patients who have failed immunosuppressive therapy that lack an HLA matched sibling donor?

HSCT using suitably matched unrelated donors is reserved for children that have failed a single course of immunosuppression or for adults who are refractory to multiple courses of ATG with or without alternative therapies such as androgens. A prospective multicenter study conducted from 1994 to 2004 in 62 patients with aplastic anemia undergoing HLA matched unrelated donor HSCT determined that 200cGy (in combination with cyclophosphamide and ATG) was the minimal effective dose of total body irradiation required to achieve sustained engraftment without inducing prohibitive toxicity. Graft failure occurred in 2%, acute GVHD (grade II–IV) in 70%, chronic GVHD in 52%, and overall survival was 61% (25). The EBMT-SAA Working Party recently reported results using a conditioning regimen substituting fludarabine for irradiation in 38 related and family mismatched donor transplants; graft rejection occurred in 18% with a two-year survival rate of 73% (26).

Recommendations. The small number of patients receiving irradiation-based regimens and the lack of randomized clinical trials precludes defining the optimal conditioning approach in this setting. Irradiation incorporated into the conditioning regimen for alternative donor transplants may facilitate engraftment (Grade 1C). Fludarabine-based conditioning may be useful for HLA matched unrelated transplants in which the recipient has a contraindication or aversion to irradiation (Grade 2C).

Paroxysmal nocturnal hemoglobinuria

Introduction

(Paroxysmal nocturnal hemoglobinuria) PNH is a rare acquired clonal disorder of hematopoietic stem cells (HSC) characterized clinically by recurrent hemolysis, a propensity for venous thrombosis, and bone marrow failure (27,28). The PNH stem cell and all its progeny lack an entire class of cell surface proteins call glycosylphosphatidylinositol anchored proteins (GPI-AP) due to a defect in the GPI anchor. The GPI-AP defect results from mutation in hematopoietic stem cells of the *PIG*-A gene located on the X chromosome. This leads to partial or complete absence in hematopoietic cells of certain GPI-linked proteins, some of which protect red blood cells (RBCs) from complement-mediated lysis (i.e., CD59 and CD55). PNH stem cells can arise and expand de novo or may be detected in the setting of acquired aplastic anemia (29).

Approaches to the treatment of PNH require patients be stratified into hypoplastic and classical subtypes (30)

Hypoplastic PNH. In patients with PNH who meet criteria for severe aplastic anemia, treatment options include allogeneic bone marrow transplantation (18), (ATG) and CSA (7), or high-dose cyclophosphamide (12). If the patient's cytopenias do not fulfill criteria for severe aplastic anemia, watchful waiting or immunosuppressive therapy may be appropriate.

Classical PNH. These patients tend to have mild to moderate cytopenias, a normocellular to hypercellular bone marrow and >60% GPI-AP-deficient granulocytes. Patients with classical PNH are at risk of thrombosis and recurrent hemolysis.

Clinical manifestations

Hemolysis. CD59 directly interacts with the membrane attack complexes (MAC) and reduces the number of MACs preventing the formation of lytic pores (31). CD55 accelerates the rate of destruction of membrane-bound C3 convertase and hence reduces the amount of cleaved C3. The reduction or complete absence of CD59 and CD55 on red blood cells enhances their susceptibility to complement-mediated lysis resulting in hemolysis.

Thrombosis. Venous thrombosis is an ominous complication with the abdominal and the cerebral veins being the most commonly involved regions. The mechanism by which thrombosis occurs is not clearly understood. In two series, most patients developing thrombosis had more than 50% PNH-type granulocytes (28,32).

Bone marrow failure. Patients who present with the clinical manifestations of PNH, including a large PNH clone, may progress to AA, although the exact frequency with which this occurs is not known. MDS may also be associated with the presence of a PNH clone in up to 20% of patients.

PNH patients, similar to those with aplastic anemia or MDS, are at increased risk for clonal progression. The incidence of leukemic transformation in PNH is lower, however, than that of MDS (33). The leukemic cells arise from the GPI anchor-deficient clone in most cases (34).

Diagnosis

GPI anchor-based assays. Monoclonal antibodies to the GPI-anchored proteins, particularly CD55 and CD59, in conjunction with flow cytometry are used for the diagnosis of PNH. Because of accelerated hemolysis of PNH-type RBCs compared with normal RBCs, the percentage of PNH granulocytes detected by flow cytometry gives a more accurate assessment of the number of PNH-type stem cells contributing to hematopoiesis.

What is the role of eculizumab in patients with PNH?

Eculizumab is a humanized monoclonal antibody against C5 that inhibits the activation of terminal components of complement. In a pilot trial, 11 patients with transfusion-dependent PNH received infusions of eculizumab (600 mg) every week for four weeks, followed one week later by a 900-mg dose and then every other week doses through week 12. The mean and median transfusion rates decreased from 2.1 and 1.8 units per patient per month to 0.6 and 0.0 units per patient per month, respectively ($p = 0.003$ for the comparison of the median rates) (35). Based on these promising results, a double-blind, randomized, placebo-controlled, multicenter, phase III trial was conducted in which 87 patients with PNH were given either placebo or eculizumab intravenously; eculizumab was given at a dose of 600 mg weekly for four weeks, followed one week later by a 900-mg dose and then 900 mg every other week through week 26. Intravascular hemolytic episodes were significantly reduced in recipients of eculizumab. Hemoglobin levels stabilized or increased and transfusion independence was achieved in 49% (21 of 43) of the patients assigned to eculizumab versus none of the 44 patients assigned to placebo ($p < 0.001$). During the study, a median of 0 units of packed red cells was administered in the eculizumab group, as compared with 10 units in the placebo group ($p < 0.001$). The most common adverse event reported for eculizumab-treated patients were headache, nasopharyngitis, back pain, and upper respiratory tract infections (36). Based on these favorable data, eculizumab gained U.S. Food and Drug Administration approval for the treatment of PNH in March 2007. A long-term followup report on the 195 trial participants who continued treatment in the multinational open-label extension study suggested the rate of thromboembolism (TE) was reduced in patients receiving eculizumab compared to the pretreatment TE rate in the same patients. The TE event rate with eculizumab treatment was 1.07 events/100 patient-years compared with 7.37 events/100 patient-years ($p < .001$) prior to eculizumab treatment (relative reduction, 85%; absolute reduction, 6.3 TE events/100 patient-years). With equalization of the duration of exposure before and during treatment for each patient, TE events were reduced from 39 events before eculizumab to 3 events during eculizumab ($p < .001$). The TE event rate in antithrombotic-treated patients (n = 103) was reduced from 10.61 to 0.62 events/100 patient-years with eculizumab treatment ($p < .001$). These results provide the first evidence that eculizumab treatment reduces the risk of clinical thromboembolism in patients with PNH (37).

Recommendation. For patients with classical PNH, eculizumab is highly effective in decreasing intravascular hemolysis reducing or eliminating the need for blood transfusions, improving the quality of life and significantly reducing the rate of thromboembolic events(Grade 1A). Eculizumab is recommended for PNH patients without bone marrow failure as an effective alternative to allogeneic HSCT (Grade 1A).

What is the role of allogeneic hematopoietic transplant in patients with PNH?

Allogeneic bone marrow transplantation can be curative for PNH although morbidity and mortality associated with the procedure can be substantial. The number of studies addressing this question is limited. The outcome of 57 consecutive allogeneic bone marrow transplants for PNH reported to the International Bone Marrow Transplant Registry between 1978 and 1995 was analyzed retrospectively. The two-year probability of survival in 48 recipients of HLA identical sibling transplants was 56% (95% confidence interval 49%–63%). The most common causes of treatment failure were graft failure and infections (38). These results indicate that bone marrow transplantation can restore normal bone marrow function in about 50% of PNH patients.

Recommendation. The recent development of eculizumab for patients with PNH offers an effective alternative therapy to transplantation. HSCT is recommended for younger patients with severe pancytopenia who have an HLA-identical sibling and in those patients with classical PNH who do not want to be committed to indefinite treatment with eculizumab (Grade 2C).

What role does prophylactic anticoagulation play in the management of patients with PNH?

In one retrospective analysis of 163 patients, the 10-year risk of thrombosis was 44% in those with large PNH clones (i.e., PNH granulocytes >50% of the total) and 5.8% in those with small clones ($p < 0.01$). Based on these observations, patients with large PNH clones without a contraindication to anticoagulation were subsequently offered warfarin prophylaxis (target INR 2.0 to 3.0); at a median follow-up of six years, there were no thrombotic episodes in the 39 patients who received warfarin prophylaxis, while the 10-year thrombosis rate was 36.5% ($p = 0.01$) in 56 patients not taking warfarin (because of either by patient or physician choice). There were only two serious bleeding episodes in more than 100 patient-years of warfarin treatment (39). Despite the limitations of the retrospective design, the results of this study suggest that primary prophylaxis may be beneficial. There are no studies of antiplatelet drugs, such as aspirin or clodiprogrel, in PNH.

Recommendations. Warfarin prophylaxis is recommended to be instituted in patients with PNH if the granulocyte clone size is >50% and the platelet count is >100,000/µL as long as no contraindications to anticoagulation exist (Grade 1C).

Table 23.2 Causes of acquired pure red cell aplasia.

Drugs	**Lymphoid malignancies**
Phenytoin	Chronic lymphocytic leukemia
Trimethoprim-sulfamethoxazole	LGL leukemia
Zidovudine	Hodgkin disease
Chlorpropamide	Non-Hodgkin lymphoma
Recombinant human erythropoietins	Multiple myeloma
Mycophenolate mofetil	
Infection	**Myeloid malignancies**
B19 parovirus	Chronic myeloid leukemia
HIV	Agnogenic myeloid metaplasia with myelofibrosis
Viral hepatitis	Prodrome to myelodysplastic syndromes
Immune disorders	**Other cancers**
Autoimmune hemolytic anemia	Thymoma (10% to 15% of cases)
Systemic lupus erythematosus	Lung
Rheumatoid arthritis	Breast
ABO-incompatible bone marrow transplantation	**Pregnancy**

LGL, large granular lymphocyte

Pure red cell aplasia

Pure red cell aplasia (PRCA) is a syndrome characterized by normochromic, normocytic anemia, reticulocytopenia (reticulocyte count <1%), and almost complete absence of erythroblasts (<0.5%) in the bone marrow. Pathophysiologically, maturation of red cell precursors is defective.

Etiology and classification

PRCA may manifest as a congenital disorder early in life or later as an acquired anemia that may be primary or secondary to a variety of neoplastic, autoimmune, or infectious diseases (Table 23.2). As with AA, the etiology of PRCA is often immune in origin. In a significant number of cases, no immune pathogenic mechanism can be established, and the disorder is classified as idiopathic.

What is the diagnostic work up for PRCA?

A bone marrow aspiration shows normal myelopoiesis, lymphopoiesis, and megakaryocytopoiesis but few if any erythroid precursors. Laboratory evaluations should be done to assess for other coexisting diseases as indicated in Table 23.2.

What are the therapeutic options for patients diagnosed with PRCA?

After the diagnosis of PRCA is confirmed, all potential offending drugs should be discontinued and any identified infection should be treated with the appropriate antimicrobial therapy. In the case of B19 parvovirus infection, the usual course is spontaneous resolution within two to three weeks. In 1989, Kurtzman et al. (40) described a 24-year-old man with a 10-year history of PRCA related to B19 infection, whose hemoglobin levels were normalized and then maintained by intravenous immunoglobulin (IVIg) infusions. Since then, IVIg have been used to treat severe anemia secondary to chronic B19 infection (Grade 1C). Patients with thymoma can be effectively treated by thymectomy; in 30% to 40% of cases, erythropoiesis returns to normal within four to eight weeks following thymectomy (Grade 1C) (41,42).

Corticosteroids have been used as immunosuppressive therapy for both primary PRCA and secondary PRCA not responding to treatment of underlying cause (41,43). Prednisone is administered orally at a dose of 1 mg/kg/d until a remission is induced. In about 40% of patients, remission usually occurs within four weeks, and continuation of treatment with prednisone longer than 12 weeks is not recommended (Grade 1C). ATG or CSA can be given as second-line therapy to patients who fail to respond to corticosteroids. In a small series, 6 of 9 steroid-refractory patients responded to ATG (44). In a retrospective study, PRCA associated with large granular lymphocytic leukemia, 28 of 47 patients treated with CSA had a hematological response that may reflect the responsiveness of the underlying disorder to CSA (45). Other drugs that have shown activity in refractory cases as evidenced mainly from case reports include the anti-CD20 monoclonal antibody rituximab (46,47), the anti-CD52 monoclonal antibody alemtuzumab (48,49), and cyclophosphamide (50). The anti-interleukin-2 receptor monoclonal antibody daclizumab was shown in a pilot study of 15 patients with transfusion-dependent idiopathic PRCA (11 patients were not responsive to previous treatment) to achieve a response rate of 40% (51). No data exist favoring one type of treatment over the other once patients have proven to be steroid refractory. The physician should consider any coexisting systemic disease, the age of the patient, the potential short- and long-term side effects, and the cost of treatment. In patients not responding to initial therapy, our choice has been to continue immunosuppression by sequential use of low-dose corticosteroids combined with CSA or ATG, high-dose intravenous IgG, anti-CD20 monoclonal antibody, daclizumab, or cytotoxic agents, which is followed if necessary by another round of immunosuppressive therapy (Grade 2C). In primary PRCA, because of their potential leukemogenic and carcinogenic effects, the use of cytotoxic agents is avoided until other means of immunosuppression are found ineffective. Relapses are usually treated with the same regimen that induced the initial remission. Cases refractory to all forms of treatment should receive regular red blood cell transfusions with iron chelation therapy to avoid organ toxicity from iron overload. Bone marrow transplantation offers potentially curative therapy in selected patients with refractory disease who have an HLA identical sibling as evidenced mainly by case reports (52) (Grade 2C).

References

1 Young NS. Acquired aplastic anemia. *Ann Intern Med.* 2002;**136**(7): 534–46.

2 Rozman C, et al. Criteria for severe aplastic anaemia. *Lancet.* 1987;**2**(8565):955–57.

3 Young NS. Acquired aplastic anemia. *JAMA.* 1999;**282**(3):271–78.

4 Zoumbos NC, et al. Interferon is a mediator of hematopoietic suppression in aplastic anemia in vitro and possibly in vivo. *Proc Natl Acad Sci USA.* 1985;**82**(1):188–92.

5 Maciejewski J, et al. Fas antigen expression on CD34+ human marrow cells is induced by interferon gamma and tumor necrosis factor alpha and potentiates cytokine-mediated hematopoietic suppression in vitro. *Blood.* 1995;**85**(11):3183–90.

6 Frickhofen N, Rosenfeld SJ. Immunosuppressive treatment of aplastic anemia with antithymocyte globulin and cyclosporine. *Semin Hematol.* 2000;**37**(1):56–68.

7 Rosenfeld S, et al. Antithymocyte globulin and cyclosporine for severe aplastic anemia: association between hematologic response and long-term outcome. *JAMA.* 2003;**289**(9):1130–35.

8 Tichelli A, et al. Repeated treatment with horse antilymphocyte globulin for severe aplastic anaemia. *Br J Haematol.* 1998;**100**(2):393–400.

9 Scheinberg P, Nunez O, Young NS. Retreatment with rabbit anti-thymocyte globulin and ciclosporin for patients with relapsed or refractory severe aplastic anaemia. *Br J Haematol.* 2006;**133**(6):622–27.

10 Tisdale JF, et al. High-dose cyclophosphamide in severe aplastic anaemia: a randomised trial. *Lancet.* 2000;**356**(9241):1554–59.

11 Brodsky RA., et al. High-dose cyclophosphamide as salvage therapy for severe aplastic anemia. *Exp Hematol.* 2004;**32**(5):435–40.

12 Brodsky RA, et al. Durable treatment-free remission after high-dose cyclophosphamide therapy for previously untreated severe aplastic anemia. *Ann Intern Med.* 2001;**135**(7):477–83.

13 Marsh J, et al. Prospective randomized multicenter study comparing cyclosporin alone versus the combination of antithymocyte globulin and cyclosporin for treatment of patients with nonsevere aplastic anemia: a report from the European Blood and Marrow Transplant (EBMT) Severe Aplastic Anaemia Working Party. *Blood.* 1999;**93**(7):2191–95.

14 Maciejewski JP, et al. Recombinant humanized anti-IL-2 receptor antibody (daclizumab) produces responses in patients with moderate aplastic anemia. *Blood.* 2003;**102**(10):3584–86.

15 Socie G, et al. Malignant tumors occurring after treatment of aplastic anemia. European Bone Marrow Transplantation-Severe Aplastic Anaemia Working Party. *N Engl J Med.* 1993;**329**(16):1152–57.

16 Young NS, Calado RT, Scheinberg P. Current concepts in the pathophysiology and treatment of aplastic anemia. *Blood.* 2006;**108**(8):2509–19.

17 Kahl C, et al. Cyclophosphamide and antithymocyte globulin as a conditioning regimen for allogeneic marrow transplantation in patients with aplastic anaemia: a long-term follow-up. *Br J Haematol.* 2005;**130**(5):747–51.

18 Storb R, et al. Cyclophosphamide and antithymocyte globulin to condition patients with aplastic anemia for allogeneic marrow transplantations: the experience in four centers. *Biol Blood Marrow Transplant.* 2001;7(1):39–44.

19 Storb R, et al. Cyclophosphamide combined with antithymocyte globulin in preparation for allogeneic marrow transplants in patients with aplastic anemia. *Blood.* 1994. **84**(3):941–49.

20 Gluckman E, et al. Bone marrow transplantation for severe aplastic anemia: influence of conditioning and graft-versus-host disease prophylaxis regimens on outcome. *Blood.* 1992;**79**(1):269–75.

21 Gluckman E, et al. Bone marrow transplantation in 107 patients with severe aplastic anemia using cyclophosphamide and thoraco-abdominal irradiation for conditioning: long-term follow-up. *Blood.* 1991;**78**(9):2451–55.

22 Srinivasan R, et al. Overcoming graft rejection in heavily transfused and allo-immunised patients with bone marrow failure syndromes using fludarabine-based haematopoietic cell transplantation. *Br J Haematol.* 2006;**133**(3):305–14.

23 Gomez-Almaguer D, et al. Allografting in patients with severe, refractory aplastic anemia using peripheral blood stem cells and a fludarabine-based conditioning regimen: the Mexican experience. *Am J Hematol.* 2006;**81**(3):157–61.

24 Kumar R, et al. Fludarabine, cyclophosphamide and horse antithymocyte globulin conditioning regimen for allogeneic peripheral blood stem cell transplantation performed in non-HEPA filter rooms for multiply transfused patients with severe aplastic anemia. *Bone Marrow Transplant.* 2006;**37**(8):745–49.

25 Deeg HJ, et al. Optimization of conditioning for marrow transplantation from unrelated donors for patients with aplastic anemia after failure of immunosuppressive therapy. *Blood.* 2006;**108**(5):1485–91.

26 Bacigalupo A, et al. Fludarabine, cyclophosphamide and anti-thymocyte globulin for alternative donor transplants in acquired severe aplastic anemia: a report from the EBMT-SAA Working Party. Bone Marrow Transplant, 2005;**36**(11):947–50.

27 Hillmen P, et al. Natural history of paroxysmal nocturnal hemoglobinuria. *N Engl J Med.* 1995;**333**(19):1253–58.

28 Moyo VM, et al. Natural history of paroxysmal nocturnal haemoglobinuria using modern diagnostic assays. *Br J Haematol.* 2004;**126**(1):133–38.

29 Nagarajan S, et al. Genetic defects underlying paroxysmal nocturnal hemoglobinuria that arises out of aplastic anemia. *Blood.* 1995;**86**(12):4656–61.

30 Brodsky, RA. New insights into paroxysmal nocturnal hemoglobinuria. *Hematol Am Soc Hematol Educ Program.* 2006:24–8.

31 Meri S, et al. Human protectin (CD59), an 18,000–20,000 MW complement lysis restricting factor, inhibits C5b-8 catalysed insertion of C9 into lipid bilayers. *Immunology.* 1990;**71**(1):1–9.

32 Nishimura J, et al. Clinical course and flow cytometric analysis of paroxysmal nocturnal hemoglobinuria in the United States and Japan. *Medicine (Baltimore).* 2004;**83**(3):193–207.

33 Graham DL, Gastineau DA. Paroxysmal nocturnal hemoglobinuria as a marker for clonal myelopathy. *Am J Med.* 1992;**93**(6):671–74.

34 Nishimura JI, et al. Analysis of PIG-A gene in a patient who developed reciprocal translocation of chromosome 12 and paroxysmal nocturnal hemoglobinuria during follow-up of aplastic anemia. *Am J Hematol.* 1996;**51**(3):229–33.

35 Hillmen P, et al. Effect of eculizumab on hemolysis and transfusion requirements in patients with paroxysmal nocturnal hemoglobinuria. *N Engl J Med.* 2004;**350**(6):552–29.

36 Hillmen P, et al. The complement inhibitor eculizumab in paroxysmal nocturnal hemoglobinuria. *N Engl J Med.* 2006;**355**(12):1233–43.

37 Hillmen, P., et al., Effect of the complement inhibitor eculizumab on thromboembolism in patients with paroxysmal nocturnal hemoglobinuria. Blood, 2007. 110(12): pp. 412–28.

38 Saso R, et al. Bone marrow transplants for paroxysmal nocturnal haemoglobinuria. *Br J Haematol.* 1999;**104**(2):392–96.

39 Hall C, Richards S, Hillmen P. Primary prophylaxis with warfarin prevents thrombosis in paroxysmal nocturnal hemoglobinuria (PNH). *Blood.* 2003;**102**(10):3587–91.

40 Kurtzman G, et al. Pure red-cell aplasia of 10 years' duration due to persistent parvovirus B19 infection and its cure with immunoglobulin therapy. *N Engl J Med.* 1989;**321**(8):519–23.

41 Marmont AM. Therapy of pure red cell aplasia. *Semin Hematol.* 1991;**28**(4):285–97.

42 Masaoka A, et al. Thymomas associated with pure red cell aplasia: histologic and follow-up studies. *Cancer.* 1989;**64**(9):1872–78.

43 Clark DA, Dessypris EN, Krantz SB. Studies on pure red cell aplasia. XI. Results of immunosuppressive treatment of 37 patients. *Blood.* 1984;**63**(2):277–86.

44 Abkowitz JL et al. Pure red cell aplasia: response to therapy with antithymocyte globulin. *Am J Hematol.* 1986;**23**(4):363–71.

45 Lacy MQ, Kurtin PJ, Tefferi A. Pure red cell aplasia: association with large granular lymphocyte leukemia and the prognostic value of cytogenetic abnormalities. *Blood.* 1996;**87**(7):3000–3006.

46 Ghazal H. Successful treatment of pure red cell aplasia with rituximab in patients with chronic lymphocytic leukemia. *Blood.* 2002;**99**(3):1092–94.

47 Zecca M, et al. Anti-CD20 monoclonal antibody for the treatment of severe, immune-mediated, pure red cell aplasia and hemolytic anemia. *Blood.* 2001;**97**(12):3995–97.

48 Willis F, et al. The effect of treatment with Campath-1H in patients with autoimmune cytopenias. *Br J Haematol.* 2001;**114**(4):891–98.

49 Ru X, Liebman HA. Successful treatment of refractory pure red cell aplasia associated with lymphoproliferative disorders with the anti-CD52 monoclonal antibody alemtuzumab (Campath-1H). *Br J Haematol.* 2003;**123**(2):278–81.

50 Yamada O, Mizoguchi H, Oshimi K. Cyclophosphamide therapy for pure red cell aplasia associated with granular lymphocyte-proliferative disorders. *Br J Haematol.* 1997;**97**(2):392–99.

51 Sloand EM, et al. Brief communication: Successful treatment of pure red-cell aplasia with an anti-interleukin-2 receptor antibody (daclizumab). *Ann Intern Med.* 2006;**144**(3):181–85.

52 Müller BU, et al. Successful treatment of refractory acquired pure red cell aplasia (PRCA) by allogeneic bone marrow transplantation. *Bone Marrow Transplant.* 1999;**23**(11):1205–7.

24 Acquired Anemias

Iron Deficiency, Cobalamin Deficiency, and Autoimmune Hemolytic Anemia

Marc S. Zumberg, Marc J. Kahn

Literature-search criteria

Evidence-based guidelines for this chapter were derived from PubMed and Ovid searches using standard search terms applicable to each clinical question. After reviewing retrieved documents, additional references were obtained from literature cited in the documents from the original literature search.

Grading evidence and recommendations

Level of evidence for each recommendation was assigned according to the Seventh American College of Chest Physicians Conference Guidelines (1).

Iron deficiency anemia

Are alternative oral iron preparations preferred over ferrous sulfate for first-line treatment of iron deficiency anemia?

Multiple preparations of oral iron are available, including oral iron salts, controlled release iron preparations, polysaccharide, and carbonyl iron preparations. As compared with ferrous salts, alternative iron preparations are claimed to be better tolerated as less iron is presented to the proximal gastrointestinal tract. Whether this leads to compromised efficacy has been debated. Most data concerning tolerance or efficacy of these products compared with iron salts are derived from small randomized trials with short-term follow-up and variable methodology (Table 24.1).

Limited data are available comparing efficacy and tolerance of different oral iron salt preparations. A randomized placebo-controlled study conducted in the 1960s, consisting of three separate substudies, compared side effects of three equivalent doses of different ferrous salt preparations (ferrous sulfate, ferrous gluconate, and ferrous fumurate) (2). The gastrointestinal side effect rate was similar between formulations but was higher with all preparations as compared with placebo ($p < 0.05$). No efficacy data were reported.

A more recent study by Wingard et al. in 56 dialysis patients receiving recombinant human erythropoietin (rhEPO) showed no difference in hemoglobin responses or side effects between ferrous sulfate, ferrous fumarate, and iron polysaccharide (3). Other small studies have shown similar rates of absorption between ferrous salts and iron polymaltose preparations (4,5).

Three randomized trials and one crossover comparative trial assessed tolerability between controlled-release iron formulations and oral ferrous sulfate (Table 24.1) (6–9). Although lower rates of gastrointestinal side effects were noted in the controlled release group in all three randomized studies, no difference in discontinuation rates were seen as compared with ferrous sulfate. Efficacy was only reported in two studies and showed no differences between the iron formulations.

Two small nonblinded, randomized studies compared polysaccharide-iron complexes and ferrous sulfate with conflicting results. One study consisting of 159 patients showed lower rates of discontinuation with the polysaccharide-iron complex, while the second showed no difference in side effects (5,10). Equivalent hemoglobin responses were noted in both studies.

Two small, randomized, double-blinded studies showed no difference in efficacy or tolerance between carbonyl iron and ferrous sulfate (11,12).

Summary

There are no significant differences in tolerability or efficacy between different formulations of oral iron salts. Controlled-release iron preparations may cause fewer gastrointestinal side effects, but discontinuation rates are similar and efficacy is comparable.

Evidence-based Hematology. Edited by Mark A. Crowther, Jeff Ginsberg, Holger J. Schünemann, Ralph M. Meyer, and Richard Lottenberg.

Table 24.1 Randomized summary of studies comparing tolerability or efficacy of oral iron preparations.*

Reference	No. patients	Comparison	Efficacy	GI tolerance	Discontinuation	Limitations
Iron Salts						
Hallberg (2)	1,496 blood donors	Various oral iron salts	X	Equivalent	Equivalent	—3 separate series —Results based on patient surveys
Wingard (3)	46 dialysis patients + rhEPO	Oral iron salts and iron polysaccharide	Equivalent	Less adverse events with iron polysaccharide	Equivalent	—Distinct patient population —Small study —Receiving rhEPO
Sustained Release						
Aronstam (6)	40 iron deficient	Sustained release vs. iron salt	Equivalent	Slightly favored sustained release	Equivalent	—Small number of patients —Single-blinded
Brock (7)	543 nonanemic	Sustained release wax matrix vs. ferrous sulfate	X	Less severe side effects with sustained release	Equivalent	—Nonanemic patients —Nonblinded —Patient surveys
Elwood (8)	521 iron deficient	Sustained release vs. iron salt	Equivalent	Equivalent	Equivalent	—Nonblinded —Disproportionate randomization
Rybo (9)	1,376 blood donors 232 pregnant	Sustained release vs. ferrous sulfate	X	Less nausea and epigastric pain with sustained release	Equivalent	—3 separate series —Results based on patient surveys
Iron Polysaccharide						
Jacobs (5)	159 iron deficient blood donors	Iron polysaccharide vs. iron salt	Equivalent	X	Favored iron polysaccharide	—Blood donors —Nonblinded
Sas (10)	60 iron deficient	Iron polysaccharide vs. iron salt	Equivalent	Equivalent	X	—Small number of patients —Statistics poorly defined —Nonblinded
Carbonyl Iron						
Devasthali (11)	49 anemic blood donors	Carbonyl iron vs. iron salt	Equivalent	Equivalent	X	—Small number of patients
Gordeuk (12)	50 blood donors with mild iron deficiency	High dose carbonyl iron vs. iron salt	Equivalent	Equivalent	X	—Small number of patients —Nonintention to treat analysis —High dropout rate

*X, data not available.

Minimal data are available comparing polysaccharide and carbonyl iron formulations to traditional iron salts.

Recommendation. Ferrous sulfate is recommended over newer iron preparations as first-line therapy of iron deficiency (Grade 2B). If ferrous sulfate is not tolerated, alternative formulations may be tried.

In patients requiring parenteral iron is ferric gluconate or iron sucrose preferred over iron dextran?

Over the past few years the U.S. Food and Drug Administration has approved intravenous ferric gluconate and intravenous iron sucrose for use in the United States. No randomized trials directly compare efficacy or side effects of iron dextran to these products. The incidence of serious life-threatening anaphylaxis with iron dextran has been reported to be 0.6%–0.7% based on a prospective study conducted between the years 1962 and 1970 in which three life-threatening reactions were documented out of 481 individuals treated (13,14). In a multicenter, randomized, crossover, double-blind, placebo-controlled prospective study, ferric gluconate was compared with placebo as well as iron dextran based on adverse event reporting from historical data obtained from four previously published studies. A serious life-threatening event rate of 0.04% was reported with ferric gluconate, which was similar to placebo but less than the 0.6% rate reported from the historical data of patients treated with iron dextran (15). In a follow-up study, no life-threatening adverse events were reported with repeated dosing of ferric gluconate in more than 13,000 doses administered (16). A retrospective review of allergic events based on manufacturer reports, World Health Organization data, and reports to the German Health Ministry and other European agencies (ferric gluconate was used primarily in Germany, Italy, and Spain) has also shown a favorable toxicity profile for ferric gluconate with 3.3 episodes per million doses as compared with 8.7 episodes per million doses with iron dextran (17). A significantly lower reported mortality rate was also noted with ferric gluconate ($p < 0.001$). Adverse event data reported to the FDA during the years 2001–2003 using the FDA Medwatch system showed absolute rates of life-threatening adverse events of 0.6, 0.9, 3.3, and 11.3 per million for iron sucrose, ferric gluconate complex, low-molecular-weight iron dextran, and high-molecular-weight iron dextran, respectively (18). A randomized study of 59 patients undergoing hemodialysis and receiving stable doses of rhEPO showed that both intravenous iron sucrose (250 mg/month) and intravenous iron gluconate (62.5 mg/week) could maintain hemoglobin levels from baseline to endpoint without anaphylactic reactions in either group (19). A single-institution five-year retrospective review included 44 intravenous iron infusions in 121 patients and noted a higher adverse event rates with iron dextran as compared with iron gluconate (20). However, in a subgroup analysis, where iron dextran was preceded by both premedications as well as a test dose, the adverse event rate was similar to iron gluconate. No anaphylaxis or serious adverse events were noted. In another retrospective, single-institution chart review 39 infusions of iron dextran were compared with 26 infusions of iron gluconate. Only a single severe reaction occurred in the iron dextran group. Mild to moderate reactions were similar between the two groups (21% vs. 23%) (21).

Recommendations. All three preparations of intravenous iron are reasonable choices for first-line parenteral iron replacement (Grade 1C). Severe life-threatening anaphylaxis is less frequent with iron sucrose or ferric gluconate as compared with iron dextran (Grade 1C+). Although ferric gluconate and iron sucrose have a lower rate of life-threatening adverse events than iron dextran, both are more costly and neither can be given as a total dose infusion. No studies were identified comparing the efficacy of these preparations.

Are there patient populations, other than hemodialysis, for which intravenous iron is preferred over oral iron as initial replacement therapy?

Randomized trials comparing the efficacy of initial treatment with oral iron as compared with intravenous iron are limited to a few specific clinical scenarios (excluding dialysis dependant renal failure) (Table 24.2).

Table 24.2 Studies comparing intravenous iron to oral iron salts in various patient populations.*

Reference	Patient characteristics	Intervention	Hb response	Ferritin response
Chronic nondialysis dependent kidney disease				
Agarwal (22)	75 iron deficient no rhEPO	Ferric gluconate vs. ferrous sulfate	Equivalent	Favored IV
Aggarwal (23)	40 severely anemic (hb < 9.5g/dL) + rhEPO	Iron dextran vs. ferrous sulfate	Favored IV	Favored IV
Charytan (24)	96 anemic + rhEPO	Iron sucrose vs. ferrous sulfate	Equivalent	Favored IV
Stoves (25)	45 anemic + rhEPO	Iron sucrose vs. ferrous sulfate	Equivalent	Favored IV
Van Wyck (26)	188 anemic + rhEPO	Iron sucrose vs. ferrous sulfate	Favored IV	Favored IV
Cancer				
Auerbach (27)	157 chemo-related anemia + rhEPO	Iron dextran vs. ferrous sulfate —Bolus and total dose IV infusion	Favored IV	Favored IV
Henry (28)	187 chemo-related anemia + rhEPO	Ferric gluconate vs. ferrous sulfate	Favored IV	Favored IV
Inflammatory Bowel Disease				
Shroeder (29)	46 anemic	Iron sucrose vs. ferrous sulfate	Equivalent	Favored IV
Pregnancy				
Al RA (31)	90 iron deficient	Iron sucrose vs. iron polymaltose	Favored IV	Favored IV
Bayoumeu (32)	50 iron deficient	Iron sucrose vs. ferrous sulfate	Equivalent	Favored IV
Singh (33)	100 iron deficient	Iron dextan vs. ferrous fumerate	Favored IV	Favored IV
Al-Mormen (34)	111 iron deficient	Iron sucrose vs. ferrous sulfate	Favored IV	Favored IV

*IV, intravenous.

Five randomized studies in patients with chronic kidney disease have been reported (22–26). The use and doses of rhEPO were variable across studies as was the preparation of intravenous iron administered and the baseline transferrin saturation and ferritin values in the inclusion criteria. All studies had short patient follow-up. The results of these studies were variable and the patient populations were heterogeneous with anemia ranging from severe to mild. Ferritin responses were improved in the intravenous iron group in all studies. Hemoglobin responses were similar in three of five studies, while two favored intravenous iron (23,26). Gastrointestinal side effects were more common in the oral iron group.

Two recent open-label randomized studies compared oral to intravenous iron in cancer patients who were also receiving rhEPO 40,000 units weekly (27,28). In the first study, both bolus and total dose infusion intravenous iron dextran groups showed superior efficacy as compared with the groups receiving no iron or oral iron (27). Quality of life as measured by the linear analogue scale assessment method was also improved in the intravenous iron group. The second study compared oral iron to intravenous ferric gluconate in nonmyeloid cancer patients undergoing chemotherapy. In an intention to treat analysis hemoglobin responses were significantly better in the intravenous arm (73% vs. 46%, $p < 0.01$) (28).

In inflammatory bowel disease (IBD), a single small prospective randomized open-label study of 46 anemic patients showed comparable increases in hemoglobin between intravenous iron sucrose and oral ferrous sulfate, although only the intravenous route led to increases in serum ferritin (29). Oral iron was poorly tolerated in this study leading to drug discontinuation in 21% of patients. In a small crossover study, clinical disease severity increased in IBD patients treated with oral as opposed to intravenous iron, although ferritin response was improved in the intravenous arm (30).

Data on postpartum iron replacement is not included in this review. In a recent study of 90 pregnant anemic patients who received either oral iron polymaltose complex or intravenous iron sucrose, hemoglobin responses were significantly higher in the intravenous iron group. No serious maternal or fetal side effects were observed in the intravenous arm. Gastrointestinal side effects were frequent in the oral arm (31). In another randomized prospective study, in 50 iron deficient anemic pregnant patients, no significant differences were noted in hemoglobin response at any time in the study, although ferritin response was greater in the intravenous iron group ($p < 0.0001$) (32). A study in Singapore compared iron dextrin to oral ferrous fumarate and noted better responses to intravenous iron both in terms of efficacy and tolerability (33). Hemoglobin and ferritin responses were improved and quicker in the intravenous arm of a Saudi Arabian study (34).

Recommendations. In non-dialysis-dependent renal disease, intravenous iron may be preferred over oral iron based on improvement in serum ferritin and possible improvement in hemoglobin (Grade 2B). Study results are confounded by different degrees of anemia and variable use of erythropoietic agents in these studies.

In cancer patients receiving rhEPO, intravenous iron is more effective than oral replacement and may be preferred over oral iron (Grade 1B).

Because of the small sample size in patients with inflammatory bowel disease, no definitive recommendations can be made concerning the efficacy of oral versus intravenous iron, although tolerance is likely better via the intravenous route (Grade 2B). Intravenous iron may be more effective than oral iron during pregnancy, although results are conflicting (Grade 2B). Oral iron is recommended as initial therapy in pregnancy, but intravenous iron can be considered for those who do not tolerate or respond to oral formulations (Grade 2C). Intravenous iron dextran is listed as category C, and iron sucrose and ferric gluconate are listed as category B for use in pregnancy.

Is the soluble tranferrin receptor-ferritin index (sTfR-F) better than the serum ferritin in diagnosing iron deficiency?

In the 1990s, the soluble transferrin receptor (sTfr) and more recently the ratio of the soluble transferrin receptor/log serum ferritin (sTfR-F) index has been proposed to be a better reflection of functional iron than traditional iron studies, including serum ferritin.

A recent prospective-controlled study in 49 patients greater than 80 years of age compared the sTfR-F index with traditional iron studies (using iron stains on bone marrow aspirate sections as the reference standard) to evaluate iron deficiency anemia. The use of the sTFR-F index increased the sensitivity for diagnosing iron deficiency anemia from 16% with standard measures to 88% in this elderly population (35). A more recent study in 121 hemodialysis patients receiving rhEPO also showed that the sTfR-F is superior to routine iron studies in predicting response to intravenous iron (36). Other studies, however, have failed to show an added benefit of sTfR-F when compared with serum ferritin. A trial of 72 patients investigating the value of sTfR-F at different phases of iron deficiency showed that the test was only sensitive in cases of advanced iron deficiency anemia as compared with earlier stages (37). Another study compared serum ferritin and sTFR-F in several heterogeneous groups of anemic patients (iron deficiency, chronic inflammation, nonhematologic malignancies) to nonanemic controls and showed no improvement with use of the sTfR-F as compared with serum ferritin in predicting bone marrow biopsy confirmed cases of iron deficiency (38). No randomized data are available comparing the ability of sTFR-F with serum ferritin in guiding the treatment of iron deficiency. In addition, the cutoff "positive" levels of sTFR-F used for predicting iron deficiency are not uniform across studies, making this literature difficult to interpret.

Recommendation. There remains no definitive evidence that the sTFR-F should replace serum ferritin in the routine diagnosis of iron deficiency (Grade 2C).

Cobalamin (B12) deficiency

What is the role of measurement of homocysteine and methylmalonic acid in the assessment of patients with presumed cobalamin deficiency?

Serum concentrations of both homocysteine and methylmalonic acid elevated in cobalamin deficiency and are considered early markers of deficiency. Because they reflect tissue levels of cobalamin, rather than serum levels, homocysteine and methylmalonic acid are considered more sensitive for deficiency in patients whose measured cobalamin levels are in the low normal (<300 pmoles/L) range.

Lindenbaum and colleagues investigated the sensitivity of methylmalonic acid and homocysteine in cobalamin-deficient patients seen at two university hospitals from 1982 to 1989 and in patients seen from 1968 to 1981 where banked serum was available (39). Four hundred thirty-four episodes of cobalamin deficiency were identified in 406 patients. Cobalamin deficiency was identified by any one of the following: low serum vitamin B-12 levels, neurologic findings, or response to cobalamin therapy. Serum methylmalonic acid and homocysteine levels were elevated in 98.4% and 95.9% of samples, respectively. Only one patient had normal metabolite levels in this study. Furthermore, among the 173 patients with cobalamin deficiency based on response to therapy, 5% had normal serum cobalamin levels. The authors concluded that normal methylmalonic acid and homocysteine levels rule out cobalamin deficiency with virtual certainty. Another prospective study of over 1,500 asymptomatic randomly screened elderly patients in the United Kingdom found that elevated homocysteine and methylmalonic acid levels could identify patients requiring cobalamin replacement, based on symptoms, when their serum cobalamin levels were borderline (150–300 pmol/L) (40). An additional study of 196 patients referred from primary care physicians for analysis of cobalamin deficiency, utilizing a combination of serum cobalamin levels, serum homocysteine, serum methylmalonic acid, gastroscopy, and serum and erythrocyte folate levels, concluded that serum cobalamin should be the first test used in the assessment of cobalamin deficiency (41). When cobalamin levels were low normal and a firm diagnosis could not be made, methylmalonic acid was the most specific diagnostic test for cobalamin deficiency.

Recommendations. For patients with cobalamin levels less than 300 pmols/L, we recommend measuring serum methylmalonic acid (Grade 1C+). Elevated (>0.35 mcmoles/L) methylmalonic acid can identify patients who require cobalamin replacement (Grade 2C).

How effective is oral cobalamin replacement for patients with cobalamin deficiency?

Because malabsorption is the most common etiology of cobalamin deficiency, cobalamin-deficient patients have traditionally been treated with parenteral replacement. However, because of mass action alone, approximately 1% of oral cobalamin can be absorbed in the intestine, even in the absence of intrinsic factor. Therefore, oral replacement may be adequate for most patients.

A randomized study of 38 newly diagnosed cobalamin-deficient patients due to a variety of etiologies, including pernicious anemia and malabsorption, revealed that 1 mg cobalamin given intramuscularly on days 1, 3, 7, 10, 14, 21, 30, 60, and 90 was inferior to 2 mg given orally for 120 days based on cobalamin ($p < 0.005$) and methylmalonic acid levels ($p < 0.05$) measured at four months (42). In each group, four patients had mild to moderate neurologic abnormalities. Despite the improved serum levels in the oral group, hematologic and neurologic responses were similar between the two groups. In addition, in a review that summarized articles identified through a MEDLINE search from 1966 to 2000 assessing oral cobalamin replacement, it was concluded that daily oral doses of 1,000 to 2,000 mcg cobalamin were adequate replacement for cobalamin-deficient patients without severe neurologic symptoms (43). The etiology of cobalamin deficiency was diverse in these studies and included pernicious anemia as well as malabsorption. Doses less than 1,000 mcg daily were noted to have variable efficacy. The authors of this study were unable to comment on the adequacy of oral cobalamin replacement for patients with severe neurologic symptoms.

Recommendations. We recommend oral cobalamin replacement as an effective alternative to parenteral therapy in patients with cobalamin deficiency without severe neurologic symptoms (Grade 1B). The oral route may be favored because of ease of administration, but compliance needs to be ensured. Patients with severe neurologic impairment were excluded from these studies, and the parenteral route continues to be recommended in this setting (Grade 2C).

Autoimmune hemolytic anemia (AIHA)

What is the role of splenectomy in corticosteroid-refractory warm antibody autoimmune hemolytic anemia (WAIHA)?

WAIHA is caused by IgG that usually binds to an Rh-related antigen. IgG-coated erythrocytes, which rarely fix complement, are cleared by macrophages in the spleen. For at least 50 years, corticosteroids have been the mainstay of therapy for patients with WAIHA, producing response rates of over 60%. Unfortunately, about a third of patients become dependent on corticosteroids to maintain an adequate hemoglobin. Because splenectomy removes the site of erythrocyte destruction, it has been used as treatment for corticosteroid-dependent patients with WAIHA.

The medical literature suggests that approximately two-thirds of patients with WAIHA respond to splenectomy (44–51). Much of this literature is derived from retrospective reviews of splenectomies done for various hematologic indications, only a minority

Table 24.3 Studies utilizing rituximab for the treatment of refractory warm antibody autoimmune hemolytic anemia (WAIHA).

Study author	Pt number	Prior splenectomy	Number of Rituximab cycles	Response rate (%)	Response duration (months)
Narat (54)	11	5	4	64	11 (median)
Shanafelt (55)	5	3	3 to 8	40	4+ and13+
Zecca (56)	15	2	2 to 4	87	7–28+
Quartier (57)	5	2	4 to 14	100	15–22+
Heidel (58)	3	No	8	100	12.5+
Ramanathan (59)	2	Yes	4	100	15+, 9+

of which were for WAIHA. In addition, patient characteristics in these studies were heterogeneous, with a significant percentage of patients having concomitant autoimmune or lymphoproliferative disorders. Early evidence for the efficacy of splenectomy comes from a single institution study of 47 patients with WAIHA treated from 1955 through 1965 (45). Twenty-eight of these patients underwent splenectomy with a 68% response rate, and 44% responders remained in remission without steroid therapy throughout the study period (45). In another retrospective review, seven patients with WAIHA underwent splenectomy; three reported excellent responses, and three good responses in which patients still required low-dose steroids for variable periods of time (46). In a retrospective review of 113 splenectomies performed for various hematologic indications, 52 patients had WAIHA (47). Four patients in this study had concomitant lymphoid malignancies, 11 had the diagnosis of Evans syndrome, and 4 were Coombs' test negative. A grouped rate of 64% excellent responses and 21% additional responses, where low prednisone was still requited, was reported. A more recent prospective series of 103 patients treated with laparoscopic splenectomy for a variety of indications, included 10 patients with WAIHA (51). In this study, the response rate, as defined by a 75% reduction in transfusion requirements, was 70%. Another small single-center retrospective series between the years 1978 and 1997 included 30 patients with WAIHA who had undergone splenectomy (52). In this study, 12 cases were considered idiopathic, while 18 patients had associated diseases. Both complete (82% vs. 18%, $p < 0.001$) and overall (100% vs. 55%, $p < 0.02$) responses were superior in the idiopathic group. In this study, partial response was defined as at least a 50% improvement in transfusion requirements for at least six months. A recent retrospective review of a prospective database of laparoscopic splenectomy identified 17 cases of WAIHA and noted a 70% response rate with a 40-month mean follow-up period (48). Although there are no published randomized trials comparing splenectomy to other forms of therapy in patients with WAIHA, expert opinion suggests that splenectomy is indicated for patients dependent on or refractory to corticosteroid therapy (53).

Recommendation. Splenectomy should be considered for patients with corticosteroid refractory or dependent WAIHA (Grade 2C).

What is the role of rituximab in WAIHA?

Rituximab is a human-murine chimeric monoclonal antibody that targets CD20 on B-lymphocytes and results in B-lymphocyte depletion. Originally used, and approved, for the treatment of lymphoid malignancies, rituximab has been administered to patients with a variety of immune diseases.

There are no randomized controlled trials in the published literature comparing rituximab with other forms of therapy in the treatment of WAIHA. The available literature consists of case reports and small case series. Only four studies, two in adults (54,55) and two in children (56,57) included five or more patients. The populations studied are heterogeneous and include both patients with idiopathic WAIHA as well as WAIHA associated with other autoimmune conditions, lymphoproliferative disorders, hepatitis, mixed warm and cold antibodies, or Evans syndrome. Studies reporting the efficacy of rituximab in patients with refractory WAIHA are summarized in Table 24.3 (54–59). Studies reporting exclusively on patients with WAIHA having underlying lymphoproliferative disorders or Evans syndrome are excluded from our review, although a proportion of patients in the included studies have these conditions (54–57). Single-patient case reports were also excluded from review. Response to therapy was generally defined as an increase in hemoglobin (>10 g/dL), decrease in lactic dehydrogenase, reversion to a negative Coombs' test, and a decrease in reticulocytosis but was variable across studies.

Recommendation. We recommend that rituximab be considered in patients with WAIHA who are resistant to corticosteroid therapy (Grade 2C). Whether rituximab should be used prior to, or reserved until after splenectomy, remains unknown.

What is the role of intravenous immunoglobulin (IVIg) in the treatment of WAIHA?

The available literature is limited to case reports and case series. The largest published study evaluating the role of IVIg in WAIHA consists of 73 cases, which include 37 prospective cases at two referral medical centers and 36 retrospective cases identified in the literature (60). Doses of IVIg varied between studies and consisted of 0.4–1.0 gm/kg daily for five to seven days. Less than half of the cases of WAIHA were considered idiopathic. A response, as defined as loss of transfusion requirement, was noted in approximately 40% of the patients but was not separated between those with idiopathic versus secondary WAIHA. A retrospective case series of seven patients treated with IVIg for a variety of hematologic disorders included two patients with WAIHA. Both patients became transfusion-independent for 10 months and one year, respectively (61). One of these patients was taking steroids concurrently. Finally, IVIg has been studied in patients with WAIHA associated with lymphoproliferative disorders. In a study of seven such patients, all patients became transfusion independent for up to four years while receiving IVIg maintenance therapy every three weeks (62). In another study four patients, two with prior splenectomy and one with NHL failing steroid therapy, received 0.2–0.4 g/kg/d of IVIG. Two patients had temporary responses and one had a sustained response (63). A recent Canadian consensus statement on the use of IVIg in various hematologic diseases concluded that IVIg is not recommended for routine use in either acute or chronic treatment of WAIHA but may be considered among the options for treatment of severe life-threatening WAIHA (64).

Recommendation. We suggest that IVIg be considered only in patients with refractory WAIHA, not as first-line therapy (Grade 2C). The optimal dose and frequency of IVIg has not been determined.

Does rituximab have a role in cold agglutinin disease (CAD)?

In CAD, hemolysis occurs as a direct result of complement-mediated lysis as well as from clearance of C3-coated erythrocytes in the liver. Treatment of CAD is primarily focused on keeping the patient warm. Splenectomy and corticosteroid therapy have limited efficacy in the treatment of CAD. Rituximab has been suggested as a less toxic first-line alternative to cytotoxic chemotherapy to treat transfusion-dependent patients with CAD.

There are no published randomized studies comparing rituximab to other therapies in the treatment of CAD. Only two case series were identified that included more than two patients (65,66). A significant number of patients were either known to have or found to have underlying lymphoproliferative disorders on subsequent bone marrow examination. Four to eight cycles were administered and response rates of 45% and 54% were noted. The remaining evidence consists of case reports, including only one or two patients. These case reports suggest effectiveness of rituximab in CAD. Because of the small sample size and the possibility of reporting bias, these studies are not included in our review.

Recommendation. Rituximab can be considered as a first-line treatment for patients with CAD and symptomatic anemia not responding to supportive measures (Grade 2B).

References

1 Guyatt G, Schunemann HJ, Cook D, et al. Applying the grades of recommendation for antithrombotic and thrombolytic therapy: the Seventh ACCP Conference on Antithrombotic and Thrombolytic Therapy. *Chest.* 2004;**126**:179S–87S.

2 Hallberg L, Ryttinger L, Solvell L. Side-effects of oral iron therapy: a double-blind study of different iron compounds in tablet form. *Acta Med Scand Suppl.* 1966;**459**:3–10.

3 Wingard RL, Parker RA, Ismail N, et al. Efficacy of oral iron therapy in patients receiving recombinant human erythropoietin. *Am J Kidney Dis.* 1995;**25**:433–39.

4 Jacobs P, Wormald LA, Gregory MC. Absorption of iron polymaltose and ferrous sulphate in rats and humans: a comparative study. *S Afr Med J.* 1979;**55**:1065–72.

5 Jacobs P, Fransman D, Coghlan P. Comparative bioavailability of ferric polymaltose and ferrous sulphate in iron-deficient blood donors. *J Clin Apher.* 1993;**8**:89–95.

6 Aronstam A, Aston DL. A comparative trial of a controlled-release iron tablet preparation ("Ferrocontin" Continus) and ferrous fumarate tablets. *Pharmatherapeutica.* 1982;**3**:263–67.

7 Brock C, Curry H, Hanna C, et al. Adverse effects of iron supplementation: a comparative trial of a wax-matrix iron preparation and conventional ferrous sulfate tablets. *Clin Ther.* 1985;**7**:568–73.

8 Elwood PC, Williams G. A comparative trial of slow-release and conventional iron preparations. *Practitioner.* 1970;**204**:812–15.

9 Rybo G, Solvell L. Side-effect studies on a new sustained release iron preparation. *Scand J Haematol.* 1971;**8**:257–64.

10 Sas G, Nemesanszky E, Brauer H, et al. On the therapeutic effects of trivalent and divalent iron in iron deficiency anaemia. *Arzneimittelforschung.* 1984;**34**:1575–79.

11 Devasthali SD, Gordeuk VR, Brittenham GM, et al. Bioavailability of carbonyl iron: a randomized, double-blind study. *Eur J Haematol.* 1991;**46**:272–78.

12 Gordeuk VR, Brittenham GM, Hughes M, et al. High-dose carbonyl iron for iron deficiency anemia: a randomized double-blind trial. *Am J Clin Nutr.* 1987;**46**:1029–34.

13 Hamstra RD, Block MH, Schocket AL. Intravenous iron dextran in clinical medicine. *JAMA.* 1980;**243**:1726–31.

14 Silverstein SB, Rodgers GM. Parenteral iron therapy options. *Am J Hematol.* 2004;**76**:74–8.

15 Michael B, Coyne DW, Fishbane S, et al. Sodium ferric gluconate complex in hemodialysis patients: adverse reactions compared to placebo and iron dextran. *Kidney Int.* 2002;**61**:1830–39.

16 Michael B, Coyne DW, Folkert VW, et al. Sodium ferric gluconate complex in haemodialysis patients: a prospective evaluation of long-term safety. *Nephrol Dial Transplant.* 2004;**19**:1576–80.

17 Faich G, Strobos J. Sodium ferric gluconate complex in sucrose: safer intravenous iron therapy than iron dextrans. *Am J Kidney Dis.* 1999;**33**:464–70.

18 Chertow GM, Mason PD, Vaage-Nilsen O, et al. Update on adverse drug events associated with parenteral iron. *Nephrol Dial Transplant.* 2006;**21**:378–82.

19 Kosch M, Bahner U, Bettger H, et al. A randomized, controlled parallel-group trial on efficacy and safety of iron sucrose (Venofer) vs iron gluconate (Ferrlecit) in haemodialysis patients treated with rHuEpo. *Nephrol Dial Transplant.* 2001;**16**:1239–44.

20 Laman CA, Silverstein SB, Rodgers GM. Parenteral iron therapy: a single institution's experience over a 5-year period. *J Natl Compr Canc Netw.* 2005;**3**:791–95.

21 Eichbaum Q, Foran S, Dzik S. Is iron gluconate really safer than iron dextran? *Blood.* 2003;**101**:3756–57.

22 Agarwal R, Rizkala AR, Bastani B, et al. A randomized controlled trial of oral versus intravenous iron in chronic kidney disease. *Am J Nephrol.* 2006;**26**:445–54.

23 Aggarwal HK, Nand N, Singh S, et al. Comparison of oral versus intravenous iron therapy in predialysis patients of chronic renal failure receiving recombinant human erythropoietin. *J Assoc Physicians India.* 2003;**51**:170–74.

24 Charytan C, Qunibi W, Bailie GR. Comparison of intravenous iron sucrose to oral iron in the treatment of anemic patients with chronic kidney disease not on dialysis. *Nephron Clin Pract.* 2005;**100**: c55–c62.

25 Stoves J, Inglis H, Newstead CG. A randomized study of oral vs intravenous iron supplementation in patients with progressive renal insufficiency treated with erythropoietin. *Nephrol Dial Transplant.* 2001;**16**:967–74.

26 Van Wyck DB, Roppolo M, Martinez CO, et al. A randomized, controlled trial comparing IV iron sucrose to oral iron in anemic patients with nondialysis-dependent CKD. *Kidney Int.* 2005;**68**:2846–56.

27 Auerbach M, Ballard H, Trout JR, et al. Intravenous iron optimizes the response to recombinant human erythropoietin in cancer patients with chemotherapy-related anemia: a multicenter, open-label, randomized trial. *J Clin Oncol.* 2004;**22**:1301–7.

28 Henry DH, Dahl NV, Auerbach M, et al. Intravenous ferric gluconate significantly improves response to epoetin alfa versus oral iron or no iron in anemic patients with cancer receiving chemotherapy. *Oncologist.* 2007;**12**:231–42.

29 Schroder O, Mickisch O, Seidler U, et al. Intravenous iron sucrose versus oral iron supplementation for the treatment of iron deficiency anemia in patients with inflammatory bowel disease—a randomized, controlled, open-label, multicenter study. *Am J Gastroenterol.* 2005;**100**:2503–9.

30 Erichsen K, Ulvik RJ, Nysaeter G, et al. Oral ferrous fumarate or intravenous iron sucrose for patients with inflammatory bowel disease. *Scand J Gastroenterol.* 2005;**40**:1058–65.

31 Al RA, Unlubilgin E, Kandemir O, et al. Intravenous versus oral iron for treatment of anemia in pregnancy: a randomized trial. *Obstet Gynecol.* 2005;**106**:1335–40.

32 Bayoumeu F, Subiran-Buisset C, Baka NE, et al. Iron therapy in iron deficiency anemia in pregnancy: intravenous route versus oral route. *Am J Obstet Gynecol.* 2002;**186**:518–22.

33 Singh K, Fong YF, Kuperan P. A comparison between intravenous iron polymaltose complex (Ferrum Hausmann) and oral ferrous fumarate in the treatment of iron deficiency anaemia in pregnancy. *Eur J Haematol.* 1998;**60**:119–24.

34 Al-Momen AK, al-Meshari A, al-Nuaim L, et al. Intravenous iron sucrose complex in the treatment of iron deficiency anemia during pregnancy. *Eur J Obstet Gynecol Reprod Biol.* 1996;**69**:121–24.

35 Rimon E, Levy S, Sapir A, et al. Diagnosis of iron deficiency anemia in the elderly by transferrin receptor-ferritin index. *Arch Intern Med.* 2002;**162**:445–49.

36 Chen YC, Hung SC, Tarng DC. Association between transferrin receptor-ferritin index and conventional measures of iron responsiveness in hemodialysis patients. *Am J Kidney Dis.* 2006;**47**:1036–44.

37 Choi JW. Sensitivity, specificity, and predictive value of serum soluble transferrin receptor at different stages of iron deficiency. *Ann Clin Lab Sci.* 2005;**35**:435–39.

38 Lee EJ, Oh EJ, Park YJ, et al. Soluble transferrin receptor (sTfR), ferritin, and sTfR/log ferritin index in anemic patients with nonhematologic malignancy and chronic inflammation. *Clin Chem.* 2002;**48**:1118–21.

39 Savage DG, Lindenbaum J, Stabler SP, et al. Sensitivity of serum methylmalonic acid and total homocysteine determinations for diagnosing cobalamin and folate deficiencies. *Am J Med.* 1994;**96**: 239–46.

40 Clarke R, Refsum H, Birks J, et al. Screening for vitamin B-12 and folate deficiency in older persons. *Am J Clin Nutr.* 2003;**77**:1241–1247.

41 Bolann BJ, Solli JD, Schneede J, et al. Evaluation of indicators of cobalamin deficiency defined as cobalamin-induced reduction in increased serum methylmalonic acid. *Clin Chem.* 2000;**46**:1744–50.

42 Kuzminski AM, Del Giacco EJ, Allen RH, et al. Effective treatment of cobalamin deficiency with oral cobalamin. *Blood.* 1998;**92**:1191–98.

43 Lane LA, Rojas-Fernandez C. Treatment of vitamin B(12)-deficiency anemia: oral versus parenteral therapy. *Ann Pharmacother.* 2002;**36**:1268–72.

44 Bowdler AJ. The role of the spleen and splenectomy in autoimmune hemolytic disease. *Semin Hematol.* 1976;**13**:335–48.

45 Allgood JW, Chaplin H Jr. Idiopathic acquired autoimmune hemolytic anemia: a review of forty-seven cases treated from 1955 through 1965. *Am J Med.* 1967;**43**:254–73.

46 Schwartz SI, Bernard RP, Adams JT, et al. Splenectomy for hematologic disorders. *Arch Surg.* 1970;**101**:338–47.

47 Coon WW. Splenectomy in the treatment of hemolytic anemia. *Arch Surg.* 1985;**120**:625–28.

48 Balague C, Targarona EM, Cerdan G, et al. Long-term outcome after laparoscopic splenectomy related to hematologic diagnosis. *Surg Endosc.* 2004;**18**:1283–87.

49 Gibson J. Autoimmune hemolytic anemia: current concepts. *Aust N Z J Med.* 1988;**18**:625–37.

50 Pirofsky B, Bardana EJ Jr. Autoimmune hemolytic anemia. II. Therapeutic aspects. *Ser Haematol.* 1974;**7**:376–85.

51 Katkhouda N, Hurwitz MB, Rivera RT, et al. Laparoscopic splenectomy: outcome and efficacy in 103 consecutive patients. *Ann Surg.* 1998;**228**:568–78.

52 Akpek G, McAneny D, Weintraub L. Comparative response to splenectomy in Coombs-positive autoimmune hemolytic anemia with or without associated disease. *Am J Hematol.* 1999;**61**:98–102.

53 King KE, Ness PM. Treatment of autoimmune hemolytic anemia. *Semin Hematol.* 2005;**42**:131–36.

54 Narat S, Gandla J, Hoffbrand AV, et al. Rituximab in the treatment of refractory autoimmune cytopenias in adults. *Haematologica.* 2005;**90**:1273–74.

55 Shanafelt TD, Madueme HL, Wolf RC, et al. Rituximab for immune cytopenia in adults: idiopathic thrombocytopenic purpura, autoimmune hemolytic anemia, and Evans syndrome. *Mayo Clin Proc.* 2003;**78**:1340–46.

56 Zecca M, Nobili B, Ramenghi U, et al. Rituximab for the treatment of refractory autoimmune hemolytic anemia in children. *Blood.* 2003;**101**:3857–61.

57 Quartier P, Brethon B, Philippet P, et al. Treatment of childhood autoimmune haemolytic anaemia with rituximab. *Lancet.* 2001;**358**: 1511–13.

58 Heidel F, Lipka DB, von AC, et al. Addition of rituximab to standard therapy improves response rate and progression-free survival in relapsed or refractory thrombotic thrombocytopenic purpura and autoimmune haemolytic anaemia. *Thromb Haemost.* 2007;**97**:228–33.

59 Ramanathan S, Koutts J, Hertzberg MS. Two cases of refractory warm autoimmune hemolytic anemia treated with rituximab. *Am J Hematol.* 2005;**78**:123–26.

60 Flores G, Cunningham-Rundles C, Newland AC, et al. Efficacy of intravenous immunoglobulin in the treatment of autoimmune hemolytic anemia: results in 73 patients. *Am J Hematol.* 1993;**44**: 237–42.

61 Sherer Y, Levy Y, Fabbrizzi F, et al. Treatment of hematologic disorders other than immune thrombocytopenic purpura with intravenous immunoglobulin (IVIg)—report of seven cases and review of the literature. *Eur J Intern Med.* 2000;**11**:85–88.

62 Besa EC. Rapid transient reversal of anemia and long-term effects of maintenance intravenous immunoglobulin for autoimmune hemolytic anemia in patients with lymphoproliferative disorders. *Am J Med.* 1988;**84**:691–98.

63 Mitchell CA, Van der Weyden MB, Firkin BG. High dose intravenous gammaglobulin in Coombs positive hemolytic anemia. *Aust N Z J Med.* 1987;**17**:290–94.

64 Anderson D, Ali K, Blanchette V, et al. Guidelines on the use of intravenous immune globulin for hematologic conditions. *Transfus Med Rev.* 2007;**21**:S9–S56.

65 Berentsen S, Ulvestad E, Gjertsen BT, et al. Rituximab for primary chronic cold agglutinin disease: a prospective study of 37 courses of therapy in 27 patients. *Blood.* 2004;**103**:2925–28.

66 Schollkopf C, Kjeldsen L, Bjerrum OW, et al. Rituximab in chronic cold agglutinin disease: a prospective study of 20 patients. *Leuk Lymphoma.* 2006;**47**:253–60.

25 Immune Thrombocytopenic Purpura

James N. George, Sara K. Vesely, George R. Buchanan

Introduction

Evaluation and management of immune thrombocytopenic purpura (ITP) in children and adults has been comprehensively reviewed for the purpose of establishing practice guidelines by the American Society of Hematology (ASH) in 1996 (1) and subsequently by the British Committee for Standards in Haematology (BCSH), a task force of the British Society for Haematology (2). The ASH guideline was developed from a systematic literature review performed in April 1994 that was supplemented by an explicit analysis of the panel's expert opinion using a modified RAND scoring system (3). A major conclusion of the ASH guideline was that there was little scientific evidence to guide clinical decisions (4,5). The BCSH guideline was also developed from a systematic literature review, completed before 2003 (2). Two additional recent practice guidelines for the evaluation and management of childhood ITP have been published: by the Associazione Italiana di Ematologia e Oncologia Pediatrica (AIEOP), based on a systematic literature review and a consensus conference by the Japanese Society of Pediatric Hematology, based on analysis of a questionnaire sent to society members (6,7).

Additional data were obtained from a literature search using Ovid software to search the MEDLINE database from 1994 (the date of our previous literature search [1]) to December 2006, using search terms for ITP (8) combined with the phrases "randomized controlled trials," "randomized clinical trials," "systematic reviews," "meta-analysis," "guidelines," and "practice guidelines" as keywords and/or MeSH to identify articles with important clinical evidence. The quality of the evidence and the strength of the recommendation were classified according to the American Thoracic Society guidelines and recommendations statement (9).

These guidelines and the additional data from our current literature search provide a basis for current clinical practice and a foundation for this chapter. Chapter organization is based on clinical questions, outlined in Table 25.1.

Evidence-based Hematology. Edited by Mark A. Crowther, Jeff Ginsberg, Holger J. Schünemann, Ralph M. Meyer, and Richard Lottenberg.

Definition

ITP was defined in the ASH guideline as "isolated thrombocytopenia with no clinically apparent associated conditions or other causes of thrombocytopenia. No specific criteria establish the diagnosis; the diagnosis relies on the exclusion of other causes of thrombocytopenia" (1). This remains the standard definition of ITP; it is critical for all considerations of evaluation and management. Although ITP is a relatively common autoimmune disorder, with an annual incidence of approximately 5 per 10^5 in children (10,11) and 2 per 10^5 in adults (12,13) as determined by population-based studies, there should always be concern for potential alternative etiologies of isolated thrombocytopenia.

Pathogenesis

What is the role of impaired platelet production in the pathogenesis of thrombocytopenia? ITP has been classically considered a result of increased platelet destruction by antiplatelet autoantibodies. This was dramatically documented many years ago by infusion of whole blood and plasma from ITP patients into normal subjects (14); increasing doses of plasma caused more severe thrombocytopenia (15). However, there is evidence that ineffective platelet production also contributes to thrombocytopenia in patients with ITP: (1) Kinetic studies with autologous ^{111}In-labeled platelets demonstrated that 16 of 17 patients with untreated ITP had normal or decreased platelet production, not the expected compensatory increase of platelet production (16). (2) Serum thrombopoietin levels are not increased in patients with ITP, in contrast to patients with aplastic anemia (17). (3) Plasma from ITP patients suppressed in vitro megakaryocyte development (18,19). (4) Megakaryocytes from ITP patients demonstrated ultrastructural features of apoptosis (20).

Table 25.1 Chapter outline: clinical questions, evidence, and recommendations.*

Definition	Data, interpretation	Evidence	Grade (Recommendation, evidence)
DIAGNOSIS			
Should a bone marrow examination be done as part of the diagnostic evaluation for ITP in children and adults?	Unnecessary for children	1 case series	Weak recommendation; very low-quality evidence
	Unnecessary for adults	1 case series	Weak recommendation; very low-quality evidence
CLINICAL COURSE			
What is the rate of development of chronic ITP in children?	Approximately two-thirds in untreated children within 6 months	Multiple case series (1)	Weak recommendation; very low-quality evidence
Do any presenting features of children with ITP predict progression to chronic disease?	Adolescents, especially girls	Case series (31)	Weak recommendation; very low-quality evidence
What is the rate of death from bleeding?	Children—about 0.2%	Systematic review (33)	Weak recommendation; low-quality evidence
	Adults—about 0.5%	2 cases series (13,34)	Weak recommendation; very low-quality evidence
MANAGEMENT			
Children			
Does initial treatment result in more rapid increase of the platelet count?	Treatment with steroids or IVIg increased platelet count more rapidly than when no treatment was administered	Randomized clinical trial (44)	Strong recommendation; moderate-quality evidence
	Treatment with IVIg more likely to raise platelet count above 20,000/μL at 48 hours than steroids	Meta-analysis (33)	Strong recommendation; high-quality evidence
	Anti-D as effective as IVIg at raising platelet count in 24 hours	Randomized clinical trial (45)	Strong recommendation; moderate-quality evidence
Does initial treatment alter the clinical course and long-term outcome?	No published data documenting that specific drug treatment decreased the rate of intracranial hemorrhage, other life-threatening bleeding, or death	No published data	No recommendation
	Suggestion that children treated with IVIg were less likely to develop chronic ITP (18% vs. 25%; $p = 0.04$)	Meta-analysis (33)	Weak recommendation; moderate-quality evidence
Adults			
Is there a threshold presenting platelet count above which patients can be safely observed without drug treatment?	Patients with platelet counts $\geq$30,000/μL had no clinically important bleeding manifestations	3 case series (13,34,49)	Weak recommendation; very low-quality evidence
When splenectomy is considered: (1) What is the rate of complete response? (2) Are there any clinical features that can predict response? (3) What is the mortality and morbidity?	(1) 66% of patients achieved a complete response	Systematic review (54)	Weak recommendation; low-quality evidence
	(2) No clinical features consistently predicted response	Systematic review (54)	Weak recommendation; low-quality evidence
	(3) Mortality for laparoscopy is 0.2%; morbidity is about 10%	Systematic review (54)	Weak recommendation; low-quality evidence
When severe thrombocytopenia persists following splenectomy, what are the outcomes with different treatments and what is the most effective treatment?	Few published cases series	Systematic review (8)	Weak recommendation; low-quality evidence
What is the evidence for efficacy of investigational agents that increase platelet production, rather than decrease accelerated platelet destruction?	AMG 531—thrombopoiesis-stimulating agent increased platelet counts	Phase I study (60)	Weak recommendation; very low-quality evidence

*ITP, immune thrombocytopenic purpura; IVIg, intravenous immunoglobulin.

The data describing ineffective thrombopoiesis in patients with ITP have assumed clinical importance in relation to new treatments directed toward increasing platelet production.

Diagnosis

The ASH guideline stated that for both children and adults "the diagnosis of ITP is based principally on the history, physical examination, complete blood count, and examination of the peripheral smear, which should exclude other causes of thrombocytopenia. Further diagnostic studies are generally not indicated in the routine work-up of patients with suspected ITP, assuming that the history, physical examination, and blood counts are compatible with the diagnosis of ITP and do not include atypical findings that are uncommon in ITP or suggest other etiologies" (1).

The definition of ITP emphasizes the diagnosis is based on the exclusion of other causes of isolated thrombocytopenia. The most common alternative diagnosis in adults with initially suspected ITP is drug-induced thrombocytopenia (13). A series of systematic reviews has critically evaluated all published reports describing patients with drug-induced thrombocytopenia through October 20, 2006 (21,22) using a priori criteria to assess the strength of evidence for the drug as the cause of thrombocytopenia. The complete database of citations and their assessment is accessible at http://w3.ouhsc.edu.platelets. One limitation of this database is that it is restricted to licensed drugs (21) and does not include foods (23) and herbal remedies (24) that may also be occult etiologies of isolated thrombocytopenia. Another limitation is that reports of potential drug-induced thrombocytopenia in children are not included (21). A drug-induced etiology may not be appreciated until repeated explicit histories are obtained. Drug-induced immune thrombocytopenia is rare in children and adolescents.

Should a bone marrow examination be done as part of the diagnostic evaluation for ITP in children and adults? The ASH guideline explicitly addressed the question of bone marrow aspiration/biopsy to establish the diagnosis of ITP in all adult patients and presented the results of the systematic analysis the panel's opinion (1). The range of opinions was revealing and reflected the absence of evidence, resulting in a conclusion of "uncertain appropriateness or necessity" with "strong disagreement"(1). In spite of the absence of evidence, the guideline recommended bone marrow examination as "appropriate," with only "moderate" panel agreement, for patients over 60 years old, because of concern for the potential alternative etiology of myelodysplasia (1). The ASH guideline also stated a routine bone marrow aspirate/biopsy is unnecessary for children (1). The publication of the ASH guideline stimulated the performance of three retrospective record reviews that supported the opinion that a bone marrow examination is not necessary for the routine diagnostic evaluation of ITP in adults (25,26) and children (27).

Platelet antibody tests were also considered to be unnecessary, based on opinion, to establish the diagnosis of ITP in all children and adults at presentation (1). Although two recent prospective studies of newly developed platelet glycoprotein-specific immunoassays for antiplatelet antibodies have concluded that they were diagnostically "useful" in adults with ITP, their sensitivities of 53% and 55% and specificities of 82% and 84% (28,29) indicate their limitations and suggest that even these newer assays are also unnecessary to establish the diagnosis of ITP.

Recommendations for diagnosis by the BCSH, AIEOP, and Japanese guidelines were similar (2,6.7).

Clinical course

Children

In children, ITP typically has an acute onset and spontaneous remission.

What is the rate of development of chronic ITP in children? Multiple case series have reported that ITP resolves in approximately two-thirds of untreated children within six months (1) and that spontaneous remissions continue to occur after six months (30).

Do any presenting features of children with ITP predict progression to chronic disease? Some case series suggest that adolescents, especially adolescent girls, have a greater risk for a chronic course, defined as a platelet count <150,000/μL at six months, similar to the clinical course of adults (31). No other presenting features have been demonstrated to predict progression to chronic ITP.

These observations form the basis for management decisions. Since most children will spontaneously recover, no drug treatment may be necessary unless clinically important bleeding occurs. If treatment is given to increase the platelet count in the absence of severe bleeding, the goal should be to minimize the intensity and duration of treatment to limit side effects, inconvenience, and cost.

What is the rate of death from bleeding? Intracranial hemorrhage is the most serious complication of ITP in children (32), but death from hemorrhage is very rare. In a recent systematic review, 3 (0.5%) of 586 children had an intracranial hemorrhage; 2 survived; the child who died from bleeding had a concomitant severe viral infection (33). This mortality rate of 0.2% in this report (33) is similar to other large case series (1).

Adults

In contrast to children, spontaneous remissions are rare in adults (1). This strengthens the consideration for disease-modifying treatment more often than in children. The clinical course of adults with ITP can be estimated from two large case series with a total of 397 consecutive patients and median follow-up durations of 10 (34) and 5 years (13). These case series document the safety of no treatment in patients with platelet counts over 30,000/μL (13,34).

What is the rate of death from bleeding? Death from bleeding (without other comorbid conditions) was rare, occurring in only 2

Table 25.2 Initial management of children with severe thrombocytopenia but minor bleeding symptoms: percentage of pediatric hematologists in the United States and United Kingdom who would manage the child with observation, without specific drug treatment.*

	1995, 1997	2000, 2001
U.S.	16%	14%
U.K.	40%	63%

*Data from audits of U.K. pediatric hematologists in 1995 (38) and 2000 (39) and questionnaires mailed to members of the American Society of Pediatric Hematology/Oncology in 1997 (42) and 2001 (43).

(0.5%) of 397 patients (13,34). However, death from complications of treatment was more common, occurring in 5 (1%) of 397 patients. At the end of follow-up in these two case series, 85% (34) and 91% (13) of patients had either a normal platelet count or an asymptomatic platelet count over 30,000/μL without treatment. These observations are important to assess the relative benefits and risks of pharmacologic therapy.

Management

Children

Initial management

The important issue for initial management of children with ITP who do not present with severe bleeding is whether to observe them and provide support without specific pharmacologic intervention or whether to intervene with specific drug treatment. The difference in initial management practice between the United States and the United Kingdom and Europe is striking (Table 25.2), reflecting the absence of clear evidence for outcomes.

United Kingdom guidelines published in 1992 (35) and German guidelines published in 1999 (36) for management of children with ITP, based on opinion, have recommended that children who present with only cutaneous bleeding (bruising, purpura, and petechiae) and little or no mucosal hemorrhage should be managed by observation alone regardless of the severity of thrombocytopenia; specific drug treatment was advised only for children with overt bleeding. The safety of this approach was then demonstrated in a prospective study of 55 consecutive, unselected children in Germany (37). Only four children who had active mucosal bleeding received drug treatment (with a three-day course of prednisone); no critical bleeding or deaths occurred (37). In the United Kingdom, an audit of pediatricians and pediatric hematologists in 1995, with a 76% response rate to questionnaires, demonstrated substantial variation in practice, with more drug treatment and use of platelet transfusions than had been recommended (38). Overall 60% of children received some form of drug treatment, approximately equal between steroids and intravenous immunoglobulin (IVIg) (38). The national audit was repeated in 2000 to assess the results of a publicity and education campaign directed at primary care physicians about the United Kingdom guidelines (35). A significant trend for more observation without specific drug treatment was noted (63% of children compared to 40% in the 1995 audit; Table 25.2) (39).

Children with a new diagnosis of ITP in the United States and Canada receive drug treatment more frequently than in the United Kingdom or Europe, based solely on the severity of thrombocytopenia, whether or not bleeding signs are present (Table 25.2). This is consistent with the ASH guideline that recommended treatment with IVIg or steroids for children with platelet counts less than 20,000/μL and only minor purpura, although this recommendation was based on only a marginal panel opinion score with moderate disagreement (1). The controversial nature of this recommendation was emphasized by the criticism that followed publication of the guideline (40,41). Practice patterns of pediatric hematologists in the United States and Canada were documented in two surveys of the membership of the American Society of Pediatric Hematology/Oncology in 1997 (42) and 2001 (43). In both surveys, in response to a hypothetical scenario of a child with severe thrombocytopenia (platelet counts, 3,000/μL and 7,000/μL) but only minor purpura, few hematologists indicated that they would observe the child without specific drug treatment: 16% (42) and 14% (43) (Table 25.2). The second survey documented increased use of anti-D as initial treatment for the hypothetical case (43). Although the difference between the practice in the United Kingdom and the United States is striking, the different methodologies of these assessments may make these two set of data difficult to compare.

Does initial treatment result in more rapid increase of the platelet count? There is firm evidence from randomized trials that treatment of children with either steroids or IVIg increases the platelet count more rapidly than when no specific treatment is administered (44). A recent systematic review and meta-analysis of randomized trials comparing steroids with IVIg for the initial treatment of children with ITP and a platelet count <20,000/μL documented that children treated with IVIg were more likely to achieve a platelet count over 20,000/μL at 48 hours (33).

A randomized trial comparing IVIg to anti-D for initial treatment of children with ITP demonstrated that anti-D at a dose of 75 μg/kg was as effective as IVIg (0.8 gm/kg) at increasing the platelet count at 24 hours (45). An expected side effect of anti-D is immune hemolysis. In this trial, hemoglobin concentrations at day 7 decreased by 2.0 gm/L in children treated with 75 μg/kg anti-D and 0.3 gm/L in children treated with IVIg (45). Anti-D also may rarely cause acute intravascular hemolysis with disseminated intravascular coagulation and acute renal failure (46).

Does initial treatment alter the clinical course and long-term outcome? Although the above data are interpreted to indicate that IVIg and anti-D are effective and appropriate treatments because children have shorter exposure to severe thrombocytopenia (33,45), no published data document that specific drug

Table 25.3 Management of adults with ITP.*

Management	Evidence	Grade (Recommendation, Evidence)
Initial management		
Observation with no specific drug treatment if platelet count >30,000/μL and no important bleeding symptoms	3 large case series: 108 of 486 patients with platelet counts >30,000/μL; median follow-up, 3–10 years (13,34,49)	Weak recommendation; very low-quality of evidence
Prednisone, 1 mg/kg/d if platelet count <30,000/μL	Many case series; no consistent data	Weak recommendation; very low-quality of evidence
Dexamethasone, 40 mg/d × 4 days platelet count <30,000/μL	1 cohort study of 125 patients; 43% responses with median follow-up of 31 months (51)	Weak recommendation; very low-quality of evidence
Splenectomy		
Response: 66% durable complete response	Systematic review identified 135 case series across 58 years and from 29 countries (54)	Weak recommendation; low-quality of evidence
Prediction of response: no preoperative features consistently predict response		Weak recommendation; low-quality of evidence
Surgical complications: 0.2%–1.0% death; 9.6%–12.9% complications		Weak recommendation; low-quality of evidence
Management of chronic refractory ITP		
Current therapies: no information is available to guide management decisions	Systematic review identified 90 articles reporting 656 patients treated with 22 therapies. Only small case series without controls; no studies compared one therapy to another or therapy to no therapy (8)	Weak recommendation; very low-quality of evidence
Investigational therapy thrombopoietin receptor agonist	Small placebo-controlled randomized clinical trial (21 patients) suggested efficacy (58)	Weak recommendation; very low-quality of evidence

*ITP, immune thrombocytopenic purpura.

treatment decreases the rate of intracranial hemorrhage, other life-threatening hemorrhage, or death in children with ITP. In fact, one retrospective study of steroid or IVIg administered to children with ITP and severe bleeding demonstrated minimal or delayed increases in the platelet count (47).

A secondary outcome of the meta-analysis of randomized trials comparing steroids with IVIg was the suggestion that children treated with IVIg were less likely to develop chronic ITP: 18% of children treated with IVIg versus 25% of children treated with steroids had a platelet count less than 150,000/μL after six months ($p = 0.04$) (33). If this observation about treatment with IVIg is reproduced and is valid, the potential mechanism is unknown.

Management of chronic ITP

For children with chronic ITP, splenectomy has been a standard treatment for the past 50 years. Complete responses, described as a normal platelet count with no additional treatment for the duration of observation, are reported in 72% of children (1). For children in whom splenectomy was contraindicated or was unsuccessful, a phase I/II clinical trial of rituximab reported a response, defined as a platelet count >50,000/μL for four consecutive weeks, in 11 (31%) of 36 patients (48). Although a limitation of this study was the short observation time of 16 weeks (48), these data documented the safety and potential efficacy of rituximab treatment for children with chronic severe ITP. Similar to management of adults (discussed below), rituximab may now be a principal treatment of chronic ITP in children, together with splenectomy, replacing less targeted and more cytotoxic immunosuppressive agents.

Adults

Initial management

Is there a threshold presenting platelet count above which patients can be safely observed without drug treatment? Large case series have supported the safety of initial management with observation, without specific treatment, for patients with platelet counts >30,000/μL and no clinically important bleeding manifestations. In three cohort studies of consecutive patients, 49 of 117 (49), 28 of 124 (34), and 31 of 245 patients (13) had platelet counts >30,000/μL, received no drug treatment, and had no significant bleeding for the duration of follow-up (median, 3–10 years) (Table 25.3).

The common practice for adults with a new diagnosis of ITP is to initiate treatment with steroids when the platelet count is <30,000/μL, even if there are no symptoms (Table 25.3) (1). The rationale for this practice is that the thrombocytopenia is assumed to be persistent and that adults, particularly older individuals, may have greater risk for bleeding than children (49) because of potential comorbidities, such as hypertension, gastrointestinal disorders, and exposure to antiplatelet medications.

Therapy is typically begun with daily oral prednisone, 1 mg/kg (Table 25.3). There is no standard of practice regarding the duration of treatment or tapering schedule. Case series suggest that approximately 80% of patients will have an increased platelet count with this treatment but that thrombocytopenia will usually recur when the prednisone is decreased or discontinued (1). A randomized trial demonstrated that IVIg (0.4 gm/kg/d for five days) was not more effective than prednisone (1 mg/kg/d) as initial treatment (50).

A recent report described 125 consecutive adult patients with an initial diagnosis of ITP and platelet count <20,000/μL who received treatment with a single four-day course of dexamethasone, 40 mg/d (51). One hundred and six patients (85%) responded with platelet counts >50,000/μL, and 53 (50%) of these patients maintained this response with no further treatment during a median of 30.5 months of follow-up (51). This regimen, adapted from treatment of multiple myeloma, has the important advantage of a well-defined and brief duration without need for tapering (Table 25.3). These results were confirmed and extended in two subsequent cohort studies (52). In the first trial, 37 previously untreated adult patients with platelet counts <20,000/μL received six cycles of dexamethasone, 40 mg/d for four days repeated every four weeks. Thirty-one (84%) responded with platelet counts >50,000/μL, 23 (62%) of whom had normal platelet counts (>150,000/μL); relapse-free survival was estimated to be 90% at 15 months and 53% at 50 months (52). In the subsequent study, 95 patients were treated with four cycles of dexamethasone given every 14 days. Seventy-four (85%) responded with platelet counts >50,000/μL and 58 of them (65%) had normal platelet counts (>150,000/μL); relapse-free survival was 81% at 15 months (52). This group (GIMEMA, or Gruppo Italiano Malattie Ematologiche dell'Adulto) is currently conducting a randomized trial comparing three cycles of high-dose dexamethasone to standard prednisone therapy (1 mg/kg/d) (52).

IVIg at a dose of 1 gm/kg/d for two days is recommended, together with high-dose parenteral glucocorticoid and platelet transfusions, for patients with severe thrombocytopenia and critical bleeding (1). There is no evidence that IVIg is more effective than glucocorticoids in the management of patients without critical bleeding.

Anti-D is also commonly used in adults to provide transient increases of the platelet count. One randomized controlled clinical trial tested the hypothesis that regular treatments with anti-D, compared with standard care with prednisone, would decrease the requirement for prednisone and avoid the need for splenectomy (53). The rationale was that with effective and sustained initial therapy, not feasible with prednisone because of side effects, a high frequency of spontaneous remissions may be revealed in adults with ITP. The results of the clinical trial were that splenectomy was not avoided; 14 (42%) of 33 patients treated with anti-D compared with 14 (38%) of 37 patients managed with steroids had a splenectomy (53). However, the regular treatments with anti-D did temporarily defer splenectomy (53).

Management of persistent ITP: splenectomy

When splenectomy is considered, what is the rate of complete response? Following failure of initial prednisone, the traditional next treatment for the past 50 years has been splenectomy. Splenectomy may be the most effective overall treatment for ITP, with 66% of patients achieving a complete response, defined as normal platelet count (>150,000/μL) despite no treatment for at least 30 days and for the duration of observation (54). These data were obtained from a systematic review of all case series of adults with splenectomy for ITP through February 2004 (Table 25.3) (54). Response to splenectomy was assessed in 47 case series describing ≥15 adult patients: 1,731 (66%) of 2,623 patients had a complete response with a median follow-up of 29 months; 1,853 (88%) of 2,116 had a complete or partial response (54). Case series that included children (who could not be distinguished from adults) were analyzed separately because children appeared to have better responses to splenectomy. In 38 case series that included up to 25% children each, the complete response rate was 72% (54). These results were consistent across 58 years of publications from 29 countries (54). Although the median relapse rate was 15%, the overall durability of the response to splenectomy was documented by the observation that there was no correlation between complete response rates and duration of follow-up when all 85 case series were analyzed (54).

When splenectomy is considered, are there any clinical features that can predict response? This systematic review also analyzed potential preoperative predictors of response; none consistently predicted the response to splenectomy (54). Among all of the prediction variables tested, younger age was most often associated with response, but an equal number of case series reported no correlation of patient age with response to splenectomy (54). These data, together with the high frequency of complete and partial responses, suggest that no preoperative parameter should contradict the decision for splenectomy when it is otherwise considered to be clinically appropriate.

What are the mortality and morbidity of splenectomy? The risks of splenectomy are significant, especially when balanced against the extremely low risk of death from bleeding in patients with ITP. Splenectomy performed by laparotomy had a 1% mortality (48 deaths in 4,955 patients), whereas splenectomy by laparoscopy had a 0.2% mortality (3 deaths in 1,301 patients) (Table 25.3) (54). The mortality rate for the laparoscopic procedure may more accurately reflect current surgical practice since the death rates in more recent case series of open and laparoscopic splenectomy are similar (54). Other postoperative complications occur in about 10% of patients following splenectomy (54). The risks of splenectomy may be even greater than these data suggest, because this systematic review (54) did not address the long-term complications of sepsis and thrombosis.

Because of concerns about complications, splenectomy for ITP is decreasing, as documented during the clinical trial of anti-D to prevent splenectomy when the frequency of splenectomy decreased from 53% (10 of 19 patients enrolled in 1997–1998) to 22% (4 of 18 patients enrolled in 1999–2000; $p = 0.06$) (53). The decreased rate of splenectomy is also apparent when the two recent large cohort studies are compared: among 152 consecutive patients diagnosed from 1974 to 1994 in the Netherlands, 78 (51%) had a splenectomy (34), whereas of 245 consecutive patients diagnosed from 1993 to 1999 in England, only 30 (12%) had a splenectomy (13).

Management of persistent ITP: rituximab

Although the decreasing frequency of splenectomy preceded the first reports of rituximab for ITP, increasing use of rituximab will probably further decrease the frequency of splenectomy. Although half of patients receiving rituximab for ITP have previously had an unsuccessful splenectomy (55) our current impression of community practice is that rituximab is being used earlier in the course of ITP, often following failure of initial prednisone treatment and before splenectomy.

To assess the efficacy and safety of rituximab for adults with ITP, a systematic review was conducted through April 2006. In 19 articles reporting 313 patients, 44% had a complete response (platelet count >150,000/μL) and 63% had a complete or partial response (platelet count >50,000/μL) (55). Essentially all of these patients had been treated with steroids, half had had a splenectomy, and many had received other treatments. However, this systematic review noted many limitations among these reports. (1) Additional drug treatments following response to rituximab were not described. (2) Small studies reporting high rates of response were overrepresented. (3) Median follow-up was only 9.5 months (55). The toxicities described in these reports were frequent and serious. Ten patients (3.7% of 306) had severe or life-threatening events and 9 (2.9%) died; 2 deaths may have been related to rituximab (55). This systematic review suggests that rituximab is not as effective as splenectomy for establishing durable complete responses, and rituximab may not in fact be safer than splenectomy (54,55).

Management of persistent ITP: other treatments

When severe thrombocytopenia persists following splenectomy, what is the most effective treatment? The enthusiasm for rituximab must in part result from patient and physician dissatisfaction with other treatments for ITP, which have usually been prescribed only after failure of glucocorticoids and splenectomy. For these patients with chronic refractory ITP (56), there has been no clear sequence of management strategies nor have there been randomized trials comparing one treatment to another, or treatment to no drug treatment.

In a systematic review of management of adults with chronic refractory ITP through September 2003, the remarkable conclusion was the surprisingly few evaluable patients who have been reported (8). For patients who most need treatment, that is, those with ITP for more than three months and platelet counts <10,000/μL despite splenectomy, there are very few reports. Only 111 patients could be identified who fulfilled these criteria among 289 articles describing 40 different therapies (Table 25.3) (8). Most other patients described in these 289 articles had less severe thrombocytopenia and may have had better responses to drug treatment or not needed it at all. This analysis emphasizes why there is no evidence to inform management of patients with severe and symptomatic thrombocytopenia following splenectomy (8). In addition to the few patients described, reported follow-up durations were short and outcomes other than platelet count responses were rarely described. For several of the seemingly successful treatments described, most or all of the patients with complete responses were reported from only one site (8). Before physicians can be confident about the best management for their patients, new approaches must be evaluated for safety as well as effectiveness in prospective cohort studies of consecutive patients as well as in randomized, controlled trials with measurements of clinical outcomes as well as platelet count responses.

Management of persistent ITP: investigational treatments

What is the evidence for efficacy of investigational agents that increase platelet production, rather than prevent accelerated platelet destruction? Since the evidence supporting the safety and effectiveness of current treatments for chronic, refractory ITP is weak, the opportunity to assess new pharmacologic approaches is strong. A new class of agents currently in development for patients is thrombopoiesis-stimulating drugs that increase platelet production rather than decrease antibody-mediated platelet destruction. The rationale for the development of these agents is the evidence that ITP is characterized by ineffective platelet production. The first agent in advanced clinical trials is AMG 531, a molecule that has no sequence homology with native thrombopoietin but binds to the thrombopoietin receptor on megakaryocytes, causing the same receptor-mediated signaling as native thrombopoietin (57). In the initial clinical trials, most ITP patients responded to doses of 1 to 3 μg/kg/week, including those with severe thrombocytopenia who had failed splenectomy and multiple other treatments (Table 25.3) (58,59). Patients enrolled in these clinical trials have subsequently been treated with adjusted doses to keep their platelet counts between 50,000 and 450,000/μL for over two years (60). In this long-term study, most patients had stable, safe platelet counts (60). One patient had diffuse reticulin formation in the marrow that resulted in discontinuation of treatment, an adverse event likely related to the increased number of marrow megakaryocytes (60). Other thrombopoiesis-stimulating agents are in development (61). It is exciting that this new class of agents may provide effective management for patients who currently are unresponsive to other treatment.

Conclusion

There are few rigorously designed clinical studies to document the long-term natural history of ITP and to guide patient evaluation and management. Therefore, recommendations are based on very limited evidence. These observations are important to emphasize the importance of further research on ITP.

References

1 George JN, Woolf SH, Raskob GE, et al. Idiopathic thrombocytopenic purpura: a practice guideline developed by explicit methods for the American Society of Hematology. *Blood.* 1996;**88**:3–40.

2 British Committee for Standards in Haematology. Guidelines for the investigation and management of idiopathic thrombocytopenic purpura in adults, children and in pregnancy. *Br J Haematol.* 2003;**120**:574–96.

3 Brook RH, Chassin M, Fink A, et al. *A method for the detailed assessment of the appropriateness of medical technologies. A RAND note.* N-3376-HHS. Santa Monica, CA: RAND Corp; 1991.

4 George JN, Davidoff F. Idiopathic thrombocytopenic purpura: lessons from a guideline. *Ann Int Med.* 1997;**126**:317–18.

5 Cook DJ, Giacomini M. The trials and tribulations of clinical practice guidelines. *JAMA.* 1999;**281**:1950–52.

6 De Mattia D, del Principe D, Del Vecchio GC, et al. Acute childhood idiopathic thrombocytopenic purpura: AIEOP consensus guidelines for diagnosis and treatment. *Haematologia.* 2000;**85**:420–24.

7 Shirahata A, Ishii E, Eguchi H, et al. Consensus guideline for diagnosis and treatment of childhood idiopathic thrombocytopenic purpura. *Int J Hematol.* 2006;**83**:29–38.

8 Vesely SK, Perdue JJ, Rizvi MA, et al. Management of adult patients with idiopathic thrombocytopenic purpura after failure of splenectomy: a systematic review. *Ann Int Med.* 2004;**140**:112–20.

9 Schunemann HJ, Jaeschke R, Cook DJ, et al. An official ATS statement: grading the quality of the evidence and strength of recommendations in ATS guidelines and recommendations. *Am J Respir Crit Care Med.* 2006;**174**:605–14.

10 Zeller B, Helgestad J, Hellebostad M, et al. Immune thrombocytopenic purpura in childhood in Norway: a prospective, population-based registration. *Pediatr Hematol Oncol.* 2000;**17**:551–58.

11 Zeller B, Rajantie J, Hedlund-Treutiger I, et al. Childhood idiopathic thrombocytopenic purpura in the Nordic countries: epidemiology and predictors of chronic disease. *Acta Paediatr.* 2005;**94**:178–84.

12 Frederiksen H, Schmidt K. The incidence of ITP in adults increases with age. *Blood.* 1999;**94**:909–13.

13 Neylon AJ, Saunders PWG, Howard MR, et al. Clinically significant newly presenting autoimmune thrombocytopenic purpura in adults: a prospective study of a population-based cohort of 245 patients. *Br J Haematol.* 2003;**122**:966–74.

14 Harrington WJ, Minnich V, Hollingsworth JW, et al. Demonstration of a thrombocytopenic factor in the blood of patients with thrombocytopenic purpura. *J Lab Clin Med.* 1951;**38**:1–10.

15 Shulman NR, Weinrach RS, Libre EP, et al. The role of the reticuloendothelial system in the pathogenesis of idiopathic thrombocytopenic purpura. *Trans Assoc Am Phys.* 1965;**78**:374–90.

16 Ballem PJ, Segal GM, Stratton JR, et al. Mechanisms of thrombocytopenia in chronic autoimmune thrombocytopenia purpura: evidence for both impaired platelet production and increased platelet clearance. *J Clin Invest.* 1987;**80**:33–40.

17 Aledort L, Hayward CPM, Chen M-G, et al. Prospective screening of 205 patients with ITP, including diagnosis, serological markers, and the relationship between platelet counts, endogenous thrombopoietin, and circulating antithrombopoietin antibodies. *Am J Hematol.* 2004;**76**:205–13.

18 Chang M, Nakagawa PA, Williams SA, et al. Immune thrombocytopenic purpura (ITP) plasma and purified ITP monoclonal autoantibodies inhibit megakaryocytopoiesis in vitro. *Blood.* 2003;**102**:887–95.

19 McMillan R, Wang L, Tomer A, et al. Suppression of in vitro megakaryocyte production by antiplatelet autoantibodies from adult patients with chronic ITP. *Blood.* 2004;**103**:1364–69.

20 Houweerzijl EJ, Blom NR, van der Want JJL, et al. Ultrastructural study shows morphologic features of apoptosis and para-apoptosis in megakaryocytes from patients with idiopathic thrombocyotpenic purpura. *Blood.* 2004;**103**:500–506.

21 George JN, Raskob GE, Shah SR, et al. Drug-induced thrombocytopenia: a systematic review of published case reports. *Ann Int Med.* 1998;**129**:886–90.

22 Li X, Swisher KK, Vesely SK, et al. Drug-induced thrombocytopenia: an updated systematic review, 2006. *Drug Safety.* 2007;**30**:185–6.

23 Arnold J, Ouwehand WH, Smith G, et al. A young woman with petechiae. *Lancet.* 1998;**352**:618.

24 Ohmori T, Nishii K, Hagihara A, et al. Acute thrombocytopenia induced by *Jui*, a traditional herbal medicine. *J Thromb Haemost.* 2004;**2**:1479–80.

25 Westerman DA, Grigg AP. The diagnosis of idiopathic thrombocytopenic purpura in adults: does bone marrow biopsy have a place? *Med J Aust.* 1999;**170**:216–17.

26 Jubelirer SJ, Harpold R. The role of the bone marrow examination in the diagnosis of immune thrombocytopenic purpura: case series and literature review. *Clin Appl Thromb Hemost.* 2002;**8**:73–76.

27 Calpin C, Dick P, Poon A, et al. Is bone marrow aspiration needed in acute childhood idiopathic thrombocytopenic purpura to rule out leukemia? *Arch Pediatr Adolesc Med.* 1998;**152**:345–47.

28 Davoren A, Bussel J, Curtis BR, et al. Prospective evaluation of a new platelet glycoprotein (GP)-specific assay (PakAuto) in the diagnosis of autoimmune thrombocytopenia (AITP). *Am J Hematol.* 2005;**78**:193–97.

29 McMillan R, Wang L, Tani P. Prospective evaluation of the immunobead assay for the diagnosis of adult chronic immune thrombocytopenic purpura (ITP). *J Thromb Haemost.* 2003;**1**:485–91.

30 Imbach P, Kuhne T, Muller D, et al. Childhood ITP: 12 months follow-up data from the prospective registry I of the intercontinental childhood ITP study group (ICIS). *Pediatr Blood Cancer.* 2006;**46**(3):351–56.

31 Lowe EJ, Buchanan GR. Idiopathic thrombocytopenic purpura diagnosed during the second decade of life. *J Pediatr.* 2002;**141**:253–58.

32 Butros LJ, Bussel JB. Intracranial hemorrhage in immune thrombocytopenia: a retrospective analysis. *J Pediatr Hematol Oncol.* 2003;**8**:660–64.

33 Beck CE, Nathan PC, Parkin PC, et al. Corticosteroids versus intravenous immune globulin for the treatment of acute immune thrombocytopenic purpura in children: a systematic review and meta-analysis of randomized controlled trials. *J Pediatr.* 2005;**147**:521–27.

34 Portielje JEA, Westendorp RGJ, Kluin-Nelemans HC, et al. Morbidity and mortality in adults with idiopathic thrombocytopenic purpura. *Blood.* 2001;**97**:2549–54.

35 Eden OB, Lilleyman JS, British Paediatric Haematology Group. Guidelines for management of idiopathic thrombocytopenic purpura. *Arch Dis Child.* 1992;**67**:1056–58.

36 Sutor AH, Dickerhoff R, Gaedicke G, et al. Hamostasiologie: Akute postinfektiose Immunthrombozytopenie im Kindesalter. In: Reinhard D, Creutzig U, Kiess W, et al., editors. *Leitlinien Kinderheilkunde und Jugendmedizin.* Munich: Urban & Fischer; 1999. p. 23–7.

37 Dickerhoff R, von Ruecker A. The clinical course of immune thrombocytopenic purpura in children who did not receive intravenous immunoglobulins or sustained prednisone treatment. *J Pediatr.* 2000;**137**:629–32.

38 Bolton-Maggs PHB, Moon I. Assessment of UK practice for management of acute childhood idiopathic thrombocytopenic purpura against published guidelines. *Lancet.* 1997;**350**:620–23.

39 Bolton-Maggs PHB, Moon I. National audit of the management of childhood idiopathic thrombocytopenic purpura against UK guidelines: closing the loop—education and re-audit demonstrate a change in practice. *Blood.* 2001;**98**:58b.

40 Buchanan GR, De Alarcon PA, Feig SA, et al. Acute idiopathic thrombocytopenic purpura—management in childhood. *Blood.* 1997;**89**:1464–65.

41 Bolton-Maggs PHB. Acute idiopathic thrombocytopenic purpura—management in childhood. *Blood.* 1997;**89**:1465.

42 Vesely SK, Buchanan GR, George JN, et al. Self-reported diagnostic and management strategies in childhood idiopathic thrombocytopenic purpura: results of a survey of practicing pediatric hematology/oncology specialists. *J Pediatr Hematol Oncol.* 2000;**22**:55–61.

43 Vesely SK, Buchanan GR, Adix L, et al. Self-reported initial management for childhood idiopathic thrombocytopenic purpura: results of a survey of members of the American Society of Pediatric Hematology/Oncology-2001. *J Pediatr Hematol Oncol.* 2003;**25**:130–33.

44 Blanchette VS, Luke B, Andrew M, et al. A prospective, randomized trial of high-dose intravenous immune globulin G therapy, oral prednisone therapy, and no therapy in childhood acute immune thrombocytopenic purpura. *J Pediatr.* 1993;**123**:989–95.

45 Tarantino MD, Young G, Bertolone SJ, et al. Single dose of anti-D immune globulin at 75 μg/kg is as effective as intravenous immune globulin at rapidly raising the platelet count in newly diagnosed immune thrombocytopenic purpura in children. *J Pediatr.* 2006;**148**:489–94.

46 Gaines AR. Disseminated intravascular coagulation associated with acute hemoglobinemia or hemoglobinuria following Rh immune globulin intravenous administration for immune thrombocytopenic purpura. *Blood.* 2005;**106**:1532–37.

47 Medeiros D, Buchanan GR. Major hemorrhage in children with idiopathic thrombocytopenic purpura: immediate response to therapy and long-term outcome. *J Pediatr.* 1998;**133**:334–39.

48 Bennett CM, Rogers ZR, Kinnamon DD, et al. Prospective phase I/II study of rituximab in childhood and adolescent chronic immune thrombocytopenic purpura. *Blood.* 2006;**107**:2639–42.

49 Cortelazzo S, Finazzi G, Buelli M, et al. High risk of severe bleeding in aged patients with chronic idiopathic thrombocytopenic purpura. *Blood.* 1991;**77**:31–33.

50 Jacobs P, Wood L, Novitzky N. Intravenous gammaglobulin has no advantages over oral corticosteroids as primary therapy for adults with immune thrombocytopenia: a prospective randomized clinical trial. *Am J Med.* 1994;**97**:55–59.

51 Cheng Y, Wong RSM, Soo YOY, et al. Initial treatment of immune thrombocytopenic purpura with high-dose dexamethasone. *N Engl J Med.* 2003;**349**:831–36.

52 Mazzucconi MG, Fazi P, Bernasconi S, et al. Therapy with high-dose dexamethasone (HD-DXM) in previously untreated patinets affected by idiopathic thormbocytopenic purpura. *Blood.* 2007;**109**:1401–7.

53 George JN, Raskob GE, Vesely SK, et al. Initial management of immune thrombocytopenic purpura in adults: a randomized controlled trial comparing intermittent anti-D with routine care. *Am J Hematol.* 2003;**74**:161–69.

54 Kojouri K, Vesely SK, Terrell DR, et al. Splenectomy for adult patients with idiopathic thrombocytopenic purpura: a systematic literature review to assess long-term platelet count responses, prediction of response, and surgical complications. *Blood.* 2004;**104**:2623–34.

55 Arnold DM, Dentali F, Crowther MA, et al. Systematic review: efficacy and safety of rituximab for adults with idiopathic thrombocytopenic purpura. *Ann Int Med.* 2007;**146**:25–33.

56 George JN. Management of patients with refractory immune thrombocytopenic purpura. *J Thromb Haemost.* 2006;**4**:1664–72.

57 Broudy VC, Lin NL. AMG531 stimulates megakaryocytopoiesis in vitro by binding to Mpl. *Cytokine.* 2004;**25**:52–60.

58 Bussel JB, Kuter DJ, George JN, et al. AMG 531, a thrombopoiesis-stimulating protein, for chronic ITP. *N Engl J Med.* 2006;**355**:1672–81.

59 Newland A, Caulier MT, Kappers-Klunne MC, et al. An open-label, unit dose-finding study of AMG 531, a novel thrombopoiesis-stimulating peptibody, in patients with immune thrombocytopenic purpura. *Br J Haematol.* 2006;**135**:547–53.

60 Kuter DJ, Bussel JB, George JN, et al. Long-term dosing of AMG 531 in thrombocytopenic patients with immune thrombocytopenic purpura: 48 week update. *Blood.* 2006;**108**:144a.

61 Bussel JB, Cheng G, Saleh MN, et al. Analysis of bleeding in patients with immune thrombocytopenic purpura (ITP): a randomized, double-blind, placebo-controlled trial of eltrombopag, an oral platelet growth factor. *Blood.* 2006;**108**:144a.

26 Neutropenia

David C. Dale

Introduction

Neutropenia is a reduction in the absolute neutrophil count (ANC) to less than $2.0 \times 10^9/L$. Mild neutropenia is defined as a count between $1.0 \times 10^9/L$ to $2.0 \times 10^9/L$. Moderate neutropenia is $0.5 \times 10^9/L$ to $1.0 \times 10^9/L$ and severe neutropenia is $<0.5 \times 10^9/L$. In most clinical situations, severe neutropenia is clearly associated with enhanced susceptibility to bacterial and fungal infections (1–3). In general, brief periods of acute severe neutropenia (one to three days) are tolerated much better than longer periods. Neutropenia, with associated lymphocytopenia and monocytopenia, is riskier than neutropenia alone. Concomitant diabetes, hepatic or renal disease, immunosuppressive therapies, catheters, breaks in the skin, and mucosal barriers enhance the risk of infections.

Each clinical question was addressed using a MEDLINE (PubMed) literature search and the quality of the evidence was graded according to the criteria of the Seventh American College of Chest Physicians Conference on Antithrombotic and Thrombolytic Therapy (4).

Causes of neutropenia

The principal causes and categories of neutropenia are listed in Table 26.1. The most common causes of acquired neutropenia—drugs, nutritional deficiencies, associated immunological, or infectious diseases—are usually not difficult to diagnose based on a complete medical history, physical examination, and routine laboratory tests.

Identifying other causes for acquired neutropenia is more challenging. In young adult females with a history of fatigue and recurrent fevers, the most frequent cause is chronic idiopathic neutropenia. The large granular lymphocytic leukemia syndrome is associated with rheumatoid arthritis, other autoimmune disorders, or as an isolated abnormality. It is diagnosed by finding increased numbers of circulating CD57+ or CD56+ lymphocytes by fluorescence activated cell sorting analysis. Myelodysplasia, aplastic anemia, marrow infiltration by tumor, and the hemophagocytic lymphohistiocytosis syndrome are usually diagnosed by bone marrow aspiration and biopsy.

There are many congenital or inherited disorders causing neutropenia (1–3). These rare syndromes divide into those involving only myeloid cells and those associated with abnormalities in many organ systems in addition to the hematapoietic system. Until recently, these syndromes were identified by their clinical phenotype; genetic diagnosis is now becoming increasingly available.

Diagnostic tests and strategies

Many aspects of the diagnosis of neutropenia have not been studied systematically. To make a diagnosis, it is critical to have enough historical and laboratory information about serial blood cell counts and ANCs to know whether the condition is acute or chronic and whether it is associated with other hematologic abnormalities. The indirect granulocyte immunofluorescence test is probably the most sensitive and specific assay for antineutrophil antibodies. Useful resources for the diagnosis of a genetic abnormality are www.genetest.org and www.ncbi.nlm.nih.gov/omim/.

The hierarchy or staging of tests to evaluate neutropenia is illustrated in Table 26.2.

Principles of Management

Acute severe neutropenia is usually managed with antibiotics, colony-stimulating factors (primarily granulocyte colony-stimulating factor [G-CSF]), or a combination of these agents. Acute febrile neutropenia is managed primarily with prompt administration of broad-spectrum antibiotics. For chronic

Evidence-based Hematology. Edited by Mark A. Crowther, Jeff Ginsberg, Holger J. Schünemann, Ralph M. Meyer, and Richard Lottenberg.

Table 26.1 Neutropenia—differential diagnosis.*

Acquired disorders of granulopoiesis
- Aplastic anemia
- Chronic idiopathic neutropenia
- Clonal myeloid stem cell disorders (MDS)
- Drugs (chemotherapy induced, dose related)
- Drugs (idiosyncratic)
- Hemophagocytic lymphohistiocytosis
- Immune/autoimmune (RA, SLE)
- Infection (EBV, parovirus, CMV, HIV, sepsis)
- Large granular lymphocytic (LGL) leukemia
- Marrow infiltration (NHL, CLL)
- Nutritional deficiency (Vitamin B-12, folic acid, copper)

Congenital/inherited disorders
- Cyclic neutropenia
- Severe congenital neutropenia
- Multilineage disorders

*MDS, myelodysplastic syndromes; RA, heumatoid arthritis; SLE, systemic lupus erythomatosus; EBV, Epstein-Barr virus; CMV, cytomegalovirus; HIV, human immunodeficiency virus; NHL, non-Hodgkin lymphoma; CLL, chronic lymphocytic leukemia.

neutropenia, no therapy may be necessary; however, patients with severe chronic neutropenia and recurrent fever and infections benefit from long-term treatment with G-CSF. Other agents, for example, corticosteroids, immunosuppressant agents, chemotherapy, neutrophil transfusions, and hematopoietic transplantation have much narrower indications in management of neutropenia.

What are the management strategies for drug-induced or idiosyncratic neutropenia?

Background

Idiosyncratic drug-induced neutropenia, also called drug-induced agranulocytosis, is an uncommon, but potentially life-threatening complication of many drugs (1–6). Patients usually present with fever, pharyngitis, and severely reduced blood neutrophil counts a few days or weeks after starting a new drug, but the presentation can vary considerably.

Criteria for the diagnosis of idiosyncratic drug-induced agranulocytosis include ANC less than $0.5 \times 10^9/L$ (with an ANC previously known to be normal), onset associated with starting a new drug and recovery of the ANC when the suspected drug is withdrawn. Recovery is usually within one month. Recurrence of agranulocytosis with a second exposure to the drug is a fourth diagnostic criterion, but rechallenge is not recommended.

In suspected cases of drug-induced agranulocytosis, all blood cell counts should be reviewed carefully. Anemia or thrombocytopenia or suspicion of an underlying hematological malignancy necessitates bone marrow examination. With drug-induced agranulocytosis, marrow cellularity is usually normal or only mildly reduced due to decreased cells of the neutrophil series. If metamyelocytes, bands, and mature neutrophils are absent, it can be predicted that marrow recovery will take longer; that is, generally more than 5 to 7 days (8–11).

Table 26.2 Hierarchy of diagnostics tests.

History and physical examination
CBC and ANC counts*
Smear and morphology
Nutritional tests vitamin B12, folate, copper, etc.
Immunological tests
Bone marrow aspirate and biopsy
Cytogenetics
Genetic testing
Neutrophil functional testing

*ANC, absolute neutrophil count; CBC, complete blood cell count.

Management Strategies

The presumed causative agent(s) should be stopped immediately (8–11). Usually patients with presumed drug-induced agranulocytosis are on multiple drugs. The decision about which drugs to withdraw may seem complex, but ordinarily as many drugs as possible should be discontinued.

Patients with fever and severe neutropenia generally should be hospitalized or very closely monitored because of the risk of bacteremia, hypotension, and septic shock (7,8). Immediate management includes broad-spectrum antibiotic treatment similar to that for febrile neutropenia in patients receiving myelotoxic chemotherapy. Patients need attentive care by skilled nurses and physicians who are careful with hand washing and conscientious in avoiding transfer of infectious agents from the environment to the patients. Specialized facilities for isolation of patients are of limited value. Antibiotics are continued until neutrophil counts improve, the patient becomes afebrile, or a specific infecting organism is identified and therapy can be appropriately modified (7–11).

The administration of hematapoietic growth factors to patients with presumed drug-induced agranulocytosis is controversial. A meta-analysis of 118 patients in published reports indicated that CSF treatment reduced the mean time for neutrophil recovery from 10 ± 8 to 7.7 ± 5.1 days for cases with initial neutrophil counts less than $0.1 \times 10^9/L$ (11). Mortality was reduced from 16% to 4.2%. A case control study involving 70 patients and two cohort studies involving 74 patients also showed significant reduction in the mean duration of severe neutropenia with treatment with G-CSF (12). By contrast, one smaller prospective randomized trial involving 24 patients with drug-induced agranulocytosis attributable to antithyroid drugs showed no benefit (13).

Overall, most recent published reports on the management of the drug-induced neutropenia suggest a benefit of the hematopoietic growth factor, G-CSF, given in conjunction with antibiotic therapy (14–16).

Recommendations

In drug-induced severe neutropenia, patients with fever should be hospitalized, and the treatment approach is similar to patients receiving myelotoxic therapy (Grade 1C). G-CSF should be administered in conjunction with antibiotic therapy (Grade 1C).

Chemotherapy-induced neutropenia

Risk factors

Combinations of myelotoxic drugs are used for treatment of most malignancies; the specific toxicities of each combination are generally established through clinical trials. Neutropenia is an important dose-limiting toxicity. Current data indicate that moderate to severe myelotoxicity occurs in about 30% to 50% of patients receiving standard dose chemotherapy in community settings in the United States (17,18). Within a population, it is difficult to predict precisely which patients will actually experience the greatest toxicity. Known risk factors are patient related (age, gender, body surface area, pretreatment levels of neutrophils and other blood cells, comorbidities such as diabetes, lung, kidney, or liver disease), treatment related (specific drugs to be administered), and cancer related (advanced disease, bone marrow involvement) (17–21). Guidelines based on analysis of risk are now available from the National Comprehensive Cancer Network (www.nccn.org) (22), the American Society of Clinical Oncology (www.jco.org) (23), and the European Organization for Research and Treatment of Cancer (www.ejconline.com) (24). The risk of severe myelotoxicity is generally greater in the first cycle of chemotherapy; almost two-thirds of episodes of febrile neutropenia in clinical practice occur in the first cycle (22,25). The physiological basis for the first-cycle risk is not completely understood.

In patients receiving combination chemotherapy, what are the roles of prophylactic antibiotics and G-CSF administration in preventing febrile neutropenia?

Efforts to ameliorate the myelotoxicity of cancer chemotherapy began five decades ago. The central problem is that all exposed surfaces of the body are the habitat for myriads of microorganisms. Infection is prevented by the integrity of skin and mucous membranes, the sweeping motions of the ciliated cells linings of the respiratory tract, and rapid responses of the immune system. Neutrophils play a critical role in the first line of defense of the innate immune system.

Decades of study of isolation of patients from the environment and administration of prophylactic antibiotics treatments have shown that it is difficult to rid the body surface of resident organisms or to prevent colonization by new ones (26). The gastrointestinal tract can be purged, but it cannot be sterilized. In addition, the antibiotics required to suppress the resident microbial flora are not palatable by most patients (26).

Prophylactic trimethoprim-sulfamethoxazole has a significant benefit to delay development of febrile neutropenia after myelotoxic drugs, based on 14 studies (27). This treatment is associated with emergence of resistant organisms and yeast infections and trimethoprim-sulfamethoxazole can also cause neutropenia (26,27). Prophylactic quinolone antibiotics also have been demonstrated to delay significantly the onset of febrile neutropenia after chemotherapy (27–29). However, this strategy is also associated with the risk of emergence of resistant organisms and is probably effective only as a short-term strategy (29,30). There are no significant differences between trimethoprim-sulfamethoxazole and quinolones (27) in clinical benefits. The number of patients that need to be treated prophylactically with antibiotics to prevent an episode of febrile neutropenia is approximately 23 and to prevent a fatality about 50 (27). Most infectious disease experts and epidemiologists recommend against the use of quinolone prophylaxis (30–32), but other experts favor antibiotic prophylaxis (27).

Randomized control trials of the hematopoietic drug factors G-CSF and granulocyte-macrophage colony stimulating factor (GM-CSF) to hasten the recovery of the marrow and the return of blood neutrophils after chemotherapy began in the late 1980s. In a pivotal trial in patients with lung cancer, Crawford et al. showed that G-CSF, begun the day following chemotherapy and continued daily for about 10 days, accelerated neutrophil recovery and reduced the occurrence of febrile neutropenia and infections by about 50% (33). The outcome of this trial, subsequent similar trials, and meta-analyses from these trials, led to widespread use of G-CSF to prevent fever and infection after chemotherapy (34). More recently, a pegylated form of G-CSF, or pegfilgrastim, has been shown to have equivalent effects with a single injection given approximately 24 hours after chemotherapy (35). If G-CSF administration is delayed until severe neutropenia has developed, the treatment effect is lost (23).

Despite years of investigation, there are relatively little data directly comparing antibiotics and colony stimulating factors. One recent randomized controlled trial of G-CSF and antibiotics compared with antibiotics alone suggests the combination may have added benefit (37). There also may be populations for which one approach is better than the other.

Recommendations

Guidelines for the appropriate use of the hematopoietic growth factors to prevent febrile neutropenia after chemotherapy are

Table 26.3 2006 guidelines for colony stimulating factors—American Study of Clinical Oncology.*

- CSF use is recommended when patientís risk of febrile neutropenia is 20% or greater, and there is no alternate equally effective regimen not requiring CSF.
- CSF use is recommended for primary prophylaxis for high-risk patients due to medical history, age, disease, or chemotherapy regimen.
- CSF use should be considered for patients with febrile neutropenia.
- CSF use is not recommended for afebrile neutropenia.

*See reference (23) for review of evidence; CSF, colony-stimulating factor.

available from the National Comprehensive Cancer Network (www.nccn.org) (22), the American Society of Clinical Oncology (www.jco.org) (23), and the European Organization for Research and Treatment of Cancer (www.ejconline.com) (24). These guidelines are briefly summarized in Table 26.3. There are currently no widely accepted evidence-based or consensus guidelines for prophylactic use of antibiotics in this setting.

Treatment of febrile neutropenia

It is standard practice to treat patients with chemotherapy-induced neutropenia and fever with broad-spectrum antibiotics at the earliest opportunity. Over the years, the antibiotics and antibiotic combinations used have evolved as new agents have been introduced and patterns of antibiotic sensitivity of the microorganisms have changed. Both single agents and a combination of agents have been shown to be effective through randomized controlled trials (32,38). Recently, oral therapy has been shown to be as effective as parenteral therapy in several trials (39,40). The general principles are to treat initially with broadly acting agents and to narrow the treatment if a pathogen is isolated in a blood culture or other ordinarily sterile fluid. Otherwise, broad-spectrum treatment is continued until neutrophils recover. Layering of agents to complete the coverage spectrum and to include fungal pathogens is a challenging problem in the management of patients with severe neutropenia, particularly when treatment is prolonged (38). The assistance of an infectious disease specialist familiar with the antibiotic pharmacokinetics and toxicities and the local sensitivities of microorganisms is important for patient management of such cases. Adjunctive treatment of febrile neutropenia with G-CSF is not standard practice, but is supported by evidence from clinical trials (23).

Recommendations

Promptly treat febrile neutropenia with broad spectrum antibiotics (Grade 1A). Oral and parenteral antibiotic regimens are equally effective, if the patient is well enough for oral treatment (Grade 1A). CSFs should not be used routinely in this setting but should be considered for patients at high risk of complications from infections (Grade 1B).

Which patients with severe chronic neutropenia benefit from G-CSF administration?

Congenital, Cyclic, and Idiopathic Neutropenia

Severe chronic neutropenia is defined as blood neutrophil counts less than 0.5×10^9/L on a continuing or intermittent basis lasting for months or years and has numerous causes (1–3).

Treatment of severe chronic neutropenia changed greatly with the discovery and development of the hematopoietic growth factors, particularly G-CSF. Beginning in the late 1980s, a series of phase II trials and then a phase III randomized control trial established the effectiveness of G-CSF for the long-term treatment of congenital, cyclic, and idiopathic neutropenia (41–43). GM-CSF is generally not used because of a lack of efficacy and greater adverse effects. Observational studies conducted by the Severe Chronic Neutropenia International Registry have shown the long-term effectiveness of G-CSF treatment for periods up to 20 years of subcutaneous treatment (44,45). For patients with cyclic and idiopathic neutropenia, G-CSF is administered at 1–3 mcg/kg/d either on a daily or alternate-day basis. In the acute phase of treatment, patients may have bone pain, headache, and other symptoms, but these are usually mild and tend to disappear with long-term therapy. Osteoporosis may be associated with G-CSF therapy by stimulating osteoclasts and the remodeling of bone. This risk appears to be relatively small; fractures and clinical consequences of osteopenia have thus far been infrequent in this population.

In patients with severe congenital neutropenia, treatment responses are less uniform. Five to 10% of patients do not respond readily to G-CSF (45). In addition, some patients with severe congenital neutropenia, particularly the less responsive patients who require higher doses of G-CSF, are at risk of evolution to myelodysplasia and acute myeloid leukemia. It appears that the primary risk is intrinsic to the marrow cells. Because of the risk of evolution to myeloid leukemia, patients with severe congenital neutropenia, both those with and without associated mutations of the ELA-2 gene or HAX-1 gene (47,48), should be followed carefully with blood counts and bone marrow examinations. Hematopoietic transplantation should be considered if there is a suitable, well-matched donor.

Recommendations

Patients with congenital neutropenia should have a bone marrow examination with cytogenetics at diagnosis and before initiation of G-CSF treatment and at yearly intervals thereafter (Grade 1C). G-CSF should be used for treatment of cyclic, congenital, and idiopathic neutropenia patients with recurrent fevers and infections (Grade 1A).

HIV-associated neutropenia

During the early years of the HIV epidemic, G-CSF and GM-CSF were widely used to treat HIV-associated neutropenia (49). Based on phase II studies, this treatment appeared to be very effective. With development of highly effective therapies for HIV, neutropenia has become much less of a concern.

Recommendation

G-CSF or GM-CSF may be effective as an aid in management of chronic neutropenia due to HIV infection (Grade 1C).

Autoimmune Neutropenia

Autoimmune neutropenia is a common diagnosis in children and some adults. The diagnosis is usually based on a finding of selective neutropenia, normal myeloid development in the marrow, and a positive test for acute-neutrophil antibodies. Many patients with proven or suspected autoimmune neutropenia require no therapy, presumably because they have a reserve of neutrophils in the marrow that can be mobilized with infections.

Recommendation

Severe autoimmune neutropenia with recurrent fevers and infections can be effectively treated with G-CSF, usually in very low doses (50) (Grade 1C).

Acknowledgments and disclosures

The assistance of Alice Meyer in the preparation of this manuscript is gratefully acknowledged.

D. C. Dale is a consultant and advisor for Amgen, Inc., Thousand Oaks, California, the manufacturer of G-CSF/filgrastim and peg-G-CSF/pegfilgrastim. He also serves as a consultant for Merck and Schering-Plough, companies manufacturing antibiotics and other therapies that may be used in the management of patients with neutropenia.

References

1 Dale DC, Liles WC. Neutrophils and monocytes: normal physiology and disorders of neutrophil and monocyte production. In: Handin RI, Lux SE, Stossel TP, editors. *Blood: principles and practice of hematology*. Philadelphia: Lippincott, Williams and Wilkins; 2003. pp. 455–82.

2 Dale DC. Nonmalignant disorders of leukocytes. In: Dale DC, Federman DD, editors. *ACP medicine 2006*. Vol 1. New York: WebMD; 2006. pp. 1097–112.

3 Dale DC. Neutropenia and neutrophilia. In: Lichtman MA, Kipps TJ, Kaushansky K, et al., editors. *Williams hematology*. 7th ed. New York: McGraw-Hill; 2006. pp. 181–91.

4 Schunemann HJ, Cook D, Grimshaw J, et al. Antithrombotic and thrombolytic therapy from evidence to application: the Seventh ACCP Conference on Antithrombotic and Thrombolytic Therapy. *Chest*. 2004;**126**:179–87.

5 International Agranulocytosis and Aplastic Anemia Study. Risk of agranulocytosis and aplastic anemia in relation to use of antithyroid drugs. *BMJ*. 1998;**297**:262–65.

6 Van der Klauw MM, Goudsmit R, Halie MR, et al. A population-based case-cohort study of drug-associated agranulocytosis. *Arch Intern Med*. 1999;**159**:369–74.

7 Andrés E, Zimmer J, Affenberger S, et al. Idiosyncratic drug-induced agranulocytosis: update of an old disorder. *Eur J Intern Med*. 2006;**17**:529–35.

8 Andrés E, Kurta JE, Maloisel F. Non-chemotherapy drug-induced agranulocytosis: experience of the Strasbourg teaching hospital (1985–2000) and review of the literature. *Clin Lab Haematol*. 2000;**24**:99–106.

9 Strom BL, Carson JL, Schinnar R, et al. Descriptive epidemiology of agranulocytosis. *Arch Intern Med*. 1992;**159**:1475–80.

10 Andrés E, Noel E, Kurtz JE, Henoun Loukili N, et al. Life-threatening idiosyncratic drug-induced aganulocytosis in elderly patients. *Drugs Aging*. 2004;**21**:427–35.

11 Beauchesne MF, Shalansky SJ. Nonchemotherapy drug-induced agranulocytosis: a review of 118 patients treated with colony-stimulating factors. *Pharmacotherapy*. 1999;**19**:299–305.

12 Sprikkelman A, de Wolf JTM, Vellenga E. Application of haematopoietic growth factors in drug-induced agranulocytosis: a review of 70 cases. *Leukemia*. 1994;**8**:2031–36.

13 Fukata S, Kuma K, Sugawara M. Granulocyte colony-stimulating factor (G-CSF) does not improve recovery from antithyroid drug-induced agranulocytosis: a prospective study. *Thyroid*. 1999;**9**:29–31.

14 Andrés E, Kurtz JE, Perrin AE, et al. The use of haematopoietic growth factors in antithyroid-related drug-induced agranulocytosis: a report of 20 patients. *Q J Med*. 2001;**94**:423–28.

15 Andrés E, Kurtz JE, Martin-Hunyadi C, et al. Non-chemotherapy drug-induced agranulocytosis in elderly patients: the effects of granulocyte colony-stimulating factor. *Am J Med*. 2002;**112**:460–64.

16 Tajiri J, Noguchi S. Antithyroid drug-induced agranulocytosis: how has granulocyte colony-stimulating factor changed therapy? *Thyroid*. 2005;**15**:292–97.

17 Dale DC, McCarter GC, Crawford J, et al. Myelotoxicity and dose intensity of chemotherapy: reporting practices from randomized clinical trials. *J Natl Compr Canc Netw*. 2003;**1**:440–54.

18 Crawford J, Dale DC, Lyman GH. Chemotherapy-induced neutropenia: risks, consequences, and new directions for its management. *Cancer*. 2004;**100**:228–37.

19 Lyman G, Dale DC, Crawford J. Incidence and predictors of low dose-intensity in adjuvant breast cancer chemotherapy: A nationwide study of community practices. *J Clin Oncol*. 2003:**21**:4524–31.

20 Wolff D, Culokova E, Poniewierski MS, et al. Predictors of chemotherapy-induced neutropenia and its complications: results from a prospective nationwide registry. *J Support Oncol*. 2005;**3**(6 Suppl 4):24–5.

21 Lyman GH, Dale DC, Friedberg J, et al. Incidence and predictors of low chemotherapy dose-intensity in aggressive non-Hodgkin's lymphoma: a nationwide study. *J Clin Oncol*. 2004;**22**:4302–11.

22 Lyman GH. Guidelines of the National Comprehensive Cancer Network on the use of myeloid growth factors with cancer chemotherapy: A review of the evidence. *J Natl Compr Canc Netw*. 2005;**3**:557–71.

23 Smith TJ, Katcheressian J, Lyman GH, et al. Update of recommendations for the use of white blood cell growth factors: an evidence-based clinical practice guideline. *J Clin Oncol*. 2006;**24**:3187–205.

24 Aapro MS, Cameron DA, Pettengell R, et al. EORTC guidelines for the use of granulocyte-colony stimulating factor to reduce the incidence of chemotherapy-induced febrile neutropenia in adult patients with lymphomas and solid tumours. *Euro J Cancer*. 2006;**42**:2433–453.

25 Crawford J, Dale DC, Culakova E, et al. First-cycle risk of chemotherapy-induced neutropenia: initial results of the ANC Registry, a prospective national study of oncology practice. Submitted; 2006.

26 Pizzo PA. Management of fever in patients with cancer and treatment-induced neutropenia. *N Engl J Med*. 1993;**328**:1323–32.

27 Gafter-Gvili A, Fraser A, Paul M, et al. Meta analysis: antibiotic prophylaxis reduces mortality in neutropenic patients. *Ann Intern Med*. 2005;**142**:979–95.

28 Bucaneve G. Micozzi A, Menichetti F, et al. Levofloxacin to prevent bacterial infection in patients with cancer and neutropenia. *N Engl J Med*. 2005;**353**:977–87.

29 Cullen M, Steven N, Billingham L, et al. Antibacterial prophylaxis after chemotherapy for solid tumors and lymphomas. *N Engl J Med*. 2005;**353**:988–98.

30 Baden LR. Prophylactic antimicrobial agents and the importance of fitness. *N Engl J Med.* 2005;**353**:1052–54.

31 Cullen M, Steven N, Billingham L, et al. Antibacterial prophylaxis reduced the incidence of fever in patients receiving chemotherapy for solid tumors or lymphoma. *ACP J Club.* 2006;**144**:42.

32 Hughes WT, Armstrong D, Body GP, et al. 2002 guidelines for the use of antimicrobial agents in neutropenic patients with cancer. *Clin Infect Dis.* 2002;**34**:730–51.

33 Crawford J, Ozer H, Stoller R, et al. Reduction by granulocyte colony-stimulating factor of fever and neutropenia induced by chemotherapy in patients with small-cell lung cancer. *N Engl J Med.* 1991;**325**: 164–70.

34 Clark OA, Lyman G, Castro AA, et al. Colony stimulating factors for chemotherapy induced febrile neutropenia. *Cochrane Database Syst Rev.* 2003;(3):CD003039.

35 Crawford J. One-per-cycle pegfiltrastim (Neulasta) for the management of chemotherapy-induced neutropenia. *Semin Oncol.* 2003;**30**: 24–30.

36 Price TH, Chatta GS, Dale DC. Effect of recombinant granulocyte colony-stimulating factor on neutrophil kinetics in normal young and elderly humans. *Blood.* 1996;**88**:335–40.

37 Timmer-Bonte JN, de Boo TM, Smith HJ, et al. Prevention of chemotherapy-induced febrile neutropenia by prophylactic antibiotics plus or minus granulocyte-stimulating factor in small cell lung cancer: a Dutch randomized phase III study. *J Clin Oncol.* 2005;**23**(31): 7974–84.

38 Sepkowitz KA. Treatment of patients with hematologic neoplasm, fever, and neutropenia. *Clin Infect Dis.* 2005;**40** Suppl 4:S253–S56.

39 Freifeld A, Marchigiani D, Walsh T, et al. A double-blind comparison of empirical oral and intravenous antibiotic therapy for low-risk febrile patients with neutropenia during cancer chemotherapy. *N Engl J Med.* 1999;**341**:305–11.

40 Kern WV. Risk assessment and treatment of low-risk patients with febrile neutropenia. *Clin Infect Dis.* 2006;**42**:533–40.

41 Bonilla MA, Gillio AP, Ruggeiro M, Kernan, et al. Effects of recombinant human granulocyte colony-stimulating factor on neutropenia in patients with congenital agranulocytosis. *N Engl J Med.* 1989;**320**:1574–80.

42 Hammond WP IV, Price TH, Souza LM, et al. Treatment of cyclic neutropenia with granulocyte colony-stimulating factor. *N Engl J Med.* 1989;**320**:1306–11.

43 Dale DC, Bonilla MA, Davis MW, et al. A randomized controlled phase III trial of recombinant human granulocyte colony-stimulating factor (filgrastim) for treatment of severe chronic neutropenia. *Blood.* 1993;**81**:2496–502.

44 Dale DC, Bolyard AA, Schwinzer BG, et al. The severe chronic neutropenia international registry: 10-yr follow-up report. *Supportive Cancer Ther.* 2006;**3**:220–31.

45 Welte K, Zeidler C, Dale DC. Severe congenital neutropenia. *Semin Hematol.* 2006;**43**:189–95.

46 Rosenberg PS, Alter BP, Bolyard AA, et al. The incidence of leukemia and mortality from sepsis in patients with severe congenital neutropenia receiving long-term G-CSF therapy. *Blood.* 2006;**107**:4628–35.

47 Dale DC. ELA2-related neutropenia [database online]. In: Gene reviews: Genetic disease online reviews at GeneTests-GeneClinics. University of Washington, Seattle; 2002. Available at http://www.geneclinics.org.

48 Klein, C, Grudzien M, Appaswamy G, et al. HAX1 deficiency causes autosomal recessive severe congenital neutropenia (Kostmann disease). *Nat Genet.* 2007;**39**(1):86–92.

49 Sloand E. Hematologic complications of HIV infection. *AIDS Rev.* 2005;**7**:187–96.

50 Dale DC, Cottle TE, Fier CJ, et al. Severe chronic neutropenia: treatment and follow-up of patients in the Severe Chronic Neutropenia International Registry. *Am J Hematol.* 2003;**72**:82–93.

27 Hypereosinophilia

Primary and Secondary

Florence Roufosse, Michel Goldman, Elie Cogan

Background

Hypereosinophilia, defined as an increase in blood eosinophilia above 500/μL, arises in a number of medical conditions (Table 27.1), among which parasitic diseases involving tissue-invasive helminths and allergic disorders, including atopy and drug reactions, are by far the most commonly observed in developing and industrialized countries, respectively (1). Once the underlying disease is identified, therapeutic options are quite straightforward. Occasionally, however, thorough evaluation fails to detect a condition known to be associated with hypereosinophilia, and diagnosis of "idiopathic" hypereosinophilic disease must be considered. Clinical manifestations in these disorders are directly related to the presence of eosinophils in tissues and organs and to the extent of their activation and resulting release of toxic substances. Different eosinophil-mediated idiopathic disorders have been defined, depending on sites of eosinophil infiltration; they may target a specific tissue or organ (e.g., eosinophilic esophagitis, chronic eosinophilic pneumonia) or cause a variety of complications in association with marked blood hypereosinophilia in "hypereosinophilic syndrome" (HES). The following chapter will deal with the latter condition, focusing on diagnostic workup and modern therapeutic strategies. Recent advances in pathogenesis will be highlighted, as well as their impact on patient management.

Definition and characteristics of HES

The most extensively used diagnostic criteria for "idiopathic" hypereosinophilic syndrome were proposed by Chusid in 1975: (1) blood eosinophilia exceeding 1,500/μL for more than six consecutive months, (2) lack of evidence for parasitic infection, allergy, or other known causes of hypereosinophilia, and (3) signs and symptoms of organ disease related to hypereosinophilia (2). More recently, experts in the field have proposed that the duration criteria be revised, integrating the rapidity with which modern diagnostic tools permit exclusion of underlying causes of hypereosinophilia, and physicians' concern about lowering eosinophil levels rapidly in patients with potentially life-threatening complications (3). The spectrum of clinical complications of HES, including cutaneous, cardiac, pulmonary, digestive, and neurological involvement, has been extensively reviewed elsewhere (4,5).

Current knowledge concerning HES disease presentations is based on case reports, single-center patient series, and expert opinion. Together with the great clinical heterogeneity within this syndrome, the methods of reporting data account for significant referral bias. The tendency for positive reporting of therapeutic success stories in orphan diseases also represents a limitation to interpreting HES literature.

Literature-search strategy

We have focused this chapter on diagnostic workup and therapy for hypereosinophilic syndromes, excluding pediatric cases and rare cases of familial hypereosinophilia. Sources from which data were derived for elaboration of this chapter include PubMed, Uptodate, and the 2005 National Institutes of Health–funded HES workshop preceding the International Eosinophil Society Congress in Bern. There are no systematic reviews regarding hypereosinophilia or hypereosinophilic syndrome in the Cochrane Library or PubMed, and the results of the only placebo-controlled clinical trial conducted to date in this disease are in press at time of writing (6).

The keywords used for extracting relevant articles from PubMed were as follows: hypereosinophilic syndrome and management<th>/<th>treatment<th>/<th>review <th>/<th> (clonal) T cell<th>/<th>clinical trial; FIP1L1; imatinib and hypereosinophilic<th>/<th>chronic eosinophilic

Evidence-based Hematology. Edited by Mark A. Crowther, Jeff Ginsberg, Holger J. Schünemann, Ralph M. Meyer, and Richard Lottenberg.

Table 27.1 Causes of hypereosinophilia.*

Diseases associated with hypereosinophilia	Eosinophil-mediated diseases
Parasitosis (mostly helminths)	Eosinophilic pneumonia (acute, chronic)
Allergic disease	Eosinophilic esophagitis
—Atopy	Eosinophilic gastrointestinal disorders
—Drug allergy	Eosinophilic fasciitis (Shulman's syndrome)
Malignancy	Eosinophilic cellulitis (Well's syndrome)
—Hematological disorders	Kimura's disease
Myeloproliferative (CML, CMML-Eo, SMCD-Eo, AML)	Angiolymphoid hyperplasia with eosinophilia
Non-myeloproliferative (HD, CTCL, PTCL, ATLL, T cell lymphoblastic lymphoma, pre-B-cell lymphoblastic leukemia)	Eosinophilic cystitis
—Solid tumors (lung, colon, cervix)	Episodic angioedema with eosinophilia (Gleich's syndrome)
Systemic immune-mediated inflammatory disorders	Hypereosinophilic syndrome
—Vasculitides (Churg-Strauss, Wegener's disease)	
—Connective tissue disorders (rheumatoid arthritis, dermatomyositis)	
Nonparasitic infections	
—HIV, HTLV	
—Scabies	
—ABPA, coccidioidomycosis	
Immunodeficiency states	
—Omenn's syndrome; HyperIgE or Job's syndrome	
Toxic	
—Eosinophilia-myalgia syndrome; Toxic oil syndrome	
Miscellaneous	
—Adrenal insufficiency	
—Cholesterol embolization	
—Irritation/Irradiation of serosal surfaces	
—Chronic GVHD	
—Psoriasis, Bullous pemphigoid	

*CML, chronic myelogenous leukemia; CMML-Eo, chronic myelomonocytic leukemia with eosinophilia; SMCD-Eo, systemic mast cell disease with eosinophilia; HD, Hodgkin disease; CTCL, cutaneous T-cell lymphoma; PTCL, peripheral T cell lymphoma; ATLL, adult T cell leukemia/lymphoma; ABPA, allergic bronchopulmonary aspergillosis; GVHD, graft versus host disease.

leukemia<th>/<th>FIP1L1<th>/<th>toxicity; mepolizumab; anti-IL-5, and human not asthma.

Grading of recommendations and evidence in this chapter is based on the guidelines proposed by the international Grading of Recommendations Assessment, Development, and Evaluation Working Group (GRADE) (American College of Chest Physicians Task Force) (7).

What diagnostic testing is indicated in patients with hypereosinophilic syndrome?

Recent studies have established that distinct molecular pathways are involved in HES subsets, and optimal patient management has become dependent on the ability to refine HES diagnosis beyond Chusid's criteria. Schematically, hypereosinophilia develops as a result of two pathogenic mechanisms; either eosinophils expand clonally in the setting of a myeloproliferative disorder involving eosinophil progenitors (M-HES) or eosinophils proliferate polyclonally in response to overproduction of eosinophil growth factors by T cells ("lymphocytic," or L-HES). Among these factors, only interleukin(IL)-5 is specific for the eosinophil lineage, displaying positive effects on differentiation and proliferation of eosinophil precursors, on eosinophil survival in the periphery, and on activation of mature eosinophils (8). $CD4^+$ T lymphocytes producing "type 2" cytokines (or "Th2" cells) represent the major source of IL-5, which is generally produced in conjunction with IL-4 and IL-13 (9).

The predominant molecular defect accounting for clonal eosinophilia in HES is an interstitial deletion spanning 800 kb on chromosome 4q12, resulting in fusion of two genes flanking this region: FIP1L1 and PDGFRα (10). The fusion gene is in-frame and encodes a FIP1LI-PDGFRα (F/P) protein with constitutive tyrosine kinase activity. The central role of this fusion gene in disease pathogenesis is supported by its disappearance in most patients successfully treated with the tyrosine kinase inhibitor imatinib mesylate (IM) (11,12). There is a striking male predominance, and anemia or thrombocytopenia, increased serum vitamin B12 levels,

Table 27.2 Practical approach to diagnosis of HES variants.

Documented myeloproliferative disorder	Documented T-cell mediated disorder
F/P rearrangement Eosinophil clonality (clonal cytogenetic abnormalities including other fusion genes involving PDGFRα, methylation patterns of X-linked genes)	Flow cytometry (CD3$^-$CD4$^+$, CD3$^+$CD4$^-$CD8$^-$, other) Clonal TCR rearrangement pattern Increased IL-5 production by PBL
Features suggestive of primitive eosinophilic expansion (myeloproliferative disorder)	**Features suggestive of reactive T–cell mediated eosinophilia**
Increased serum vitamin B12 (>1,000 pg/mL) Circulating myeloid precusors Dysplastic eosinophils on peripheral smear Anemia, Thrombocytopenia Splenomegaly, hepatomegaly Myelofibrosis Marrow hypercellularity (>80%) with left shift in maturation Increased serum tryptase	Increased serum IgE Polyclonal hypergammaglobulinemia Predominant eczema, urticaria, angioedema Marked corticosteroid-sensitivity History of atopy Increased serum TARC*

* TARC, thymus and activation-regulated chemokine

mucosal ulcerations, endomyocardial fibrosis, and splenomegaly are most frequently observed in affected patients (11–13), although a number of other complications, including dermatitis, pulmonary infiltrates, and peripheral neuropathy, have been reported. Overall, natural disease course and prognosis in F/P$^+$ HES patients is poor, with a high prevalence of disease-related morbidity and death due to development of cardiac complications and blastic transformation (11,14).

Besides F/P$^+$ patients, some HES patients present features of myeloproliferative disease, although eosinophil clonality is not evident. In the minority of cases, investigators have been able to demonstrate existence of other fusion genes involving PDGFRα (15,16). For other patients, experts participating in a workshop dedicated to HES have agreed that patients be classified as M-HES when at least 4 of 8 "myeloproliferative" criteria are fulfilled (Table 27.2) (3).

L-HES is defined as a primitive lymphocytic disorder characterized by nonmalignant expansion of a T cell population producing IL-5. Clonal Th2-like cells bearing a CD3$^-$CD4$^+$(CD2$^+$TCR$\alpha\beta^-$) surface phenotype are most frequently involved (17–21). The molecular basis of this unique entity has been characterized extensively (20,22). CD3$^-$CD4$^+$-associated disease affects females at least as much as males, and cutaneous manifestations, including pruritus, eczema, erythroderma, urticaria, and angioedema, generally dominate the clinical picture, whereas endomyocardial fibrosis is a rare complication despite high eosinophil levels (20). Serum IgE levels are often increased and polyclonal IgG or IgM hypergammaglobulinemia may be observed (20,21). Although patients with CD3$^-$CD4$^+$ cells rarely experience life-threatening end-organ damage and have better short-term prognosis compared with F/P$^+$ patients, some may develop peripheral T cell lymphoma bearing the same phenotype many years after diagnosis (20).

In addition to CD3$^-$CD4$^+$ T cell–mediated disease, increased IL-5 production by T cells with unusual phenotypes, such as CD3$^+$CD4$^-$CD8$^-$ T cells, or T cells with abnormal staining intensity for CD2, CD4, CD6, or CD7 antigens, has been reported by independent groups (23,24).

Despite active research in the field, molecular mechanisms of disease remain elusive in more than half of HES patients. Using modern diagnostic tools in expert hands, it is still unclear whether they present primitive or reactive eosinophilia; for these patients, the term "idiopathic" HES therefore remains appropriate.

Recommendations

Given the major therapeutic impact of detecting the 4q12 deletion, it is recommended that patients fulfilling HES criteria be evaluated for its occurrence whenever possible, by reverse transcriptase polymerase chain reaction (RT-PCR) or fluorescent in situ hybridization (FISH) using probes for the CHIC2 locus (located between the FIP1L1 and PDGFRα genes on chromosome 4q12) (25), on blood or bone marrow (Grade 1A). Nested PCR is preferred to single-round PCR and to FISH, as the level of fusion gene expression is low in some patients, and it may be missed by the latter methods (26).

Investigation of circulating (and eventually bone marrow-derived) T-cell phenotype by flow cytometry (Grade 1B), and TCR gene rearrangement patterns using both Southern Blot (for TCRβ) and PCR amplification (for TCR-β and -γ) is recommended (Grade 1B). However, clonal TCR rearrangement patterns in absence of an abnormal T cell phenotype may be observed in healthy subjects, and even in some patients with clear-cut F/P-associated disease (12) and are not necessarily indicative of T cell–mediated disease. Demonstration of IL-5 overproduction by T cells is more convincing but less readily available to clinicians and can therefore not be systematically recommended at this time (Grade 2B).

Identification of accessible and reproducible biomarkers for diagnosis of HES variants would be valuable for clinicians. One study has shown that increased serum tryptase levels (>11.5 ng/mL) in nine HES patients was associated with presence of myeloproliferative features, response to therapy with IM (6/6 treated patients), and presence of the F/P fusion (5/5 tested patients), whereas four patients with normal serum tryptase tested negative for the fusion (14). In another study, serum levels of thymus and activation-regulated chemokine (TARC), which can be measured by a commercially available ELISA kit, were shown to be about 100-fold higher in 13 L-HES patients compared with 19 healthy subjects, subjects with atopic (n = 14) or parasitic (n = 4) disease, and four HES patients with no evidence of T cell–mediated disease (27). Although the preliminary results are encouraging, these potential biomarkers for F/P-HES and L-HES remain investigational until the sensitivity, specificity, and discriminatory cutoff values have been assessed in a large-scale and representative patient cohort (Grade 2C).

What is the therapy for F/P-associated HES?

Imatinib mesylate is a small molecule that occupies the adenosine triphosphate (ATP)-binding site in the kinase moiety of fusion genes involving abl, c-kit, PDGFRα and PDGFRβ, thereby inhibiting kinase autophosphorylation and phosphorylation of downstream substrates involved in cell survival and proliferation (28). The tyrosine kinase activity of the F/P fusion is 100-fold more sensitive to IM than the CML-associated bcr-abl fusion in vitro (10), explaining that F/P$^+$ patients respond to extremely low doses of this agent (often less than 100 mg/d).

Reports on treatment of F/P-associated disease with IM are numerous, and it is difficult to assess precisely how many patients have been treated thus because of overlapping patient series. In a comprehensive literature review of HES patients treated with IM published in 2006, 31 patients were F/P$^+$ and all presented a complete response to IM (29). Indeed, among F/P$^+$ patients, no cases of primary resistance to IM have been reported to date and response to treatment is both rapid (generally within a week) and dramatic in terms of controlling eosinophil levels (10–13,30). Although most clinical and hematological complications of hypereosinophilia can be reversed by IM in F/P$^+$ patients, impact of therapy on signs and symptoms of endomyocardial fibrosis may be disappointing (11,12), underscoring the importance of initiating therapy as early as possible.

Cytogenetic remission can be achieved in a majority of patients with the F/P fusion, within a period ranging from one month to over a year (11,12,26,30). Several groups have observed recurrence of the fusion transcript after interruption of IM in such patients (26,31). Although reintroduction of IM was again followed by cytogenetic remission, one study showed that the dose of IM required had to be increased compared to the initial treatment, to maintain remission in some cases (31), suggesting that treatment interruption may decrease overall sensitivity of cells bearing the F/P fusion to IM. More concerning is the relapse of hypereosinophilia during treatment with IM in two patients, associated with appearance of a T674I point mutation in the PDGFRα ATP-binding site, similar to the T315I mutation observed in patients with CML that become refractory to IM (10,32). Alternative tyrosine kinase inhibitors are being developed and tested in vitro on cells expressing the IM-resistant mutated F/P.

IM is generally well tolerated, and side effects including nausea, myalgia, fluid retention, and neutropenia are rarely observed at the doses used to control HES. However, development of acute congestive heart failure shortly after initiation has been reported in a few patients, presumably related to overwhelming release of cytotoxic mediators by targeted eosinophils within the myocardium (33,34). This complication was associated with increased serum troponin levels and could be reversed by timely administration of corticosteroids (CS). One study has shown that IM-induced mitochondrial dysfunction in cardiomyocytes is responsible for development of left ventricular dysfunction in CML patients several months after initiation of therapy (400–800 mg/d) (35). It therefore appears reasonable to pay close attention to cardiac function in HES patients treated with IM.

Recommendations

Timely administration of IM is recommended in all F/P$^+$ patients (Grade 1A). There is some controversy on the initial dose. Some investigators recommend 400 mg/d, arguing that higher doses could prevent emergence of mutated IM-resistant F/P$^+$ cells (3). We recommend an initial dose of 100 mg/d, provided this ensures rapid biological remission (within two weeks), as well as cytogenetic remission within six to nine months. If not, the dose should be increased up to 400 mg/d. It has been recommended that the dose of IM used for F/P$^+$ patients be adjusted to ensure cytogenetic remission to decrease the risk of acquired resistance to treatment (3,26) (Grade 1C).

Serum troponin level should be measured prior to initiation of therapy, and we recommend performing an echocardiogram if this hasn't been done in the previous 3 months (Grade 1C). If either test is suggestive of cardiac involvement, administration of CS immediately prior to IM is recommended (Grade 1C). The only data available on dose and duration of CS for this indication are for one patient who had developed acute heart failure within days after starting IM and who was subsequently successfully rechallenged with this agent along with 60 mg prednisone (PDN) for the first three days, followed by progressive tapering (33). It is reasonable to administer 1 mg PDN per kilogram per day for the first week of treatment (36), during which time eosinophil levels drop most rapidly. Furthermore, serum troponin levels should be measured during the first days of treatment, during which eosinophil levels decrease rapidly, even in patients with no evidence of cardiac involvement prior to IM, to detect development of acute cardiomyopathy (Grade 1C). Serial measurements every 2 days for the first week of treatment or until eosinophil counts are controlled should detect this early complication of imatinib therapy.

What is the therapy for F/P-negative HES?

Corticosteroids remain first-line therapy in the majority of HES cases, excluding F/P$^+$ patients. The proportion of CS-responders has not been evaluated recently, and response rates before discovery of the F/P fusion (37,38) (approximately one-third complete CS-responses and one-third partial responses) cannot be extended to the F/P$^-$ population, which is overall more likely to respond. Despite the widespread use of CS for HES and other organ-specific, eosinophil-mediated disorders, no studies have evaluated the optimal starting dose or tapering regimen following remission. The CS dose required to maintain disease control is highly variable from one patient to another and even for a given patient over time. Long-term use of CS is associated with a number of side effects that will not be detailed here. Therapeutic strategies therefore aim to minimize overall CS exposure, by introducing CS-sparing agents whenever the dose of CS required to control disease is considered unacceptable.

The compounds used for CS-sparing purposes and those used as second-line therapy for CS nonresponders are the same, and for most, their use has been inspired from treatment of chronic myeloproliferative disorders (4). With the recent exception of the anti-IL-5 mAb mepolizumab, none of these agents has been evaluated for HES treatment in controlled clinical trials (6).

Hydroxyurea (HU) is a commonly used agent for HES, generally at doses between 0.5–2 g/d (37,38). Clinical efficacy is delayed because it acts centrally while leaving peripheral eosinophils intact. Patients that respond to <1 g/d generally tolerate therapy, but hematological and gastrointestinal toxicities may be an issue at higher doses. Theoretically, this compound would appear more useful for treating patients with myeloproliferative features; however, it effectively lowered eosinophil levels in one patient with a CD3$^-$CD4$^+$ clone (39). It has proven useful in individual cases to associate low-dose HU with other compounds such as interferon-alpha (IFN-α) (40), combining efficacy while reducing side effects of each molecule.

Interferon-alpha has been shown to control disease and induce cytogenetic remission in HES patients with chromosomal abnormalities and features of aggressive myeloproliferative disease (41,42). Importantly, some patients have experienced durable remission after treatment interruption, suggesting that IFN-α may be curative in some cases. This immunomodulatory agent targets both eosinophils and T cells, making it an interesting choice for all disease variants. The dose required for disease control is very variable but is generally between 7 and 14 million units/week (3). Effects on eosinophilia are delayed, and poor tolerance is common as the dose increases. Use of the pegylated form may improve patient comfort (only one weekly injection, less side effects), while conserving efficacy (3).

Imatinib mesylate is efficacious in a subset of patients that do not harbor the F/P fusion (10,29), suggesting involvement of other IM-sensitive tyrosine kinases in this disorder. In very few cases, other fusion genes involving PDGFRα have been detected, and these patients respond dramatically to IM, similar to those with the F/P fusion (15,16). However, in the absence of a demonstrated cytogenetic defect targeting an IM-sensitive kinase, clinical responses appear to be less spectacular (response often delayed, and only partial remissions), and generally require higher doses of IM (29,30,43). Characteristics of F/P$^-$ HES patients that would benefit from IM remain elusive. A retrospective review of 94 published cases of HES treated with IM has indicated that male sex and splenomegaly are associated with a higher probability of a complete response, whereas patients with isolated or predominant cutaneous manifestations are less likely to respond (29). IM has proven ineffective for controlling L-HES in three patients (33,43,44).

Monoclonal anti-IL-5 antibodies target eosinophils by binding to IL-5 and preventing its ligation to the IL-5R α-chain expressed on the eosinophil membrane (45,46). Several open-label studies evaluating effects of intravenous anti-IL-5 mAb in HES patients showed a rapid decline of blood eosinophil counts shortly after administration, associated with improvement of a range of clinical manifestations (47–50). Eosinophil depletion and clinical benefit in response to 750 mg intravenous mepolizumab, the anti-IL-5 mAb produced by GlaxoSmithKline, can be surprisingly long-lasting (48). Efficacy of mepolizumab as a CS-sparing agent in CS-responsive F/P$^-$ HES patients has just recently been confirmed in the setting of a randomized double-blind, placebo-controlled clinical trial (6). In this study, patients were stabilized on CS monotherapy (ranging from 20 to 60 mg PDN or PDN-equivalent per day) before randomization to two treatment arms, one with intravenous mepolizumab 750 mg, and the other with intravenous saline solution (placebo), both administered every four weeks for a period of 36 weeks. The primary endpoint, i.e. maintenance of disease control with 10 mg PDN or less per day for a period of at least 8 consecutive weeks, was achieved in a significantly higher proportion of patients in the active treatment arm than in the placebo arm (36/43 or 84% versus 18/42 or 43%, respectively, $p < 0.001$). The difference between treatment arms was even more significant in patients requiring more than 30 mg PDN per day at baseline (10/13 or 77% in the active treatment group versus 1/12 or 8% in the placebo group, $p < 0.001$), indicating that benefit of treatment with mepolizumab is particularly marked in patients with more severe disease. A significant difference in the daily dose of PDN required to stabilize disease at study completion was observed (6.2 ± 1.9 mg in the active treatment group versus 21.8 ± 1.9 mg in the placebo group, $p < 0.001$). Exploratory and post-hoc analyses showed a significant difference in the proportion of patients that were successfully and durably tapered off CS until completion of the study (47% in the active treatment group versus 5% in the placebo group). Importantly, mepolizumab was shown to be well tolerated and safe in this short-term study; long-term safety

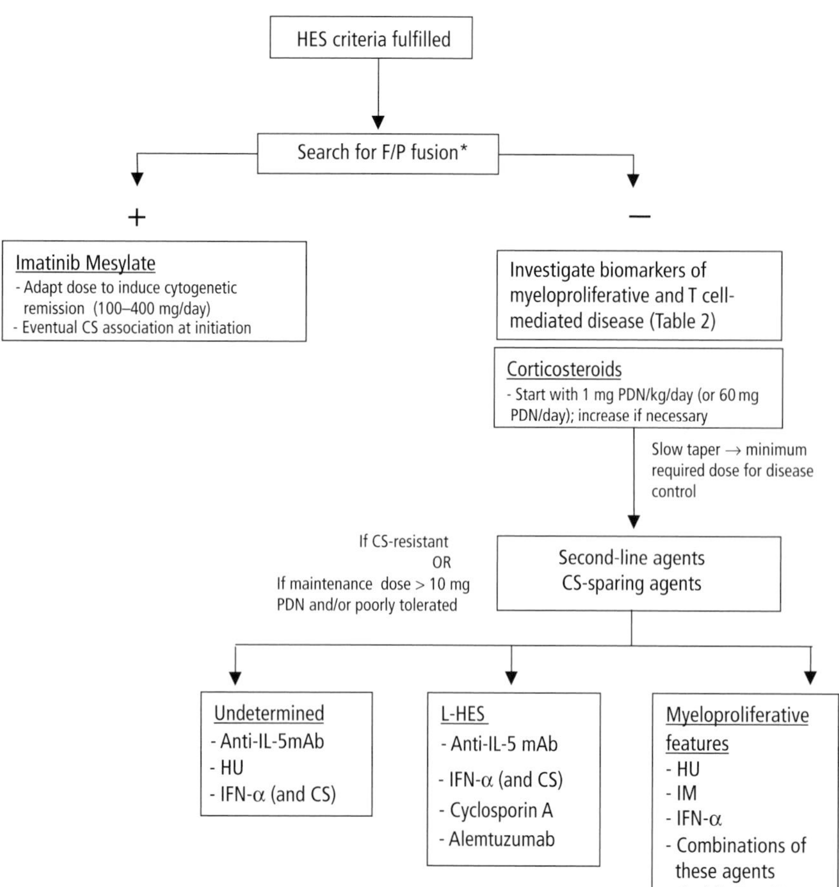

Figure 27.1 Suggested algorithm for management of patients with definite HES.

*Depending on the delay before results are obtained and clinical complications of hypereosinophilia (e.g., microvascular thrombosis, cardiac involvement), it may be necessary to initiate corticosteroids in the meantime (1 mg PDN/kg/d or more).

is currently being evaluated in an open extension of this clinical trial.

Several other agents have been successfully administered to small numbers of HES patients, including vincristine, cyclosporin A, and alemtuzumab, an anti-CD52 mAb (3). Vincristine may be useful for rapid lowering of eosinophil levels in patients with marked leukocytosis (>100,000/μL) and in pediatric cases; Cyclosporin A has been used as a CS-sparing agent in patients with an "allergic" profile; and alemtuzumab was shown to be effective in two patients with refractory HES, one of whom had $CD3^-CD4^+$ T cell–mediated disease (51).

Recommendations

Corticosteroids should be initiated as first-line therapy, at a dose of 1 mg PDN per kilogram per day (or 60 mg/d) and eosinophil levels monitored closely (Grade 1C). In the absence of a rapid response, it may prove useful to administer CS at higher doses for a few days intravenously (e.g. 3–10 mg per kilogram per day). In CS-resistant patients, alternative therapy with second-line agents should be introduced rapidly, especially in patients with life-threatening complications. For patients who do respond to CS, the dose should then be tapered carefully while monitoring eosinophil levels and clinical manifestations to reach the minimal dose required to maintain disease control. If the maintenance dose is more than 10 mg PDN-equivalent per day, addition of a CS-sparing agent should be considered to reduce long-term toxicity.

Although there are currently little data on pathogenesis-oriented approaches to choice of the second-line or CS-sparing agent for a given F/P^- patient, it appears reasonable to take biological and clinical features of disease into account (Figure 27.1; Table 27.2). For patients with clear-cut L-HES or typically associated clinical features, we recommend anti-IL-5 mAb (Grade 1A) or IFN-α combined with CS (Grade 2C). Cyclosporin A and alemtuzumab may represent other alternatives (Grade 2C), whereas IM is not considered a therapeutic option for this variant (Grade 1C). For patients with features of myeloproliferative disease (Table 27.2), we recommend HU, IFN-α, IM or various combinations of these agents (all Grade 1C), anti-IL-5 (Grade 2A). The ranking of IM with regard to the other more classical agents in this setting is debated. Some investigators consider that combined male sex, increased serum vitamin B12 and tryptase levels, circulating myeloid precursors, anemia and thrombocytopenia, splenomegaly, and endomyocardial and marrow fibrosis should prompt a short trial with IM at 400 mg/d before considering other second-line agents (3), given the fact that some patients with an F/P rearrangement remain undetected by PCR and FISH (Grade 2C). In absence of a response to 400 mg/d within four weeks, IM should be withdrawn (Grade 1B). Others recommend trying IM only when CS, HU, and IFN-α have failed. Finally, for patients lacking features of myeloproliferative or T cell–mediated disease, the recommended alternatives include anti-IL-5 (Grade 1A), HU (Grade 1C), and IFN-α (Grade 2C).

In conclusion, at most, half of HES patients can be classified according to well-documented pathogenic mechanisms with a high level of precision. Administration of IM as first-line therapy for F/P^+ patients is widely recommended, although no controlled clinical trial has substantiated this recommendation to date. For F/P^- patients, only mepolizumab has recently been proven highly effective in lowering eosinophil levels and controlling disease, allowing CS tapering, in the setting of a well-conducted clinical trial. Efficacy of other agents classically used for HES, and ranking of therapeutic alternatives according to clinical profiles, have not yet been evaluated in this population.

References

1 Weller P. Causes of eosinophilia [online database]. uptodate.com; 2006.

2 Chusid MJ, Dale DC, West BC, et al. The hypereosinophilic syndrome: analysis of fourteen cases with review of the literature. *Medicine (Baltimore).* 1975;**54**:1–27.

3 Klion AD, Bochner BS, Gleich GJ, et al. Approaches to the treatment of hypereosinophilic syndromes: a workshop summary report. *J Allergy Clin Immunol.* 2006;**117**:1292–302.

4 Weller PF, Bubley GJ. The idiopathic hypereosinophilic syndrome. *Blood.* 1994;**83**:2759–79.

5 Klion A, Weller P. Idiopathic and other hypereosinophilic syndromes [online database]. uptodate.com; 2007.

6 Rothenberg ME, Klion AD, Roufosse FE, et al. Corticosteroid reduction and clinical control in patients with hypereosinophilic syndrome treated with mepolizumab, an anti-interleukin-5 monoclonal antibody. *New Engl J Med.* 2008; **358**:1215–28.

7 Guyatt G, Gutterman D, Baumann MH, et al. Grading strength of recommendations and quality of evidence in clinical guidelines: report from an american college of chest physicians task force. *Chest.* 2006;**129**: 174–81.

8 Rothenberg ME, Hogan SP. The eosinophil. *Annu Rev Immunol.* 2006;**24**:147–74.

9 Romagnani S. Th1 and Th2 in human diseases. *Clin Immunol Immunopathol.* 1996;**80**:225–35.

10 Cools J, DeAngelo DJ, Gotlib J, et al. A tyrosine kinase created by fusion of the PDGFRA and FIP1L1 genes as a therapeutic target of imatinib in idiopathic hypereosinophilic syndrome. *N Engl J Med.* 2003;**348**:1201–14.

11 Vandenberghe P, Wlodarska I, Michaux L, et al. Clinical and molecular features of FIP1L1-PDFGRA (+) chronic eosinophilic leukemias. *Leukemia.* 2004;**18**:734–42.

12 Klion AD, Robyn J, Akin C, et al. Molecular remission and reversal of myelofibrosis in response to imatinib mesylate treatment in patients with the myeloproliferative variant of hypereosinophilic syndrome. *Blood.* 2004;**103**:473–78.

13 Gleich GJ, Leiferman KM, Pardanani A, et al. Treatment of hypereosinophilic syndrome with imatinib mesilate. *Lancet.* 2002;**359**: 1577–78.

14 Klion AD, Noel P, Akin C, et al. Elevated serum tryptase levels identify a subset of patients with a myeloproliferative variant of idiopathic hypereosinophilic syndrome associated with tissue fibrosis, poor prognosis, and imatinib responsiveness. *Blood.* 2003;**101**:4660–66.

15 Score J, Curtis C, Waghorn K. Identification of a novel imatinib responsive KIF5B-PDGFRA fusion gene following screening for PDGFRA overexpression in patients with hypereosinophilia. *Leukemia.* 2006;**20**:827–32.

16 Curtis CE, Grand FH, Musto P, et al. Two novel imatinib-responsive PDGFRA fusion genes in chronic eosinophilic leukaemia. *Br J Haematol.* 2007; **138**:77–81.

17 Bank I, Amariglio N, Reshef A, et al. The hypereosinophilic syndrome associated with CD4+CD3- helper type 2 (Th2) lymphocytes. *Leuk Lymphoma.* 2001;**42**:123–33.

18 Brugnoni D, Airo P, Rossi G, et al. A case of hypereosinophilic syndrome is associated with the expansion of a CD3-CD4+ T-cell population able to secrete large amounts of interleukin-5. *Blood.* 1996;**87**:1416–22.

19 Cogan E, Schandene L, Crusiaux A, et al. Brief report: clonal proliferation of type 2 helper T cells in a man with the hypereosinophilic syndrome. *N Engl J Med.* 1994;**330**:535–38.

20 Roufosse F, Cogan E, Goldman M. Lymphocytic variant hypereosinophilic syndromes. *Immunol Allergy Clin North Am.* 2007;**27**:389–413.

21 Roufosse F, Schandene L, Sibille C, et al. Clonal Th2 lymphocytes in patients with the idiopathic hypereosinophilic syndrome. *Br J Haematol.* 2000;**109**:540–48.

22 Ravoet M, Sibille C, Roufosse F, et al. 6q- is an early and persistent chromosomal aberration in $CD3^-CD4^+$ T-cell clones associated with the lymphocytic variant of hypereosinophilic syndrome. *Haematologica.* 2005;**90**:753–65.

23 Kitano K, Ichikawa N, Shimodaira S, et al. Eosinophilia associated with clonal T-cell proliferation. *Leuk Lymphoma.* 1997;**27**:335–42.

24 Simon HU, Plotz SG, Dummer R, et al. Abnormal clones of T cells producing interleukin-5 in idiopathic eosinophilia. *N Engl J Med.* 1999;**341**:1112–20.

25 Pardanani A, Ketterling RP, Brockman SR, et al. CHIC2 deletion, a surrogate for FIP1L1-PDGFRA fusion, occurs in systemic mastocytosis associated with eosinophilia and predicts response to imatinib mesylate therapy. *Blood.* 2003;**102**:3093–96.

26 Jovanovic JV, Score J, Waghorn K, et al. Low-dose imatinib mesylate leads to rapid induction of major molecular responses and achievement of complete molecular remission in FIP1L1-PDGFRA positive chronic eosinophilic leukemia. *Blood.* 2007; **109**:4635–40.

27 de Lavareille A, Roufosse F, Schmid-Grendelmeier P, et al. High serum thymus and activation-regulated chemokine levels in the lymphocytic variant of the hypereosinophilic syndrome. *J Allergy Clin Immunol.* 2002;**110**:476–79.

28 Savage, DG, Antman KH. Imatinib mesylate—a new oral targeted therapy. *N Engl J Med.* 2002;**346**:683–93.

29 Muller AM, Martens UM, Hofmann SC, et al. Imatinib mesylate as a novel treatment option for hypereosinophilic syndrome: two case reports and a comprehensive review of the literature. *Ann Hematol.* 2006;**85**:1–16.

30 Pardanani A, Brockman SR, Paternoster SF, et al. FIP1L1-PDGFRA fusion: prevalence and clinicopathologic correlates in 89 consecutive patients with moderate to severe eosinophilia. *Blood.* 2004;**104**:3038–45.

31 Klion AD, Robyn J, Maric I, et al. Relapse following discontinuation of imatinib mesylate therapy for FIP1L1/PDGFRA-positive chronic eosinophilic leukemia: implications for optimal dosing. *Blood.* 2007;**110**:3552–6.

32 von Bubnoff N, Sandherr M, Schlimok G, et al. Myeloid blast crisis evolving during imatinib treatment of an FIP1L1-PDGFR alpha-positive chronic myeloproliferative disease with prominent eosinophilia. *Leukemia.* 2005;**19**:286–87.

33 Pardanani A, Reeder T, Porrata LF, et al. Imatinib therapy for hypereosinophilic syndrome and other eosinophilic disorders. *Blood.* 2003;**1**:3391–97.

34 Pitini V, Arrigo C, Azzarello D, et al. Serum concentration of cardiac Troponin T in patients with hypereosinophilic syndrome treated with imatinib is predictive of adverse outcomes. *Blood.* 2003;**102**:3456–57.

35 Kerkela R, Grazette L, Yacobi R, et al. Cardiotoxicity of the cancer therapeutic agent imatinib mesylate. *Nat Med.* 2006;**12**:908–16.

36 Fletcher S, Bain B. Diagnosis and treatment of hypereosinophilic syndromes. *Curr Opin Hematol.* 2007;**14**:37–42.

37 Parrillo JE, Fauci, AS, Wolff SM. Therapy of the hypereosinophilic syndrome. *Ann Intern Med.* 1978;**89**:167–72.

38 Fauci AS, Harley JB, Roberts WC. NIH conference. The idiopathic hypereosinophilic syndrome. Clinical, pathophysiologic, and therapeutic considerations. *Ann Intern Med.* 1982;**97**:78–92.

39 Sugimoto K, Tamayose K, Sasaki M, et al. More than 13 years of hypereosinophila associated with clonal CD3-CD4+ lymphocytosis of TH2/TH0 type. *Int J Hematol.* 2002;**75**:281–284.

40 Butterfield JH. Interferon treatment for hypereosinophilic syndromes and systemic mastocytosis. *Acta Haematol.* 2005;**114**:26–40.

41 Butterfield JH, Gleich GJ. Interferon-alpha treatment of six patients with the idiopathic hypereosinophilic syndrome. *Ann Intern Med.* 1994;**121**:648–53.

42 Malbrain ML, Van den Bergh H, Zachee P. Further evidence for the clonal nature of the idiopathic hypereosinophilic syndrome: complete haematological and cytogenetic remission induced by interferon-alpha in a case with a unique chromosomal abnormality. *Br J Haematol.* 1996;**92**:176–83.

43 Musto P, Falcone A, Sanpaolo G. Heterogeneity of response to imatinib-mesylate (glivec) in patients with hypereosinophilic syndrome: implications for dosing and pathogenesis. *Leuk Lymphoma.* 2004;**45**:1219–22.

44 Vaklavas C, Tefferi A, Butterfield J, et al. 'Idiopathic' eosinophilia with an Occult T-cell clone: Prevalence and clinical course. *Leuk Res.* 2007;**31**:691–4.

45 Kay AB, Klion AD. Anti-interleukin-5 therapy for asthma and hypereosinophilic syndrome. *Immunol Allergy Clin North Am.* 2004;**24**:645–66, vii.

46 Sutton SA, Assa'ad AH, Rothenberg ME. Anti-IL-5 and hypereosinophilic syndromes. *Clin Immunol.* 2005;**115**:51–60.

47 Klion AD, Law MA, Noel P. Safety and efficacy of the monoclonal anti-interleukin-5 antibody SCH55700 in the treatment of patients with hypereosinophilic syndrome. *Blood.* 2004;**103**:2939–41.

48 Plotz SG, Simon HU, Darsow U, et al. Use of an anti-interleukin-5 antibody in the hypereosinophilic syndrome with eosinophilic dermatitis. *N Engl J Med.* 2003;**349**:2334–39.

49 Garrett JK, Jameson SC, Thomson B, et al. Anti-interleukin-5 (mepolizumab) therapy for hypereosinophilic syndromes. *J Allergy Clin Immunol.* 2004;**113**:115–19.

50 Roufosse F, Goldman M, Cogan E. Hypereosinophilic syndromes: a novel therapeutic indication for tyrosine kinase inhibitors and IL-5 antagonists. *Drug Discov Today Thera Strateg.* 2006;**3**:55–61.

51 Pitini V, Teti D, Arrigo C. Alemtuzumab therapy for refractory idiopathic hypereosinophilic syndrome with abnormal T cells: a case report. *Br J Haematol.* 2004;**127**:477.

28 Porphyrias

Gagan Sood, Karl E. Anderson

Porphyrias result from enzymatic defects in the heme biosynthetic pathway and present with neurovisceral or photocutaneous symptoms due to accumulated intermediates (1). Sensitive and specific laboratory methods are available for diagnosis. Effective treatments have been developed, and their use is supported mostly by observational studies and strong scientific rationale, but because of the rarity of these diseases, randomized controlled trials are lacking. This review poses clinically relevant questions as the basis for summarizing diagnostic and treatment recommendations for the four acute porphyrias, porphyria cutanea tarda (PCT), erythropoietic protoporphyria (EPP), and congenital erythropoietic porphyria CEP). A systematic literature review used MEDLINE (PubMed version), EMBASE (dialog version), and Cochrane Library data from 1966 to January 2007. The search included all human studies in English on diagnosis and treatment of porphyrias in all age groups and countries and all study designs, including observational and randomized controlled studies. The quality of the evidence was graded according to the Grading of Recommendations Assessment, Development, and Evaluation Working Group (GRADE) definitions as proposed by a recent American College of Chest Physicians Task Force report (2).

Diagnosis of porphyrias

Porphyrias are classified as erythropoietic or hepatic based on the major site of initial accumulation of pathway intermediates or as acute or cutaneous based on major clinical characteristics (Table 28.1). Very different specific and sensitive laboratory tests are available for screening for the acute and cutaneous porphyrias

Acute porphyrias

The four acute porphyrias (standard abbreviations shown in Table 28.1) cause acute attacks of neurological symptoms that can be life threatening and require prompt diagnosis and treatment.

Evidence-based Hematology. Edited by Mark A. Crowther, Jeff Ginsberg, Holger J. Schünemann, Ralph M. Meyer, and Richard Lottenberg.

Diagnosis of the acute attack

What is the evidence that demonstration of a substantial increase in urinary porphobilinogen is sensitive and specific for diagnosis of acute porphyrias?

Rapid detection of increased urinary porphobilinogen (PBG) by a method such as the Trace PBG kit (Trace America/Trace Diagnostics, Louisville, CO) (3) is important for prompt diagnosis of acute porphyrias. Detection of a substantial increase in PBG in a spot urine sample provides a quick diagnosis of the three most common acute porphyrias, acute intermittant porphyria (AIP), hereditary copophyria (HCP), and variegate porphyria (VP) and avoids delay from collecting a 24-hour urine and shipping to an off-site laboratory. A negative result makes an acute attack of porphyria very unlikely. The sample should be saved for later confirmation of the positive or negative PBG result and to measure δ-aminolevulinic acid (ALA), to detect very rare cases of ALA dehydratase porphyria (ADP) and porphyrins (which remain elevated in some cases of HCP and VP after ALA and PBG have fallen to normal). If PBG is substantially elevated, treatment of the attack can begin while further testing is in progress. Sensitivity and specificity of a kit for semiquantitative assessment of urinary PBG is much higher than the older Watson Schwartz test (4).

In a study of 196 patients with AIP and their families, urinary PBG was elevated (20- to 50-fold greater than reference values) in all patients during acute attacks, and in two-thirds of patients in remission. Erythrocyte PBG deaminase activity was decreased in 84% of AIP patients but also in 23% of healthy subjects reflecting overlap between the ranges for AIP and normals (5).

Second-line tests, which are essential to differentiate AIP, HCP, and VP and to diagnose ADP, lack specificity, and their use for initial screening may reveal nonspecific abnormalities and lead to an incorrect diagnosis of porphyria (3). Fecal porphyrins are normal or minimally increased in AIP but substantially increased in HCP (marked predominance of coproporphyrin III) and VP (predominance of both coproporphyrin III and protoporphyrin). Plasma porphyrins are increased in VP, with a characteristic fluorescence peak at neutral pH (6,7). Urinary coproporphyrins are usually more elevated in HCP and VP than in AIP. ADP causes substantial

Table 28.1 Classification of the human porphyrias, the underlying enzyme deficiencies, modes of inheritance, and increases in porphyrin precursors and porphyrins that are most important for laboratory diagnosis.

	Classification		Deficient enzyme	Inheritance	Increased porphyrin precursors and/or porphyrins*			
	Erythropoietic	Hepatic			Urine	Plasma	Erythrocytes	Stool
Acute porphyrias								
ALAD[†] Porphyria (ADP)		+	ALAD	AR	ALA, coproporphyrin III	—	Zn protoporphyrin	
Acute intermittent porphyria (AIP)		+	PBGD	AD	ALA, PBG, uroporphyrin	—	—	
Acute and cutaneous porphyrias[†]								
Hereditary coproporphyria (HCP)[‡]		+	CPO	AD	ALA, PBG, uroporphyrin, coproporphyrin III	—	—	Coproporphyrin III
Variegate porphyria (VP)[‡]		+	PPO	AD	ALA, PBG, uroporphyrin, coproporphyrin III	Porphyrin covalently bound to protein[§]	—	Coproporphyrin III, protoporphyrin
Cutaneous porphyrias								
Congenital erythropoietic porphyria (CEP)	+		UROS	AR	Uroporphyrin I, coproporphyrin I			Coproporphyrin I
Porphyria cutanea tarda (PCT)		+	UROD	AD	Uroporphyrin, coproporphyrin	Uroporphyrin, coproporphyrin	—	Isocoproporphyrin
Hepatoerythropoietic porphyria (HEP)	+	+	UROD	AR	Uroporphyrin, coproporphyrin	Uroporphyrin, coproporphyrin	Zn protoporphyrin	Isocopro-porphyrin
Erythropoietic protoporphyria (EPP)	+		FECH[¶]	AD	—	Protoporphyrin	Free protoporphyrin	Protoporphyrin

*Substantial increases that are most important for diagnosis.

[†]Abbreviations and alternate names: ALA, 5-aminolevulinic acid; PBG, porphobilinogen; ALAD, ALA dehydratase, also known as PBG synthase; PBGD, PBG deaminase, also known as hydroxymethylbilane synthase; UROS, uroporphyrinogen III synthase, also known as uroporphyrinogen III cosynthase; UROD, uroporphyrinogen decarboxylase; CPO, coproporphyrinogen oxidase; PPO, protoporphyrinogen oxidase; FECH, ferrochelatase; AD, autosomal dominant; AR, autosomal recessive.

[‡]These acute porphyrias are also classified as cutaneous, because they may present with blistering skin lesions resembling porphyria cutanea tarda.

[§]Detected by fluorescence spectroscopy of diluted plasma at neutral pH.

[¶]In most families, expressed disease results from inheritance of a null mutation from one parent and a low-expression normal allele caused by a common intronic polymorphism from the other parent.

increases in urinary ALA and coproporphyrin and erythrocyte protoporphyrin (Table 28.1).

Decreased erythrocyte PBG deaminase (PBGD) helps confirm a diagnosis of AIP. However, a mutation in or near exon 1 of the PBGD gene may cause a deficiency of the housekeeping but not the erythroid enzyme (1). The erythrocyte enzyme is also age-sensitive (8) and may be falsely normal in very ill patients with increased erythropoiesis. Assays for the mitochondrial enzymes that are deficient in HCP and VP are technically challenging.

Cases of acute porphyrias should be confirmed by mutation analysis, which greatly facilitates detection of other gene carriers in a family (1,9). Mutational analysis is available in United States through the Department of Human Genetics at Mount Sinai Medical Center, New York (3).

Recurrent attacks of porphyria are diagnosed on clinical grounds, and it is not necessary to document increases in ALA and PBG with each attack (3).

Levels of ALA, PBG, and porphyrins decrease with recovery from an attack and may become normal with prolonged clinical latency. In HCP and VP, ALA and PBG levels are less markedly increased and may decrease more rapidly after an acute attack. Prior hemin therapy often normalizes these levels (usually transiently) and decreases the likelihood of positive findings.

If erythrocyte PBG deaminase activity is low in a case of AIP, relatives can be tested by that method. The preferred approach is to identify the disease-related mutation in a well-documented index case and then screen family members for that mutation. Biochemical testing can follow to assess the degree of disease expression (3).

Recommendations

- All major medical centers should be prepared to screen patients for elevated PBG using spot urine samples by a rapid method (Grade 1C).
- Second-line biochemical testing should differentiate the type of acute porphyria, and the diagnosis should be finally confirmed by mutation analysis (Grade 1C).
- Measurement of erythrocyte PBGD activity is part of second-line testing, and if the activity is low in an index case, this can be used to detect asymptomatic carriers of the enzyme deficiency in the family (Grade 1C).
- Mutation analysis should be done after the type of acute porphyria is established by biochemical testing, and the identified mutation can be looked for in other family members (Grade 1C).

Diagnosis of porphyrias causing blistering cutaneous porphyrias

Which tests are sensitive and specific for diagnosis of porphyrias that cause blistering skin lesions?

PCT, the most common porphyria, usually presents in middle or late adult life with blisters on the backs of the hands and other sun-exposed areas. VP and much less commonly HCP can cause identical skin manifestations. The total plasma porphyrin concentration is substantially elevated in all porphyrias that cause blistering skin lesions. PCT is confirmed by finding substantial increases in uroporphyrin and heptacarboxylporphyrin in urine or plasma or an increase in isocoproporphyrin in feces. But urinary porphyrin measurements are not preferred for screening because elevations, especially in coproporphyrin, lack specificity. VP can be rapidly differentiated from PCT by a fluorescence scan of porphyrins in diluted plasma (6,7). Fecal porphyrin increases are much greater in VP and HCP than in PCT. Patients with pseudoporphyria have PCT-like skin lesions but no significant elevations in plasma total porphyrins.

CEP, also known as Günther disease may present as nonimmune hydrops (10) or in early childhood with severe skin blistering, which over time is often complicated by infection and mutilation. Uroporphyrin I and coproporphyrin I are markedly elevated in bone marrow, erythrocytes, plasma, urine, and feces. Milder cases in adults may resemble PCT and may be due to myelodysplasia and expansion of a clone of erythroid cells harboring a somatic UROS mutation (11). A case of CEP in a child due to a GATA mutation was recently described (12).

In HEP, the autosomal recessive form of familial (type 2) PCT, the predominant porphyrins in plasma and urine are uroporphyrin and heptacarboxylporphyrin, and zinc protoporphyrin is increased in erythrocytes.

Recommendations

- The preferred screening test for porphyrias that cause blistering skin lesions is measurement of the total plasma porphyrin concentration (Grade 1C).
- Second-line testing readily differentiates the several types of porphyria that cause blistering skin lesions (Grade 1C).

Erythropoietic protoporphyria

In patients with cutaneous photosensitivity that suggest erythropoietic protoporphyria, which tests are sensitive and specific for diagnosis of this condition?

EPP, the third most common porphyria and the most common in children, causes nonblistering photosensitivity that differs from all other cutaneous porphyrias. Plasma porphyrins are increased but often to a lesser degree than in other cutaneous porphyrias. EPP is most reliably screened for by measuring total erythrocyte protoporphyrin, which includes both zinc protoporphyrin and metal-free protoporphyrin. Increased erythrocyte zinc protoporphyrin occurs in many conditions affecting erythrocytes (iron deficiency, thalassemia, lead poisoning, etc.). A substantial increase in metal-free protoporphyrin is specific for EPP. Most patients have inherited a ferrochelatase (FECH) null mutation from one parent and a low-expression FECH polymorphism from the other. This common polymorphism by itself has no phenotype, even when homozygous. In a recently described variant, FECH activity is normal, and both free and zinc protoporphyrin are increased in erythrocytes (13). In these cases, a genetic defect in iron delivery to normal FECH is postulated. Rare late-onset cases of EPP may be associated with myelodysplastic syndromes and expansion of a clone of hematopoietic cells with deletion of one *FECH* allele (14).

Recommendations

- Measurement of erythrocyte protoporphyrin is the preferred method of screening for EPP (Grade 1C), although plasma porphyrins are also elevated in most cases.
- The diagnosis is confirmed by finding a predominant increase in erythrocyte metal-free protoporphyrin.
- Mutation analysis facilitates family screening and genetic counseling.

Treatment of acute porphyrias

Neurovisceral symptoms are treated in the same manner in all four acute porphyrias but have been most studied in AIP and VP.

Hemin therapy

In patients with documented acute porphyria who present with an acute attack, what is the evidence that hemin is effective?

Hemin is the generic name that includes lyophilized hematin (heme hydroxide, available in the United States as Panhematin®, Ovation Pharmaceuticals, Deerfield, IL) and for heme arginate (available in Europe and South Africa as Normosang®, Orphan Europe, Paris, France). By repressing the induction of the rate-limiting hepatic enzyme δ-aminolevulinic acid synthase 1 (ALAS1), hemin addresses an important aspect of the underlying pathophysiology of the acute porphyrias. Intravenous infusion of hematin was first shown in 1971 to decrease ALA and PBG in a severe case of AIP (15). Experience by 1979 included 32 published cases and 45 courses of treatment and indicated that a biochemical response was consistent but clinical improvement was less predictable (16). A single randomized controlled trial comparing heme arginate and placebo in nine patients treated at different times with heme arginate and placebo showed striking biochemical improvement with hemin and trends favoring clinical efficacy that were not statistically significant (17). This study was underpowered, included a limited number of clinical endpoints, and treatment was delayed for two days after hospitalization. Later published experience indicates that clinical response to hemin is frequent if given early in an attack but less evident after extensive neuropathic damage has developed. For example, in a series in France and Finland, heme arginate was started within 24 hours of admission for treatment of 51 attacks in 22 patients, and within four days in 49 attacks (73% and 96%, respectively). All patients responded, and hospitalization was seven days or less in 90% of cases (18). Although adequately powered randomized clinical trials were not conducted, hemin was the first drug approved for marketing in the United States under the Orphan Drug Act. The standard regimen for hemin treatment is 3–4 mg/kg of body weight infused intravenously once daily for four days, or longer for more severe attacks or if treatment is delayed (3).

Instability of hematin in solution was found to account for the occurrence of infusion site phlebitis in up to 50% of infusions into peripheral veins (19) and, even more commonly, a transient anticoagulant effect that is seldom clinically manifest (20,21). Degradation of hemin can be prevented by preparing hemin as heme arginate (22) or reconstituting hematin with albumin (21), which reduces the risk of both phlebitis and transient anticoagulation and may enhance efficacy (21). Rare adverse events have included circulatory collapse and hemolysis after hematin (23,24) and anaphylaxis after heme arginate (25). A fourfold excessive dose of hematin caused gross hematinuria and acute, reversible renal impairment in one patient (26).

Recommendation

Hemin therapy is recommended for acute attacks of porphyria supported by numerous reports of a biochemical response and clinical effectiveness documented in case series (Grade 1C).

Carbohydrate loading

In patients with documented acute porphyria who present with an acute attack, what is the evidence that carbohydrate loading is effective?

Induction of hepatic ALAS1 is enhanced by fasting and repressed by carbohydrate loading in animals and in patients with acute porphyria (27,28), and these effects are mediated by the peroxisome proliferator-activated receptor γ coactivator 1α (PGC-1 α) (29). Early case studies suggested benefit from carbohydrate loading in AIP (27,28). In seven patients with AIP, urine ALA and PBG increased with low-calorie diets and decreased with a high carbohydrate diet (27). Favorable biochemical and clinical responses to a high carbohydrate diet were observed in 10 of 14 patients (30). In another series of 32 courses of treatment of patients with acute hepatic porphyrias, high-carbohydrate diet (450–500 gm/d) resulted in biochemical and clinical improvement in most patients, although details of their clinical presentation and responses were not provided (31). These and other studies of carbohydrate loading have included small numbers of patients that were heterogeneous in clinical severity. There have been no randomized trials comparing carbohydrate loading to placebo or hemin, but there is a consensus that this treatment may be beneficial for mild attacks and that many patients with more severe attacks will respond to hemin after failing to respond to carbohydrate loading (16,31). The standard intravenous regimen is 10% glucose for a total of at least 300 gm daily, with amounts up to 500 g daily being possibly more effective (3). However, the large fluid volumes required may increase the risk of hyponatremia. Patients without vomiting, ileus, or abdominal distension may be given oral sucrose, glucose polymers, or carbohydrate-rich foods.

Recommendation

Intravenous glucose loading is recommended only for early treatment of mild attacks (e.g., mild pain and nausea, no motor neuropathy, hyponatremia, or seizures, Grade 2C).

Cimetidine

In patients with documented acute porphyria who present with an acute attack, what is the evidence that cimetidine is effective?

Cimetidine is a well-known inhibitor of hepatic CYPs and was shown to prevent experimental forms of porphyria induced by chemical agents that are activated by these enzymes (32). This mechanism is not highly relevant to human acute porphyrias. Biochemical and clinical improvement has been reported with oral cimetidine in several individual patients (33), and subsequently intravenous administration of 900–1,200 mg cimetidine daily resulted in clinical and biochemical improvement in four patients (34). But the scientific rationale and clinical evidence are not sufficient to recommend use of cimetidine in acute porphyria at this time.

Recommendation

• Based on current evidence, cimetidine is not recommended (Grade 2C).

Supportive, symptomatic, and other treatment

In patients with documented acute porphyria who present with an acute attack, what is the evidence that supportive therapies are effective?

Supportive and symptomatic treatment of pain, nausea, vomiting and electrolyte imbalances that occurs during acute attacks is essential (3), but the evidence is from clinical observations rather than controlled studies.

Pain in the abdomen, chest, back, and extremities usually requires a narcotic analgesic. Nausea and vomiting are treated with a phenothiazine or ondansetron. Phenothiazines are also useful for tremors, increased sweating, restlessness, insomnia, disorientation, hallucinations, and paranoia. Porphyria is an approved treatment indication for chlorpromazine, but published evidence is limited (35,36). Dosing recommended in product labeling is considered excessive and prolonged treatment is seldom if ever indicated. Agitation and anxiety can be treated with low doses of benzodiazepines. Tachycardia and hypertension, if severe or symptomatic, may be treated cautiously with a β-adrenergic blocker such as propranolol. Acute depression may require a serotonin reuptake inhibitor or other antidepressant (3). Hyponatremia may cause seizures and be due to hypothalamic involvement and inappropriate antidiuretic hormone secretion. Seizures in the absence of hyponatremia may be an acute neurological manifestation of porphyria. Most anticonvulsants are unsafe; clonazepam may be less harmful than others; gabapentin and probably vigabatrin are safe.

AIP improved markedly both clinically and biochemically after liver transplantation in one reported case (37), and this may become an option for severe cases that do not respond to established therapies.

A double-blind placebo controlled study of recombinant human PBG deaminase infused intravenously for 48 hours had a marked lowering effect on PBG (but not ALA and porphyrins) in both latent AIP and during acute attacks, but was not clinically beneficial (38). Enzyme replacement in hepatocytes may be accomplished in the future and be more effective.

Recommendations

• Opioid analgesics, phenothiazines, β-adrenergic blockers, and other drugs are important for treatment of severe symptoms, until these improve with specific therapies (Grade 1C).

• Liver transplantation is not generally recommended at this time (Grade 1C).

Early detection of hepatocellular carcinoma

Chronic elevations in AST and ALT are common in AIP, HCP and VP, and the risk of hepatocellular carcinoma, not associated with elevations in serum α-fetoprotein, is increased (39,40).

Recommendation

• Screening by ultrasound or another suitable imaging technique is suggested yearly after age 40 (Grade 2C).

Prevention of recurrent attacks

Some patients continue to have acute attacks or chronic symptoms even with avoidance of harmful drugs and dietary indiscretions. Long-term oral carbohydrate loading is seldom of value and may lead to undesirable weight gain. Frequent premenstrual attacks can be prevented by administration of a GnRH analogue with low-dose estrogen add-back if effective; this approach is reversible and usually preferable to surgical oophorectomy (41). Prophylactic infusions of hemin may also be effective in preventing frequent attacks, but published experience is limited (42).

Recommendations

• A GnRH analogue is recommended for prevention of attacks recurring frequently and confined to the luteal phase of the menstrual cycle (Grade 1B).

• A trial of hemin infusions at timed intervals (e.g., weekly) is recommended for prevention of frequent noncyclic attacks (Grade 2C).

Treatment of congenital erythropoietic porphyria

Treatment of CEP primarily involves protection of skin from sunlight and treatment of infections to avoid mutilation. Oral β-carotene may be of some value. Severe, transfusion-dependent cases may benefit from splenectomy. A long-term, high-level transfusion regimen with or without hydroxyurea may help to suppress erythropoiesis and decrease porphyrin production and photosensitivity (43). Other treatment approaches have included oral activated charcoal, which adsorbs porphyrins in the intestine and prevents their reabsorption, plasmapheresis, and intravenous hemin (44,45). Bone marrow or stem cell transplantation has markedly reduced porphyrin levels and photosensitivity and increased long-term survival (46–49).

Recommendation

• Bone marrow or stem cell transplantation should be considered especially for severe, transfusion-dependent cases (Grade 1C).

Treatment of porphyria cutanea tarda

Removal of susceptibility factors such as alcohol, estrogens, or smoking is beneficial, but improvement is likely to be slow without treatment by phlebotomy or low-dose chloroquine or hydroxychloroquine. Treatment of hepatitis C, which is commonly associated with PCT, is seldom urgent, can interfere with treatment of PCT by phlebotomy, and is therefore best postponed until PCT is in remission (50).

Repeated phlebotomy

In patients with documented PCT, what is the evidence that repeated phlebotomies are effective?

PCT is an iron-dependent disease, and the scientific rationale for its treatment by phlebotomy, which depletes hepatic iron and interrupts formation of an inhibitor of UROD, is strong. This is the most widely recommended treatment for PCT, based on multiple case series rather than randomized controlled trials. For example, 18 of 20 patients treated by phlebotomy responded both biochemically and clinically, and remission persisted more than one year in 14 cases (51). In another study, clinical and partial biochemical remission was observed in all 44 patients treated by phlebotomy and in only 2 of 12 who had no active intervention. Fifteen of 41 patients who underwent phlebotomy relapsed biochemically during 3–10 years of follow-up, and remission was achieved with reinstitution of phlebotomies (52). Later studies established that response is best monitored by serum ferritin and plasma porphyrin levels. Phlebotomies at about two-week intervals are continued until the serum ferritin is reduced to ~20 ng/mL, without producing significant anemia (53,54). Porphyrin levels decrease to normal in parallel but more slowly, and development of new skin lesions ceases (50).

Recommendation

Repeated phlebotomy is recommended for treatment of PCT, especially in patients with substantial iron overload and/or genetic hemochromatosis (Grade 1C).

Low-dose 4-aminoquinolines

In patients with documented PCT, what is the evidence that treatment with low-dose hydroxychloroquine or chloroquine is effective?

Use of low doses of these 4-aminoquinoline antimalarial drugs as an alternative treatment is supported by numerous case series, but randomized controlled trials are lacking. The mechanism for the effects of these drugs in PCT is uncertain (55). Standard dosing induces acute hepatocellular damage, releases the excess porphyrins stored in the liver, increases plasma and urinary porphyrins and photosensitivity, and is then followed by remission of the porphyria. These troublesome side effects are largely avoided with a very low dose regimen (100 mg of hydroxychloroquine or 125 mg of chloroquine twice weekly), which is continued until porphyrin levels have been normal for least several months (56,57). The risk of retinal damage is very low, but ophthalmologic evaluation is advisable before treatment.

Low-dose chloroquine achieved symptomatic and biochemical remission in all four patients reported by Felscher and coworkers (58). Additional small case series supported the beneficial effect of chloroquine (59,60). Treatment of 30 patients with hydroxychloroquine (200 mg twice weekly — a higher dose than generally recommended) was more effective than phlebotomy in 31 patients, but the efficacy of phlebotomy was unexpectedly low in this series (61). Chloroquine is reported to be ineffective in patients with PCT and hemochromatosis (HFE genotype C282Y/C282Y) (62).

Recommendation

• A low-dose regimen of one of the antimalarial 4-aminoquinolines is recommended as an alternative treatment of PCT when phlebotomy is contraindicated or poorly tolerated (Grade 1C).

Treatment of erythropoietic protoporphyria

In patients with established EPP, what is the evidence that β-carotene is effective in partially controlling symptoms?

Most patients with EPP have life-long photosensitivity due to increases in circulating porphyrin levels. Avoidance of sunlight and use of tightly woven clothing designed for photosensitive individuals is important. Reflectant sunscreens containing zinc oxide or titanium dioxide are more effective in protecting against long-wave ultraviolet light (UV-A) than are conventional sunscreens (63). Sunscreens that include both UV-A and UV-B protection are also useful.

β-carotene was shown to prevent hematoporphyrin-induced photosensitivity in experimental animals and was then studied in EPP. Oral β-carotene 120 to 180 mg daily for one to three months improved tolerance to sunlight in the majority of 53 patients in an uncontrolled trial, in which serum carotene levels were maintained between 600 and 800 mg/dL. There were no untoward side effects except for mild carotenoderma (64). A later controlled trial showed no benefit compared with placebo (65). Some patients find this drug to be partially effective in improving sunlight tolerance.

Oral cysteine was reported to be safe and more effective than placebo in ameliorating photosensitivity in a double-blind crossover study of 16 patients with EPP (66). Narrow-band UV-B phototherapy can increase skin pigmentation and has been used effectively in individual cases (67).

Recommendation

• Topical reflectant sunscreens containing zinc oxide or titanium dioxide, oral β-carotene (Solatene®, Tishcon), or cysteine and narrow-band UV-B phototherapy are recommended for improving tolerance to sunlight and may be partially beneficial in some patients (Grade 2C).

Treatment of protoporphyric hepatopathy

Severe protoporphyric liver disease, which develops in less than 5% of patients, is accompanied by higher than usual circulating porphyrin levels and enhanced photosensitivity and may be further complicated by motor neuropathy resembling that seen in acute porphyrias (68,69). Spontaneous resolution may occur, especially if a reversible cause of liver dysfunction, such as viral hepatitis or alcohol, is contributing (70,71).

Treatment must be individualized and controlled observations are lacking. A combination of plasmapheresis, intravenous hemin (72,73), ursodeoxycholic acid (74,75), cholestyramine (76), and vitamin E is currently recommended, each based on limited studies that suggested effectiveness in one or a few patients. Transfusions for anemia should be considered to suppress erythropoiesis and protoporphyrin accumulation. Red cell exchange has also been advocated (77). Splenectomy may be beneficial when EPP is complicated by hemolysis and splenomegaly (78,79). Recurrent liver damage in 20 patients was common after liver transplantation (65%) but survival (85% at one year and 69% at five years) was comparable to that with other forms of liver disease (80). Sequential liver and bone marrow transplantation was recently successful in a child with EPP and may be the treatment of choice for severe protoporphyric liver disease in the future (81).

Recommendations

• Plasmapheresis, intravenous hemin, ursodeoxycholic acid, cholestyramine, and vitamin E or combinations of these interventions should be considered for treatment of severe protoporphyric hepatopathy (Grade 2C). If there is no improvement, liver transplantation should be considered (Grade 1C).

References

1 Anderson KE, Sassa S, Bishop DF, et al. Disorders of heme biosynthesis: X-linked sideroblastic anemias and the porphyrias. In: Scriver CR, Beaudet AL, Sly WS, et al., editors. *The metabolic and molecular basis of inherited disease.* 8th ed. Vol II. New York: McGraw-Hill; 2001. pp. 2991–3062.

2 Guyatt G, Gutterman D, Baumann MH, et al. Grading strength of recommendations and quality of evidence in clinical guidelines: report from an American College of Chest Physicians Task Force. *Chest.* 2006;**129**(1):174–81.

3 Anderson KE, Bloomer JR, Bonkovsky HL, et al. Recommendations for the diagnosis and treatment of the acute porphyrias. *Ann Intern Med.* 2005;**142**(6):439–50.

4 Deacon AC, Peters TJ. Identification of acute porphyria: evaluation of a commercial screening test for urinary porphobilinogen. *Ann Clin Biochem.* 1998;**35**(Pt 6):726–32.

5 Kauppinen R, von und zu Fraunberg M. Molecular and biochemical studies of acute intermittent porphyria in 196 patients and their families. *Clin Chem.* 2002;**48**(11):1891–900.

6 Poh-Fitzpatrick MB. A plasma porphyrin fluorescence marker for variegate porphyria. *Arch Dermatol.* 1980;**116**:543–47.

7 Hift RJ, Davidson BP, van der Hooft C, et al. Plasma fluorescence scanning and fecal porphyrin analysis for the diagnosis of variegate porphyria: precise determination of sensitivity and specificity with detection of protoporphyrinogen oxidase mutations as a reference standard. *Clin Chem.* 2004;**50**(5):915–23.

8 Anderson KE, Sassa S, Peterson CM, et al. Increased erythrocyte uroporphyrinogen-I-synthetase, δ-aminolevulinic acid dehydratase and protoporphyrin in hemolytic anemias. *Am J Med.* 1977;**63**:359–64.

9 Akagi R, Inoue R, Muranaka S, et al. Dual gene defects involving δ-aminolaevulinate dehydratase and coproporphyrinogen oxidase in a porphyria patient [erratum appears in *Br J Haematol.* 2006;**132**(5):662]. *Br J Haematol.* 2006;**132**:237–43.

10 Verstraeten L, Van Regemorter N, Pardou A, et al. Biochemical diagnosis of a fatal case of Gunther's disease in a newborn with hydrops-fetalis. *Eur J Clin Chem Clin Biochem.* 1993;**31**:121–28.

11 Sassa S, Akagi R, Nishitani C, et al. Late-onset porphyrias: what are they? *Cell Mol Biol (Noisy-le-grand).* 2002;**48**(1):97–101.

12 Phillips JD, Steensma DP, Pulsipher MA, et al. Congenital erythropoietic porphyria due to a mutation in GATA1: the first trans-acting mutation causative for a human porphyria. *Blood.* 2007;**109**(6):2618–21.

13 Wilson JHP, Edixhoven-Bosdijk A, Koole-Lesuis R, et al. A new variant or erythropoietic protoporphyria with normal ferrochelatase activity [abstract]. *Physiol Res.* 2003;**52**:29S.

14 Goodwin RG, Kell WJ, Laidler P, et al. Photosensitivity and acute liver injury in myeloproliferative disorder secondary to late-onset protoporphyria caused by deletion of a ferrochelatase gene in hematopoietic cells. *Blood.* 2006;**107**(1):60–62.

15 Bonkowsky HL, Tschudy DP, Collins A, et al. Repression of the overproduction of porphyrin precursors in acute intermittent porphyria by intravenous infusions of hematin. *Proc Natl Acad Sci USA.* 1971;**8**:2725–29.

16 McColl KEL, Moore MR, Thompson GG, et al. Treatment with haematin in acute hepatic porphyria. *Q J Med.* 1981;**198**:161–74.

17 Herrick AL, McColl KEL, Moore MR, et al. Controlled trial of haem arginate in acute hepatic porphyria. *Lancet.* 1989;**1**:1295–97.

18 Mustajoki P, Nordmann Y. Early administration of heme arginate for acute porphyric attacks. *Arch Int Med.* 1993;**153**:2004–8.

19 Simionatto CS, Cabel R, Jones RL, et al. Thrombophlebitis and disturbed hemostasis following administration of intravenous hematin in normal volunteers. *Am J Med.* 1988;**85**:538–40.

20 Green D, Reynolds N, Klein J, et al. The inactivation of hemostatic factors by hematin. *J Lab Clin Med.* 1983;**102**:361–69.

21 Anderson KE, Bonkovsky HL, Bloomer JR, et al. Reconstitution of hematin for intravenous infusion. *Ann Intern Med.* 2006;**144**(7):537–38.

22 Tenhunen R, Tokola O, Lindén IB: Haem arginate: a new stable haem compound. *J Pharm Pharmacol.* 1987;**39**:780–86.

23 Khanderia U. Circulatory collapse associated with hemin therapy for acute intermittent porphyria. *Clin Pharm.* 1986;**5**:690–92.

24 Petersen JM, Pierach CA. Hematin-induced hemolysis in acute porphyria [letter to editor]. *Ann Intern Med.* 1984;**101**(6):877–88.

25 Daimon M, Susa S, Igarashi M, et al. Administration of heme arginate, but not hematin, caused anaphylactic shock. *Am J Med.* 2001;**110**(3):240.

26 Jeelani Dhar G, Bossenmaier I, Cardinal R, et al. Transitory renal failure following rapid administration of a relatively large amount of hematin in a patient with acute intermittent porphyria in clinical remission. *Acta Med Scand.* 1978;**203**:437–43.

27 Welland FH, Hellman ES, Gaddis EM, et al. Factors affecting the excretion of porphyrin precursors by patients with acute intermittent porphyria. 1. The effects of diet. *Metabolism.* 1964;**13**:232–50.

28 Bonkowsky HL, Collins A, Doherty JM, et al. The glucose effect in rat liver: studies of δ-aminolevulinate synthetase and tyrosine aminotransferase. *Biochim Biophys Acta.* 1973;**320**:561–76.

29 Handschin C, Lin J, Rhee J, et al. Nutritional regulation of hepatic heme biosynthesis and porphyria through PGC-1alpha. *Cell.* 2005;**122**(4):505–15.

30 Stein JA, Tschudy DP. Acute intermittent porphyria: a clinical and biochemical study of 46 patients. *Medicine.* 1970;**49**:1–16.

31 Doss M, Sixel-Dietrich F, Verspohl F. "Glucose effect" and rate limiting function of uroporphyrinogen synthase on porphyrin metabolism in hepatocyte culture: relationship with human acute hepatic porphyrias. *J Clin Chem Clin Biochem.* 1985;**23**(9):505–13.

32 Marcus DL, Nadel H, Lew G, et al. Cimetidine suppresses chemically induced experimental hepatic porphyria. *Am J Med Sci.* 1990;**300**:214–17.

33 Horie Y, Norimoto M, Tajima F, et al. Clinical usefulness of cimetidine treatment for acute relapse in intermittent porphyria. *Clin Chim Acta.* 1995;**234**(1–2):171–75.

34 Cherem JH, Malagon J, Nellen H. Cimetidine and acute intermittent porphyria. *Ann Intern Med.* 2005;**143**(9):694–95.

35 Melby JC, Street JP, Watson CJ. Chlorpromazine in the treatment of porphyria. *J Am Med Assoc.* 1956;**162**(3):174–78.

36 Calvy GL, Leeper RD, Monaco RN, et al. Intermittent acute porphyria treated with chlorpromazine. *N Engl J Med.* 1957;**256**(7):309–11.

37 Soonawalla ZF, Orug T, Badminton MN, et al. Liver transplantation as a cure for acute intermittent porphyria. *Lancet.* 2004;**363**(9410):705–6.

38 Sardh E, Rejkjaer L, Harper P, et al. First clinical trial of I.V. rhPBGD in healthy subjects with and without diagnosed manifest acute intermittent porphyria (AIP) [abstract]. *Physiol Res.* 2003;**52**:23S.

39 Andant C, Puy H, Bogard C, et al. Hepatocellular carcinoma in patients with acute hepatic porphyria: frequency of occurrence and related factors. *J Hepatol.* 2000;**32**(6):933–39.

40 Sardh E, Harper P, Andersson D. Clinical, biochemical and pathohistological aspects in 12 patients with acute porphyria and hepatocellular carcinoma. In: Meissner P, editor. *Porphyrins and porphyrias.* Cape Town; p. 39.

41 Anderson KE, Spitz IM, Bardin CW, et al. A GnRH analogue prevents cyclical attacks of porphyria. *Arch Int Med.* 1990;**150**:1469–74.

42 Anderson KE, Collins S. Open-label study of hemin for acute porphyria: clinical practice implications. *Am J Med.* 2006;**119**(9):801, e19–24.

43 Guarini L, Piomelli S, Poh-Fitzpatrick MB. Hydroxyurea in congenital erythropoietic porphyria [letter]. *N Engl J Med.* 1994;**330**:1091–92.

44 Watson CJ, Bossenmaier I, Cardinal R, et al. Repression by hematin of porphyrin biosynthesis in erythrocyte precursors in congenital erythropoietic porphyria. *Proc Natl Acad Sci USA.* 1974;**71**:278–82.

45 Rank JM, Straka JG, Weimer MK, et al. Hematin therapy in late onset congenital erythropoietic porphyria. *Br J Haematol.* 1990;**75**(4):617–18.

46 Zix-Kieffer I, Langer B, Eyer D, et al. Successful cord blood stem cell transplantation for congenital erythropoietic porphyria (Gunther's disease). *Bone Marrow Transplant.* 1996;**18**(1):217–20.

47 Thomas C, Ged C, Nordmann Y, et al. Correction of congenital erythropoietic porphyria by bone marrow transplantation. *J Pediatr.* 1996;**129**(3):453–56.

48 Tezcan I, Xu W, Gurgey A, et al. Congenital erythropoietic porphyria successfully treated by allogeneic bone marrow transplantation. *Blood.* 1998;**92**(11):4053–58.

49 Dupuis-Girod S, Akkari V, Ged C, et al. Successful match-unrelated donor bone marrow transplantation for congenital erythropoietic porphyria (Gunther disease). *Eur J Pediatr.* 2005;**164**(2):104–7.

50 Anderson KE. The porphyrias. In: Boyer T, Wright T, Manns M, editors. *Zakim and Boyer's hepatology: a textbook of liver diseases.* Philadelphia: Elsevier; 2006. pp. 1391–32.

51 Epstein JH, Redeker AG. Porphyria cutanea tardo; a study of the effect of phlebotomy. *N Engl J Med.* 1968;**279**(24):1301–4.

52 Lundvall O. Phlebotomy treatment of porphyria cutanea tarda. *Acta Derm Venereol Suppl (Stockh).* 1982;**100**:107–18.

53 Rocchi E, Gibertini P, Cassanelli M, et al. Serum ferritin in the assessment of liver iron overload and iron removal therapy in porphyria cutanea tarda. *J Lab Clin Med.* 1986;**107**:36–42.

54 Ratnaike S, Blake D, Campbell D, et al. Plasma ferritin levels as a guide to the treatment of porphyria cutanea tarda by venesection. *Australas J Dermatol.* 1988;**29**:3–7.

55 Egger NG, Goeger DE, Anderson KE. Effects of chloroquine in hematoporphyrin-treated animals. *Chem Biol Interact.* 1996;**102**:69–78.

56 Ashton RE, Hawk JLM, Magnus IA. Low-dose oral chloroquine in the treatment of porphyria cutanea tarda. *Br J Dermatol.* 1984;**3**:609–13.

57 Valls V, Ena J, Enriquez-De-Salamanca R. Low-dose oral chloroquine in patients with porphyria cutanea tarda and low-moderate iron overload. *J Dermatol Sci.* 1994;**7**(3):169–75.

58 Felsher BF, Redeker AG. Effect of chloroquine on hepatic uroporphyrin metabolism in patients with porphyria cutanea tarda. *Medicine.* 1966;**45**:575–83.

59 Vogler WR, Galambos JT, Olansky S. Biochemical effects of chloroquine therapy in porphyria cutanea tarda. *Am J Med.* 1970;**49**:316–21.

60 Malkinson FD, Levitt L. Hydroxychloroquine treatment of porphyria cutanea tarda. *Arch Dermat.* 1980;**116**:1147–50.

61 Cainelli T, Padova CD, Marchesi L, et al. Hydroxychloroquine versus phlebotomy in the treatment of porphyria cutanea tarda. *Br J Dermat.* 1983;**108**:593–600.

62 Stolzel U, Kostler E, Schuppan D, et al. Hemochromatosis (HFE) gene mutations and response to chloroquine in porphyria cutanea tarda. *Arch Dermatol.* 2003;**139**(3):309–13.

63 Kaye ET, Levin JA, Blank IH, et al. Efficiency of opaque photoprotective agents in the visible light range. *Arch Dermatol.* 1991;**127**(3):351–55.

64 Mathews-Roth MM, Pathak MA, Fitzpatrick TB, et al. β-carotene as an oral photoprotective agent in erythropoietic protoporhyria. *JAMA.* 1974;**228**:1004–8.

65 Corbett MF, Herxheimer A, Magnus IA, et al. The long term treatment with beta-carotene in erythropoietic protoporphyria: a controlled trial. *Br J Dermatol.* 1977;**97**(6):655–62.

66 Mathews-Roth MM, Rosner B, Benfell K, et al. A double-blind study of cysteine photoprotection in erythropoietic protoporphyria. *Photodermatol Photoimmunol Photomed.* 1994;**10**(6):244–48.

67 Warren LJ, George S. Erythropoietic protoporphyria treated with narrow-band (TL-01) UVB phototherapy. *Australas J Dermatol.* 1998;**39**(3):179–82.

68 Muley SA, Midani HA, Rank JM, et al. Neuropathy in erythropoietic protoporphyrias. *Neurology*. 1998;**51**(1):262–65.
69 Key NS, Rank JM, Freese D, et al. Hemolytic anemia in protoporphyria: possible precipitating role of liver failure and photic stress. *Am J Hemat.* 1992;**39**:202–7.
70 Bonkovsky HL, Schned AR. Fatal liver failure in protoporphyria: synergism between ethanol excess and the genetic defect. *Gastroenterology.* 1986;**90**:191–201.
71 Poh-Fitzpatrick MB, Whitlock RT, Lefkowitch JH. Changes in protoporphyrin distribution dynamics during liver failure and recovery in a patient with protoporphyria and Epstein-Barr viral hepatitis. *Am J Med.* 1986;**80**:943–50.
72 Bloomer JR, Pierach CA. Effect of hematin administration to patients with protoporphyria and liver disease. *Hepatology.* 1982;**2**:817–21.
73 Do KD, Banner BF, Katz E, et al. Benefits of chronic plasmapheresis and intravenous heme-albumin in erythropoietic protoporphyria after orthotopic liver transplantation. *Transplantation.* 2002;**73**(3):469–72.
74 Pirlich M, Lochs H, Schmidt HH. Liver cirrhosis in erythropoietic protoporphyria: improvement of liver function with ursodeoxycholic acid. *Am J Gastroenterol.* 2001;**96**(12):3468–69.
75 Gross U, Frank M, Doss MO. Hepatic complications of erythropoietic protoporphyria. *Photodermatol Photoimmunol Photomed.* 1998;**14**(2):52–7.
76 McCullough AJ, Barron D, Mullen KD, et al. Fecal protoporphyria excretion in erythropoietic protoporphyria: effect of Cholestyramine and bile acid feeding. *Gastroenterology.* 1988;**94**:177–81.
77 Eichbaum QG, Dzik WH, Chung RT, et al. Red blood cell exchange transfusion in two patients with advanced erythropoietic protoporphyria. *Transfusion.* 2005;**45**(2):208–13.
78 Porter FS, Lowe BA. Congenital erythropoietic protoporphyria. I. Case reports, clinical studies and porphyrin analyses in two brothers. *Blood.* 1963;**22**:521–31.
79 Lamon JM, Poh-Fitzpatrick MB, Lamola AA, et al. Hepatic protoporphyrin production in human protoporphyria: effects of intravenous hematin and analysis of erythrocyte protoporphyrin distribution. *Gastroenterology.* 1980;**79**:115–25.
80 McGuire BM, Bonkovsky HL, Carithers RL Jr, et al. Liver transplantation for erythropoietic protoporphyria liver disease. *Liver Transpl.* 2005;**11**(12):1590–96.
81 Rand EB, Bunin N, Cochran W, et al. Sequential liver and bone marrow transplantation for treatment of erythropoietic protoporphyria. *Pediatrics.* 2006;**118**(6):e1896–99.

29 Membrane and Enzyme Abnormalities of the Erythrocyte

Patrick G. Gallagher, Ernest Beutler

Introduction

Hemolytic anemias due to abnormalities of the erythrocyte membrane and enzymatic defects are well-described disorders. Strategies used in the management of these disorders have not been subjected to randomized control trials but instead are based on small trials, retrospective reviews, and clinical experience. This chapter addresses several important topics in the clinical care of patients with these disorders, including when should splenectomy be performed in patients with hereditary spherocytosis. For each question, a systematic literature review in MEDLINE (PubMed) and Cochrane Library databases April 2007, including only English-language citations, was performed and quality of the reported evidence graded as described (1). No meta-analyses or randomized controlled trials were found. A single systematic review, as well as textbook chapters, published reviews, and original reports were examined.

Where possible, evidence-based recommendations are made for the diagnosis and management of erythrocyte membrane and enzyme abnormalities. Grading of the quality of evidence and strengths of recommendations in this chapter are based on the guidelines proposed by the international Grading of Recommendations Assessment, Development, and Evaluation Working Group (GRADE) adopting the modification used by the American College of Chest Physicians that merges the very low and low categories of quality of evidence (see chapter 1).

What is the best way to diagnose hereditary spherocytosis?

The history

The diagnosis of hereditary spherocytosis (HS) generally is straightforward. Usually, there is a positive family history of HS, a dominantly inherited hemolytic anemia, or splenectomy, or cholecystectomy in childhood or early adulthood (2). However, cases of de novo and recessively inherited HS occur, probably at a greater frequency than typically thought. Signs and symptoms associated with chronic or intermittent hemolysis such as pallor, jaundice, and splenomegaly may be present.

Other inherited and acquired disorders, such as immune hemolytic disease, thermal burns, and Heinz body anemias, are associated with spherocytosis (Table 29.1) (3). In most of these conditions, spherocytes are but one of several types of abnormal erythrocytes, and additional historical data such as onset later in life, recent prescription of various medications such as methyldopa, or symptoms attributable to malignancy or connective tissue disease, are elicited. Additional laboratory features, such as a positive antiglobulin reaction in immune hemolytic disease, may also be present.

Laboratory diagnosis

The classic laboratory features of HS include variable degrees of anemia, reticulocytosis, increased mean corpuscular hemoglobin concentration (MCHC), spherocytes on the peripheral blood smear, hyperbilirubinemia, and an abnormal osmotic fragility test. Guidelines for the diagnosis and management have been published (4).

The blood film

Spherocytic erythrocyte morphology is characteristic but not diagnostic of HS (4). Spherocytes are easily identified on blood film by their characteristic shape. They lack central pallor, their mean cell diameter is decreased, and they appear more intensely hemoglobinized. In mild cases of HS, the blood film may appear normal because the loss of surface area may be too small to be appreciated. In severe cases, numerous small, dense spherocytes and poikilocytes are seen. Specific morphologic findings, including pincered, stomatocytic (band 3 mutation), or acanthocytic (β-spectrin mutation) spherocytes have been correlated with specific membrane mutations. These findings, however, are not diagnostic.

Evidence-based Hematology. Edited by Mark A. Crowther, Jeff Ginsberg, Holger J. Schünemann, Ralph M. Meyer, and Richard Lottenberg.

Table 29.1 Disorders with spherocytes on blood film.

Hereditary spherocytosis
Autoimmune hemolytic anemias (warm-reacting antibodies)
Liver disease
Thermal injuries
Microangiopathic and macroangiopathic hemolytic anemias
Clostridial septicemia
Transfusion reactions with hemolysis
Poisoning with certain snake, spider, and Hymenoptera venoms
Severe hypophosphatemia
ABO blood group incompatibility (in neonates)
Heinz body anemias

Erythrocyte indices

Erythrocyte indices typically demonstrate a normal or borderline low mean corpuscular volume despite increased numbers of reticulocytes, reflecting membrane loss and dehydration. The mean MCHC is usually increased ($\geq$35 g/dL) due to mild cellular dehydration (5). Examination of the indices by automated cell counters has been used as screening tests for HS. An MCHC greater than 35.4 g/dL combined with a red cell distribution width greater than 14 has a sensitivity of 63% and a specificity of 100% (6). Another screening method performed by laser-based cell counters provides a histogram of hyperdense erythrocytes (MCHC >40 g/dL) claimed to identify nearly all HS patients (7–9), especially when combined with an elevated MCHC (10). Unfortunately, most clinical laboratories do not report these data.

Osmotic fragility testing

The osmotic fragility (OF) test, which measures the in vitro lysis of red blood cells suspended in solutions of decreasing osmolarity, is frequently used in the diagnosis of HS (11,12).

Because of their decreased membrane surface area relative to cell volume, spherocytes are unable to withstand the introduction of small amounts of free water that occurs when they are placed in increasingly hypotonic saline solutions. As a consequence, they hemolyze more readily than normal erythrocytes at any saline concentration. Hemolysis is determined by measuring the amount of hemoglobin released from red cells into the extracellular fluid.

The fresh OF test detects circulating spherocytes, erythrocytes that have been conditioned by the spleen. Fresh OF testing suffers from lack of sensitivity and specificity because, in many cases, reduced surface area is balanced by a reduction in volume due to cell dehydration (13). The incubated OF test, which is performed after incubating cells 18 to 24 hours at 37 °C, is more sensitive than fresh OF testing. Under these conditions, essentially all erythrocytes lose membrane. However, the process is markedly accelerated in HS erythrocytes with hemolysis of HS cells complete at saline concentrations that cause little or no lysis of normal cells. The osmotic fragility correlates well with the magnitude of spherocytosis but not with hemoglobin concentration. The sensitivity of the incubated osmotic fragility test may be outweighed by a loss of its specificity, that is, spherocytes due to any cause (Table 29.1) exhibit abnormal incubated OF. A normal OF does not exclude the diagnosis of HS as up to 20% of patients with HS lack circulating spherocytes, and the test may be normal in the patients with iron deficiency, obstructive jaundice, and those recovering from aplastic crisis.

The relative contributions of cell surface area deficiency and dehydration can be accurately determined by osmotic gradient ectacytometry, available only in research laboratories (10).

Autohemolysis and other tests

Red blood cell autohemolysis, the spontaneous hemolysis of red blood cells incubated under sterile conditions without glucose, was previously advocated as a sensitive test for the detection of HS. Other tests described in the literature, for example, the glycerol lysis test, the pink test, cryohemolysis, and the skeleton gelation test, like the OF, suffer from lack of sensitivity and specificity (3).

Flow cytometric analysis of eosin-5-maleimide (EMA) binding to erythrocytes, a reflection of the relative amounts of the integral membrane proteins band 3 and Rh-related proteins, has been explored as a screening test for HS. Simple and rapidly performed, it has not been widely used or validated, but initial studies suggest it has high sensitivity and specificity (92.7% and 99.1%, respectively, in one small study) (14,15). Like OF and cryohemolysis, non-HS variants may be detected such as other membrane abnormalities, abnormalities of erythrocyte hydration, and some variants of dyserythropoietic anemia.

Molecular studies

Specialized testing such as quantitation of major erythrocyte membrane proteins via sodium dodecyl sulfate-polyacrylamide gel electrophoresis reveals an abnormality in up to two-thirds of patients. However, it is cumbersome to perform and not commercially available. It is likely to be beneficial only in unusual or diagnostically challenging cases. Similarly, detection of the causative mutation, either utilizing mutation screening tools or direct DNA sequence analyses, is cumbersome, expensive, and not readily available (2,3).

Recommendations

There is no specific "HS test." Clinicians are advised to combine historical, clinical, and laboratory findings when evaluating a potential HS patient, utilizing the best-available combination of laboratory tests as indicated. When historical data and physical findings suggest HS in a patient with DAT-negative hemolytic anemia, findings of spherocytes on blood film and an MCHC $\geq$35 provide a high index of suspicion for HS. Additional confirmatory testing, for example, incubated osmotic fragility, EMA binding studies, or analyses of dense cells, should be sought (Grade 1C). Molecular testing is rarely indicated except in unusual cases, such as the transfusion-dependent patient.

What is the best approach to a patient with a suspected erythrocyte enzyme defect?

The history

Erythrocyte enzyme deficiencies may occur occasionally secondary to neoplasia or poisoning with copper; however, most patients with hemolytic anemia due to enzyme defects have inherited enzyme deficiencies. Since the enzyme defect has been present for the lifetime of the patient, a history of long-standing anemia can often be elicited, and there may be a history of neonatal icterus. However, the absence of a positive history by no means eliminates the possibility that an inherited deficiency is present. In glucose-6-phosphate dehydrogenase (G6PD) deficiency, in particular, there is often no prior history of anemia because the red cell life span is usually normal until the erythrocyte encounters an oxidative stress, such as that produced by the administration of drugs, ingestion of fava beans, or certain infections. Such events in the history may provide an important clue regarding the cause of hemolysis. The presence of anemia may also be unapparent in some cases because the hemolysis may be well compensated. The problem does not become apparent in such patients until an aplastic crisis occurs, usually because of an infection by parvovirus or other infectious agent. In this instance, reticulocytosis, usually an important marker of hemolysis, will be absent.

A family history of an unusual anemia can be very helpful. The existence of gall bladder disease or splenectomy may provide a valuable clue in this regard. If siblings of the patient are affected but the parents are free of the disease, then transmission is autosomal recessive, the mode of transmission of most of the red cell enzyme defects. There are two red cell enzyme deficiencies that are transmitted as X-linked disorders, G6PD deficiency and phosphoglycerate kinase deficiency. Increased adenosine deaminase activity is the only enzymopathy inherited in an autosomal dominant fashion, and this disorder is so rare that we know of only four kindreds that have ever been encountered. Dominant inheritance is characteristic of other erythrocyte disorders associated with hemolytic anemia, such as hemoglobinopathies and membrane defects. Accordingly, little is gained by performing enzyme panels when a family history reveals autosomal dominant inheritance.

Laboratory diagnosis

The blood film

Examination of the blood film yields information of value at low cost, but it is important to recognize its limitations. The appearance of the film will often confirm that the patient has hemolytic anemia by revealing the presence of polychromasia and anisocytosis. It is particularly useful in establishing diagnoses other than an enzyme deficiency, thereby preventing wasted effort attempting to define an enzyme deficiency. The very definition of nonspherocytic hereditary hemolytic anemia implies normality of red cell morphology. The only morphologic finding that can be considered to be of diagnostic value in the differential diagnosis of red cell enzyme deficiencies is the basophilic stippling that is characteristic of pyrimidine 5′-nucleotidase deficiency. However, considerable confusion has been engendered by descriptions of morphologic features mistakenly regarded to be characteristic of other red cell enzyme deficiencies. For example, many hematologists have the mistaken idea that extensive spiculation of red cells is characteristic of pyruvate kinase deficiency. This misconception is probably based on a 1964 publication (16) in which such an association was documented. Although occasional contracted, dense, spiculated cells may sometimes be seen on the blood film of a pyruvate kinase deficient patient (17), they are quite nonspecific and of little diagnostic value. Similarly, bite cells, erythrocytes in which denatured, precipitated hemoglobin has been pitted by the spleen can result from oxidative injury to hemoglobin by drugs as occurs in G6PD deficiency or by the denaturation of unstable mutant hemoglobins.

The autohemolysis test

Introduced by Selwyn in Dacie (18) in 1954 before any meaningful studies of red cell metabolism had been performed in patients with hemolytic anemia, it is quite remarkable that the autohemolysis test is occasionally still performed. It has been clear for decades that it has no diagnostic value (19).

Screening tests

With the discovery of G6PD deficiency, a plethora of screening tests were developed for this disorder. The G6PD reaction:

$$\text{Glucose-6-P} + \text{NADP}^+ \rightarrow \text{6-phosphogluconolactone} + \text{NADPH} + \text{H}^+$$

reduces $NADP^+$ to NADPH, and earlier generations of these tests depend on linking the NADPH formed to a visible substance—a dye or hemoglobin. However, the formation of NADPH or NADH can be observed directly because they fluoresce in the visible spectrum when illuminated with long-wave ultraviolet light. A series of simple-to-perform screening tests based on this principle have been devised. They can be implemented without the need for any equipment other than an inexpensive long-wave ultraviolet lamp. This type of test is available for the detection of the enzyme deficiencies enumerated in Table 29.2 (20–27).

The diagnosis of pyrimidine 5′-nucleotidase deficiency can be achieved by making use of the difference between the ultraviolet absorption spectrum of pyrimidine and purine nucleotides (28).

Enzyme assays

In some instances, a screening test is adequate to establish the diagnosis. For example, the fluorescent screening test for G6PD deficiency applied to males establishes very clearly whether the deficiency exists. However, the detection of heterozygotes for X-linked disorders is difficult because of X inactivation: the red cells

Table 29.2 Fluorescent screening tests for red cell enzyme deficiencies that cause hereditary nonspherocytic hemolytic anemia.

Enzyme Deficiency	References
Glucosephosphate isomerase (GPI)	(20,21)
Triosephosphate isomerase (TPI)	(20,22)
Pyruvate kinase (PK)	(20,23)
Glucose-6-P dehydrogenase (G6PD)	(20,24–27)

represent a mosaic of cells, some of which are enzyme deficient while others are normal. The deficient cells, like the cells of male hemizygotes, are susceptible to hemolysis. In the case of G6PD deficiency, even quantitative enzyme assays are not sufficiently sensitive to enable the detection of heterozygotes with a high degree of reliability. To detect heterozygotes with confidence, DNA analysis is the method of choice. An integrated series of enzyme assays has been developed (29) for the quantitation of red cell enzymes (20,30,31), and these methods are used almost universally for the performance of red cell enzyme assays.

DNA analysis

Mutation detection by DNA analysis is complementary to the performance of enzyme assays in the diagnosis of red cell enzyme deficiencies. Table 29.3 summarizes the advantages and disadvantages of the enzymatic and DNA approach. With the technological advances of the past few years, complete sequencing of the coding regions and of the promoter of individual genes is quite readily carried out. However, without foreknowledge of which gene is of interest, gene sequencing is an impractical primary approach today. When sequencing the DNA encoding a red cell enzyme, it is prudent to start seeking common, known mutations. Thus, a European patient with possible pyruvate kinase deficiency is most likely to have the common C1529A mutation (32), while a patient with Gypsy ancestry is likely to have a deletion of exon 10 (33).

In most cases, complete sequencing of the coding region and in the promoter will reveal the pathogenic mutation. However, when no mutation is found, enzyme deficiency is not ruled out with absolute certainty. It is always possible that the gene is not transcribed because of the action of some distant DNA element, such as an enhancer. Moreover, sequencing the coding regions will often not reveal aberrant splicing. Isolation of mRNA from erythroid cells is difficult, since only sparse amounts are present, and these only in reticulocytes. Even when a mutation is found, one cannot always be certain that it does not represent a benign polymorphism or family mutation that has no functional effect. Only when the discovered mutation has been associated with disease in previously studied families can one feel reasonably secure about the relationship between the genotype and disease phenotype.

Table 29.3 Advantages and disadvantages of enzyme assays and DNA analysis in the diagnosis of nonspherocytic hemolytic anemia.

Advantage	Enzyme assay	DNA analysis
Suitable as a "panel" of many enzymes	Yes	No
Finds all mutations in a given enzyme	Yes	No
Gives definite "Yes" or "No" result	No	Yes
Stability of sample	Low	High
Availability of quality control samples	Only of normals	Yes
Useful in transfused patients	No	Yes
Suitable for prenatal diagnosis	No	Yes

Recommendations

In summary, testing for disorders of erythrocyte enzymes requires careful consideration of historical, clinical, and laboratory findings. Where indicated, screening tests, specific enzyme assays, or molecular diagnostic studies should be pursued, using the best available studies (Grade 2C).

Role of splenectomy in hereditary spherocytosis

Treatment

Splenectomy is a permanently curative therapy in HS, with hemoglobin rising and jaundice fading within days, eliminating both the need for transfusion and the risk of aplastic crisis (2,3). Postsplenectomy, normal to high-normal values for reticulocytes, and serum bilirubin reflect an ongoing but modest increase in red cell turnover. Microspherocytosis persists, and chronic leukocytosis and thrombocytosis are expected consequences. Removal of the spleen also prevents development of gallstones and symptomatic biliary tract disease, as well as the need for biliary tract surgery.

Risks

On the basis of the previous observations, for years splenectomy was recommended for all patients with HS regardless of the degree of anemia, gall bladder disease, or other symptomatology. Concerns about overwhelming postsplenectomy infection (OPSI), the emergence of penicillin-resistant pneumococci, and increased risk of cardiovascular disease have tempered these recommendations.

OPSI, particularly due to encapsulated organisms, such as *Streptococcus pneumoniae*, *Neisseria meningitides*, and *Haemophilus influenzae*, can rapidly lead to fatal sepsis (34). The risk of OPSI appears to be greatest in children under five years of age and in the first few years postsplenectomy, but it can occur at any age and decades after splenectomy. The true incidence of this grave complication is unknown. Numerous studies have addressed this issue (34–39). However, many have serious methodologic failings, such as retrospective data collection, no or poorly chosen controls, mixtures of patient populations, for example, variability in postsplenectomy vaccination, postsplenectomy antibiotic use, have clouded their interpretation. In adults, the incidence of OPSI has been estimated at 0.2 to 0.5/100 person-years of follow-up, with a death rate of ~0.1/100 person-years (36). These rates may overestimate the current risk of sepsis, since many studies included patients who underwent splenectomy before the introduction of pneumococcal, *H. influenzae*, and meningococcal vaccines. The introduction of these vaccines and the promotion of early antibiotic therapy for febrile children who have had a splenectomy have led to decreases in the incidence of OPSI (40).

Several reports indicate an increased rate of thrombotic complications, pulmonary hypertension, and cardiovascular disease years after splenectomy for HS (41–46). The degree of risk for any of these complications is not defined.

Recommendations

The benefits and risks detailed should be considered and discussed between healthcare providers, patient, and family when considering splenectomy (4). Additional considerations include distance from medical care in case of a febrile illness or whether the individual lives in or travels to countries where parasitic diseases such as malaria or babesiosis occur and splenectomy may pose additional risk. There are no studies to guide practice. Expert opinions (2–4) have suggested splenectomy for all HS patients with severe spherocytosis and all patients who suffer from significant signs or symptoms of anemia, including growth failure, skeletal changes, leg ulcers, and extramedullary hematopoietic tumors (Grade 2C). Because the risk of OPSI is highest in infancy and childhood, it is preferable to defer splenectomy until at least six years of age (Grade 1C). Other candidates for splenectomy are older HS patients who suffer vascular compromise of vital organs. Whether patients with moderate HS and compensated, asymptomatic anemia should have a splenectomy remains controversial. Patients with mild HS and compensated hemolysis can be followed carefully and referred for splenectomy if clinically indicated. The treatment of patients with mild to moderate HS and gallstones is also debatable, particularly since new treatments for cholelithiasis lower the risk of this complication.

Postsplenectomy Management

Patient education, particularly regarding prompt intervention during febrile illnesses, is a critical part of postsplenectomy management.

Many prescribe daily prophylactic penicillin or amoxicillin to HS patients postsplenectomy. Duration of antibiotic therapy is unknown, and randomized control trials are not available. Some prescribe antibiotics throughout childhood and adolescence, or in adults, for two to five years postsplenectomy. Others recommend lifelong prophylaxis (2). Issues of patient compliance and the emergence of antibiotic resistance bacteria, particularly penicillin-resistant *S. pneumoniae* have led to reconsideration of these recommendations. Studies to address these issues are urgently needed.

Prophylaxis of thrombotic complications with aspirin, anticoagulants, or other agents has not been evaluated in HS.

Recommendations

Patients and, if children, their parents, should be counseled concerning postsplenectomy infectious risks. If the patient is a child, it appears reasonable to treat with prophylactic antibiotics for two to five years postsplenectomy (Grade 1C). Expert opinions on whether to continue antibiotics after this time and whether to prescribe prophylactic antibiotics for teenagers and adults postsplenectomy differ (Grade 2C). There are no studies to guide therapy, thus decisions must be made in consideration of the patient and their individual circumstances (e.g., distance from medical care, occupation—that is, schoolteacher, healthcare worker—attendance at day care, residence, or travel in endemic areas of, malaria).

References

1 Guyatt G, Gutterman D, Baumann MH, et al. Grading strength of recommendations and quality of evidence in clinical guidelines: report from an American College of Chest Physicians task force. *Chest.* 2006;**129**(1):174–81.

2 Eber S, Lux SE. Hereditary spherocytosis—defects in proteins that connect the membrane skeleton to the lipid bilayer. *Semin Hematol.* 2004;**41**(2):118–41.

3 Gallagher PG, Lux SE. Disorders of the erythrocyte membrane. In: Nathan DG, Orkin SH, editors. *Hematology of infancy and childhood.* 6th ed. Philadelphia: WB Saunders; 2003. pp. 560–684.

4 Bolton-Maggs PH, Stevens RF, Dodd NJ, et al. Guidelines for the diagnosis and management of hereditary spherocytosis. *Br J Haematol.* 2004;**126**(4):455–74.

5 Mackinney AA Jr, Morton NE, Kosower NS, et al. Ascertaining genetic carriers of hereditary spherocytosis by statistical analysis of multiple laboratory tests. *J Clin Invest.* 1962;**41**:554–67.

6 Michaels LA, Cohen AR, Zhao H, et al. Screening for hereditary spherocytosis by use of automated erythrocyte indexes. *J Pediatr.* 1997;**130**(6):957–60.

7 Gilsanz F, Ricard MP, Millan I. Diagnosis of hereditary spherocytosis with dual-angle differential light scattering. *Am J Clin Pathol.* 1993;**100**(2):119–22.

8 Pati AR, Patton WN, Harris RI. The use of the technicon H1 in the diagnosis of hereditary spherocytosis. *Clin Lab Haematol.* 1989;**11**(1):27–30.

9 Ricard MP, Gilsanz F. Assessment of the severity of hereditary spherocytosis using routine haematological data obtained with dual angle laser scattering cytometry. *Clin Lab Haematol.* 1996;**18**(2):75–78.

10 Cynober T, Mohandas N, Tchernia G. Red cell abnormalities in hereditary spherocytosis: relevance to diagnosis and understanding of the variable expression of clinical severity. *J Lab Clin Med.* 1996;**128**(3):259–69.

11 Godal HC, Nyvold N, Rustad A. The osmotic fragility of red blood cells: a re-evaluation of technical conditions. *Scand J Haematol.* 1979;**23**(1):55–58.

12 Parpart AK, Lorenz PB, Parpart ER, et al. The osmotic resistance (fragility) of human red cells. *J Clin Invest.* 1947;**26**:636.

13 Dacie JV, Lewis SM, Luzatto L. Investigation of the hereditary haemolytic anaemias: membrane and enzyme abnormalities. In: Dacie JV, Lewis SM, editors. *Practical haematology*. Edinburgh: Churchill Livingstone; 1991. pp. 195–225.

14 King MJ, Smythe JS, Mushens R. Eosin-5-maleimide binding to band 3 and Rh-related proteins forms the basis of a screening test for hereditary spherocytosis. *Br J Haematol*. 2004;**124**(1):106–13.

15 Stoya G, Gruhn B, Vogelsang H, et al. Flow cytometry as a diagnostic tool for hereditary spherocytosis. *Acta Haematol*. 2006;**116**(3): 186–91.

16 Oski FA, Nathan DG, Sidel VW, et al. Extreme hemolysis and red-cell distortion in erythrocyte pyruvate kinase deficiency. I. Morphology, erythrokinetics and family enzyme studies. *N Engl J Med*. 1964;**270**: 1023–30.

17 Tanaka KR, Paglia DE. Pyruvate kinase deficiency. *Semin Hematol*. 1971;**8**(4):367–96.

18 Selwyn JG, Dacie JV. Autohemolysis and other changes resulting from the incubation in vitro of red cells from patients with congenital hemolytic anemia. *Blood*. 1954;**9**(5):414–38.

19 Beutler E. Why has the autohemolysis test not gone the way of the cephalin flocculation test [editorial]? *Blood*. 1978;**51**(1):109–10.

20 Beutler E. *Red cell metabolism: a manual of biochemical methods*. New York: Grune & Stratton; 1984.

21 Blume KG, Beutler E. Detection of glucose-phosphate isomerase deficiency by a screening procedure. *Blood*. 1972;**39**(5):685–87.

22 Kaplan JC, Shore N, Beutler E. The rapid detection of triose phosphate isomerase deficiency. *Tech Bull Regist Med Technol*. 1968;**38**(10):274–76.

23 Beutler E. A series of new screening procedures for pyruvate kinase deficiency, glucose-6-phosphate dehydrogenase deficiency, and glutathione reductase deficiency. *Blood*. 1966;**28**(4):553–62.

24 Beutler E, Mitchell M. Special modifications of the fluorescent screening method for glucose-6-phosphate dehydrogenase deficiency. *Blood*. 1968;**32**(5):816–18.

25 Jiang J, Ma X, Song C, et al. Using the fluorescence spot test for neonatal screening of G6PD deficiency. *Southeast Asian J Trop Med Public Health*. 2003;**34** Suppl 3:140–42.

26 Meissner PE, Coulibaly B, Mandi G, et al. Diagnosis of red cell G6PD deficiency in rural Burkina Faso: comparison of a rapid fluorescent enzyme test on filter paper with polymerase chain reaction based genotyping. *Br J Haematol*. 2005;**131**(3):395–59.

27 Simkins RA, Culp KM. A simple, rapid fluorometric assay for the determination of glucose 6-phosphate dehydrogenase activity in dried blood spot specimens. *Southeast Asian J Trop Med Public Health*. 1999;**30** Suppl 2:84–86.

28 Valentine WN, Fink K, Paglia DE, et al. Hereditary hemolytic anemia with human erythrocyte pyrimidine 5'-nucleotidase deficiency. *J Clin Invest*. 1974;**54**(4):866–79.

29 Beutler E. *Methods in hematology: red cell metabolism*. Beutler E, editor. Edinburgh: Churchill Livingston; 1986.

30 Beutler E. Erythrocyte enzyme assays. In: Beutler E, Lichtman MA, Coller BS, et al., editors. *Hematology*. New York: McGraw-Hill; 1995. p. L45–L46.

31 Beutler E, Blume KG, Kaplan JC, et al. International Committee for Standardization in Haematology: recommended methods for red-cell enzyme analysis. *Br J Haematol*. 1977;**35**(2):331–40.

32 Baronciani L, Beutler E. Analysis of pyruvate kinase-deficiency mutations that produce nonspherocytic hemolytic anemia. *Proc Natl Acad Sci USA*. 1993;**90**(9):4324–27.

33 Baronciani L, Beutler E. Molecular study of pyruvate kinase deficient patients with hereditary nonspherocytic hemolytic anemia. *J Clin Invest*. 1995;**95**(4):1702–9.

34 Hansen K, Singer DB. Asplenic-hyposplenic overwhelming sepsis: post-splenectomy sepsis revisited. *Pediatr Dev Pathol*. 2001;**4**(2):105–21.

35 Green JB, Shackford SR, Sise MJ, Fridlund P. Late septic complications in adults following splenectomy for trauma: a prospective analysis in 144 patients. *J Trauma*. 1986;**26**(11):999–1004.

36 Schwartz PE, Sterioff S, Mucha P, et al. Postsplenectomy sepsis and mortality in adults. *JAMA*. 1982;**248**(18):2279–83.

37 Eber SW, Langendorfer CM, Ditzig M, et al. Frequency of very late fatal sepsis after splenectomy for hereditary spherocytosis: impact of insufficient antibody response to pneumococcal infection. *Ann Hematol*. 1999;**78**(11):524–28.

38 Schilling RF. Hereditary spherocytosis: a study of splenectomized persons. *Semin Hematol*. 1976;**13**(3):169–76.

39 Schilling RF. Estimating the risk for sepsis after splenectomy in hereditary spherocytosis. *Ann Intern Med*. 1995;**122**(3):187–88.

40 Konradsen HB, Henrichsen J. Pneumococcal infections in splenectomized children are preventable. *Acta Paediatr Scand*. 1991;**80**(4):423–27.

41 Hayag-Barin JE, Smith RE, Tucker FC Jr. Hereditary spherocytosis, thrombocytosis, and chronic pulmonary emboli: a case report and review of the literature. *Am J Hematol*. 1998;**57**(1):82–4.

42 Hoeper MM, Niedermeyer J, Hoffmeyer F, et al. Pulmonary hypertension after splenectomy? *Ann Intern Med* 1999;**130**(6):506–9.

43 Jardine DL, Laing AD. Delayed pulmonary hypertension following splenectomy for congenital spherocytosis. *Intern Med J*. 2004;**34**(4):214–16.

44 Schilling RF. Spherocytosis, splenectomy, strokes, and heat attacks. *Lancet*. 1997;**350**(9092):1677–78.

45 Verresen D, De Backer W, Van Meerbeeck J, et al. Spherocytosis and pulmonary hypertension coincidental occurrence or causal relationship? *Eur Respir J*. 1991;**4**(5):629–31.

46 Robinette CD, Fraumeni JF Jr. Splenectomy and subsequent mortality in veterans of the 1939–45 war. *Lancet*. 1977;**2**(8029):127–29.

30 Sickle Cell Disease

Richard Lottenberg, Sally C. Davies

Background

Sickle cell disease (SCD) is characterized by hemolytic anemia and vaso-occlusion. Genotypes include hemoglobin (Hb) SS (typically identified as sickle cell anemia) and compound heterozygotes (e.g., Hb SC and Hb S/β thalassemia). Few randomized controlled trials (RCTs) have been performed addressing management of patients with SCD, but they have had major impact on current clinical practice and in decreasing mortality (see Table 30.1) (1–7). Studies have focused on patients with Hb SS or HbSβ^0 thalassemia. Prospective clinical trial data on other subtypes are lacking. The overall approach to preventive therapies and management of complications has been largely guided by observational studies or the opinions of experts. We have focused this chapter on questions of high relevance to physicians caring for patients in settings outside of medical centers specializing in SCD. The approach may have to be different in developing and transition countries.

Literature-search strategy and grading the evidence

Literature searches were performed using MEDLINE, the Cochrane Collaboration Cystic Fibrosis and Genetic Disorders Group, and the National Guidelines Clearinghouse. The quality of evidence was evaluated using Grading of Recommendations Assessment, Development, and Evaluation Working Group (GRADE) criteria according to the American College of Chest Physicians Task Force Recommendations (8).

Evidence-based Hematology. Edited by Mark A. Crowther, Jeff Ginsberg, Holger J. Schünemann, Ralph M. Meyer, and Richard Lottenberg.
 ISBN: 978-1-4051-5747-6.

In patients with SCD, what is the appropriate primary stroke prevention strategy?

Introduction

The prevalence of cerebral vascular disease in children with SCD identified by imaging studies is as high as 64%. Silent brain infarction occurs in approximately 20% and clinical stroke in 10% of patients with sickle cell anemia. The majority of these events are due to occlusive vasculopathy affecting major intracranial arteries. Increased blood velocity in the terminal portion of the internal carotid or middle cerebral artery measured with transcranial Doppler (TCD) has been demonstrated to be associated with an increased risk of initial stroke (9).

Evidence

The Stroke Prevention Trial in Sickle Cell Anemia (STOP), a multicenter RCT initiated in 1994, tested whether transfusion can prevent stroke in sickle cell anemia (6). Children ages 2–16 years of age at high risk for stroke (as defined by TCD time average maximal mean velocity ≥200 cm/sec of the internal carotid or middle cerebral artery determined on two exams) were randomized to standard care or chronic transfusion to reduce and maintain Hb S concentration below 30%. Interim analysis at a median follow-up of 21.1 months revealed 11/63 patients in the standard care arm had a stroke compared with 1/67 in the transfusion arm (relative risk (RR) 0.10; 95% confidence interval (CI) 0.01–0.73), resulting in an number needed to treat of 11 to prevent one stroke per year (3). The trial was terminated in 1997, and all participants were recommended to receive chronic transfusion. The randomized Optimizing Primary Stroke Prevention in Sickle Cell Anemia (STOP 2) Trial was designed to determine the consequences of discontinuing chronic transfusions (7). Children ages 5–20 years from the STOP trial who received transfusions for at least 30 months and demonstrated reversion of TCD velocities into the low-risk range were randomized to discontinue or continue transfusion. TCD was performed at 12-week intervals. Interim analysis in 2004

Table 30.1 Major randomized clinical trials in sickle cell disease.

Clinical trial	Outcome
Penicillin prophylaxis in sickle cell disease (1)	Oral penicillin greatly reduces the incidence of invasive pneumococcal infections
Prophylactic Penicillin Study II (2)	Discontinuation of penicillin prophylaxis can be can be considered at age 5 years
Multicenter Study of Hydroxyurea in Sickle Cell Anemia (3)	Hydroxyurea reduces the frequency of painful episodes, acute chest syndrome, transfusions, hospitalizations
Preoperative Transfusion in Sickle Cell Disease (4)	Simple blood transfusion to increase the Hb level to 10 g/dL is as effective as exchange transfusion to reduce Hb S to 30%
Prophylactic transfusion in pregnancy (5)	Prophylactic blood transfusion to increase the Hb level to 10 g/dL compared with transfusion for Hb <6 g/dL or for emergent indications did not improve obstetrical or perinatal outcomes
Stroke prevention trial in sickle cell anemia (6)	Children at risk for stroke on the basis of an abnormally elevated transcranial Doppler velocity benefit from prophylactic blood transfusions
Optimizing primary stroke prevention in sickle cell anemia (7)	Prophylactic transfusions for patients with high-risk transcranial Doppler cannot be stopped safely at 30 months

revealed 14/41 of the patients on the discontinuation arm reverted to high-risk TCD results and 2 patients had strokes as compared with 38 patients on the continuation arm not experiencing either event ($p < 0.001$) (7). The conclusion was that transfusion could not be safely stopped after 30 months, and the optimal duration remains unknown. The frequency of retesting children with normal TCD examinations (velocity $\leq$170 cm/sec) or treatment of children with "conditional" TCD results (velocity of 171–199 cm/sec) has not been evaluated in clinical trials. There have been no prospective studies of adults with SCD using TCD examination to determine stroke risk (10). Recent guidelines from the American Heart Association/American Stroke Association Stroke Council recommend adults with sickle cell disease should be evaluated for risk factors and managed similar to the general population (11).

Recommendations

Children with sickle cell anemia aged 2–16 should be screened using TCD equipment meeting the specifications used in the STOP trials (Grade 1A). Children with high-risk TCD examinations confirmed with a repeat study should be considered for a chronic transfusion program to maintain the hemoglobin S level below 30% (Grade 1A). The benefit must be weighed against risks and burdens of chronic transfusion, particularly if adequate iron chelation therapy cannot be accomplished. The timing of rescreening children with normal or conditional TCD results has not been established but extensive data from the screening phase of STOP have been published, which provide guidance for the clinician in terms of risk of conversion to abnormal based on age and prior TCD results (12) (Grade 1C). TCD screening of adults with SCD is not recommended, and risk factor modification, as for patients without hemoglobinopathies, should be instituted (Grade 1C).

For patients with SCD who have experienced stroke in childhood, what is the duration of maintaining chronic blood transfusion?

Introduction

A retrospective case series in the 1970s revealed that the majority of children with stroke not receiving transfusions experienced a recurrent event within the following year (13). Reduction in stroke recurrence by chronic transfusion is supported by several observational studies (14–16). A goal of maintaining the hemoglobin S concentration below 30% has been accepted as standard practice based on these studies. The acceptability of reducing the intensity after four years to target Hb S to 50% is supported by a case series of 15 patients demonstrating no recurrent events with median follow-up of seven years (17).

Evidence

There are no controlled clinical trials addressing the optimal duration of transfusion for secondary stroke prevention. In a prospective case series of 10 patients transfused for 5 to 12 years, there was a 50% incidence of recurrence within 12 months of stopping transfusion (18). In a retrospective case series of 9 patients discontinuing transfusion, there were no recurrences with a median follow-up of 7.2 months; however, several patients had been placed on hydroxyurea during the period of observation (19). Chronic transfusion does not completely protect against recurrent ischemic events.

A retrospective review of 60 patients receiving transfusions with a median follow-up of three years revealed a recurrence rate of 4.2 strokes/100 patient-years (20). A retrospective analysis of 137 children maintained on transfusions to target hemoglobin S levels below 30%–50% revealed a recurrence rate of 2.2 strokes/year with 1,390 patient-years of follow-up (21). The highest incidence was within two years of the initial event. The lack of a concomitant medical illness at the time of initial stroke was identified as a major risk factor for recurrent ischemic cerebrovascular events. In a retrospective single institution case series of children maintained on chronic transfusion, the occurrence of moyamoya syndrome was identified as a risk factor for recurrent neurological events (22). Hydroxyurea combined with phlebotomy has been examined in a pilot study as an alternative approach to chronic transfusion for stroke prevention. Ware et al. evaluated a cohort of 35 children who had been on a chronic transfusion program for a mean duration of 4.2 years before being switched to hydroxyurea (23). The initial group of 15 patients with abrupt discontinuance of transfusion followed by starting hydroxyurea had an incidence of 5.7 strokes/100 patient-years. Subsequently, 20 patients were placed on hydroxyurea while receiving transfusions, which were stopped after reaching what was identified as the maximum-tolerated hydroxyurea dose; the recurrence rate for this subgroup was 3.6 /100 patient-years, which is higher than that observed for chronic transfusion (21). A RCT in children with sickle cell anemia, sponsored by the National Institutes of Health (NIH), is under way to compare hydroxyurea and phlebotomy with transfusion for secondary stroke prevention (24). There have not been prospective studies addressing the management of patients with the initial stroke occurring in adulthood.

Recommendations

Children experiencing stroke should receive chronic transfusions with a target hemoglobin S level at 30% (Grade 1B). Efficacy of reducing the intensity of transfusion has not been addressed in clinical trials. Indefinite transfusion into adult years is recommended; however, adverse effects (e.g., iron overload with inadequate chelation therapy, red cell alloimmunization) and patient preferences need to be taken into consideration (Grade 1C). Hydroxyurea therapy should be considered for patients unable to be maintained on a chronic transfusion program (Grade 2B).

What are the indications for preoperative red blood cell transfusion in SCD?

Introduction

Retrospective observational studies from the 1970s and 1980s indicate that patients with sickle cell disease have poorer surgical outcomes compared with the general population. Acute chest syndrome has been identified as the leading cause of mortality (25). Analysis of data from the Cooperative Study of Sickle Cell Disease revealed preoperative transfusion resulted in a reduction in complications (26). There is consensus that meticulous perioperative management is imperative with attention to fluid management and oxygenation and particular attention to postoperative measures to prevent respiratory complications (27).

Evidence

A U.S. multicenter RCT addressed the intensity of preoperative transfusion for Hb SS patients (4). Patients were randomized to a conservative approach using additive transfusion raising Hb level to 10 g/dL or aggressive transfusion to decrease the HbS level to less than 30% (57% received exchange transfusions) and analyzed by the intention-to-treat principle. Surgical procedures were grouped as low risk (e.g., inguinal hernia), medium risk (e.g., intra-abdominal procedures), or high risk, (e.g., intracranial procedures), according to a scoring system of the American Society of Anesthesiologists. The study enrolled 551 patients with 75% below age 20 and 25% of the procedures considered low risk. The results demonstrated that serious complications were no more prevalent in the conservative transfusion group (35%) than in the aggressive transfusion group (31%). Acute chest syndrome occurred in 10% of the conservative arm and 11% of the aggressive arm, 7% of participants in the aggressive regimen group had infections, which was 2% higher, although not significantly different in statistical terms, from the additive transfusion group (odds ratio [OR] 1.49; 95% CI 0.76–2.94). There was a significant difference in alloimmunization that occurred in 10% of the aggressive transfusion group but in only 5% of the conservative transfusion group (OR 2.34; 95% CI 1.22–4.49). Hemolysis, delayed or immediate, was seen in 6% of participants in the aggressive regimen group and 1% in the conservative regimen group (OR 4.97; 95% CI 1.67–14.78). The average inpatient stay in both groups was eight days. Data on patients undergoing cholecystectomy were reported separately, however, an additional 37 patients not receiving transfusion and 97 transfused patients not enrolled in the RCT were included in the analysis (28). A complication rate for 364 patients was 39% with a higher incidence in the nontransfused patients. The only RCT comparing no transfusion to preoperative transfusion (additive or exchange) in patients with SCD has never been published in a peer-reviewed journal (29). In that study, 369 patients were enrolled over a five-year period. Although not significantly different, the transfusion group developed more painful episodes (OR 1.62; 95% CI 0.38–6.88), neurological complications (OR 8.85; 95% CI 0.47–165.63), and respiratory complications (OR 1.36; 95% CI 0.42–4.37). There was no significant difference in the incidence of perioperative infection between groups, and data on surgical complications and alloimmunization were not reported. Attempts to contact the authors by the Cochrane Collaboration for follow-up proved unsuccessful.

A recent retrospective analysis of 13 adult patients (10 with Hb SS) undergoing laparoscopic cholecystectomy without preoperative transfusion, however, with administration of operative continuous positive airway pressure resulted in one postoperative acute chest syndrome and no painful episodes (30). A retrospective analysis of 28 children with Hb SS undergoing 38 minor procedures with general anesthesia and not receiving preoperative transfusion demonstrated a 15% incidence of minor complications with no occurrence of acute chest syndrome (31). Buck and colleagues performed a prospective survey on the use of preoperative transfusion for 127 procedures in 114 patients with SCD in 21 English hospitals (32). The majority of patients with Hb SS/Sβ^0 thalassemia were transfused (70%) compared with only 15% of the patients with Hb SC/ Sβ^+ thalassemia. Moderate/high-risk procedures was a predictor of postoperative complications (OR 4.9; 95% CI 1.32–18) while preoperative transfusion was not (OR 1.7; 95% CI 0.52–6) demonstrating the lack of clear benefit of transfusion in this observational study. An additional nonrandomized study of 92 patients with Hb SC demonstrated complications associated with intra-abdominal procedures occurred in 35% of patients not transfused compared with none in the patients transfused (33).

Recommendations

In the absence of an adequate RCT comparing transfusion to no transfusion, the following recommendations are provided for management of patients with SCD receiving general anesthesia. All individuals with Hb SS undergoing moderate- to high-risk procedures should be considered for preoperative transfusions (Grade 1C). Most patients can be prepared using additive red cell transfusion with a goal to reach an Hb level of 10 g/dL (Grade 1B). A more aggressive approach to reduce the Hb S level <30% should be considered for older adults or patients with pulmonary or cardiac disease (Grade 2C). Management without using preoperative transfusion appears safe for younger uncomplicated patients undergoing low-risk procedures (Grade 2C). Clinical trials to guide management of patients with Hb SC or Hb Sβ^+ thalassemia are lacking. Patients with Hb SC undergoing intra-abdominal procedures should be considered for preoperative transfusion (Grade 2C).

What are the indications for hydroxyurea therapy in SCD?

Introduction

Hydroxyurea is the only medication approved by the U.S. Food and Drug Administration to treat SCD. The exact mechanism(s) of action resulting in beneficial effects in SCD is not known. In addition to increasing fetal hemoglobin levels, hydroxyurea improves erythrocyte hydration, decreases erythrocyte adhesion to vascular endothelium, and enhances generation of nitric oxide. It also reduces the white blood cell count. In the Multicenter Study of Hydroxyurea in Sickle Cell Anemia (MSH), there was a correlation between the neutrophil count and frequency of crises suggesting a possible benefit of a decrease in neutrophils related to the cytotoxic effect of the medication (34).

Evidence

The MSH was a U.S. RCT that enrolled 299 adults with three or more painful episodes per year (3). Adequate results were obtained after a planned interim analysis with mean follow-up period of 21 months. Hydroxyurea treatment produced a reduction in average crisis rate as compared with placebo (weighted mean difference −2.80; 95% CI −4.74 to −0.86). The treatment group also had reductions in the occurrence of acute chest syndrome (RR 0.44; 95% CI 0.28–0.68), and fewer patients underwent red cell transfusions (RR 0.67; 95% CI 0.52–0.87). There were no observed differences in the occurrence of stroke (RR 0.64; 95% CI 0.11–3.80) or mortality (RR 0.48; 95% CI 0.09–2.60) although the trial lacked the power to detect a difference in these outcomes. There were similar rates for new leg ulcers (RR 0.85; 95% CI 0.44–1.64) and avascular necrosis of femur and humerus (RR 0.97; 95% CI 0.39–2.37). Neutropenia ($<2{,}500 \times 10^9$/L) was reported in 79% of the treatment group, but there were no reports of associated infection. Other possible adverse effects of hydroxyurea, including hair loss, skin rash, fever, and gastrointestinal disturbance, were not significantly different between hydroxyurea and placebo. A nine-year follow-up of the MSH cohort showed a survival advantage for patients continuing to take hydroxyurea, although the observational design and the uncontrolled crossover of patients following reported evidence of benefit reduces the strength of this finding (35). In addition, there was evidence for continuing benefit for patients on hydroxyurea with a reduction in pain episodes and acute chest syndrome and no increased incidence of cancer. A Belgian randomized crossover study of 22 pediatric patients with six-month assignment to hydroxyurea and placebo demonstrated a reduction in frequency and number of days of hospitalization for patients while on hydroxyurea (36). The treatment of a limited number of patients with Hb Sβ^+thalassemia and Hb SC with hydroxyurea has been reported in retrospective case series (37,38). Prospective clinical trials are needed to determine efficacy in patients with these genotypes. Several observational studies of hydroxyurea therapy in children with SCD have demonstrated tolerability, hematological response, and lack of major side effects (39–43). A phase I/II trial in children age 5 to 15 years of hydroxyurea titrated to maximum-tolerated dose demonstrated similar hematologic responses as observed in adults and no major adverse effects (40). Long-term follow-up of hydroxyurea therapy in children is not available. A NIH-sponsored RCT is under way to address whether hydroxyurea therapy can prevent organ damage in infants with sickle cell anemia (44).

Recommendations

Hydroxyurea therapy is indicated for adult patients with Hb SS and Hb S/β^0 thalassemia experiencing frequent moderate-severe painful episodes (Grade 1A). Hydroxyurea is recommended for patients with Hb SS experiencing severe or recurrent acute chest syndrome or symptomatic anemia (Grade 1B). Adult patients with Hb Sβ^+ thalassemia or Hb SC experiencing frequent painful episodes or recurrent acute chest syndrome may benefit from hydroxyurea (Grade 2B). Hydroxyurea can be considered for children with SCD experiencing frequent severe painful episodes despite optimal management (Grade 1B). Informed consent should be obtained and close monitoring of clinical and laboratory parameters is required (Grade 1C). No recommendations can be made for use of hydroxyurea in infants at this time.

In patients with SCD what is the optimal screening strategy for pulmonary hypertension?

Introduction

In both retrospective and prospective case series, pulmonary hypertension has been identified in 20% to 35% of adult patients with SCD. Pulmonary hypertension is associated with hemolysis, systemic hypertension, renal disease, skin ulcers, and mortality (45,46). Proven therapies in patients with idiopathic pulmonary arterial hypertension (who do not have SCD) have not been adequately studied for efficacy and safety in the sickle cell population. However, small case series of patients with SCD with various agents, including arginine and sildenafil, have provided encouraging short-term results (47,48). There are no published prospective randomized clinical trials in this patient population; nevertheless, experts in the field recommend screening patients with SCD for pulmonary hypertension.

Evidence

Pulmonary hypertension is defined as a resting mean pulmonary artery pressure >25 mm Hg or >30 mm Hg during exercise. Systolic pulmonary artery pressure (SPAP) can be estimated by the presence and extent of the tricuspid regurgitant jet velocity measured by Doppler echocardiography. For patients in the general population with evidence of pulmonary hypertension identified by echocardiogram, right heart catheterization is recommended to confirm the diagnosis (49,50). Transthoracic Doppler echocardiography has been found to be an acceptable screening technique in patients with SCD with one group reporting analyzable tricuspid regurgitant flow data in 87% of patients (48). In a prospective NIH cohort study of 195 adult patients (mean age 36 years), pulmonary hypertension was defined as a tricuspid regurgitant jet (TRJ) velocity ≥2.5 m/sec (SPAP of at least 30 mm Hg) (51). Right heart catheterization verified the finding of elevated SPAP in 17/18 using this criterion. In another single-institution observational study of 60 adult patients, pulmonary hypertension was diagnosed based on SPAP derived from TRJ velocity and adjusted for age, sex, and body mass index (52). Correlation with cardiac catheterization was not reported. In a subsequent report, repeat echocardiographic studies were obtained on a subset of 43 patients and after a mean follow-up of 3.0 years 13% of SCD patients with no previous evidence of pulmonary hypertension developed pulmonary hypertension by echocardiographic criteria (46). In contrast to the general population, even mild degrees of pulmonary artery systolic pressure elevations are associated with poor outcomes for patients with SCD, with multiple studies showing increased mortality for affected patients (RR 10.1; CI 2.2–47.0 in the NIH study). The timing of performing the echocardiogram affects the results. Machado et al. evaluated 25 patients in steady state and subsequently during a vaso-occlusive crisis (53). A significant increase in the pulmonary artery pressures as determined by echocardiogram was observed during acute painful episodes ($p < 0.0001$). In an additional 21 patients, exercise-induced elevation of pulmonary artery pressure was demonstrated by right heart catheterization ($p < 0.001$).

Although no prospective clinical trial data are available, right heart catheterization has been suggested for patients with TRJ velocity >2.9 M/sec representing moderate-severe pulmonary hypertension in this population (54). Despite the limited data available on the subsequent incidence of pulmonary hypertension in patients with initial echocardiograms demonstrating TRJ velocity values <2.5 M/sec, repeat screening at one- to three-year intervals has been recommended (46,54). Prospective cohort studies are limited to the adult population; however, two single-institution retrospective studies of children or adolescents evaluated with echocardiograms revealed a 26% incidence of pulmonary hypertension using the criteria of TRJ velocity ≥2.5 M/sec (55,56). Longitudinal studies of children with pulmonary hypertension have not been reported, and the clinical consequences of the finding of elevated TRJ velocity in this group of patients are unknown.

Recommendations

Screening for pulmonary hypertension with transthoracic echocardiogram should be considered for all adult patients with SCD (Grade 1C). Data are lacking at this time to provide guidelines on the evaluation of children. The screening should preferably be performed in the resting steady state and avoided during an acute vaso-occlusive episode or acute chest syndrome. Suggested echocardiographic diagnostic criteria for pulmonary hypertension in SCD are peak TRJ velocity of ≥2.5 M/sec or use of a nomogram based on age, sex, and body mass index (Grade 1B). Right heart catheterization as in the general population is required to establish the diagnosis of pulmonary hypertension (Grade 1C). A TRJ velocity cutoff value of >2.9 M/sec has been recommended for selection of patients to undergo right heart catheterization (Grade 1C). For patients with echocardiograms demonstrating TRJ velocity <2.5 M/sec repeat studies are recommended every one to three years (Grade 2C).

Acknowledgments

We thank Drs. Robert Adams, Kenneth Ataga, Michael DeBaun, Mark Gladwin, and Russell Ware for helpful discussions on recommendations.

References

1 Gaston MH, Verter JI, Woods G, et al. Prophylaxis with oral penicillin in children with sickle cell anemia: a randomized trial. *N Engl J Med.* 1986;**314**:1593–99.

2 Falletta JM, Woods GM, Verter JI, et al. Discontinuing penicillin prophylaxis in children with sickle cell anemia. Prophylactic Penicillin Study II. *J Pediatr.* 1995;**127**:685–90.

3 Charache S, Terrin ML, Moore RD, et al. Effect of hydroxyurea on the frequency of painful crises in sickle cell anemia: investigators of the Multicenter Study of Hydroxyurea in Sickle Cell Anemia. *N Engl J Med.* 1995;**332**:1317–22.

4 Vichinsky EP, Haberkern CM, Neumayr L, et al. A comparison of conservative and aggressive transfusion regimens in the perioperative management of sickle cell disease. The Preoperative Transfusion in Sickle Cell Disease Study Group. *N Engl J Med.* 1995;**333**:206–13.

5 Koshy M, Burd L, Wallace D, et al. Prophylactic red-cell transfusions in pregnant patients with sickle cell disease: a randomized cooperative study. *N Engl J Med.* 1988;**319**:1447–52.

6 Adams RJ, McKie VC, Hsu L, et al. Prevention of a first stroke by transfusions in children with sickle cell anemia and abnormal results on transcranial Doppler ultrasonography. *N Engl J Med.* 1998;**339**:5–11.

7 Adams RJ, Brambilla D. Discontinuing prophylactic transfusions used to prevent stroke in sickle cell disease. *N Engl J Med.* 2005;**353**:2769–78.

8 Guyatt G, Gutterman D, Baumann MH, et al. Grading strength of recommendations and quality of evidence in clinical guidelines: report from an American College of Chest Physicians Task Force. *Chest.* 2006;**129**:174–81.

9 Adams R, McKie V, Nichols F, et al. The use of transcranial ultrasonography to predict stroke in sickle cell disease. *N Engl J Med.* 1992;**326**:605–610.

10 Valadi N, Silva GS, Bowman LS, et al. Transcranial Doppler ultrasonography in adults with sickle cell disease. *Neurology.* 2006;**67**:572–74.

11 Goldstein LB, Adams R, Alberts MJ, et al. Primary prevention of ischemic stroke: a guideline from the American Heart Association/American Stroke Association Stroke Council: cosponsored by the Atherosclerotic Peripheral Vascular Disease Interdisciplinary Working Group; Cardiovascular Nursing Council; Clinical Cardiology Council; Nutrition, Physical Activity, and Metabolism Council; and the Quality of Care and Outcomes Research Interdisciplinary Working Group. *Circulation.* 2006;**113**:e873–e923.

12 Adams RJ, Brambilla DJ, Granger S, et al. Stroke and conversion to high risk in children screened with transcranial Doppler ultrasound during the STOP study. *Blood* 2004;**103**:3689–94.

13 Powars D, Wilson B, Imbus C, et al. The natural history of stroke in sickle cell disease. *Am J Med.* 1978;**65**:461–71.

14 Sarnaik S, Soorya D, Kim J, et al. Periodic transfusions for sickle cell anemia and CNS infarction. *Am J Dis Child.* 1979;**133**:1254–57.

15 Russell MO, Goldberg HI, Hodson A, et al. Effect of transfusion therapy on arteriographic abnormalities and on recurrence of stroke in sickle cell disease. *Blood.* 1984;**63**:162–69.

16 Wilimas J, Goff JR, Anderson HR Jr, et al. Efficacy of transfusion therapy for one to two years in patients with sickle cell disease and cerebrovascular accidents. *J Pediatr.* 1980;**96**:205–8.

17 Cohen AR, Martin MB, Silber JH, et al. A modified transfusion program for prevention of stroke in sickle cell disease. *Blood.* 1992;**79**:1657–61.

18 Wang WC, Kovnar EH, Tonkin IL, et al. High risk of recurrent stroke after discontinuance of five to twelve years of transfusion therapy in patients with sickle cell disease. *J Pediatr.* 1991;**118**:377–82.

19 Rana S, Houston PE, Surana N, et al. Discontinuation of long-term transfusion therapy in patients with sickle cell disease and stroke. *J Pediatr.* 1997;**131**:757–60.

20 Pegelow CH, Adams RJ, McKie V, et al. Risk of recurrent stroke in patients with sickle cell disease treated with erythrocyte transfusions. *J Pediatr.* 1995;**126**:896–99.

21 Scothorn DJ, Price C, Schwartz D, et al. Risk of recurrent stroke in children with sickle cell disease receiving blood transfusion therapy for at least five years after initial stroke. *J Pediatr.* 2002;**140**:348–54.

22 Dobson SR, Holden KR, Nietert PJ, et al. Moyamoya syndrome in childhood sickle cell disease: a predictive factor for recurrent cerebrovascular events. *Blood.* 2002;**99**:3144–50.

23 Ware RE, Zimmerman SA, Sylvestre PB, et al. Prevention of secondary stroke and resolution of transfusional iron overload in children with sickle cell anemia using hydroxyurea and phlebotomy. *J Pediatr.* 2004;**145**:346–52.

24 http://clinicaltrials.gov/ct/gui/show/NCT00122980 [cited 15 May 2007].

25 Platt OS, Brambilla DJ, Rosse WF, et al. Mortality in sickle cell disease. Life expectancy and risk factors for early death. *N Engl J Med.* 1994;**330**:1639–44.

26 Koshy M, Weiner SJ, Miller ST, et al. Surgery and anesthesia in sickle cell disease. Cooperative Study of Sickle Cell Diseases. *Blood.* 1995;**86**:3676–84.

27 National Institute of Health, National Heart Lung and Blood Institute. The Management of Sickle Cell Disease. 4th ed.; 2002. NIH Publication No. 02-2117.

28 Haberkern CM, Neumayr LD, Orringer EP, et al. Cholecystectomy in sickle cell anemia patients: perioperative outcome of 364 cases from the National Preoperative Transfusion Study. Preoperative Transfusion in Sickle Cell Disease Study Group. *Blood.* 1997;**89**:1533–42.

29 Al-Jaouni, Al-Muhayawi S, Qari M, et al. The safety of avoiding transfusion preoperatively in patients with sickle cell hemoglobinopathies [abstract]. *Blood.* 2002;**100**:21b.

30 Leff DR, Kaura T, Agarwal T, et al. A nontransfusional perioperative management regimen for patients with sickle cell disease undergoing laparoscopic cholecystectomy. *Surg Endosc.* 2007;**21**(7):1117–21. E-pub 2006.

31 Fu T, Corrigan NJ, Quinn CT, et al. Minor elective surgical procedures using general anesthesia in children with sickle cell anemia without pre-operative blood transfusion. *Pediatr Blood Cancer.* 2005;45: 43–47.

32 Buck J, Casbard A, Llewelyn C, et al. Preoperative transfusion in sickle cell disease: a survey of practice in England. *Eur J Haematol.* 2005;**75**: 14–21.

33 Neumayr L, Koshy M, Haberkern C, et al. Surgery in patients with hemoglobin SC disease: preoperative transfusion in Sickle Cell Disease Study Group. *Am J Hematol.* 1998;**57**:101–8.

34 Charache S, Barton FB, Moore RD, et al. Hydroxyurea and sickle cell anemia. Clinical utility of a myelosuppressive "switching" agent. The Multicenter Study of Hydroxyurea in Sickle Cell Anemia. *Medicine (Baltimore).* 1996;**75**:300–26.

35 Steinberg MH, Barton F, Castro O, et al. Effect of hydroxyurea on mortality and morbidity in adult sickle cell anemia: risks and benefits up to 9 years of treatment. *JAMA.* 2003;**289**:1645–51.

36 Ferster A, Vermylen C, Cornu G, et al. Hydroxyurea for treatment of severe sickle cell anemia: a pediatric clinical trial. *Blood.* 1996;**88**:1960–64.

37 Loukopoulos D, Voskaridou E, Kalotychou V, et al. Reduction of the clinical severity of sickle cell/beta-thalassemia with hydroxyurea: the experience of a single center in Greece. *Blood Cells Mol Dis.* 2000;**26**: 453–66.

38 Miller MK, Zimmerman SA, Schultz WH, et al. Hydroxyurea therapy for pediatric patients with hemoglobin SC disease. *J Pediatr Hematol Oncol.* 2001;**23**:306–8.

39 Scott JP, Hillery CA, Brown ER, et al. Hydroxyurea therapy in children severely affected with sickle cell disease. *J Pediatr.* 1996;**128**:820–28.

40 Kinney TR, Helms RW, O'Branski EE, et al. Safety of hydroxyurea in children with sickle cell anemia: results of the HUG-KIDS study, a phase I/II trial. Pediatric Hydroxyurea Group. *Blood.* 1999;**94**:1550–54.

41 Zimmerman SA, Schultz WH, Davis JS, et al. Sustained long-term hematologic efficacy of hydroxyurea at maximum tolerated dose in children with sickle cell disease. *Blood.* 2004;**103**:2039–45.

42 Gulbis B, Haberman D, Dufour D, et al. Hydroxyurea for sickle cell disease in children and for prevention of cerebrovascular events: the Belgian experience. *Blood.* 2005;**105**:2685–90.

43 de Montalembert M, Brousse V, Elie C, et al. Long-term hydroxyurea treatment in children with sickle cell disease: tolerance and clinical outcomes. *Haematologica.* 2006;**91**:125–28.

44 http://clinical trials.gov/ct/show/NCT00006400 [cited 15 May 2007].

45 Castro O, Hoque M, Brown BD. Pulmonary hypertension in sickle cell disease: cardiac catheterization results and survival. *Blood.* 2003;**101**:1257–61.

46 Ataga KI, Moore CG, Jones S, et al. Pulmonary hypertension in patients with sickle cell disease: a longitudinal study. *Br J Haematol.* 2006;**134**:109–15.

47 Morris CR, Morris SM Jr, Hagar W, et al. Arginine therapy: a new treatment for pulmonary hypertension in sickle cell disease? *Am J Respir Crit Care Med.* 2003;**168**:63–9.

48 Machado RF, Martyr S, Kato GJ, et al. Sildenafil therapy in patients with sickle cell disease and pulmonary hypertension. *Br J Haematol.* 2005;130:445–53.

49 McGoon M, Gutterman D, Steen V, et al. Screening, early detection, and diagnosis of pulmonary arterial hypertension: ACCP evidence-based clinical practice guidelines. *Chest.* 2004;**126**:14S–34S.

50 Rubin LJ, Badesch DB. Evaluation and management of the patient with pulmonary arterial hypertension. *Ann Intern Med.* 2005;**143**:282–92.

51 Gladwin MT, Sachdev V, Jison ML, et al. Pulmonary hypertension as a risk factor for death in patients with sickle cell disease. *N Engl J Med.* 2004;**350**:886–95.

52 Ataga KI, Sood N, De GG, et al. Pulmonary hypertension in sickle cell disease. *Am J Med.* 2004;**117**:665–69.

53 Machado RF, Kyle MA, Martyr S, et al. Severity of pulmonary hypertension during vaso-occlusive pain crisis and exercise in patients with sickle cell disease. *Br J Haematol.* 2007;**136**:319–25.

54 Machado RF, Castro O. Sickle cell disease-associate pulmonary hypertension: overview of clinical manifestations and emerging therapeutic options. *Adv Pulm Hypertens.* 2007;**6**:16–22.

55 Ambrusko SJ, Gunawardena S, Sakara A, et al. Elevation of tricuspid regurgitant jet velocity, a marker for pulmonary hypertension in children with sickle cell disease. *Pediatr Blood Cancer.* 2006;**47**:907–13.

56 Suell MN, Bezold LI, Okcu MF, et al. Increased pulmonary artery pressures among adolescents with sickle cell disease. *J Pediatr Hematol Oncol.* 2005;**27**:654–58.

31 Evidence-based Treatment of Thalassemia Major

Isaac Odame, Deborah Rund

Introduction

This chapter will review the evidence-based findings on the treatment of transfusion-dependent β-thalassemia major, which is the most serious form of the disease.

Thalassemia major is a serious life-threatening disease, which is one of the world's most common single gene disorders. Approximately 100,000 transfusion-dependent patients will be born each year worldwide, most of these in underdeveloped countries where conducting controlled clinical trials is challenging. By comparison, only about 1,000 thalassemia major patients reside within the United States and several thousand more in Western Europe (mostly Italy and Greece). Thus in the countries with the resources for conducting clinical trials, there is a relatively small number of patients. As a result, there are few randomized clinical trials in the management of thalassemia, while observational studies conducted over long periods of time are the rule.

Literature-search strategy

The following databases were searched: *Cochrane Database of Systematic Reviews, BMJ Clinical Evidence, National Guidelines Clearinghouse* (United States), Center for Reviews and Dissemination (York, United Kingdom). In addition, PubMed was searched using "thalassemia AND randomized clinical trials." Other keyword combinations that were used include "thalassemia" plus an additional keyword relevant to the specific clinical question: transfusion, chelation, splenectomy, bone marrow transplantation, and fetal hemoglobin.

Evidence-based Hematology. Edited by Mark A. Crowther, Jeff Ginsberg, Holger J. Schünemann, Ralph M. Meyer, and Richard Lottenberg.

Grading of evidence and recommendations

Grading of the quality of evidence and strengths of recommendations in this chapter are based on the guidelines proposed by the international Grading of Recommendations Assessment, Development, and Evaluation Working Group (GRADE) adopting the modification used by the American College of Chest Physicians that merges the very low and low categories of quality of evidence (see chapter 1) (1).

In patients on chronic transfusion therapy, what is the target hemoglobin that should be maintained?

Untransfused patients will inevitably die within the first year or two of life. Hypertransfusion, first published in Italian by Orsini in 1961, was the first major advancement in the treatment of thalassemia. Orsini noted that regularly transfused children fared better in appearance and function. Several years later, Piomelli began transfusing patients to maintain hemoglobin level of 95 to 100 g/L to eliminate hypoxia and suppress endogenous erythropoiesis (2). This prevented the bony deformities and extramedullary hematopoiesis associated with the disease. The absence of controlled trials notwithstanding, there is overwhelming clinical evidence that transfusion benefits thalassemia major (improved survival and quality of life). All transfused patients had longer life span, better cosmetic effects, and less hepatosplenomegaly than historical controls who were only transfused in extremis. Hypertransfusion has become standard therapy for thalassemia major. Subsequently, a debate ensued regarding the level of pretransfusion hemoglobin that should be maintained (ranging from 80 to 90 to as high as 110 to 120 g/L). The high versus low cutoff points for transfusion were evaluated as described in Table 31.1 (2–7).There has, however, never been a trial formally evaluating the benefits of transfusion or comparing the effects of maintaining a particular

Table 31.1 Evaluation of optimal pretransfusion hemoglobin level.

Reference	Number of patients/ study type	Target Hb (g/L)/Hct levels	Outcomes
Propper et al., 1980 (3)	20 single-center prospective observational + laboratory	Hct over 35% (35%–44.7%)	Initial increase followed by no change in transfusion requirement. Decrease in plasma volume. Ferrokinetics showed decreased iron turnover.
Masera et al., 1982 (4)	11 single-center retrospective observational	First maintained baseline of 102, then raised to baseline of 123	No difference in transfusion requirement according to pretransfusion Hb level.
Gabutti et al., 1982 (5)	392 multicenter prospective observational	Hb between 95 and 140	No difference in transfusion requirement according to pretransfusion hemoglobin. Lower transfusion requirement in splenectomized patients.
Rebulla and Modell, 1991 (6)	3,468 multicenter retrospective observational	Hb between 90 and 134	1. Increased blood requirement with higher hemoglobin maintenance, particularly in nonsplenectomized patients. 2. Alloimmunization more frequent with later age at first transfusion. Use of filters reduces alloimmunization in regularly transfused patients. 3. 1.1% of units caused a transfusion reaction. 4. Disturbance of growth and puberty is a sign of iron overload.
Piomelli, 1995 (2)	Summary of several observational studies	Hb between 95 and 100	No need to maintain hemoglobin higher than 9.5 to ensure normal growth. Reduced iron loading with less frequent transfusions.
Cazzola et al., 1995 (7)	52 single-center prospective observational + laboratory	Hb between 86 and 109	Baseline Hb of 9–10 adequately suppresses endogenous erythropoiesis

level of hemoglobin. All of the studies in 31.1 are observational reports.

The question requiring clarification was the level of pretransfusion hemoglobin necessary to achieve the maximum clinical response while minimizing transfusional iron overload. While initial results were conflicting (Table 31.1), ultimately, it was demonstrated that maintaining a pretransfusion hemoglobin level of 90–95 g/L resulted in a lower transfusion requirement and less iron loading, with satisfactory clinical response (prevention of thalassemic facies and normal growth pattern). At the time, there were no more sophisticated techniques, and furthermore, the patients did not survive to adulthood, so that they did not develop the problems associated with the older thalassemia patient. Maintaining a higher hemoglobin level did not result in any demonstrable clinical improvement but resulted in a higher transfusion requirement, with more iron loading.

Recommendation

Hypertransfusion to maintain a pretransfusion hemoglobin level of 90–95 g/L is recommended for all transfusion dependent patients with β-thalassemia major (Grade 1B).

What is optimal iron chelation therapy for patients on chronic transfusion?

The use of regular transfusions for thalassemia major results in iron overload, which still accounts for about 70% of the deaths of thalassemia major patients, hence the need for iron chelation therapy (8). Chelation therapy has been proven to be unequivocally effective in reducing mortality and morbidity (9). Three drugs are currently in use for the removal of excess iron (see Chapter 22). Each drug has its advantages and disadvantages (10).

Deferiprone has the highest rate of side effects reported thus far, though less information about long-term toxicity is available for deferasirox. The efficacy of these various drugs will be summarized.

Before reviewing the evidence for efficacy, consider the different means of evaluating body iron stores, since most studies of chelation report serial assessment of body iron stores rather than just mortality, which is a late and hopefully preventable outcome. There are a number of measurable endpoints to determine changes in body iron status (see Chapter 22). All of these have varying degrees of reliability and validity (11). The interpretation of clinical trials of chelators may not be comparable since the endpoints are not the same. Thus, while chelation prolongs life by reducing cardiac mortality (9,12), it is more difficult to compare the outcomes of trials using different chelators, or combinations of chelators.

Desferrioxamine

Roberts et al. performed a systematic review of clinical trials on desferrioxamine (DFO) published as of April 2004 (9). Of the 45 trials, 33 were excluded for various reasons (not randomized or not properly randomized, outcome measures not relevant, etc.). The eight trials, involving 334 patients in Canada, Italy, the United States, Lebanon, England, and India, either compared DFO with placebo, DFO with another chelating agent, or different schedules of DFO administration. The primary outcome measure was mortality, and secondary outcomes varied, including evidence of reduced end-organ damage, cardiac failure, endocrine disease, surrogate markers of end-organ damage, and histological evidence of hepatic fibrosis. The analysis concluded that DFO significantly reduced iron overload compared with placebo. Comparing DFO with deferiprone or different DFO schedules, there were no significant differences in measures of iron overload. However, compliance was a problem with DFO. Adverse events were significantly less likely with DFO than with deferiprone (9).

Deferiprone

Deferiprone initially was heralded as a relief from the burden of parenteral infusions of DFO. Furthermore, deferiprone is significantly less costly and more available in the underdeveloped world where thalassemia is most prevalent. Because of the reduced ratio of iron molecules per molecule of drug (three molecules of deferiprone are needed to bind one iron molecule, compared with a 1:1 binding ratio of DFO to iron) (11), it was initially feared that deferiprone would be insufficiently effective, at tolerated doses, to achieve net negative iron balance. However, the ultimate iron chelation needs of any patient reflect the amount of transfusion given and the amount of iron absorbed from the diet. Some patients may be adequately and safely chelated with deferiprone if they can tolerate the necessary dose (13,14). Deferiprone has been successfully used for nearly two decades by many patients who are unable to tolerate DFO.

Deferasirox

The newest chelating agent is deferasirox, an oral agent that appears highly promising in recent clinical trials. The U.S. Food and Drug Administration approved this drug in 2005, and since then it has been approved in over 70 countries worldwide for chelation in patients with thalassemia major. Following the initial report of the drug's efficacy (15), phase II and phase III trials were reported (16,17). This oral agent seems to possess favorable biochemical and safety profiles when administered to several hundred patients for one or more years. Its pharmacokinetic characteristics enable once-daily dosing. This drug would allow noncompliant patients not receiving any chelation therapy to receive the life-saving benefit of this treatment. However, this drug is still quite new and has no long-term safety or efficacy data. Nor is there any data directly comparing its efficacy with other chelators. Thus, while promising, some caution needs to be exercised in the use of this drug, and long-term monitoring of efficacy and side effects is mandatory.

Desferrioxamine and deferiprone combinations

Two significant conceptual advances have recently influenced the approaches to iron chelation therapy. The first relates to the different chemical characteristics of the chelators and their ability to achieve the clinically important endpoint of reducing mortality. From the practical standpoint of compliance and ease of administration, practitioners began administering a combination of DFO and deferiprone.

This regimen was attractive because of the hypothesis that the combination would be more efficient at chelating iron than either drug alone, the so-called shuttle hypothesis (18). Iron removed from tissues by the "low-capacity, higher-tissue permeability" chelator (deferiprone) would be transferred in the circulation to the "high-capacity, lower-tissue permeability" chelator (DFO). This hypothesis is supported by animal and in vitro models (19) and has provided the foundation for studies of combined chelation (see below).

The second concept, which has revolutionized the approach to chelation therapy, is the recognition of the differing abilities of chelators to remove iron from various tissues. This was initially documented as a poor correlation between cardiac iron measured by MRI and iron measured by liver biopsy (10). This has been resolved as representing a kinetic phenomenon due to the different rates of iron removal from these two tissues and reflects basic differences in the tissue permeability of these drugs (10), which ultimately affects their efficiency. While liver iron content has been the classical measure of chelation efficiency, reduced cardiac mortality (which seems to be more effectively achieved using deferiprone compared with DFO) is the desired endpoint. This was demonstrated by reduced cardiac mortality in patients treated with deferiprone as compared with DFO, in a retrospective observational report of 516 patients (8). A recent randomized one-year-long trial of 61 patients found lower myocardial iron using MRI in patients treated with deferiprone only compared with DFO

(20). These two new concepts have resulted in reports of combination chelator therapy, summarized in Table 31.2. None of these are prospective randomized trials, and all the studies used different dosing schedules (21–26).

Recommendations

Some form of iron chelation therapy is strongly recommended for all patients with transfusion dependent thalassemia major (Grade 1A). The drug of choice will depend partially on licensing usage permitted in each country (See also discussion in Chapter 22). On the basis of current evidence, subcutaneous DFO is the drug of choice for patients able to tolerate the drug and whose compliance is good (Grade 1A). Deferiprone may be recommended for patients unable to tolerate DFO (Grade 1B) and for patients whose compliance with DFO is inadequate to prevent end-organ damage from iron overload. Deferiprone's greater efficacy in removing cardiac iron is significant, but its higher toxicity profile at clinically effective doses must be considered. However, the drug is not licensed in North America; therefore, its use is limited to countries in which it is available. Combination chelation therapy with DFO and deferiprone may be the optimal chelation regimen of the future, but the dosing and schedules have yet to be defined (Grade 2B). We now have three to four years safety data to recommend deferasirox in patients intolerant of DFO. However, all clinicians need to monitor for long-term side effects. This is the only orally effective iron chelator licensed in North America, and therefore its use may be warranted in patients who have no other alternative for chelation (Grade 1B).

What are the indications for splenectomy in transfused patients?

Progressive splenomegaly in patients with β-thalassemia major aggravates anemia and increases transfusion requirements, with acceleration of transfusional iron loading. The current practice of timely and appropriate initiation of a blood transfusion program in early childhood has been associated with later onset of splenomegaly, and the resulting hypersplenism, in patients than in the past. Consequently, splenectomy is less commonly required nowadays. However, even with current transfusion protocols, most patients will develop splenomegaly with increasing age. The potential benefits of splenectomy (reduced transfusion requirements, associated with reduced iron loading and reduced burden on patient and family) must be weighed against risks of postsplenectomy infection and thrombosis.

Benefits of splenectomy

Modell established the initial criteria for splenectomy based on a retrospective study of 116 patients aged 1–23 years (27). When splenectomy was performed in patients with "transfusion quotient" (observed blood consumption divided by the expected consumption obtained from standard curve based on studies of splenectomized patients) greater than 1.5–2.0, permanent reduction in transfusion requirements was achieved in all but 3 of 58 splenectomized patients. Cohen et al. conducted a prospective nonrandomized study of 65 homozygous β-thalassemia patients aged 3 to 28 years, 42 with intact spleens and 23 at least six months after splenectomy. Eleven of the patients were studied at least six months before and after splenectomy. They observed average packed cells requirement of 230 mL/kg/year in unsplenectomized patients compared with 129 mL/kg/year ($p < 0.001$) in the splenectomized to maintain pretransfusion hemoglobin 80–100 g/L (28). Other groups using more intensive hypertransfusion protocols have reported similar results. Graziano et al. went further, in a retrospective study of 79 patients with β-thalassemia major aged 1–29 years (46 with intact spleens and 33 splenectomized), to show that the ability to achieve iron balance with deferoxamine was a function of transfusion requirements; splenectomized patients with lower transfusion requirements achieved negative iron balance, whereas the nonsplenectomized did not (29). There is evidence from several observational studies that transfusion requirements can be consistently decreased by splenectomy if requirements exceed 200–220 mL of red cells/kg/year (this equates to 250–275 ml/kg/year of blood bank supplied packed cells with hematocrit of 60%) (6,30).

Risks of splenectomy

A review of the MEDLINE database for the period 1966–1996 from 78 studies involving 19,680 splenectomized individuals found fully documented information in 6,942 cases (including 293 with thalassemia major, 207 with sickle cell disease, and 628 with Hodgkin's lymphoma) with median follow-up of 6.9 years. The highest rates of infection (8.2%) and mortality (5.1%) were observed among patients with β-thalassemia major (31). The infection risk can be minimized by appropriate immunization and effective post-splenectomy antimicrobial prophylaxis (32). In a large multicenter (56 tertiary centers in eight countries) retrospective study of 8,860 patients (6,670 with thalassemia major and 2,190 thalassemia intermedia) with mean age of 30 years venous thromboembolic events were far more prevalent in transfusion-independent patients with thalassemia intermedia (4%) than in patients with transfusion-dependent thalassemia major (0.9%) (33). In both groups, the highest prevalence occurred in splenectomized patients. The observation that thrombotic events are more frequent in β-thalassemia patients who have not received regular transfusions or in splenectomized thalassemic patients provides strong support for the procoagulant activity of damaged red cells.

Recommendation

Splenectomy is recommended in patients with β-thalassemia major, aged 5 years or more, who require blood transfusion in excess of 250–275 mL of packed red cell/kg/year, as it reduces transfusion requirements resulting in reduced iron loading (Grade 1C). In these patients, the benefits of splenectomy outweigh the risks of infection (minimized by immunization and antimicrobial prophylaxis) and thrombosis. The presence of persistent significant

Table 31.2 Combined desferrioxamine and deferiprone therapy.

Authors, year, reference	No. of Pts	DFO dose	Deferiprone dose	Outcome measured	Results	Comments
Wonke et al., 1998 (21)	13	Various doses and schedules	75–100 mg/kg	Serum ferritin Urinary iron excretion	Additive effect of combined therapy	
Mourad et al., 2003 (22)	25 (11 combined, 14 DFO)	2 gm/d for 8–12 hours, 2 days/week	75 mg/kg	Serum ferritin Urinary iron excretion	Additive effect of combined therapy compared with DFO alone	
Alymara et al., 2004 (23)	36	40–50 mg/kg 4–6 days/week	60 mg/kg for 6 days/week	Serum ferritin Urinary iron excretion	Effective chelation using combination	
Origa et al., 2005 (24)	79	40±10 mg/kg 2–6 days/week	70–80 mg/kg	Serum ferritin Urinary iron excretion liver iron by SQUID LV ejection fraction	Effective chelation using combined therapy Improved LV function with combined therapy	3 patients developed agranulocytosis
Galanello et al., 2006 (25)	60	36±6 mg/kg/d for 2 days/week or same dose for 5–7 days/week	25 mg/kg 3 times a day, 5 days/week with DFO	Serum ferritin Liver iron by SQUID	Equally effective chelation on both arms	
Kattamis et al., 2006 (26)	50	30–55 mg/kg, 3 days/week	25 mg/kg every 8 hrs for 4 days/week and at beginning of and 2 hours before completion of DFO infusion 3 days/weekd	Serum ferritin Urinary iron excretion Liver iron by MRI Cardiac shortening fraction	Ferritin decreased Shortening fraction increased Liver iron decrease	2 patients developed agranulocytosis

DFO, desferrioxamine.

leucopenia or thrombocytopenia, a late sign of hypersplenism, should be considered indicators for splenectomy (Grade 1C).

What is the role of hematopoietic stem cell transplantation in the management of patients with transfusion-dependent β-thalassemia major?

With more than 1,600 transplants performed worldwide, hematopoietic stem cell transplantation (HSCT) has been established as the only currently available curative approach. However, HSCT is associated with non-negligible morbidity and mortality. These risks have to considered because of the significant improvements achieved with conventional medical management. Progress made in the development of conditioning regimens, donor identification and selection, and alternative sources of hematopoietic stem cells have, to some degree, reduced the limitation posed by the scarcity of HLA matched and related donors. As there are no controlled trials of HSCT and conventional medical therapy for thalassemia major, the decision to proceed to HSCT is difficult for clinicians, patients, and their families.

Transplants from HLA-identical related donors

The best results have been achieved in Pesaro, Italy, with related HSCT in young patients with lowest risk (class 1), categorized according to three risk factors: (1) hepatomegaly >2 cm, presence of portal fibrosis in liver biopsy and irregular chelation history (class 1 has none, class 2 one or two, and class 3 has all risk factors) with overall survival, thalassemia-free survival, nonrejection mortality, and rejection of 97%, 93%, 3%, and 4%, respectively (34–36). Reports from centers outside Italy have generally shown inferior results, although, lately, similar results have been reported in some centers (37,38). Acute graft-versus-host disease (GVHD) of grade II–IV has been reported in 30% and chronic GVHD in 15% of patients younger than 17 years. The previously reported poor results in patients in the highest risk category (class 3), with extensive liver damage from iron overload, have significantly improved with a modified preparative regimen in patients younger than 17 years of age (39). Among these patients, using the modified preparative regimen, overall survival, thalassemia-free survival and rejection rates were 93%, 85%, and 8%, respectively. Outcomes in patients older than 17 years are not as good, even in centers with the most experience, with overall survival, thalassemia-free survival, nonrejection mortality, and rejection rates of 66%, 62%, 37%, and 4%, respectively (40). These outcomes, together with the late effects of HSCT on fertility and growth, should be weighed against outcomes of conventional medical therapy. In the absence of controlled trials, comparisons between the two modalities of therapy are difficult, particularly considering the recent progress made with effective and less burdensome oral chelators.

Transplants from HLA-unrelated donors

There has been a steady increase in the number of unrelated-donor HSCTs in a variety of disorders, mainly due to the increase in number of volunteer donors and better standards of donor identification and selection using DNA methods. Among class 1 and 2 patients with β-thalassemia major, treated with unrelated-donor HSCT in a multicenter series from Italy, overall survival, disease-free survival, rejection, and mortality rates were 96.7%, 80%, 20%, and 3.3 %, respectively (41). For class 3 patients, the outcomes were inferior, with rates of 65.2%, 54.5%, 10.8%, and 34%, respectively. Recently, a Thai group has published results of their experience with 49 consecutive patients with thalassemia major from 1992 to 2005, indicating no differences in engraftment, frequency of acute and chronic GVHD, rejection rate, performance status, two-year thalassemia-free survival, and two-year mortality rates between 21 patients who received unrelated-donor HSCT and 28 who received related-donor HSCT (42). However, this was not a comparison study, and the characteristics of patients in the treatment arms were not matched. While these results look promising, particularly for the lower-risk category (class 1 and 2) of younger patients, the wider application of this approach is limited by the inferior outcomes for patients with severe complications of iron overload, coupled with the long waiting times for donor identification.

Cord blood transplantation

The use of related or unrelated umbilical-cord blood further increases the donor pool of hematopoietic stem cells. In comparison to bone marrow transplantation (BMT), the main clinical advantage of cord blood transplant (CBT) is the lower risk of grade II–IV acute and chronic GVHD. However, this advantage is largely offset by high rates of nonengraftment and secondary rejection. In a recent study by the Eurocord consortium, 7 of 33 patients, mainly children with thalassemia in class 1 and 2, rejected their grafts (43,44). These graft failures have been partially explained with the observation that CBT recipients generally receive one log less stem cells than BMT. Thus, larger numbers of transplanted cord cells need to be administered to sustain hematopoiesis and prevent graft rejection. In the future, CBT may be more successful if stem cells can be expanded ex vivo.

Recommendations

HSCT should be considered for patients younger than 17 years with HLA-identical related donors, especially those in whom compliance with chelation therapy is poor, chronic transfusion is hampered by multiple red cell alloantibodies or reliable medical treatment is unavailable (Grade 1C). For all patients with HLA-identical donors, we recommend referral for consideration of HSCT to ensure that children and families can make properly informed choices about treatment options. For patients without related donors, unrelated donor transplantation may be an option in patients under 17 years of age who are poorly compliant with conventional therapy but do not yet show severe complications of iron overload (Grade 2C). CBT cannot be recommended for patients in the entire age spectrum of 1–17 years. CBT can be considered in younger patients for whom stem cell dose is adequate (Grade 1C). We, therefore, recommend that discussion for possible cord blood stem cell harvesting (as a source of donor cells for future transplant in the affected child) should be initiated if the mother of a child with β-thalassemia major becomes pregnant.

What role do fetal hemoglobin-inducing therapies have in the management of β-thalassemia major?

The β-thalassemia syndromes are characterized by deficiency of β-globin chains and excess of α-globin chains, resulting in erythrocyte membrane damage and accelerated apoptosis of early erythroid progenitors in the bone marrow. In patients with thalassemia trait and thalassemia intermedia, the non-α:α-globin chain ratio approximates 50%, resulting in transfusion independence and milder clinical course. Thus, in β-thalassemia, pharmacologically induced increase in γ-globin chains would be expected to decrease globin chain imbalance with consequent amelioration of clinical manifestations (45,46). This has provided the impetus for the development of targeted therapies for the treatment of β-thalassemia.

5-Azacytidine and decitabine

5-Azacytidine, an inhibitor of DNA methyltransferase, was the first drug to be investigated as an Hb F-inducing agent (47). Although limited studies with 5-azacytidine in a few patients documented clinical response in eliminating transfusion requirements or raising hemoglobin significantly in nontransfused patients, the development of this drug was interrupted because of concerns about potential carcinogenicity. More recently, studies of decitabine, an analogue of 5-azacytidine, demonstrated significant increase in Hb F levels in 100% of patients with sickle cell disease who were unresponsive to hydroxyurea (48). But no controlled studies with decitabine have been reported in patients with transfusion-dependent β-thalassemia major.

Hydroxyurea

Hydroxyurea (HU), an S-phase specific chemotherapeutic agent, has been used in several clinical trails, showing substantial benefits in a subgroup of patients with sickle cell disease (49). However, HU has had little or no impact on the clinical course of patients with β-thalassemia major, except in individuals who have the *Xmn1* polymorphism at −158 in the Gγ-globin gene promoter and in a subgroup of patients with Hb E/β^0-thalassemia. In two observational studies of 178 Iranian patients aged 1–33 years with transfusion-dependent β-thalassemia, the presence of T/T homozygosity for the *Xmn1* polymorphism was highly predictive of good response to HU (50,51). Studies in patients with Hb E/β^0-thalassemia have shown that HU treatment can prevent or delay transfusions in those who present with late onset symptomatic anemia (52,53).

Butyrate (short-chain fatty acids)

Butyrate, a short-chain fatty acid (SCFA) and an inhibitor of histone deacetylases, increases γ-globin gene expression by increasing histone acetylation at their promoters. Although significant improvement of anemia has resulted from pulsed administration of arginine butyrate in patients with β-thalassemia, profound anemia persists in the majority of patients (54).

Erythropoietin

Chemotherapeutic agents that stimulate Hb F production (5-azacytdine, decitabine, hydroxyurea) inhibit cell proliferation and cause cell growth arrest, which in turn promotes apoptosis. This may account for the muted clinical responses when employing these agents in patients with β-thalassemia (54,55). The combined use of butyrate and erythropoietin (that stimulates red cell production, decreases apoptosis, and prolongs red cell survival) in limited pilot studies, has demonstrated responses in a subset of patients, particularly in those with low levels of endogenous erythropoietin (54).

Short-chain fatty acid derivatives

Recently, the search for short-chain fatty acid derivatives (SCFAD) that are orally active in inducing Hb F expression and able to increase red cell proliferation and decrease cellular apoptosis has yielded novel agents (54). These agents have more favorable pharmocokinetics than the SCFAs and are more promising candidates for targeted treatment of β-thalassemia. Clinical trials involving these SCFAD compounds are yet to be reported.

Recommendations

Hydroxyurea can be recommended in patients with hemoglobin E/β^0-thalassemia, particularly those homozygous for the *Xmn1* polymorphism (Grade 1C). Alternative currently available fetal hemoglobin-inducing agents should be considered investigational interventions and cannot be recommended.

References

1 Guyatt G, Gutterman D, Baumann MH, Addrizzo-Harris D, Hylek EM, Phillips B, Raskob G, Lewis SZ, Schunemann H. Grading strength of recommendations and quality of evidence in clinical guidelines: report from an American College of Chest Physicians Task Force. *Chest.* 2006;**129**(1):174–81.

2 Piomelli S. The management of patients with Cooley's anemia: transfusions and splenectomy. *Semin Hematol.* 1995;**32**(4):262–68.

3 Propper RD, Button LN, Nathan DG. New approaches to the transfusion management of thalassemia. *Blood.* 1980;**55**(1):55–60.

4 Masera G, Terzoli S, Avanzini A, et al. Evaluation of the supertransfusion regimen in homozygous beta-thalassaemia children. *Br J Haematol.* 1982;**52**(1):111–13.

5 Gabutti V, Piga A, Nicola P, et al. Haemoglobin levels and blood requirement in thalassaemia. *Arch Dis Child.* 1982;**57**(2):156–58.

6 Rebulla P, Modell B. Transfusion requirements and effects in patients with thalassaemia major. Cooleycare Programme. *Lancet.* 1991;**337**(8736):277–80.

7 Cazzola M, De Stefano P, Ponchio L, et al. Relationship between transfusion regimen and suppression of erythropoiesis in beta-thalassaemia major. *Br J Haematol.* 1995;**89**(3):473–78.

8 Borgna-Pignatti C, Cappellini MD, De Stefano P, et al. Cardiac morbidity and mortality in deferoxamine- or deferiprone-treated patients with thalassemia major. *Blood.* 2006;**107**(9):3733–37.

9 Roberts DJ, Rees D, Howard J. Desferrioxamine mesylate for managing transfusional iron overload in people with transfusion-dependent thalassaemia. *Cochrane Database Syst Rev.* 2005;4:CD004450.

10 Neufeld EJ. Oral chelators deferasirox and deferiprone for transfusional iron overload in thalassemia major: new data, new questions. *Blood.* 2006;**107**(9):3436–41.

11 Hershko CM, Link GM, Konijn AM, et al. Iron chelation therapy. *Curr Hematol Rep.* 2005;**4**(2):110–16.

12 Wolfe L, Olivieri N, Sallan D, et al. Prevention of cardiac disease by subcutaneous deferoxamine in patients with thalassemia major. *N Engl J Med.* 1985;**312**(25):1600–603.

13 Ceci A, Baiardi P, Felisi M, et al. The safety and effectiveness of deferiprone in a large-scale, 3-year study in Italian patients. *Br J Haematol.* 2002;**118**(1):330–36.

14 Victor Hoffbrand A. Deferiprone therapy for transfusional iron overload. *Best Pract Res Clin Haematol.* 2005;**18**(2):299–317.

15 Nisbet-Brown E, Olivieri NF, Giardina PJ, et al. Effectiveness and safety of ICL670 in iron-loaded patients with thalassaemia: a randomised, double-blind, placebo-controlled, dose-escalation trial. *Lancet.* 2003;**361**(9369):1597–602.

16 Piga A, Galanello R, Forni GL, et al. Randomized phase II trial of deferasirox (Exjade, ICL670), a once-daily, orally-administered iron chelator, in comparison to deferoxamine in thalassemia patients with transfusional iron overload. *Haematologica.* 2006;**91**(7):873–80.

17 Cappellini MD, Cohen A, Piga A, et al. A phase 3 study of deferasirox (ICL670), a once-daily oral iron chelator, in patients with beta-thalassemia. *Blood.* 2006;**107**(9):3455–62.

18 Giardina PJ, Grady RW. Chelation therapy in beta-thalassemia: an optimistic update. *Semin Hematol.* 2001;**38**(4):360–66.

19 Link G, Konijn AM, Breuer W, et al. Exploring the "iron shuttle" hypothesis in chelation therapy: effects of combined deferoxamine and deferiprone treatment in hypertransfused rats with labeled iron stores and in iron-loaded rat heart cells in culture. *J Lab Clin Med.* 2001;**138**(2):130–38.

20 Pennell DJ, Berdoukas V, Karagiorga M, et al. Randomized controlled trial of deferiprone or deferoxamine in beta-thalassemia major patients with asymptomatic myocardial siderosis. *Blood.* 2006;**107**(9):3738–44.

21 Wonke B, Wright C, Hoffbrand AV. Combined therapy with deferiprone and desferrioxamine. *Br J Haematol.* 1998;**103**(2):361–64.

22 Mourad FH, Hoffbrand AV, Sheikh-Taha M, et al. Comparison between desferrioxamine and combined therapy with desferrioxamine and deferiprone in iron overloaded thalassaemia patients. *Br J Haematol.* 2003;**121**(1):187–89.

23 Alymara V, Bourantas D, Chaidos A, et al. Effectiveness and safety of combined iron-chelation therapy with deferoxamine and deferiprone. *Hematol J.* 2004;**5**(6):475–79.

24 Origa R, Bina P, Agus A, Crobu G, et al. Combined therapy with deferiprone and desferrioxamine in thalassemia major. *Haematologica.* 2005;**90**(10):1309–14.

25 Galanello R, Kattamis A, Piga A, et al. A prospective randomized controlled trial on the safety and efficacy of alternating deferoxamine and deferiprone in the treatment of iron overload in patients with thalassemia major. *Haematologica* 2005;**91**(9):1241–43.

26 Kattamis A, Ladis V, Berdousi H, et al. Iron chelation treatment with combined therapy with deferiprone and deferioxamine: a 12-month trial. *Blood Cells Mol Dis.* 2006;**36**(1):21–25.

27 Modell B. Total management of thalassaemia major. *Arch Dis Child.* 1977;**52**:489–500.

28 Cohen A, Markenson AL, Schwartz E. Transfusion requirements and splenectomy in thalassemia major. *J Pediatr.* 1980;**97**(1):100–102.

29 Graziano JH, Piomelli S, Hilgartner M, et al. Chelation therapy in β-thalassemia major: the role of splenectomy in achieving iron balance. *J Pediatr.* 1981;**99**(5):695–99.

30 Cohen A, Gayer R, Mizanin J. Long-term effect of splenectomy on transfusion requirements in thalassemia major. *Am J Hematol.* 1989;30:254–56.

31 Bisharat N, Omari H, Lavi I, et al. Risk of infection and death among post-splenectomy patients. *J Infect.* 2001;**43**:182–86.

32 Davies JM, Barnes R, Milligan D. Update on guidelines for the prevention and treatment of infection in patients with absent or dysfunctional spleen. *Clin Med.* 2002;**2**(5):440–43.

33 Cappelini MD, Grespi E, Cassinerio E, et al. Coagulation and splenectomy: an overview. *Ann N Y Acad Sci.* 2005;**1054**:317–24.

34 Lucarelli G, Galimberti M, Polchi P, et al. Bone marrow transplantation in patients with thalassemia. *N Engl J Med.* 1990;**322**:417–21.

35 Lucarelli G, Galimberti M, Polchi P, et al. Marrow transplantation in patients with thalassemia responsive to iron chelation. *N Engl J Med.* 1993;**329**:840–44.

36 Galimberti M, Polchi P, Angelucci E, et al. Bone marrow transplantation in thalassemia: the experience of Pesaro. *Bone Marrow Transplant.* 1997;**19**:45–47.

37 Walters MC, Sullivan KM, O'Reilly RJ, et al. Bone marrow transplant for thalassemia: the USA experience. *Am J Pediatr Oncol.* 1994;**16**: 11–17.

38 Lawson SE, Roberts IAG, Amrolia P, et al. Bone marrow transplantation for β-thalassaemia major: the UK experience in two pediatric centers. *Br J Haematol.* 2003;**120**:289–95.

39 Sodani P, Gaziev D, Polchi P, et al. New approach to bone marrow transplantation in patients with class 3 thalassemia aged younger than 17 years. *Blood.* 2004;**104**:1201–3.

40 Graziev J, Sodani P, Polchi P, et al. Bone marrow transplantation in adults with thalassemia. Treatment and long-term follow-up. *Ann NY Acad Sci.* 2005;1054:196–205.

41 La Nasa G, Giardini C, Argiolu F, et al. Unrelated donor bone marrow transplantation for thalassemia: the effect of extended haplotypes. *Blood.* 2002;**99**:4350–56.

42 Hongeng S, Pakakasama S, Chuansumrit A, et al. Outcomes of transplantation with related- and unrelated-donor stem cells in children with severe thalassemia. *Biol Blood Marrow Transplant.* 2006;**12**:683–87.

43 Locatelli F, Rocha V, Reed W, et al. Related umbilical cord blood transplantation in patients with thalassemia and sickle cell disease. *Blood.* 2003;**101**:2137–43.

44 Locatelli F, De Stefano P. Innovative approaches to hemopoietic stem cell transplantation for patients with thalassemia. *Haematologica.* 2005;**90**(12):1592–94.

45 Steinberg MH, Rogers GP. Pharmacological modulation of fetal hemoglobin. *Medicine.* 2001;**80**:328–44.

46 Atweh GF, Loukopoulos D. Pharmacological induction of fetal hemoglobin in sickle cell disease and β-thalassemia. *Semin Hematol.* 2001;**38**:367–73.

47 DeSimone J, Heller P, Hall L, et al. 5-azacytidine stimulates fetal hemoglobin synthesis in anemic baboons. *Proc Natl Acad Sci U S A.* 1982;**79**:4428–31.

48 Koshy M, Dorn L, Bresller L, et al. 2-Deoxy 5-azacytidine and fetal hemoglobin induction in sickle cell anemia. *Blood.* 2000;**96**:2379–84.

49 Charache S, Terrin ML, Moore RD, et al. Effect of hydroxyurea on the frequency of painful crisis in sickle cell anemia. Investigators of the Multicenter Study of Hydroxyurea in Sickle Cell Anemia. *N Engl J Med.* 1995;**332**:1317–22.

50 Alebouyeh M, Moussavi F, Haddad-Deylami H, et al. Hydroxyurea in the treatment of major β-thalassemia and importance of genetic screening. *Ann Hematol.* 2004;**83**:430–33.

51 Yavarian M, Karimi M, Bakker E, et al. Response to hydroxyurea treatment in Iranian transfusion-dependent β-thalassemia patients. *Haematologica.* 2004;**89**(10):1172–78.

52 Fucharoen S, Siritanaratkul N, Winichagoon P, et al. Hydroxyurea increases Hemoglobin F levels and improves effectiveness of erythropoiesis in β-thalassemia/hemoglobin E disease. *Blood.* 1996;**87**(3):887–92.

53 Singer S, Kuypers F, Olivieri N, et al. Fetal haemoglobin augmentation in E/β0 thalassaemia: clinical and haematological outcome. *Br J Haematol.* 2005;**131**:378–88.

54 Perrine SP, Castaneda SA, Boosalis MS, et al. Induction of fetal globin in β-thalassemia: cellular obstacles and molecular progress. *Ann NY Acad Sci.* 2005;**1054**:257–65.

55 Fathallah H, Sutton M, Atweh GF. Pharmacological induction of fetal hemoglobin: why havent we been more successful in thalassemia? *Ann NY Acad Sci.* 2005;**1054**:228–37.

4 Malignant Hematologic Disorders

Ralph M. Meyer

32 Acute Lymphoblastic Leukemia in Adults

Stephen Couban, Andrea Kew

Introduction

This chapter will focus on the treatment of adult acute lymphoblastic leukemia (ALL). Although ALL is the most common acute leukemia in children, it only accounts for approximately 20% of adult acute leukemias. The prognosis of adult ALL has steadily improved with current therapies. However, in contrast to children with ALL, adults have a much less favorable prognosis with long-term leukemia-free survival (LFS) of only 25%–50% (1).

Questions

What is the optimal induction therapy for adolescents with ALL?
What is the role of stem cell transplantation for adults with ALL?
What is the role of tyrosine kinase inhibitors in adults with Philadelphia chromosome positive ALL?

Literature-search strategy and inclusions

The literature search was conducted through PUBMED using the search terms "acute lymphoblastic leukemia" together with terms appropriate to each question as described within each section. These searches were inclusive of articles published in English before September 2006. Grading of the quality of evidence and strengths of recommendations in this chapter are based on the guidelines proposed by the international Grading of Recommendations Assessment, Development, and Evaluation Working Group (GRADE) adopting the modification used by the American College of Chest Physicians that merges the "very low" and "low" categories of quality of evidence (see chapter 1).

Evidence-based Hematology. Edited by Mark A. Crowther, Jeff Ginsberg, Holger J. Schünemann, Ralph M. Meyer, and Richard Lottenberg.

What is the optimal induction therapy for adolescents with ALL?

Additional search terms included "adolescents" AND "treatment." Article titles were screened for those that compared treatment of adolescents with pediatric and adult protocols. Two relevant articles and subsequently two relevant abstracts were identified and are included for review. All studies were retrospective cohort comparisons. No randomized controlled trials address this question. There is growing evidence that older adolescents achieve better outcomes when treated with pediatric as opposed to adult protocols. The four studies identified all found better outcomes with pediatric protocols. Boissel et al. compared adolescents (15–20 years of age) enrolled in the pediatric FRALLE-93 and adult LALA-94 protocols (2). They found that adolescents treated on the pediatric protocol had better complete remission (CR) rates (94% versus 83%) and five-year event-free survival (EFS) (67% versus 41%) compared with adolescents treated on the adult protocol. The only significant difference between the two groups was age (median 15.9 versus 17.9 years in the FRALLE-93 and LALA-94 protocols, respectively); otherwise, the groups were similar. On multivariate analysis, the only prognostic factors identified for EFS were the white blood count and the treatment protocol. Different drug regimens and differences in dose intensity likely contribute to the superiority of the pediatric protocols; the FRALLE-93 protocol used more prednisone, vinca alkaloid and L-asparaginase than the LALA-94 protocol. The Children's Cancer Group and the Cancer and Leukemia Group B reported similar findings in adolescents treated on pediatric versus adult protocols with six-year EFS of 64% versus 38%, respectively (3), as did the Dutch Childhood Oncology Group and adult Dutch-Belgian Hemato-Oncology Cooperative Study Group with five-year EFS of 69% versus 34% (4). A similar Italian study comparing Associazione Italiana Ematologia Oncologia Pediatrica protocols to Gruppo Italiano Malattie Ematologiche dell'Adulto protocols also found an advantage of 2-year EFS of 80% versus 71% for adolescents treated with pediatric rather than adult protocols (5).

There are several potential explanations for these findings. First, ALL is the most common hematological malignancy found in children and thus pediatric oncologists have more experience with the treatment of ALL than do adult oncologists. Most children with ALL are treated on clinical trials so an adolescent referred to a pediatric oncologist may be more likely to be treated on a clinical trial than an adolescent referred to an adult oncologist. In a compelling editorial published in the *Journal of Clinical Oncology*, Charles Schiffer comments that "pediatricians administer these treatments with a military precision on the basis of a near-religious conviction about the necessity of maintaining prescribed dose and schedule come hell, high water, birthdays, Bastille Day or Christmas" (6). The role of the primary caregiver in the pediatric setting, which is typically the mother, is believed to be important; this person may actually influence adherence to treatment protocols (7). Finally, pediatric protocols tend to use more steroids, L-asparaginase, and vinca alkaloids, which may contribute to the superiority of these regimens.

Recently, the Dana-Farber Pediatric ALL Consortium, a group of collaborating pediatric centers, has joined adult institutions to form a Dana-Farber Combined Adult/PediatricALL Consortium and has begun to treat children and adults with ALL with similar protocols in the hope of achieving better outcomes in adults with ALL.

Recommendation

Adolescents and young adults should be treated with dose-intense regimens that are identical to those received by pediatric patients (Grade 1C)

What is the role of stem cell transplantation for adults with ALL?

Additional search terms included "transplant" AND "adult" and used the meta-analysis limit. One relevant meta-analysis was identified. Subsequent searches used the additional search terms "transplant" AND "adult" AND "autologous" and used the randomized clinical trial limit. Trials that compared autologous transplantation to chemotherapy or allogeneic transplantation were chosen.

The potential benefits of stem cell transplantation (SCT) in adult ALL include the ability to use myeloablative conditioning in an attempt to eradicate the leukemic clone and to leverage a graft-versus-leukemia (GVL) effect. There are several observations that support evidence for a GVL effect in ALL: (i) higher relapse rates are observed in patients who undergo syngeneic transplantation compared with allogeneic transplantation; (ii) there is also a higher risk of relapse in recipients of T cell–depleted grafts; (iii) transplantation recipients who develop graft-versus-host disease have a reduced risk of relapse; and (iv) donor lymphocyte infusions (DLI) can induce remissions in recipients who relapse after transplantation (8). These observations will be described in more detail, and then the clinical data evaluating the role of transplantation will be reviewed.

The GVL effect may be less robust in ALL compared with myeloid malignancies. In a study comparing syngeneic to allogeneic transplantation, a difference in relapse rates was not detected with three-year probabilities of relapse of 36% compared with 26%, respectively ($p = 0.1$). In contrast, significant differences in relapse were observed in patients with both acute myeloid leukemia (52% versus 16%) and chronic myeloid leukemia (40% versus 7%) (9). The design and the reduced statistical power of these comparisons limit the strength of conclusions. Several studies of DLI are in ALL, but the patient numbers are small, and it is difficult to draw definitive conclusions. One study evaluating DLI in recurrent ALL after transplantation included data from 27 transplant centers in the European Group for Blood and Marrow Transplantation. There were no remissions in 12 patients with ALL who had failed to respond to intensive chemotherapy or in patients who received DLI as sole therapy. In nine patients who had chemotherapy-induced remission, DLI failed to achieve a sustainable remission in six of nine patients (10). In a similar North American study, 25 transplantation centers were surveyed about their use of DLI. In 11 patients with ALL, two achieved remission (11). The French Society of Bone Marrow Transplantation analyzed 121 patients who had received allogeneic transplantation for Philadelphia chromosome positive ALL. Nine patients received DLI after relapse; five responded, but only two had prolonged remissions of greater than 9 and 12 months (12). Two smaller studies reported more success with DLI. Slavin et al. reported responses in four out of six patients with a median survival of greater than two years (13) and Tzeng et al. reported complete remission in two out of three ALL patients; they were leukemia-free at 9 and 7 months at the time of publication (14). Though there appears to be a modest GVL effect in ALL, it is certainly less striking than in myeloid malignancies.

The role of SCT in ALL will be discussed by considering the clinical data evidence related to four main areas: (1) sibling allogeneic SCT in first complete remission (CR1), (2) SCT in second complete remission (CR2) and refractory disease, (3) transplantation using matched, unrelated donors, and (4) autologous SCT.

A recent meta-analysis was performed to determine the efficacy of transplantation as postremission therapy for adults in CR1 (15). Eligible studies prospectively offered allogeneic SCT to all patients in CR1 with a suitable donor and offered autologous SCT or chemotherapy to all others, provided data for an intention-to-treat analysis based on donor availability and assessed outcomes in terms of overall survival (OS); the principle of these trials is referred to as "genetic randomization." Seven trials met eligibility criteria and four included only patients with high-risk ALL. One study included matched, unrelated donors. The range of compliance with allogeneic transplantation ranged from 68% to 96%, and the range of compliance with autologous transplantation in the no-donor groups ranged from 9% to 81%. The summary hazard ratio (HR) for OS for the no-donor versus the donor group was 1.29 (95% confidence interval [CI], 1.02–1.63, $p = 0.037$). In patients with high-risk disease, the summary HR for OS was 1.42 (95% CI, 1.06–1.90, $p = 0.019$). This meta-analysis provides clear evidence that allogeneic SCT in CR1 is the treatment of choice. However, this benefit in standard-risk disease remained uncertain as most studies focused on high-risk patients. To address this population, a large trial using the principle of genetic randomization was conducted by the Medical Research Council (MRC) and Eastern Cooperative Oncology Group (ECOG) to determine the efficacy of allogeneic SCT for patients with standard-risk ALL. The results have been published in abstract form (this citation became available subsequent to completing the structured literature search) and demonstrate a survival advantage for standard-risk patients undergoing transplantation in CR1 with a five-year OS of 63% in the donor group versus 51% in the no donor group ($p < 0.05$) (16).

Unfortunately, many patients with ALL who achieve a first remission will subsequently relapse. Although patients may achieve a second remission with chemotherapy, most will subsequently progress without further treatment. Data evaluating allogeneic transplantation for these patients come from case series reports and show that long-term leukemia-free survival (LFS) is achieved in approximately 20%–40% of patients. Barrett et al. reported on 391 patients transplanted in second CR; this study included both adults and children. The five-year LFS was 26% and five-year probability of relapse was 52% (17). Wingard et al. reported on 74 patients (both adults and children) with high-risk ALL (18 in CR1, 36 in CR2, 16 in CR3, and 4 in CR4). For patients in CR2, the five-year event-free survival (EFS) was 43%. Patients in CR3 had five-year EFS of 25% and none of the patients in CR4 survived (18). Less than one-quarter of patients in a transplantable age group have an HLA matched sibling donor. Thus, use of alternatives such as a matched, unrelated donor is a reasonable option. The majority of data evaluating matched, unrelated transplantation in ALL are from registries. The most applicable study is from Cornelissen et al., which reviewed data from the National Marrow Donor Program (19). They report results of 127 patients with poor-risk ALL who underwent transplantation from a matched, unrelated donor. In CR1, the four-year OS was 32%. Relapse mortality and transplantation related mortality (TRM) were 6% and 54%, respectively. Survival was significantly worse for patients undergoing transplantation beyond CR1 and in those with primary induction failure; TRM was substantial with a cumulative incidence of 61%. The authors comment that outcomes using matched, unrelated donors may be improved by reducing the interval between diagnosis and transplant to avoid the cumulative toxicities of treatment. Autologous SCT has also been investigated as postremission therapy for adult ALL. Autologous transplantation is thought to have a role based on the theory that preparative conditioning contributes significantly to the "cure" of ALL and successful transplantation does not rely greatly on the GVL effect because the GVL effect is less pronounced than in myeloid malignancies. However, the overall long-term LFS of patients undergoing autologous transplantation in CR1 is approximately 30%–50%, which is similar to chemotherapy alone. The French Group on Therapy for Adult Acute Lymphoblastic Leukemia conducted the first randomized trial of autologous SCT compared with chemotherapy for postremission treatment in patients who were not eligible for allogeneic SCT (20). A difference in the three-year OS was not detected between the two arms; 49% in the autologous SCT arm versus 42% in the chemotherapy arm. Recently, an individual database overview of the last three trials from the LALA group was reported (21); again, no survival advantage for autologous SCT compared with chemotherapy was detected with a 10-year OS of 30% and 22%, respectively ($p = 0.48$). Interestingly, the recently published abstract of the prospective trial conducted by the MRC and ECOG reveals superior EFS with chemotherapy compared with autologous transplantation (16).

Recommendations

1. Allogeneic transplantation using stem cells from a matched sibling donor is recommended for adult patients with high and standard-risk ALL who achieve a first remission (Grade 2A).
2. Allogeneic transplantation using stem cells from a matched sibling or unrelated donor is recommended for adult patients with relapsed ALL who achieve a second remission (Grade 1C).
3. Autologous transplantation is not recommended for adult patients with ALL (Grade 1C).

What is the role of tyrosine kinase inhibitors in adults with philadelphia chromosome positive ALL?

"Imatinib" was included as an additional search term. Using the randomized controlled trial limit, only one article was identified. Therefore, selected case series were also reviewed. Article titles and abstracts were reviewed for articles that used imatinib in relapsed and *de novo* ALL as well as in combination with transplantation. The Philadelphia chromosome is the result of a translocation between chromosomes 9 and 21 with the creation of a fusion gene, *bcr-abl*. The *bcr-abl* gene yields a constitutively active tyrosine kinase that acts through multiple signaling pathways that contribute to leukemogenesis. Though relatively rare in childhood ALL, the Philadelphia chromosome is the most common cytogenetic abnormality in adults with a clear increase in incidence with advancing age (22). The prognosis for Ph+ ALL is grim with long-term DFS of less than 10%. Because of the success of the tyrosine kinase inhibitor, imatinib, in chronic myeloid leukemia, it has been studied in the treatment of Ph+ ALL. Initial studies were performed in patients with relapsed or refractory disease; more recently, imatinib has been considered as part of initial therapy and in conjunction with SCT. The quality of data available testing imatinib in adult Ph+ ALL is limited; most studies are phase II trials.

Several small studies evaluating imatinib as a single agent in patients with relapsed or refractory ALL show poor results. Ottman et al. reported on 48 patients with relapsed or refractory Ph+ ALL (23). Only 19% had a complete hematologic response (CHR), with a median time to progression of 2.2 months and median OS of

4.9 months. Drucker et al. reported only 4 CHRs in 20 patients with relapsed Ph+ ALL or CML with lymphoid blast crisis and all but 1 patient subsequently relapsed (24).

Imatinib has been used in initial therapy of Ph+ ALL, both as a single agent and in combination with induction chemotherapy. Thomas et al., recently reported an update of a cohort comparison evaluating the combination of hyperCVAD and imatinib for Ph+ ALL; of 43 evaluable patients with active disease, 91% achieved CR with a three-year DFS of 55% compared with 14% with hyperCVAD alone (25). The Japan Adult Leukemia Study Group (JALSG) found similar results with the use of imatinib in combination with induction and consolidation chemotherapy. They report on 80 patients with newly diagnosed Ph+ ALL and achieved CR in 96% with a one-year EFS and OS of 60% and 76%, respectively (26). Compared with the historic controls from the JALSG ALL93 study, both EFS and OS were significantly better. However, in patients who were subsequently treated with allogeneic SCT, no survival advantage in the group that received imatinib was detected. The authors comment that treatment with imatinib may result in more patients having the opportunity for transplantation because of higher remission rates. Wassman et al. (27) have compared imatinib in combination with chemotherapy in two different schedules as initial therapy for Ph+ ALL; 92 patients were treated with imatinib concurrently or alternating with standard induction-consolidation chemotherapy and while both strategies were feasible, there was a significantly higher rate of CR with the concurrent administration schedule (27).

Imatinib has been used as a single agent in newly diagnosed elderly patients with Ph+ ALL as an alternative to standard induction chemotherapy. In the one randomized trial identified for this section, induction chemotherapy was compared with imatinib. Preliminary results published in abstract form describe that of the 12 patients allocated to imatinib, 92% achieved a CR compared to only 53% assigned to chemotherapy (28). At the time of abstract publication, follow-up was less than five months so it is unknown if the responses will be durable.

Ph+ ALL is generally considered an absolute indication for allogeneic SCT. Thus, there is also considerable interest in the effect of imatinib therapy in combination with SCT. Lee et al. reported a prospective, phase II study testing the effect of combining imatinib with conventional chemotherapy before allogeneic SCT. They compared 29 patients treated with imatinib to 33 historical controls. There was a significant advantage in probability of relapse (3.8% versus 45.7%) and DFS (78.1% versus 38.7%) favoring the imatinib group with no difference in TRM detected (29). Minimal residual disease after SCT is associated with a significant risk of relapse. Wassman et al. (30) reported successful use of imatinib in this setting with the achievement of molecular remission in 52% of patients with a 12-month DFS of 91% in patients in remission compared with 8% in patients who remained positive for MRD (30).

There are now emerging phase I studies of the new tyrosine kinase inhibitors, dasatinib, and nilotinib, in Ph+ ALL with encouraging results. It will be interesting to study these agents in larger trials to determine their effects in the treatment of Ph+ ALL.

Recommendations

1. Imatinib is recommended in combination with chemotherapy for patients with Philadelphia chromosome-positive ALL (Grade 1C).

2. Treatment with imatinib as a single agent should be considered for older ALL patients who are not candidates for standard chemotherapy (Grade 2B).

References

1 Jabbour EJ, Faderl S, Kantarjian HM. Adult acute lymphoblastic leukemia. *Mayo Clin Proc.* 2005;**80**:1517–27.

2 Boissel N, Auclerc M-F, Lheritier V, et al. Should adolescents with acute lymphoblastic leukemia be treated as old children or young adults? Comparison of the French FRALLE-93 and LALA-94 trials. *J Clin Oncol.* 2003;**21**:774–80.

3 Stock W, Sather H, Dodge RK, et al. Outcome of adolescents and young adults with ALL: A comparison of Children's Cancer Group (CCG) and Cancer and Leukemia Group B (CALGB) regimens. *Blood.* 2000;**96**:467a.

4 deBont JM, van der Holt B, Dekker AW, et al. Significant difference in outcome for adolescents with acute lymphoblastic leukemia treated on pediatric vs adult protocols in the Netherlands. *Leukemia.* 2004;**18**:2032–35.

5 Testi AM, Valsecchi MG, Conter V, et al. Difference in outcome of adolescents with acute lymphoblastic leukemia (ALL) enrolled in pediatric (AIEOP) and adult (GIMEMA) protocols. *Blood.* 2004;**104**:539a.

6 Schiffer CA. Differences in outcome in adolescents with acute lymphoblastic leukemia: a consequence of better regimens? Better doctors? Both? *J Clin* Oncol. 2003;**21**:760–61.

7 Sallon SE. Myths and lessons from the adult/pediatric interface in acute lymphoblastic leukemia. *ASH Educ Book.* 2006:128–32.

8 Soiffer RJ. *Stem cell transplantation for hematologic malignancies.* Totowa, NJ: Humana Press; 2004.

9 Gale PG, Horowitz MM, Ash RC, et al. Identical-twin bone marrow transplants for leukemia. *Ann Intern Med.* 1994;**120**:646–52.

10 Kolb HJ, Schattenberg A, Goldman JM, et al. Graft-versus-leukemia effect of donor lymphocyte transfusions in marrow grafted patients. European Group for Blood and Marrow Transplantation Working Party Chronic Leukemia. *Blood.* 1995;**86**:2041–50.

11 Collins RH, Shpilberg O, Drobyski WR, et al. Donor leukocyte infusions in 140 patients with relapsed malignancy after allogeneic bone marrow transplantation. *J Clin Oncol.* 1997;**15**:433–44.

12 Esperou H, Boiron JM, Cayuela JM, et al. A potential graft-versus-leukemia effect after allogeneic hematopoietic stem cell transplantation for patients with Philadelphia chromosome-positive acute lymphoblastic leukemia: results from the French Bone Marrow Transplantation Society. *Bone Marrow Transplantation.* 2003;**31**:909–18.

13 Slavin S, Naparstek E, Nagler A, et al. Allogeneic cell therapy with donor peripheral blood cells and recombinant human interleukin-2 to treat leukemia relapse after allogeneic bone marrow transplantation. *Blood.* 1996;**87**:2195–204.

14 Tzeng CH, Lin JS, Lee JC, et al. Transfusion of donor peripheral blood buffy coat cells as effective treatment for relapsed acute leukemia after

transplantation of allogeneic bone marrow or peripheral blood stem cells from the same donor. *Transfusion.* 1996;**36**:685–90.

15 Yanada M, Matsuo K, Suzuki T, et al. Allogeneic hematopoietic stem cell trasplantation as part of postremission therapy improves survival for adult patients with high-risk acute lymphoblastic leukemia: a metaanalysis. *Cancer.* 2006;**106**:2657–63.

16 Rowe JM, Buck G, Fielding A, et al. In adults with standard-risk acute lymphoblastic leukemia (ALL) the greatest benefit is achieved from an allogeneic transplant in first complete remission (CR) and an autologous transplant is less effective than conventional consolidation/maintenance chemotherapy: final results of the international ALL trial (MRC UKALL/ECOG E2993). *Blood.* 2006;**108**:5a.

17 Barrett AJ, Horowitz MM, Gale PG, et al. Marrow transplantation for acute lymphoblastic leukemia: factors affecting relapse and survival. *Blood.* 1989;**74**:862–71.

18 Wingard JR, Piantadosi S, Santos GW, et al. Allogenic bone marrow transplantation for patients with high-risk acute lymphoblastic leukemia. *J Clin Oncol.* 1990;**8**:820–30.

19 Cornelissen JJ, Carston M, Kollman C, et al. Unrelated marrow transplantation for adult patients with poor-risk acute lymphoblastic leukemia: strong graft-versus-leukemia effect and risk factors determining outcome. *Blood.* 2001;**97**:1572–77.

20 Fiere D, Lepage E, Sebban C, et al. Adult acute lymphoblastic leukemia: a multicentric randomized trial testing bone marrow transplantation as postremission therapy. *J Clin Oncol.* 1993;**11**:1990–2001.

21 Dhédin N, Dombret H, Thomas X, et al. Autologous stem cell transplantation in adults with acute lymphoblastic leukemia in first complete remission: analysis of the LALA-85, -87, and -94 trials. *Leukemia.* 2006;**20**:336–44.

22 Secker-Walker LM, Craig JM, Hawkins JM, et al. Philadelphia positive acute lymphoblastic leukemia in adults: age distribution, BCR breakpoint and prognostic significance. *Leukemia.* 1991;**5**:196–99.

23 Ottmann OG, Druker BJ, Sawyers CL, et al. A phase 2 study of imatinib in patients with relapsed or refractory Philadelphia chromosome-positive acute lymphoid leukemias. *Blood.* 2002;**100**:1965–71.

24 Druker BJ, Sawyers CL, Kantarjian H, et al. Activity of a specific inhibitor of the BCR-ABL tyrosine kinase in the blast crisis of chronic myeloid leukemia and acute lymphoblastic leukemia with the Philadelphia chromosome. *N Engl J Med.* 2001;**344**:1038–42.

25 Thomas DA, Kantarjian HM, Cortes J, et al. Outcome with the Hyper-CVAD and Imatinib Mesylate Regimen as Frontline Therapy for Adult Philadelphia (Ph) Positive Acute Lymphocytic Leukemia (ALL). *Blood.* 2006;**108**:87a.

26 Yanada M, Takeuchi J, Sugiura I, et al. High complete remission rate and promising outcome by combination of imatinib and chemotherapy for newly diagnosed BCR-ABL-positive acute lymphoblastic leukemia: a phase II study by the Japan Adult Leukemia Study Group. *J Clin Oncol.* 2006;**24**:460–66.

27 Wassman B, Pfeifer H, Goekbuget N, et al. Alternating versus concurrent schedules of imatinib and chemotherapy as front-line therapy for Philadelphia-positive acute lymphoblastic leukemia (Ph+ ALL). *Blood.* 2006;**108**:1469–77.

28 Ottmann OG, Wassmann B, Goekbuget N, et al. A randomized phase II study comparing Imatinib with chemotherapy as induction therapy in elderly patients with newly diagnosed Philadelphia-positive acute lymphoid leukemias (Ph+ALL). *Hematol J.* 2004;**5**:S112.

29 Lee S, Kim YJ, Min CK, et al. The effect of first-line imatinib interim therapy on the outcome of allogeneic stem cell transplantation in adults with newly diagnosed Philadelphia chromosome-positive acute lymphoblastic leukemia. *Blood.* 2005;**105**:3449–57.

30 Wassmann B, Pfeifer H, Stadler M, et al. Early molecular response to posttransplant imatinib determines outcome in MRD-positive Philadelphia-positive acute lymphoblastic leukemia (Ph+ALL). *Blood.* 2005;**106**:458–63.

33 Acute Myeloid Leukemia in Adults

Remission Induction Therapy

Cara A. Rosenbaum, Richard A. Larson

Introduction

Acute myeloid leukemia (AML) results from the malignant transformation of a bone marrow (myeloid) progenitor cell or stem cell, which is the normal precursor for granulocytes, erythrocytes, and megakaryocytes. The traditional classification of the acute leukemias has relied on morphologic description, reflecting the predominant cell type present within the bone marrow population and relating that cell to its normal hematopoietic counterpart. This system was based solely on light-microscopic evaluation of routinely stained blood and marrow smears, supplemented by a limited number of cytochemical procedures. In 2001, a committee of the World Health Organization described a comprehensive classification scheme that utilizes morphology, immunophenotyping, etiology, and cytogenetics and more clearly distinguishes between AML and other myeloproliferative disorders (Table 33.1). A diagnosis of AML is established when 20% or more of the nucleated marrow cells are blast cells (1).

Clonal chromosomal abnormalities can be detected in most cases of AML (1,2). Particular abnormalities correlate with specific morphologic subtypes and clinical profiles (1–3). These cytogenetic abnormalities are somatic (rather than germ line) mutations that frequently result from translocations of chromosomal DNA, resulting in new (abnormal) protein products from the resultant fusion genes. It is assumed that the protein products from these fusion genes are responsible for the cellular dysregulation that leads to the malignant state. Such recurring chromosomal abnormalities are critical in determining therapeutic strategy and have provided important independent information regarding response to therapy and overall prognosis (see Table 33.2). Genes known to affect the outcome in patients with AML include *FLT3*, *KIT*, *CEBPA*, *BAALC*, *ERG*, *MLL*, and *NPM1* (4,5).

Evidence-based Hematology. Edited by Mark A. Crowther, Jeff Ginsberg, Holger J. Schünemann, Ralph M. Meyer, and Richard Lottenberg.

It is strongly recommended that cytogenetic analysis be performed before initiation of therapy on every newly diagnosed patient because studies of the prognostic significance of recurring cytogenetic abnormalities in AML have yielded consistently similar results (1–3). Thus, in many centers, plans for postremission therapy rely heavily on cytogenetic analysis at diagnosis. Cytogenetic data have been used to map chromosomal breakpoints at a molecular level, allowing for the use of more sensitive techniques, including probes for fluorescence in situ hybridization and primers for reverse transcriptase polymerase chain reaction. However, both of these methods test only for specific, defined genetic mutations and are not used initially for general screening or for a comprehensive evaluation.

The goal of remission induction chemotherapy is the rapid restoration of normal bone marrow function. The term *complete remission* (CR) is reserved for patients who have full recovery of normal peripheral blood counts and bone marrow cellularity, with less than 5% residual blast cells. Induction therapy aims to reduce the total-body leukemia cell population from approximately 10^{12} cells to below the cytologically detectable level of about 10^9 cells. It is thus assumed that even in CR, a substantial burden of leukemia cells persists undetected, leading to relapse within a few weeks or months if no further therapy were administered.

Questions

1. Which remission induction regimens give the best outcomes?
   a. What is the optimum anthracycline agent and dose?
   b. What is the role of cytarabine dose?
2. What is the role of adding other agents to "7 + 3"?
3. What is the role of multiple courses of induction therapy?
4. What is the role of myeloid growth factors in the initial treatment of AML?

Literature-search strategy and inclusions

Both PubMed and MEDLINE databases were searched from March 1, 1979, to October 10, 2006, using the search terms "acute myeloid

Table 33.1 World Health Organization classification of acute myeloid leukemia (AML).

AML with recurrent genetic abnormalities:
- AML with t(8;21)(q22;q22); AML/ETO
- AML with abnormal bone marrow eosinophils and inv(16)(p13q22) or t(16;16)(q22;p13); CBFß/MYH11
- Acute promyelocytic leukemia with t(15;17)(q22;q12); PML/RARα and variants
- AML with 11q23 (MLL) abnormalities

AML with multilineage dysplasia:
- Following myleodysplastic syndrome (MDS) or MDS/myeloproliferative disorder
- Without antecedent MDS

Therapy-related myeloid leukemia (t-AML and t-MDS):
- Alkylating agent-related
- Topoisomerase type II inhibitor-related

AML not otherwise categorized:
- AML minimally differentiated (FAB M0)
- AML without maturation (FAB M1)
- AML with maturation (FAB M2)
- Acute myelomonocytic leukemia (FAB M4)
- Acute monoblastic and monocytic leukemia (FAB M5)
- Acute erythroid leukemia (FAB M6)
- Acute megakaryoblastic leukemia (FAB M7)
- Acute basophilic leukemia
- Acute panmyelosis with myelofibrosis

Myeloid sarcoma

leukemia," "induction therapy," "post-remission therapy," "stem cell transplantation," and "bone marrow transplantation" limited to human trials and English language. Various subject headings for AML were used in the MEDLINE search, including "acute myelogenous leukemia," "acute myelocytic leukemia," and "AML." The 2006 Cochrane Library was also searched for relevant articles.

The evidence described in this review is drawn primarily from large randomized controlled trials (RCTs) conducted within the past two decades, systematic reviews, and available practice guidelines. Comprehensive guidelines have been previously published (6,7), and Table 33.3 provides a list of Web-based sites where further information and guidelines can be readily accessed.

Grading of the quality of evidence and strengths of recommendations in this chapter are based on the guidelines proposed by the international Grading of Recommendations Assessment, Development, and Evaluation Working Group (GRADE) adopting the modification used by the American College of Chest Physicians that merges the very low and low categories of quality of evidence (see chapter 1).

Which remission induction regimens give the best outcomes?

The most common remission induction regimen used in patients with AML is cytarabine given by continuous intravenous infusion daily for seven days plus an anthracycline such as daunorubicin given daily for three days (the "7+3" regimen). Depending on age and patient selection, 50% to 80% of patients achieve CR (8). By the 1980s, Preisler et al. had demonstrated an overall CR rate of 66% using the 7+3 regimen; patients less than 60 years old without a history of prior malignancy had an 80% CR rate (9). The Cancer and Leukemia Group B (CALGB) demonstrated that a 7+3 regimen with infusional cytarabine was superior to bolus cytarabine and to other combination schedules such as "5+2" (10). Studies that altered the 7+3 regimen by extending the cytarabine schedule to "10+3" or by adding 6-thioguanine to 7+3 (TAD or DAT) did not significantly improve CR rates (11). Thus, these early trials all contributed to the standardization of the 7+3 induction regimen.

Table 33.2 Cytogenetic/molecular subsets in acute myeloid leukemia, treatment, and outcomes.

Karyotype [mutation]	Complete remission rate	Remission duration	Treatment approach
t(8;21)(q22;q22) [*AML1/ETO*]	High	Long	Standard induction with cytarabine and an anthracycline; intensive consolidation with several courses of high-dose cytarabine
inv(16)(p13;q22) or t(16;16)(p13;q22) [*CBFβ/MYH11*]	High	Long	Standard induction with cytarabine and an anthracycline; intensive consolidation with several courses of high-dose cytarabine
t(15;17)(q22;q11–12) [*PML/RARα*]	High	Long	All-trans-retinoic acid together with an anthracycline for induction; arsenic trioxide for consolidation and to treat relapse
t(9;11)(p22;q23) [*AF9/MLL*]	High	Intermediate	Standard induction and intensive consolidation with high-dose cytarabine; reserve stem cell transplantation for second remission for most t(9;11) patients
Normal karyotype with *NPM1* mutation	High	Long	Standard induction and consolidation. No advantage to alloHCT in CR1
del(5q), +13, +8, −7, inv 3, del(12p), t(9;22), other t(11q23), or complex abnormalities	Low	Short	New induction regimens, including use of growth factors during or after chemotherapy, or modulators of drug resistance; perform stem cell transplantation in first complete remission

Table 33.3 Web sites and comprehensive guidelines on the management of AML in adults.

The British Committee for Standards in Haematology (BCSH)	www.bcsh-guidelines.com
National Comprehensive Cancer Network (NCCN) Version 1.2006	www.nccn.org
The National Institute for Clinical Excellence	www.nice.org
CancerBACUP	www.cancerbacup.org.uk
Leukaemia Research Fund	www.lrf.org.uk
Leukaemia Care Society	www.leukaemiacare.org
National Cancer Institute	www.cancer.gov
People Living with Cancer (ASCO)	www.plwc.org

What is the optimum anthracycline agent and dose?

Anthracycline dose intensification was examined in a three-arm randomized trial comparing 45 mg/m^2 and 30 mg/m^2 of daunorubicin to 30 mg/m^2 of doxorubicin, each given as part of a 7+3 regimen (12). The higher dose of daunorubicin yielded a significantly higher CR rate, although for patients over the age of 60, a daunorubicin dose of 30 mg/m^2 was found to be less toxic. A randomized trial by the Eastern Cooperative Oncology Group (ECOG) is currently examining dose intensification of daunorubicin to 90 mg/m^2 compared to 45 mg/m^2 in patients less than 60 years. Pharmacologic advantages of idarubicin during remission induction include its rapid uptake by cells based on its lipid solubility and the fact that its major metabolite is an active compound. Superiority of idarubicin over daunorubicin, when combined with cytarabine, was first demonstrated by higher CR rates and overall survival (OS) in a single center, randomized trial (13). Later, multicenter trials (see Table 33.4) showed that certain subgroups such as patients with hyperleukocytosis (e.g., white blood cell [WBC] count >50,000/μL) achieve CR more frequently with idarubicin compared to daunorubicin (14). This same study demonstrated longer remission durations and OS with idarubicin, but only younger patients had higher CR rates. Other randomized trials have demonstrated increased CR rates with idarubicin but no significant differences in remission duration or OS (15). A meta-analysis of individual patient data was published by the AML Collaborative Group comparing idarubicin with daunorubicin and other anthracycline agents during induction. Among 1,052 patients analyzed from five different trials, no significant benefit was found in DFS, although a difference in CR rate (62.4% vs. 53.2%) and five-year OS (13% vs. 9%) was found in favor of idarubicin (16). The benefit in terms of CR rate with idarubicin was observed only in younger patients. Because therapeutically equivalent doses of idarubicin and daunorubicin were not compared in these studies and long-term outcomes were heterogeneous, idarubicin cannot be considered superior to daunorubicin when used in induction.

Mitoxantrone is a synthetic anthracycline analogue (anthracenedione) that has also been compared with daunorubicin for its effectiveness in induction therapy together with cytarabine. Randomized trials have compared these two agents in both younger and older adult populations (Table 33.4). Although early trials showed differences in CR rates, OS, and remission duration favoring mitoxantrone, the differences were not statistically significant, and later trials failed to show any benefit of mitoxantrone over daunorubicin for induction therapy (17,18). Mitoxantrone may have less cumulative cardiotoxicity than daunorubicin but cannot be strongly recommended over daunorubicin for induction therapy.

What is the role of cytarabine dose?

Modulating the dose intensity of cytarabine in induction was first studied by the CALGB, comparing 200 mg/m^2 with the standard 100 mg/m^2 dose, given by continuous infusion for seven days together with 45 mg/m^2 of daunorubicin for three days (19). Among all randomized patients less than 60 years old, no differences in rates of CR, DFS, or OS were seen. Treatment-related toxicities, including deaths during induction, were more common with the higher dose of cytarabine. However, younger patients with a performance status of zero had improved survival with the higher cytarabine dose. A single-center study compared intermediate dose (500 mg/m^2) cytarabine given every 12 hours for 12 doses to conventional dose (200 mg/m^2) cytarabine given by continuous infusion for seven days, each together with 60 mg/m^2 of daunorubicin for three days (Table 33.4); no significant differences in remission rate, remission duration, or survival were found (20). There were no differences in treatment-related toxicities between the two groups.

High-dose cytarabine regimens (HiDAC; 2–3 g/m^2 given for 6–12 doses) were first developed for patients with relapsed AML but later moved into the setting of frontline therapy. When three days of HiDAC were given immediately following standard 7+3 induction, a CR rate of 89% was observed in a single-center trial (21). However, this favorable outcome was not subsequently confirmed in phase II trials performed by large cooperative groups. As noted in Table 33.4, the Southwest Oncology Group (SWOG) and the Australian Leukemia Study Group (ALSG) conducted studies comparing 2 g/m^2 or 3 g/m^2 of cytarabine, respectively, to the standard-dose cytarabine (7+3) regimen; etoposide was also added to each arm in the ALSG study (22–24). No differences in CR rates or OS were demonstrated, although the SWOG study showed a marginal improvement in DFS for patients <65 years receiving HiDAC, while the ALSG study demonstrated a significantly better relapse-free survival (RFS) and remission duration in patients ≤60 years receiving HiDAC. In the SWOG study, induction with HiDAC was associated with significantly increased deaths and neurologic toxicity, while the ALSG showed no significant difference in induction fatalities or CNS toxicity. The ALSG trial was limited to patients 60 years or younger, and the younger patients within

Table 33.4 Patient characteristics and treatment outcomes for randomized controlled trials comparing induction therapies in adults with AML.*

Author (reference) study	Study type	Quality of evidence (grade)	Regimen	No. of pts	Exclusion criteria	Median age (eligible age or range)	Pretreatment WBC (K/μL) (median)	Pretreatment characteristics	CR (%)	Induction death rate (%)	Med F/U (mo)	DFS/RFS/ remission duration (Med)	OS (Med)
Berman (13) 1991	SC	A	A + I(5 + 3) A + D(5 + 3)	Total:120 60 60	MDS or secondary leukemia	36 (17–60) 41 (19–60)	10.3 17.9	t(8;21)&inv(16) 5% 7%	80% 58% $p = 0.005$	7% 7%	30	Not reported	19.7 mo 13.5 mo $p = 0.025$
Wiernik (14) 1992	MC	A	A + I(7 + 3) A + D(7 + 3)	Total: 208 97 111	Prior malignancy or chemo/XRT	56 (>17) 55 (>17)	7.9 10.6	Prior MDS/RAEB 10% 5%	70% 59% NS	22% 22%	Not stated	RD 9.4 mos 8.4 mos $p = 0.021$	12.9 mo 8.7 mo $p = 0.038$
Vogler (15) 1992	MC	A	A + I(7 + 3) A + D(7 + 3)	Total: 218 105 113	None	60 (>14) 61 (>14)	8.1 6.5	Antecedent MDS/RAEB 16% 13%	71% 58% $p = 0.032$	17% 22%	Not stated	RD 433 days 328 days NS	9.9 mo 9.2 mo NS
Arlin (17) 1990	MC	A	A + M(7 + 3) A + D(7 + 3)	Total: 200 98 102	Prior hematologic malignancy or chemo/XRT	60 (>15) 60 (>15)	36%>20 32%>20	NS	63% 53% NS	14% 13%	Not stated	RD 240 days 198 days NS	10.9 mo 8.2 mo NS
Schiller (20) 1992	SC	A	SDAC IDAC	Total: 101 51 50	t-AML	47 (17–75) 48 (19–75)	5 12.5	Abnormal cytogenetics 37% 36%	71% 74% NS	10% 14%	32	4 y DFS 20% 28% NS	4 y OS 25% 37% NS
Weick (22) SWOG, 1996	MC	A	SDAC HiDAC	Total: 665† 493 172	None	45 (15–64) 50 (17–64)	18 16.3	t-AML/MDS included	58%‡ 55% NS	5% 14% $p = 0.0033$	55	4 y RFS‡ 21% 33% NS§	4 y OS‡ 22% 32% NS
Bishop (23) ALSG, 1996	MC	A	7 + 3 + 7 HiDAC + 3 + 7	Total: 301 152 149	Prior chemo/MDS/other malignancy	39 (15–60) 43 (15–60)	9.7 10.9	Fav/Unfav cytogenetics‖ 30%/16% 28%/10%	74% 71% NS	11% 18% NS	68	5 y RFS/RD 25%/12mo 48%/46mo $p = 0.007/0.0007$	5 y OS 25% 33% NS

*SC, single center; MC, multicenter; A + I, AraC + idarubicin; A + D, AraC + daunorubicin; A + M, AraC + mitoxantrone; NS, not significant; Med, median; mo = months; NS = not stated; DFS, disease-free survival; RFS, relapse-free survival; RD, Remission duration; OS, Overall survival; XRT, irradiation; t-AML, therapy-related AML; F/U, follow-up

(13) A + I = cytarabine 25 mg/m^2 IV bolus followed by 200 mg/m^2/d continuous infusion (CIVI) for 5 days and idarubicin 12 mg/m^2 /d for 3 days; A + D = cytarabine as above and daunorubicin 50 mg/m^2/d for 3 days.

(14) A + I = cytarabine 100 mg/m^2/d for 7 days by CIVI and idarubicin 13 mg/m^2/d for 3 days; A + D = cytarabine as above and daunorubicin 45 mg/m^2/d for 3 days.

(15) A + I = cytarabine 100 mg/m^2/d CIVI for 7 days and idarubicin 12 mg/m^2/d for 3 days; A + D = cytarabine as above and daunorubicin 45 mg/m^2/d for 3 days.

(17) A + M = cytarabine 100 mg/m^2/d CIVI for 7 days and mitoxantrone 12 mg/m^2/d for 3 days; A + D = cytarabine as above and daunorubicin 45 mg/m2/d for 3 days.

(20) SDAC = standard dose cytarabine (200 mg/m^2/d) CIVI for 7 days and 60 mg/m^2/d daunorubicin for 3 days; IDAC = intermediate dose cytarabine (500 mg/m^2) intravenously every 12 hours for 12 doses and daunorubicin as above.

(22) SDAC = 200 mg/m^2/d for 7 days by CIVI and daunorubicin 45 mg/m^2/d for 3 days; HiDAC = 2g/m$_2$ intravenously every 12 hours for 12 doses and daunorubicin as above.

†A separate analysis was reported on 58 patients, not included in the cohort of 665 patients, randomized to induction with 3 g/m^2 of cytarabine plus daunorubicin: CR 59%, 4y RFS 29%, 4y OS 28%.

‡Outcomes listed for age group <50 years; corresponding outcomes for age group 50–64 are SDAC = CR 53%, 4y RFS 9%, 4y OS 11%; HiDAC = CR 45%, 4y RFS 21%, 4y OS 13%.

§4y RFS advantage seen with HiDAC for total cohort of 665 patients ($p = 0.049$); no significant difference found when age group <50 was considered separately.

(23) 7 + 3 + 7 = cytarabine 100 mg/m^2 for 7 days by CIVI with 50 mg/m^2/d daunorubicin for 3 days and etoposide 75 mg/m^2/d for 7 days; HiDAC + 3 + 7 = 3 g/m^2 cytarabine every 12 hours on days 1,3,5,7 for 8 doses with daunorubicin and etoposide at same dose and schedule as above.

‖Based on 102 7 + 3 + 7 patients and 101 HiDAC + 3 + 7 patients with valid cytogenetics available. Favorable cytogenetics include t(8;21), inv(16), t(15;17); unfavorable cytogenetics include -5/5q-,-7/7q- and complex (>4 abnormalities).

this age group demonstrated higher response rates and lower toxicity (23–24). A systematic review comparing the above trials and a third trial with HiDAC given in a double-induction strategy by the German AML Cooperative Group (AMLCG) highlighted the improved RFS and OS associated with HiDAC given in induction (25,26). However, no consistent effect was seen with CR rates, and conclusions drawn from this review are likely valid only for adults younger than 60 years with de novo AML due to the restricted inclusion criteria in these trials. Controversy persists as to whether the increased toxicity of HiDAC during induction is justified by the longer DFS despite a lack of improvement in CR rate. An alternative strategy is to reserve this more intensive antileukemia therapy for the postremission period when patients are generally better able to tolerate it (see Chapter 34).

Recommendations

1. The standard treatment regimen for adult patients with AML is the 7 + 3 regimen (Grade 1A).
2. When daunorubicin is used as the anthracycline agent within 7 + 3, the dose is 45–60 mg/m^2 (Grade 1A).
3. When using the 7 + 3 regimen, there is insufficient evidence to support a choice of idarubicin or mitoxantrone as a superior anthracycline agent in comparison with daunorubicin (Grade 2A).
4. The use of HiDAC in induction therapy cannot be strongly recommended given inconsistencies in observed outcomes, risks of toxicity, and the option to include this therapy as postinduction treatment (Grade 2A).

What is the role of adding other agents to 7 + 3?

The addition of etoposide to standard dose cytarabine and daunorubicin in induction was examined in two large randomized trials in the 1990s. The first was an ALSG trial, which included patients up to 70 years of age (see Table 33.5); patients were randomized between standard 7 + 3 induction and cytarabine (ara-C), daunorubicin, and etoposide (ADE) (27). No significant differences in CR rates or OS were seen although patients less than 55 years analyzed as a subgroup did have significantly better 5- and 10-year survival rates in the ADE arm. The Medical Research Council (MRC) AML-10 trial compared ADE with daunorubicin, ara-C, and thioguanine (DAT) during induction in patients less than 55 years (28). All patients received two courses of induction therapy, regardless of whether they had achieved a CR following the first induction cycle. No differences were found between the two groups in CR rates, DFS, or OS; CR rates of 81% and 83%, respectively, and six-year OS rates of 40% in both arms were demonstrated. Analysis of survival by age subgroups failed to show any benefit for etoposide.

Valspodar (PSC-833), an inhibitor of the P-glycoprotein cell membrane drug efflux pump, expressed in approximately 75% of patients with de novo AML over 55 years, has been studied in combination with ADE during induction by the CALGB (29). No differences were found in the rates of CR, DFS, or OS between ADE arms with and without PSC-833 (Table 33.5). Burnett et al. recently reported preliminary results from the MRC AML15 trial, revealing a significantly improved DFS without a higher rate of toxicities in the induction arm receiving gemtuzumab ozogamicin (Mylotarg), although no overall survival difference was seen (30). A current SWOG/CALGB intergroup trial is examining the addition of a single dose of Mylotarg on day 4 of induction to standard cytarabine and daunorubicin in patients aged ≤60 years, followed by HiDAC consolidation, with a subsequent randomization to additional Mylotarg versus no further therapy.

Recommendations

1. There is insufficient evidence to support adding etoposide to the 7 + 3 regimen (Grade 2A).
2. Current evidence indicates that valspodar (PSC-833) does not improve outcomes in patients receiving ADE, and is therefore not recommended (Grade 1B).

What is the role of multiple courses of induction therapy?

Intensification of induction therapy was tested in trials by the German AMLCG, which incorporated HiDAC into a double-induction regimen (Table 33.5). In a prospective clinical trial, 725 patients received an initial course of TAD, followed by a second induction course starting promptly on day 21 with randomization to repeat the TAD course or to receive a course of HiDAC with mitoxantrone (HAM) (25). No differences in CR rates, five-year RFS, or five-year OS were found in the study population overall. Subgroup analysis showed that patients with poor prognostic factors, such as high-residual blasts in the day 16 bone marrow exam, high LDH levels at diagnosis, and unfavorable karyotypes, had improved outcomes with the TAD-HAM double-induction regimen compared with the TAD-TAD regimen. The AMLCG also tested whether additional intensification could be given during induction and compared TAD-HAM double induction with HAM-HAM (31). As no differences in toxicities or outcomes were found between the two arms or within subgroup analyses, the authors concluded that additional upfront intensification is not beneficial during induction.

Recommendation

There is insufficient evidence to support additional upfront intensification beyond standard induction therapy (Grade 2A).

What is the role of myeloid growth factors in the initial treatment of AML?

A number of RCTs have been conducted in AML patients examining the effects of myeloid growth factors such as granulocyte colony-stimulating factor (G-CSF, filgrastim), glycosylated G-CSF (lenograstim), and granulocyte-macrophage

Table 33.5 Patient Characteristics and treatment outcomes for randomized controlled trials comparing induction therapies in adults with AML, continued.

Author (reference) study	Quality of evidence (grade)	Regimen	No. of pts	Exclusion criteria	Median age (range)	Pretreatment WBC (K/μL) median (range)	Pretreatment characteristics	CR (%)	Induction death rate (%)	Med F/U (y)	DFS/RFS/ remission duration (median)	OS (median)
Bishop (27) ALSG, 1990	A	 7 + 3 7 + 3 + 7 (ADE)	total 264 132 132	Prior MDS or other malignancy	(15–70) (15–70)	44% ≥20 35% ≥20	Not stated	56% 59% NS	Not stated	9.6	5 y RFS/RD 18%/12mo 36%/18mo $p = 0.04/0.008$	9 mo 13 mo NS
Hann (28) MRC AML10, 1997	A	 DAT x 2 ADE x 2	total1857 929 928	None	(0–55) (0–55)	12% ≥100 12% ≥100	2° AML/fav/unfav karyotype 7%/17%/6% 7%/17%/6%	81% 83% NS	8% 9%	6	6 y DFS 42% 43% NS	6 y OS 40% 40% NS
Kolitz (29) CALGB19808, 2005	A	 ADE ADEP	total 296 149 147	Prior MDS or t-AML	45 (<60) 45 (<60)	Not stated	Not stated	77% 78% NS	7% 7%	2.2	DFS 19 mo 15 mo NS	21 mo 20 mo NS
Buchner (25) AMLCG 1999	A	 TAD-TAD TAD-HAM	total 725 360 365	Prior chemo, XRT,MDS, hematologic disorder	44 (16–60) 44 (16–60)	17.2 (0.1–405) 21 (0.5–331)	Fav/unfav karyotype* 6%/4% 7%/3%	65% 71% NS	18% 14% NS	5	5 y RFS 29% 35% NS	5 y OS 30% 32% NS
Buchner (31) AMLCG 2006	A	 TAD-HAM HAM-HAM	total 840† 430 410	None	60 (16–85) 60 (16–85)	44% >20 43% >20	2° AML/fav/unfav karyotype‡ 4%/3%/5% 5%/3%/5%	71% 68% NS	12% 14% NS	3	3 y RD 45% 49% NS	3 y OS 44% 40% NS

See note to Table 33.4 for abbreviations.

(27) 7 + 3 = 100 mg/m^2/d cytarabine by CIVI for 7 days and daunorubicin 50 mg/m^2/d for 3 days; 7 + 3 + 7 = cytarabine and daunorubicin as above plus etoposide 75 mg/m^2/d for 7 days.

(28) DAT = daunorubicin 50 mg/m^2 slow intravenous push on days 1,3,5, cytarabine 100 mg/m^2 every 12 hours on days 1–10 (days 1–8 during second induction course), 6-thioguanine 100 mg/m^2 every 12 hours orally on days 1–10 (days 1–8 during course no. 2); ADE = daunorubicin and cytarabine as above and etoposide 100 mg/m^2 1-hour infusion on days 1–5 (cytarabine days 1–8 only during second induction course). Second course of DAT and ADE given whether CR achieved or not.

(29) ADE = cytarabine 100 mg/m^2/d CIVI for 7 days and daunorubicin 90 mg/m^2/d and etoposide 100 mg/m^2/d for 3 days; ADEP = cytarabine as above, daunorubicin 40 mg/m^2/d and etoposide 40 mg/m^2/d each for 3 days and PSC833 loading dose 2.8 mg/kg IV over 2 hours followed by 10 mg/m^2 CIVI over 72 hours on days 1–3.

(25) TAD = cytarabine 100 mg/m^2/d CIVI for 2 days and subsequently by 30-min infusion every 12 hours on days 3–8, daunorubicin 60 mg/m^2/d on days 3–5, 6-thioguanine 100 mg/m^2/d orally every 12 hours on days 3–9. Second induction course starting on day 21 randomized to repeat TAD or HAM = 3g/m^2 cytarabine by 3-hour infusion every 12 hours on days 1-3 with 10 mg/m^2/d mitoxantrone on days 3–5.

*Based on 172 TAD-TAD and 171 TAD-HAM patients with available cytogenetics. Favorable karyotype include t(8;21), inv(16), t(15;17); unfavorable karyotype include loss/deletion of 5 or 7, 11q23, and complex karyotype.

(31) TAD and HAM regimens as described above except patients ≥60 years received 1 g/m^2 cytarabine by 3-hour infusion every 12 hours on days 1–3 in place of 3 g/m^2.

†Table lists total number of patients and outcome data for age group <60 years only. Corresponding outcomes for age group ≥60 years are TAD-HAM = CR 53%, 3 y RD 17%, 3 y OS 18%; HAM-HAM = CR 53%, 3 y, RD 28%, 3 y OS 19%.

‡Favorable cytogenetics include t(8;21), inv(16), or t(16;16); unfavorable cytogenetics include loss or deletion of chromosomes 5 or 7, chromosome 3(q21q26) abnormalities, 11q23, or complex karyotype (≥3 abnormalities).

colony-stimulating factor (GM-CSF, sargramostim and molgramostim) (see Table 33.6). The objective of many of these trials was to determine whether a reduction in the duration of neutropenia would improve outcomes (CR rates and OS) by decreasing early mortality when CSFs are given following intensive myelosuppressive chemotherapy. Since AML cells express receptors for CSFs, additional studies tested the effect of "priming," or the sensitization of AML cells to chemotherapy by coadministration of CSFs together with induction therapy. The majority of growth factor trials have been conducted in older patient populations since they suffer the highest rate of treatment-related mortality and have the poorest overall response rates.

It is difficult to compare directly the outcomes from one trial to the next because of variation in the specific growth factor used, sample size, patient population, timing of randomization, and timing of growth factor administration. Nevertheless, the statistically significant reduction in the duration of neutropenia following CSF administration seen in all of these trials has rarely translated into a measurable clinical benefit, either when used as supportive care or when given therapeutically for "priming."

An early randomized trial reported by the ECOG demonstrated a benefit from the use of sargramostim after both induction and consolidation therapy for patients 56 to 70 years old with a more rapid neutrophil recovery and a reduction in morbidity from severe infections (32). Median survival was also doubled in the sargramostim arm although CR rates and treatment-related mortality were similar between the two arms. The CALGB conducted a larger randomized trial examining molgramostim given after standard induction chemotherapy in patients 60 years or older (33). The statistically significant shortening of the median duration of neutropenia by two days did not lead to a higher CR rate, longer survival, or lower treatment-related mortality.

A study in which lenograstim was given after induction in older patients demonstrated a shortened duration of neutropenia and higher CR rates in the lenograstim arm but no improvement in treatment-related mortality or OS (34). The differentiating effects of CSFs may lead to concealment of AML cells by the increased number of neutrophils produced from G-CSF stimulation in patients who have residual disease, thereby increasing the observed CR rate (35).

Increasing the cytotoxic effects of chemotherapy by using CSFs to stimulate AML blasts into the S-phase of the cell cycle remains unproven. Early randomized trials with concurrent GM-CSF and induction chemotherapy showed no improvement in CR, DFS, or OS, although one study by the GOELAM group showed improved survival in a subset of patients 55–64 years old (36).

The EORTC/HOVON group evaluated CSF priming by administering molgramostim concurrently with induction therapy in older patients; there was a decrease in duration of neutropenia but no other significant effects on outcome (37). This and other trials in which molgramostim was coadministered with chemotherapy for a priming effect demonstrated that chemosensitivity is not increased based on equivalent CR rates, DFS, and OS in both arms (36–38). A French trial randomized patients to 4 arms to receive molgramostim either during, during and after, or only after completion of chemotherapy versus not at all (38). There was no significant difference in CR rates between the groups randomized to receive the CSF during induction or not (59% vs. 62%). The groups randomized to receive molgramostim after chemotherapy had significantly worse CR rates (47% vs. 75%; $p = 0.008$) and four-year event-free survival, but no differences in OS were found. An ECOG study examined priming with sargramostim administered 48 hours before the start of chemotherapy and found no improvement in responses compared to a placebo arm (39). In addition, a detrimental effect was observed when this cytokine was given before induction chemotherapy.

Two recent large trials studied priming with lenograstim (40,41). The HOVON group randomized 640 young and middle-aged adults to receive lenograstim or not, concurrently with two courses of induction therapy; the G-CSF was discontinued at completion of chemotherapy (40). The duration of neutropenia (median on both arms, 30 days) lasted up to twice as long compared with other trials, but granulocyte recovery eventually occurred. Significantly improved DFS was seen in the G-CSF group overall, but a statistically significant benefit in OS was observed only for patients with standard-risk features. The authors attributed the lack of an improved CR rate to the increased early death rate observed on the lenograstim arm (17% vs. 10.5%; $p = 0.02$).

A priming study conducted by the EORTC/GIMEMA in older patients compared 4 groups of patients receiving lenograstim during, during and after, or after completion of chemotherapy vs not at all (41). Although an improved CR rate was found in the groups randomized to receive lenograstim during induction, no differences in DFS or OS were observed in either of the groups receiving lenograstim for priming or after induction. In contrast to the HOVON study, which demonstrated improved survival rates in the subgroup of standard-risk patients, this trial identified no particular cytogenetic subgroup benefiting from priming with lenograstim. The authors suggested that their three-drug induction regimen, compared to the two-drug regimens used in prior priming trials, may have contributed to an improved CR rate. However, because of the lack of benefit in long-term outcomes, they did not recommend CSF administration in induction for older patients apart from use in supportive care. An expert panel consensus report did not recommend the use of CSFs for priming in younger or older AML patients based on a lack of survival benefit (42).

Recommendations

1. Apart from hastening neutrophil recovery, the lack of other clinical benefits provides evidence that routine prophylactic use of myeloid growth factors after remission induction cannot be recommended (42–44) (Grade 1A).

2. Consistent with an expert panel consensus report (41), the use of CSFs for priming in younger or older AML patients is not recommended based on the lack of survival benefit (Grade 1A).

Table 33.6 Randomized controlled trials of colony stimulating factors (CSFs) used in induction and consolidation therapies in adults with AML.

Author (reference) study	Quality of evidence (grade)	No. of patients	Age range, years (median)	CSF	Induction or consolidation	Day CSF started during chemotherapy cycle	Priming effect assessed	Median days of neutropenia ($<500/\mu$ L); CSF/placebo	Treatment-related mortality (%); CSF/placebo	CR(%); CSF/placebo	Remission duration; CSF/placebo	Survival; CSF/placebo
Rowe (32) ECOG E1490, 1995	A	117	56–70 (64)	Sargramostim	Induction and consolidation	11	No	13/17[†] $p = 0.001$	6/15 NS	60/44 NS	DFS (median, mo) 8.5/9.6 NS	Median, mo 10.6/4.8 $p = 0.048$
Stone (33) CALGB 8923, 1995	A	388	$\geq$ 60 (69)	Molgramostim	Induction	8	No	15/17 $p= 0.02$	20/16[‡] NS	51/54 NS	(median, mo) 8.2/10.4 NS	Median, mo 8.4/10.8 NS
Dombret (34) 1995	A	173	64–83 (71)	Lenograstim	Induction	9	No	(ANC$\leq$1,000/μ L) 21/27 $p < 0.001$	23/27 NS	70/47 $p = 0.002$	NS	1 y (%) 45/40 NS
Godwin (43) SWOG 9031, 1998	A	211	56–88 (68)	Filgrastim	Induction and consolidation	11	No	24/27 $p = 0.014$	20/19 NS	41/50 NS	RFS (median, mo) 8/9 NS	Median, mo 6/9 NS
Heil (44) 1997	A	521	16–89 (54)	Filgrastim	Induction and consolidation	8	No	20/25 $p = 0.0001$	8/9.5 NS	69/68 NS	DFS (median, mo) 10.1/9.4 NS	Median, mo 12.5/14 NS
Harrousseau (45) GOELAM, 2000	A	194	15–60 (46)	Filgrastim	Consolidation (C1,C2) only	7	No	C1:12/19, $p < 0.001$ C2:20/28, $p < 0.001$	C1:2/2 C2:3.5/3.7 NS	N/A	2 y DFS (%) 47/43 NS	2 y (%) 64/63 NS
Witz (36) GOELAM, 1998	A	232	55–75 (66)	Molgramostim	Induction	1	Yes	24/29 $p = 0.0001$	18/15.5 NS	63/60.5 NS	2 y DFS (%) 48/21 $p = 0.003$	2 y (%) 39/27 NS[§]
Lowenberg (37) EORTC /HOVON, 1997	B (not blinded)	318	61–88 (68)	Molgramostim	Induction	0	Yes	23/25 $p = 0.0002$	14/13 NS	56/55 NS	2 y DFS (%) 15/19 NS	2 y (%) 22/22 NS
Zittoun (38) EORTC, 1996	B (not blinded)	102	17–59 (44)	Molgramostim	Induction	Arm 1: None Arm 2: 0–7 Arm 3: 8–28 Arm 4: 0–28	Yes	Arm 1: 24.5 Arm 2: 22.2 Arm 3: 22.0 Arm 4: 19.5 NS	Arm 1: 7.7 Arm 2: 4.0 Arm 3: 3.7 Arm 4: 8.3 NS	Arm 1:77 Arm 2:72 Arm 3:48 Arm 4:46[‖]	4 y EFS 3&4<1&2 $p = 0.02$ 1&3 = 2&4 NS	NS
Rowe (39) ECOG, 2004	A	235	>56 (68)	Sargramostim	Induction and consolidation	48 hours prior	Yes	Not stated	26/17 NS	38/40 NS	DFS (median, mo) 6.9/5.1, NS	Median, mo 5.3/8.5 NS
Lowenberg (40) HOVON, 2003	A	640	18–60 (44)	Lenograstim	Induction	0	Yes	Ind 1:30/30 Ind 2:26/25 NS	17/10.5 $p = 0.02$	79/83 NS	4 y DFS (%) 42/33 $p = 0.02$	4 y (%)[¶] 40/35 NS
Amadori (41) EORTC/ GIMEMA, 2005	B (not blinded)	722	61–80 (68)	Lenograstim	Induction	Arm 1: None Arm 2: 1–7 Arm 3: 8–28 Arm 4: 1–28	Yes	Arm 3&4: 20 Arm 1&2: 25 $p< 0.001$	Arm 1: 13.7 Arm 2: 11.1 Arm 3: 17.8 Arm 4: 11.6	Arm 1:49 Arm 2:52 Arm 3:48 Arm 4:64[#]	3 y DFS (%) Arms 1/2/3/4: 22/18/19/15 NS	3 y (%) Arms 1/2/3/4: 15/18/14.4/7.6 NS

CSF, colony stimulating factor; mo = months; NS, not significant; Rem Dur, remission duration; DFS, disease-free survival; RFS, relapse-free survival; OS, = overall survival; EFS = event-free survival.

[†] Outcomes reported for induction treatment only; no significant difference in neutrophil recovery between the two groups in consolidation therapy.

[‡] Excludes early induction deaths occurring before initiation of GM-CSF.

[§] Subgroup analysis of patients aged 55 to 64 showed a significant improvement in OS in the GM-CSF arm ($p = 0.014$).

[‖] 2 × 2 factorial analysis reveals higher CR rate after one or two courses between groups 1&2 vs. 3&4 (randomized postinduction day 8 + to no CSF vs. molgramostim, respectively (75% vs. 47%, $p = 0.008$)); no significant difference for CR rates between groups 1&3 and 2&4 (randomized during induction to no CSF vs. molgramostim, 62% vs. 59%, respectively).

[¶] Subgroup analysis of patients with standard risk AML as defined by lack of favorable characteristics (t(8;21), inv16, or t(16;16) and wbc $<20{,}000/\mu$L) and lack of unfavorable characteristics (monosomies or deletions of chromosome 5 or 7, $\geq$4 unrelated cytogenetic clones, t(6;9), chromosome 3q or 11q abnormalities, secondary or t-AML) showed a significant difference in 4 y OS in favor of the arm receiving G-CSF (45% vs. 35% ($p = 0.02$)).

[#] 2 × 2 factorial analysis reveals higher CR rate between groups 2&4 and 1&3 (randomized during induction to receive lenograstim vs. no CSF, respectively (58.3% vs. 48.6%, $p = 0.009$)); no significant difference for CR rates between groups 3&4 and 1&2 (randomized to receive lenograstim vs. no CSF postinduction, 50.6% vs. 56.4%, respectively).

References

1 Jaffe ES, Harris NL, Stein H, et al., editors. *World Health Organization classification of tumours. Pathology and genetics of tumours of haematopoietic and lymphoid tissues.* Lyon: IARC Press; 2001.

2 Byrd JC, Mrozek K, Dodge RK, et al. Pretreatment cytogenetic abnormalities are predictive of induction success, cumulative incidence of relapse, and overall survival in adult patients with de novo acute myeloid leukemia: results from Cancer and Leukemia Group B (CALGB 8461). *Blood.* 2002;**100**:4325–36.

3 Mrozek K, Heerema NA, Bloomfield CD. Cytogentics in acute leukemia. *Blood Rev.* 2004;**18**:115–36.

4 Paschka P, Marcucci G, Ruppert AS, et al. Adverse prognostic significance of *KIT* mutations in adult acute myeloid leukemia with inv(16) and t(8;21): a Cancer and Leukemia Group B study. *J Clin Oncol.* 2006;**24**:3904–11.

5 Mrozek K, Marcucci G, Paschka P, et al. Clinical relevance of mutations and gene-expression changes in adult acute myeloid leukemia with normal cytogenetics: are we ready for a prognostically prioritized molecular classification? *Blood.* 2007;**109**:431–48.

6 Milligan DW, Grimwade D, Cullis JO, et al. Guidelines on the management of acute myeloid leukaemia in adults. *Br J Haematol.* 2006;**135**:450–74.

7 Acute Myeloid Leukemia. Clinical practice guidelines in oncology [Version 1.2006]. National Comprehensive Cancer Network, Inc. Available at: http://www.nccn.org.

8 Kolitz JE. Current therapeutic strategies for acute myeloid leukaemia. *Br J Haematol.* 2006;**134**:555–72.

9 Preisler HD, Rustum Y, Henderson ES, et al. Treatment of acute nonlymphocytic leukemia: use of anthracycline-cytarabine arabinoside induction therapy and comparison of two maintenance regimens. *Blood.* 1979;**53**:455.

10 Rai KR, Holland JF, Glidewell OJ, et al. Treatment of acute myelocytic leukemia: a study by Cancer and Leukemia Group B. *Blood.* 1981;**58**:1203.

11 Preisler HD, Davis RB, Hirschner J, et al. Comparison of three remission induction regimens and two postinduction strategies for the treatment of acute nonlymphocytic leukemia: a Cancer and Leukemia Group B study. *Blood.* 1987;**69**:1441–49.

12 Yates J, Glidewell O, Wiernik P, et al. Cytarabine arabinoside with daunorubicin or adriamycin for therapy of acute myelocytic leukemia: a CALBG study. *Blood.* 1982;**60**:454.

13 Berman E, Heller G, Santorsa J, et al. Results of a randomized trial comparing idarubicin and cytarabine arabinoside with daunorubicin and cytarabine arabinoside in adult patients with newly diagnosed acute myelogenous leukemia. *Blood.* 1991;**77**:1666–74.

14 Wiernik PH, Banks P, Case DC, et al. Cytarabine plus idarubicin or daunorubicin as induction and consolidation therapy for previously untreated adult patients with acute myeloid leukemia. *Blood.* 1992;**79**:313–19.

15 Vogler WR, Velez-Garcia E, Weiner RS, et al. A phase III trial comparing idarubicin and daunorubicin in acute myelogenous leukemia. *J Clin Oncol.* 1992;**10**:1103.

16 The AML Collaborative Study Group. A systematic collaborative overview of randomized trials comparing idarubicin with daunorubicin (or other anthracyclines) as induction therapy for acute myeloid leukemia. *Br J Hematol.* 1998;**103**:100–109.

17 Arlin Z, Case DC, Moore J, et al. Randomized multicenter trial of cytosine arabinoside with mitoxantrone or daunorubicin in previously untreated patients with acute nonlymphocytic leukemia. *Leukemia.* 1990;**4**:177–83.

18 Burnett AK, Goldstone AH, Milligan DW, et al. Daunorubicin versus mitoxantrone as induction for AML in younger patients given intensive induction chemotherapy: preliminary results of MRC AML-12 trial. *Br J of Haematol.* 1999;**105** Suppl 1:154a.

19 Dillman RO, Davis RB, Green MR, et al. A comparative study of two different doses of cytarabine for acute myeloid leukemia: a phase III trial of Cancer and Leukemia Group B. *Blood.* 1991;**78**:2520–26.

20 Schiller G, Gajewski J, Nimer S, et al. A randomized study of intermediate versus conventional-dose cytarabine as intensive induction for acute myelogenous leukemia. *Br J Hematol.* 1992;**81**:170–77.

21 Mitus AJ, Miller KB, Schenkein DP, et al. Improved survival for patients with acute myelogenous leukemia. *J Clin Oncol.* 1995;**13**:560.

22 Weick JK, Kopecky KJ, Appelbaum FR, et al. A randomized investigation of high-dose versus standard-dose cytosine arabinoside with daunorubicin in patients with previously untreated acute myeloid leukemia: a Southwest Oncology Group study. *Blood.* 1996;**88**:2841-51.

23 Bishop JF, Matthews JP, Young GA, et al. A randomized study of high-dose cytarabine in induction in acute myeloid leukemia. *Blood.* 1996;**87**:1710–17.

24 Bishop JF, Matthews JP, Young GA, et al. Intensified induction chemotherapy with high-dose cytarabine and etoposide for acute myeloid leukemia: a review and updated results of the Australian Leukemia Study Group. *Leuk Lymphoma.* 1998;**28**:315–27.

25 Buchner T, Hiddemann W, Wormann B, et al. Double induction strategy for acute myeloid leukemia: the effect of high-dose cytarabine with mitoxantrone instead of standard-dose cytarabine with daunorubicin and 6-thioguanine: a randomized trial by the German AML Cooperative Group. *Blood.* 1999;**93**:4116–24.

26 Kern W, Estey EH. High-dose cytosine arabinoside in the treatment of acute myeloid leukemia. *Cancer.* 2006;**107**:116–24.

27 Bishop JF, Lowenthal RM, Joshua D, et al. Etoposide in acute nonlymphocytic leukemia. Australian Leukemia Study Group. *Blood.* 1990;**75**:27–32.

28 Hann IM, Stevens RF, Goldstone A, et al. Randomized comparison of DAT versus ADE as induction chemotherapy in children and younger adults with acute myeloid leukemia: results of the Medical Research Council's 10th AML Trial (MRC AML 10). *Blood.* 1997;**89**:2311–18.

29 Kolitz JE, George SL, Marcucci G, et al. A randomized comparison of induction therapy for untreated acute myeloid leukemia (AML) in patients <60 years using P-glycoprotein (Pgp) modulation with Valspodar (PSC833): preliminary results of Cancer and Leukemia Group B Study 19808 [abstract]. *Blood.* 2005;**106**:407.

30 Burnett AK, Kell WJ, Milligan AD, et al. The addition of gemtuzumab ozogamicin to induction chemotherapy for AML improves disease free survival without extra toxicity: preliminary analysis of 1115 patients in the MRC AML15 trial [abstract]. *Blood.* 2006;**108**:3.

31 Buchner T, Berdel WE, Schoch C. et al. Double induction containing either two courses or one course of high-dose cytarabine plus mitoxantrone and postremission therapy by either autologous stem-cell transplantation or by prolonged maintenance for acute myeloid leukemia. *J Clin Oncol.* 2006;**24**:2480–89.

32 Rowe JM, Andersen JW, Mazza JJ, et al. A randomized placebo-controlled phase III study of granulocyte-macrophage colony-stimulating factor in adult patients (>55 to 70 years of age) with acute myelogenous leukemia: a study of the Eastern Cooperative Oncology Group (E1490). *Blood.* 1995;**86**:457–62.

33 Stone RM, Berg DT, George SL, et al. Granulocyte-macrophage colony-stimulating factor after initial chemotherapy for elderly patients with primary acute myelogenous leukemia. *N Engl J Med.* 1995;**332**:1671–77.

34 Dombret H, Chastang C, Fenaux P, et al. A controlled study of recombinant human granulocyte colony-stimulating factor in elderly patients after treatment for acute myelogenous leukemia. *N Engl J Med.* 1995;**332**:1678–83.

35 Schiffer C. Hematopoietic growth factors as adjuncts to the treatment of acute myeloid leukemia. *Blood.* 1996;**88**:3675–85.

36 Witz F, Sadoun A, Perrin MC, et al. A placebo-controlled study of recombinant human granulocyte-macrophage colony-stimulating factor administered during and after induction treatment for de novo acute myelogenous leukemia in elderly patients. *Blood.* 1998;**91**:2722–30.

37 Lowenberg B, Suciu S, Archimbaud E, et al. Use of recombinant granulocyte-macrophage colony-stimulating factor during and after remission induction chemotherapy in patients aged 61 years and older with acute myeloid leukemia (AML): final report of AML-11, a phase III randomized study of the Leukemia Cooperative Group of European Organization for the Research and Treatment of Cancer (EORTC-LCG) and the Dutch Belgian Hemato-Oncology Cooperative Group (HOVON). *Blood.* 1997;**90**:2952–61.

38 Zittoun R, Suciu S, Mandelli F, et al. Granulocyte-macrophage colony-stimulating factor associated with induction treatment of acute myelogenous leukemia: a randomized trial by the European Organization for Research and Treatment of Cancer Leukemia Cooperative Group. *J Clin Oncol.* 1996;**14**:2150–59.

39 Rowe JM, Neuberg D, Friedenberg W, et al. A phase 3 study of three induction regimens and of priming with GM-CSF in older adults with myeloid leukemia: a trial by the Eastern Cooperative Oncology Group. *Blood.* 2004;**103**:479–85.

40 Lowenberg B, Van Putten, W, Theobald M, et al. Effect of priming with granulocyte colony-stimulating factor on the outcome of chemotherapy for acute myeloid leukemia. *N Engl J Med.* 2003;**349**:743–52.

41 Amadori S, Suciu S, Jehn U, et al. Use of glycosylated recombinant human G-CSF (lenograstim) during and/or after induction chemotherapy in patients 61 years of age and older with acute myeloid leukemia: final results of AML-13, a randomized phase-3 study. *Blood.* 2005;**106**:27–34.

42 Smith TJ, Khatcheressian J, Lyman GH, et al. 2006 update of recommendations for the use of white blood cell growth factors: an evidence-based clinical practice guideline. *J Clin Oncol.* 2006;**24**:3187–205.

43 Godwin JE, Kopecky KJ, Head DR, et al. A double-blind placebo-controlled trail of granulocyte colony-stimulating factor in elderly patients with previously untreated acute myeloid leukemia: a Southwest Oncology Group Study (9031). *Blood.* 1998;**91**:3607–15.

44 Heil G, Hoelzer D, Sanz MA, et al. A randomized, double-blind, placebo-controlled, phase III study of filgrastim in remission induction and consolidation therapy for adults with de novo acute myeloid leukemia. *Blood.* 1997;**90**:4710–18.

45 Harrousseau JL, Witz B, Lioure B, et al. Granulocyte colony-stimulating factor after intensive consolidation chemotherapy in acute myeloid leukemia: results of a randomized trial of the Groupe Ouest-Est Leucemies Aigues Myeloblastiques. *J Clin Oncol.* 2000;**18**:780–87.

34 Acute Myeloid Leukemia in Adults

Postremission Therapy

Cara A. Rosenbaum, Richard A. Larson

Introduction

Additional treatment after successful remission induction is mandatory to cure acute myeloid leukemia (AML). The median disease-free interval for patients who receive no additional therapy is approximately four months. When several courses of consolidation chemotherapy are given, by repeating treatment that is of similar intensity to that used in induction for one or more cycles, survival at four years is about 40% for young and middle-aged adults. High-dose cytarabine (HiDAC) provides the best survival for good and intermediate-risk patients. Maintenance therapy with relatively nonmyelosuppressive doses of cytotoxic drugs appears to have limited benefit. Many studies evaluating allogeneic or autologous hematopoietic cell transplantation (HCT) for AML patients in first complete remission (CR1) are nonrandomized, and many are retrospective. Considerable selection bias is generated by the delay between remission induction and transplantation and by the entry requirement for good performance status for most trials. Prospective, randomized controlled trials (RCTs) comparing HCT with intensive consolidation chemotherapy have failed to show a clear survival advantage (Table 34.1).

Questions

1. What role does intensified chemotherapy play in consolidation?
2. What is the role of allogeneic HCT in first complete remission (CR1)?
3. How does autologous HCT compare with chemotherapy as a strategy to consolidate first remissions?
4. Is there a role for maintenance chemotherapy in the treatment of AML?

Evidence-based Hematology. Edited by Mark A. Crowther, Jeff Ginsberg, Holger J. Schünemann, Ralph M. Meyer, and Richard Lottenberg.

Literature-search strategy and inclusions

As described in chapter 33, searches were conducted of PubMed and MEDLINE databases from March 1, 1979, to October 10, 2006, and the 2006 Cochrane Library. A list of Web-based sites where further information and guidelines can be readily accessed is shown in Table 33.3 of chapter 33.

Grading of the quality of evidence and strengths of recommendations in this chapter are based on the guidelines proposed by the international Grading of Recommendations Assessment, Development, and Evaluation Working Group (GRADE) adopting the modification used by the American College of Chest Physicians that merges the very low and low categories of quality of evidence (see chapter 1).

What role does intensified chemotherapy play in consolidation?

Consolidation therapy has been shown to result in significantly longer survival compared with maintenance therapy alone, with survival at two to three years, ranging between 35% and 50% in adults less than 60 years. In the Eastern Cooperative Oncology Group (ECOG) trial reported by Cassileth et al., all patients in CR1 who lacked a donor for allogeneic HCT (alloHCT) were randomized to receive either a single consolidation course with HiDAC or two years of continuous maintenance therapy (1). Event-free and overall (OS) survivals were superior following either HiDAC or alloHCT compared to maintenance therapy alone.

In the 1980s, RCTs comparing multiple courses of HiDAC consolidation to standard or intermediate-dose cytarabine were conducted to determine whether intensified postremission therapy prolonged survival (2,3). A landmark study (CALGB 8525), enrolled 1,088 adults who received a standard 7+3 induction regimen (3); 596 CR1 patients were then randomized to four courses of cytarabine at either standard or intermediate doses (100 mg/m^2/d or 400 mg/m^2/d, respectively) for five days by continuous infusion or 3 g/m^2 by three-hour infusion every 12 hours on days 1, 3, and 5. In patients 60 years or less, there was a highly significant difference in disease-free survival (DFS): 44% at four years in the HiDAC group compared with 29% and 24% in the intermediate and standard-dose groups, respectively; OS was also significantly different: 52% at 4 years versus 40% and 35% in the HiDAC, intermediate, and standard-dose groups, respectively. Treatment-related mortality was 5% and 6% in the HiDAC and intermediate-dose groups, respectively, compared with 1% in the standard-dose group. Survival rates for patients 60 years or less who received HiDAC in this study were comparable to those reported with alloHCT in CR1. Importantly, only 29% of patients over 60 years could tolerate four courses of HiDAC, in part due to neurotoxicity. The DFS at four years in this age group was 16% or less in all three cytarabine-dose groups. In a follow-up CALGB RCT, sequential consolidation courses of two-drug chemotherapy regimens, consisting of one course of HiDAC followed by etoposide plus cyclophosphamide and a third course of diaziquone plus mitoxantrone demonstrated equivalent DFS and OS rates compared with three courses of HiDAC given alone for patients 60 years or less (4).

The question of whether sequential HiDAC courses given in both induction and consolidation improved outcomes compared with HiDAC administered only in induction was examined by the Australasian Leukaemia and Lymphoma Group (5). All patients received ICE (idarubicin, HiDAC, and etoposide) for induction, and patients achieving CR were randomized to receive either a second cycle of ICE postremission or a similar regimen containing standard-dose cytarabine. No differences were seen between the two arms in terms of treatment-related mortality or relapse-free survival (RFS). The authors concluded that further HiDAC therapy given during consolidation after HiDAC administered in induction does not improve survival.

A number of RCTs have shown a survival advantage from intensive postremission chemotherapy with HiDAC among specific subgroups. In the CALGB 8525 study, 285 patients with centrally reviewed karyotypes were randomized to receive postremission therapy with high, intermediate, or standard-dose cytarabine (6). Patients were categorized to 1 of 3 cytogenetic groups: core binding factor (CBF) karyotypes [t(8;21), inv(16), or t(16;16)]; normal karyotype; or other abnormal karyotype. The five-year continuous complete remission (CCR) rate was 50%, 32%, and 15% among the three cytogenetic risk groups, respectively. The impact of cytarabine dose on CCR at five years was most marked in the CBF group (78%, 57%, and 16% in patients receiving 3 g/m^2, 400 mg/m^2, and 100 mg/m^2, respectively). Patients with a normal karyotype had the next greatest impact seen from cytarabine dose on CCR at five years (40%, 37%, and 20%, respectively). No effect of cytarabine dose was found in patients with other cytogenetic abnormalities.

Further studies have evaluated the optimal number of HiDAC consolidation courses for patients with CBF AML (7,8). A retrospective CALGB study of 50 patients with t(8;21) (q22;q22) who received either a single course of HiDAC (plus additional consolidation therapy) or $\geq$3 cycles of HiDAC reported that outcomes, including OS were all significantly inferior in patients receiving a single HiDAC course compared with multiple courses (7). Similar findings were seen in a study of 48 patients with either inv(16) or t(16;16) karyotypes (8). The cumulative incidence of relapse (CIR) was significantly lower (43% vs. 70% at five years) and RFS was significantly higher in patients receiving multiple HiDAC courses. However, OS at five years did not differ, in part due to the successful use of HCT to rescue patients with relapsed inv(16) AML.

A meta-analysis performed in adults with CBF AML [t(8;21 and inv(16)] treated with various postremission therapies in eight prospective German AML Intergroup trials, however, did not confirm the above findings of the CALGB studies (9). Among both CBF AML subtypes, no impact of the total dose of cytarabine on RFS was found by intention-to-treat analysis. Among patients with t(8;21) AML, no difference was seen between those receiving intensive chemotherapy with HiDAC or autologous HCT (autoHCT) in postremission. There were also no differences seen among patients with inv(16) receiving chemotherapy, autoHCT, or alloHCT.

Recommendations

1. Overall, evidence exists demonstrating that patients with favorable or normal cytogenetics derive more benefit from intensive consolidation chemotherapy with one or more courses of HiDAC compared with standard consolidation regimens. However, the heterogeneity in findings between intergroup studies leads to only a weak recommendation (Grade 2A).

2. Neither HiDAC nor other postremission chemotherapy regimens have been shown to benefit patients with unfavorable karyotypes (Grade 1A).

What is the role of allogeneic HCT in CR1?

Allogeneic transplantation emerged as a treatment option for postremission therapy in the early 1980s but was restricted to patients 45 years or less with an HLAidentical sibling (10). Many considered alloHCT the preferred consolidation modality for younger patients in CR1, yielding fewer relapses compared to chemotherapy alone and DFS rates of 45%–65% (11–13). AutoHCT was implemented in the 1980s as an alternative myeloablative option for patients without an HLA identical donor (14). After two decades, controversy still remains regarding the overall best postremission therapy even though many prospective trials have compared the three postremission modalities: intensive chemotherapy, autoHCT, and alloHCT (Table 34.1). A lack of consensus derives partly from the fact that the benefits of each modality as well as their toxicities vary greatly by cytogenetic risk group and age.

Major difficulties exist in comparing data between prospective postremission therapy trials, which have led to contradictory results of trials that might otherwise appear to be of similar design. Factors contributing to these contradictions include different induction, consolidation, and pretransplant conditioning therapies, varying remission durations before HCT, lack of cytogenetic data, low proportion of patients who actually receive the intended HCT

Table 34.1 Comparison of patient characteristics and treatment outcomes for RCTs evaluating postremission chemotherapy, autologous, and allogeneic HCT in adults with AML in first remission.[a]

Author (reference) study	Quality of evidence (grade)	No. of patients by treatment regimen[b]	Therapy received by randomization					Median age/(range) at time of therapy	Pretransplant therapies no. of courses		TRM	Med. Follow-up (mo)	Relapse Risk (y)	DFS (y)	Significance level DFS (intention to treat)		OS	Significance level OS (intention to treat)	
			TBI	CY	BU	MEL	Hi-DAC		Induct	Consol[c] (Ara-C dose)					Donor vs. No donor	Auto vs. Chemo		Donor vs. No donor	Auto vs. Chemo
Reiffers (10)	B (low no. of	Total 58											3 y	2.5 y					
BGMT 84,	patients; no	Allo BMT 23	√	√				27.5 (15–42)	1–2	1	20%	32	22%	61%	$p < 0.015$	$p = 0.06$	Not	NS	NS
1989	OS)	Auto BMT[d] 15				√		31.5 (17–47)		SDAC	5%		59%	41%	(actually	(actually	stated		
		Chemo 20					√[e]	36.5 (15–50)			5%		82%	16%	treated)	treated)			
Reiffers (18)	A	Total 113											3 y	3 y			3 y		
BGMT 87,		Allo BMT 36	√	√	√[g]			32 (15–45)	1–2	1	11%	Not	24%	67%	$p < 0.05$[i]	NS	65%	NS	NS
1996		Auto SCT 39			√	√	√[h]	34 (15–45)[i]		SDAC	5%	stated	45%	51%			56%		
		Chemo[f] 38					√[h]				0%		58%	42%			55%		
Zittoun (17)	A	Total 422											4 y	4 y			4 y		
GIMEMA/		Allo BMT 168	√	√	√[g]			(11–45)	1–2	1	17%	Not	24%	55%	Significant	$p = 0.05$	59%	NS	NS
EORTC, 1995		Auto BMT 128	√	√	√[g]			(11–59)		IDAC	9%	stated	41%	48%	(p value not		56%		
		Chemo 126					√	(11–59)			7%		57%	30%	stated)		46%		
Harousseau	A	Total 252											4 y	4 y			4 y		
(16) GOELAM,		Allo BMT 88	√	√	√[g]			(15–40)	1–2	1[j]	22%	62	37%	44%	NS	NS	53%	NS	NS
1997		Auto BMT 86		√	√		√	(15–50)		HiDAC	7%		Not	44%			50%		
		Chemo 78					√	(15–50)			3%		stated	40%			55%		
Cassileth (11)	A	Total 346											4 y	4 y			4 y		
ECOG CALGB/		Allo BMT 113		√	√			(16–55)	1–2	1	21%	48	29%	43%	NS	NS	46%	NS	$p = 0.05$
SWOG, 1998		Auto BMT 116		√	√			(16–55)		SDAC	14%		48%	35%			43%		(chemo> auto)
		Chemo 117					√	(16–55)			3%		61%	35%			52%		
Burnett(21)	A	Total 1287								2			7 y	7 y			7 y		
MRC AML 10,		Allo BMT 419	√	√				(0–55)	2	(1 SDAC & 1	19%	80	36%	50%	$p = 0.001$	N/A	55%	NS	N/A
2002		Auto BMT /No Rx 868[k]	√	√				(0–55)		IDAC)	9%		52%	42%			50%		

Tsimberidou	B (low no. of	Total 100[l]											3 y[n]			3 y		
(15) 2003	patients)	Allo SCT 21				√[m]	(15–49)	2	1	10%	55	Not	73%	$p = 0.01$[o]	NS	73%	$p = 0.05$[o]	NS
		Auto SCT 19		√	√	√[m]	45 (15–60)		HiDAC	not		stated	42%			58%		
		Chemo 15				√	44 (15–60)			stated			33%			46%		
Suciu (13)	A	Total 734										4 y	4 y			4 y		
EORTC/		Allo SCT 293	√	√	√[g]		35 (15–45)	1–2	1	17%	48	30%	52%	$p = 0.044$	N/A	58%	NS	N/A
GIMEMA, 2003		Auto SCT 441	√	√	√[g]		33 (15–45)		IDAC	5%		53%	42%			51%		

[a] Allo/AutoBMT/SCT, allogeneic/autologous bone marrow/stem cell transplant; SDAC/IDAC/HiDAC, standard/intermediate/high-dose Ara-C; TRM, treatment-related mortality; NS, not significant; DFS, disease-free survival; OS, overall survival; FFS, failure-free survival; SC, subcutaneous; TBI, total body irradiation; CY, cyclophosphamide; BU, busulfan; MEL, melphalan; N/A, not available.

[b] No. of patients and results are reported according to "intention to treat"; actual no. of patients receiving assigned treatment and corresponding DFS/OS (if stated) are as follows for each study (patients treated – total/allo/auto/chemo): Reiffers '89 (52/20/12/20), 2.5 y DFS = 66%/41%/16%; Reiffers '96 (93/33/33/38), 3 y DFS= 73%/51%/42%, 3 y OS = not stated/56%/55%; Zittoun (343/144/95/104); Harrousseau (219/73/75/71), 4 y DFS= 50%/48%/43%, 4 y OS = 55%/52%/59%; Cassileth (261/92/63/106), 4 y DFS = 47%/45%/not stated, 4 y OS = 48%/55%/not stated; Tsimberidou (49/15/19/15), FFS and OS not stated; Suciu (448/202/246/-), 4 y DFS =~62%/~52%.

[c] Consolidation chemotherapy given to all patients unless specified prior to genetic randomization and true randomization of no donor group; standard dose Ara-C equivalent to 50–200 mg/m^2 SQ q12h or continuous infusion for 5–7 days with daunorubicin or idarubicin for 2 days, or amsacrine and etoposide for 5 days; Intermediate dose Ara-C= 500–1,000 mg/m^2 q12h for either 3 or 6 consecutive days with amsacrine, daunorubicin, mitoxantrone, or idarubicin (Ara-C dose reduced in Zittoun study given high incidence of lethal infections); HiDAC = high-dose Ara-C= 3 g/m^2 q12 h days 1 through 4 or for days 1,3, and 5 either alone or with idarubicin or rubidizone.

[d] Tandem autologous BMTs performed.

[e] HiDAC given for one cycle as part of a 4-month intensive sequential chemotherapy (ISC) regimen; VP-16, amsacrine, SDAC, daunorubicin, 6-MP, vincristine, MTX, prednisone, and cranial irradiation given.

[f] 2 y maintenance chemotherapy given with standard dose Ara-C and daunorubicin alternating with 6-MP and MTX after receiving one cycle of HiDAC intensification.

[g] Patients either received a conditioning regimen of CY and TBI or CY and BU.

[h] Both ASCT and maintenance chemotherapy arms received one cycle of HiDAC intensification prior to randomization.

[i] The outcome of the alloBMT arm was compared to that of 60 patients without an HLA identical sibling donor who were randomized to either ASCT or chemotherapy; median age and age range given is for this "no donor" group.

[j] Only patients entering randomization received HiDAC; allogeneic BMT patients received one standard chemotherapy course first.

[k] Analyses provided between donor and no donor arms only; 200 out of 868 patients actually received an autoBMT; other patients initially randomized to receive no further treatment after 4 cycles of induction/consolidation chemotherapy.

[l] Total no. also includes nonrandomized patients with "better prognosis" cytogenetics who received a second course of HiDAC for consolidation and were not included in randomization between ASCT and chemotherapy groups.

[m] Allogeneic and autologous transplant patients received one course of HiDAC in CR before randomization, the conditioning regimen given to alloHCT patients was not reported; autoHCT patients received CY and BU as conditioning; chemotherapy alone group received a second course of HiDAC.

[n] FFS (failure-free survival) is not DFS.

[o] Significant difference seen in the "intermediate" prognosis cytogenetic group only (normal karyotype, +8 or less than 3 numerical abnormalities but not including chromosomes 5 or 7 abnormalities).

or randomized therapy, and analyses performed according to treatment actually given and not by intention-to-treat.

Typically, induction therapies in these trials consisted of one to two cycles of standard-dose cytarabine with an anthracycline; two induction cycles were required in one of the trials (15). Among the chemotherapy arms of the trials, HiDAC was administered for consolidation in various schedules sequenced with a variety of agents or given alone (10,11,15–18). At least one cycle of HiDAC intensification was administered to all patients in both the autoHCT and chemotherapy arms in three of the trials (15,16,18). In the BGMT-87 trial, patients randomized to the chemotherapy arm received two years of maintenance therapy following a single course of HiDAC consolidation (18). The conditioning regimens used for autoHCT also differed and number of autoHCTs performed varied. For example, in the BGMT-84 trial, patients randomized to the autoHCT arm received tandem transplants, while most other trials administered a single autoHCT (10). AlloHCT conditioning regimens were fairly similar among trials, with patients receiving either total body irradiation or busulfan-based therapies.

Comparing survival rates among trials is also problematic because of the varied remission duration lengths prior to randomization. An inherent selection bias is introduced in many trials due to the delay between achieving CR1 and the date of HCT. The initial date used for determining OS differs between studies. In the BGMT-84 and -87 trials, the date of initial diagnosis was used (10,18), while in the GOELAM-97 trial, the HLA-typing date was used (16). OS was calculated based on CR date in the ECOG 1998 and GIMEMA-EORTC 1995 trials (11,17).

In a recent Cochrane meta-analysis, the respective roles of intensive chemotherapy, autoHCT, and alloHCT as postremission modalities were compared among the trials outlined above along with other major prospective trials (19). The potential benefit from alloHCT was considered in light of biologic randomization by "donor versus no donor" analyses, with the no donor subgroup composed of both autoHCT and chemotherapy arms. The authors concluded that for the average patient in CR1 insufficient evidence currently exists to make strong recommendations regarding optimal postremission therapy as most trials did not include pretreatment cytogenetic stratification, and compliance with HCT was low such that only half of patients actually received their allocated HCT.

The meta-analysis demonstrated a significantly decreased risk of relapse with alloHCT (27%) compared with autoHCT (46%) and intensive chemotherapy (62%). Donor versus no donor comparison yielded consistent results for risk of relapse (34% vs. 54%, respectively). Fewer relapses were also observed with autoHCT compared with chemotherapy alone (41% vs. 54%, respectively). However, treatment-related mortality was eight times higher with alloHCT compared with chemotherapy (22% vs. 4%, respectively), and three times higher with autoHCT compared with chemotherapy (11% vs. 4%, respectively). These differences translated into improved DFS and OS at two years following alloHCT due to fewer relapses and deaths, but at five years, this benefit was lost due to the high-transplantation-related mortality. Similarly, donor versus no donor analyses performed at two years demonstrated DFS and OS advantages with alloHCT compared with autoHCT or chemotherapy, but this advantage disappeared in the five-year analyses. Comparison between HCT modalities revealed no difference in DFS rates between alloHCT and autoHCT at any time point but higher DFS rates at two years for both alloHCT and autoHCT compared with chemotherapy alone. However, this advantage did not remain at five years with either HCT modality.

Only two studies included in the meta-analysis compared postremission therapies among subgroups stratified by cytogenetic risk, but no conclusions were drawn as these studies could not be pooled (20-21). In an RCT conducted by SWOG/ECOG, superior OS rates were observed among patients with favorable karyotypes receiving alloHCT or autoHCT compared with patients receiving chemotherapy alone, although outcomes in the latter group were unexpectedly poor (20). Patients with unfavorable karyotypes derived the most benefit from alloHCT. In the MRC AML-10 trial, only the standard-risk group with normal karyotypes and less than 15% blasts in the marrow after one induction course demonstrated a DFS and OS advantage with alloHCT (21). In a German study, patients considered standard-risk with normal karyotypes and a rapid early response to induction (<5% blasts in the day 15 bone marrow) underwent alloHCT if an HLA matched sibling was available; otherwise, they were randomized to receive HiDAC or an autoHCT (22). No significant OS difference was seen in a donor versus no donor comparison although the donor group demonstrated higher RFS rates (56% vs. 36%; $p =$ NS).

The BGMT analyzed data from four RCTs with over 1,000 patients to determine the impact of early alloHCT in CR1 with regard to cytogenetic classification and other prognostic factors (23). No survival differences were found comparing donor versus no donor groups as a whole. Three subpopulations emerged, however, when survival outcomes were analyzed based on karyotype, FAB subtype, number of induction courses needed to achieve CR1, and initial white blood cell count. Among low-, intermediate-, and high-risk cytogenetic subgroups, an OS advantage with alloHCT was found in the intermediate-risk group, composed mostly of patients with normal karyotypes or other cytogenetic features not falling within a favorable or unfavorable cytogenetic risk group. For low- and high-risk cytogenetic groups, patient numbers were limited and no advantage with alloHCT in CR1 was found.

A meta-analysis of five studies comprising 3,100 patients sought to further determine the efficacy of alloHCT in CR1 among cytogenetic risk groups (24). All risk groups combined, alloHCT yielded an equivalent OS benefit to that reported in the Cochrane meta-analysis, although the effect of alloHCT was found to differ depending on cytogenetic stratification, similar to the BGMT report. The overall benefit of alloHCT was greatest in the poor-risk group, while no benefit was detected for the favorable-risk group. Evaluation of the intermediate cytogenetic risk group suggested that the beneficial effect of alloHCT demonstrated for the whole population also applied to this specific subgroup. One limitation of this meta-analysis is that definitions of cytogenetic risk were not uniform across studies with several inconsistencies existing within the intermediate and poor-risk cytogenetic categories. A further consideration pertaining to all studies is that 25%–35% of patients across all cytogenetic risk groups have a high-risk molecular mutation with an internal tandem duplication within the *FLT3* gene; the role of HCT in this subgroup is undefined at present (25,26).

Recommendations

1. Strong evidence exists supporting the use of alloHCT in CR1 using an HLA-matched sibling donor for patients with unfavorable cytogenetics and high-risk features (Grade 1A).

2. There is less evidence to support the use of alloHCT in CR1 for patients with favorable or intermediate-risk karyotypes (Grade 2B).

How does autologous HCT compare with chemotherapy as a strategy to consolidate first remissions?

The role of autoHCT as consolidation therapy in CR1 has been examined across different risk groups in many of the studies described above as well as in prospective RCTs comparing autoHCT to chemotherapy alone or versus no further therapy (Table 34.1). Five of the previously described RCTs report the outcomes of patients who lacked an HLA matched sibling donor and were thus randomized to receive an autoHCT versus chemotherapy alone (10,11,16–18). For OS, one trial reported a trend favoring autoHCT (17), while two trials reported trends favoring chemotherapy alone (11,16). Three of the five trials also reported trends in DFS favoring autoHCT over chemotherapy (10,17–18).

In two RCTs, autoHCT following consolidation therapy was compared with no further therapy (27–28). In the MRC AML-10 trial, four courses of standard and intermediate-dose cytarabine were given for consolidation, and patients who lacked an HLA matched sibling donor were further randomized to autoHCT or no further therapy (27); the relapse rate was significantly lower in the autoHCT arm (37% vs. 58%, respectively), resulting in superior DFS at seven years (53% vs. 40%). However, no difference in OS was detected at seven years (57% vs. 45%) due in part to the transplant-related mortality. The authors concluded that autoHCT following consolidation chemotherapy in CR1 leads to improved DFS in all age and risk groups evaluated. In good-risk patients, however, autoHCT may be reserved until CR2 given its success as a salvage therapy. A HOVON/SAKK trial also assessed whether autoHCT following consolidation improved survival in CR1 (28). Following three courses of intensive chemotherapy with standard and intermediate-dose cytarabine, patients were randomized to autoHCT or no further treatment. No differences in relapse rate or DFS were observed between the two treatment arms, although a trend toward improved OS was observed in the no treatment arm due to fewer deaths compared to the transplant-related mortalities.

The question of whether autoHCT in CR1 offers a survival advantage to patients without an HLA matched sibling donor compared chemotherapy alone or no further therapy was also the subject of two meta-analyses (29-30). Nathan et al. performed a meta-analysis of six RCTs (29); while DFS at four years was significantly higher in patients receiving autoHCT, no difference in OS was seen due to higher treatment-related mortality rates. Thus, they concluded that routine use of autoHCT over chemotherapy in CR1 should not be recommended, and, instead, this option should be reserved patients in CR2. In contrast, a meta-analysis by Levi et al. analyzed death and relapse rates from the identical six trials but concluded that autoHCT should be offered to every patient in CR1 without an HLA matched related donor (30), based on the lower event rate and superior DFS.

Several RCTs have evaluated the role of auto HCT among prognostic subgroups. Based on the MRC AML-10 trial, Burnett et al. recommended delaying autoHCT in favorable risk patients until CR2 (27). In a German trial, patients with CBF or normal karyotypes without an HLA matched sibling and with good response to induction therapy (<5% blasts in a day 15 bone marrow) were randomized to HiDAC or autoHCT for consolidation (22). No survival differences (59% and 62%, respectively, at 63 months) were detected, but autoHCT was recommended because of lower rates of treatment-related toxicity. The CALGB compared outcomes in cytogenetically normal patients who received either HiDAC or autoHCT for consolidation (31). Over a series of studies, patients had received either one cycle of HiDAC followed by sequential courses of two-drug chemotherapy regimens, three cycles of HiDAC, four cycles of intermediate-dose cytarabine (IDAC) or HiDAC, or high-dose chemotherapy followed by autoHCT. Patients who received either four cycles of IDAC/HiDAC or autoHCT had improved DFS and less relapses compared with patients receiving three or fewer cycles of HiDAC with additional non-cross-resistant chemotherapy agents.

The value of intensive consolidation chemotherapy before HCT in CR1 was examined retrospectively in the International Bone Marrow Transplant Registry (32,33). Among 431 patients receiving alloHCT in CR1, no survival benefit was observed with prior administration of standard or high-dose cytarabine compared with proceeding directly to HCT (32). In the setting of autoHCT, the registry data suggested that DFS and OS rates at five years were significantly higher in patients who received one to two cycles of standard or high-dose cytarabine prior to autoHCT, with similar outcomes seen between patients receiving either standard or high doses (33).

Recommendations

1. The role of autoHCT as a therapeutic modality in CR1 remains controversial and may better serve as a salvage therapy after relapse (Grade 2B).

2. Given the additional graft-versus-leukemia effect associated with alloHCT, additional postremission consolidation chemotherapy (to provide a leukemia-free graft) appears to be more important if patients are to undergo autoHCT rather than an alloHCT (Grade 1C).

Is there a role for maintenance chemotherapy in the treatment of AML?

Extended maintenance chemotherapy as postremission therapy in AML has been studied prospectively since the early 1960s. Conflicting data have arisen from these trials, and the value of maintenance therapy in prolonging disease-free survival remains unclear. An early trial conducted by the German AMLCG demonstrated that monthly maintenance therapy in CR1 was associated with a significantly higher CCR rate at 30 months compared with standard-dose consolidation therapy without maintenance (34). A SWOG study also showed a significantly prolonged DFS, but not OS, among patients without a donor who were randomized to receive late intensification plus monthly maintenance therapy versus late intensification alone (35). In contrast, one study failed to show a difference in remission duration or relapse rate between groups randomized to receive monthly maintenance versus no further therapy following consolidation with intermediate-dose cytarabine (36). The Japan Adult Leukemia Study Group AML-97 study likewise found no difference in DFS or OS between patients receiving three courses of standard-dose consolidation plus six maintenance courses compared to those receiving four courses of standard-dose consolidation therapy without maintenance (37).

The optimal duration of maintenance therapy has also been studied prospectively with contradictory findings. A small RCT, which examined a short (6 months) versus long (15 months) duration of maintenance therapy, failed to show a survival difference between the two arms (38). In contrast, the Japanese AML-87 study randomized patients to 4 or 12 maintenance courses and demonstrated significantly prolonged DFS in patients receiving the longer maintenance course (39).

Whether maintenance therapy after intensified induction offers improved outcomes compared with HiDAC given sequentially both for induction and consolidation was examined prospectively by the German AMLCG (40); RFS was superior in poor-risk patients ($p = 0.006$) but not in good-risk patients who received monthly maintenance therapy following intensified induction compared with patients who received sequential HiDAC for induction and consolidation without maintenance. In another RCT conducted by the German AMLCG, 840 patients less than 60 years of age were allocated, before receiving any therapy, to receive prolonged maintenance therapy or myeloablative therapy followed by autoHCT after receiving single versus double HiDAC induction courses (41). Only 51% of those assigned to maintenance therapy and 24% of those assigned to autoHST received their assigned therapy; no differences in outcomes observed. Thus, overall, benefits have not been detected with additional maintenance therapy in patients who receive intensified postinduction treatment.

Recommendation

Maintenance therapy cannot be recommended unless patients are unable to tolerate more intensive postremission therapy (Grade 1A).

References

1 Cassileth PA, Lynch E, Hines JD, et al. Varying intensity of postremission therapy in acute myeloid leukemia. *Blood.* 1992;**79**:1924–30.

2 Jehn U, Zittoun R, Suciu S, et al. A randomized comparison of intensive maintenance treatment for adult acute myelogenous leukemia using either cyclic alternating drugs or repeated courses of the induction-type chemotherapy: AML-6 trial of the EORTC Leukemia Cooperative Group. *Haematol Blood Transfus.* 1990;**33**:277–84.

3 Mayer RJ, Davis RB, Schiffer CA, et al. Intensive postremission chemotherapy in adults with acute myeloid leukemia. Cancer and Leukemia Group B. *N Engl J Med.* 1994;**331**:896–903.

4 Moore JO, George SL, Dodge RK, et al. Sequential multiagent chemotherapy is not superior to high-dose cytarabine alone as postremission intensification therapy for acute myeloid leukemia in adults under 60 years of age: Cancer and Leukemia Group B Study 9222. *Blood.* 2005;**105**:3420–27.

5 Bradstock KF, Matthews JP, Lowenthal RM, et al. A randomized trial of high-versus conventional-dose cytarabine in consolidation chemotherapy for adult de novo acute myeloid leukemia in first remission after induction therapy containing high-dose cytarabine. *Blood.* 2005;**105**:481–88.

6 Bloomfield CD, Lawrence D, Byrd JC, et al. Frequency of prolonged remission duration after high-dose cytarabine intensification in acute myeloid leukemia varies by cytogenetic subtype. *Cancer Res.* 1998;**58**:4173–79.

7 Byrd JC, Dodge RK, Carroll A, et al. Patients with t(8;21)(q22;q22) and acute myeloid leukemia have superior failure-free and overall survival when repetitive cycles of high-dose cytarabine are administered. *J Clin Oncol.* 1999;**17**:3767–75.

8 Byrd JC, Ruppert AS, Mrozek K, et al. Repetitive cycles of high-dose cytarabine benefit patients with acute myeloid leukemia and inv(16)(p13q22) or t(16;16)(p13;q22): results from CALGB 8461. *J Clin Oncol.* 2004;**22**:1087–94.

9 Schlenk RF, Benner A, Krauter J, et al. Individual patient data-based meta-analysis of patients aged 16–60 years with core binding factor acute myeloid leukemia: a survey of the German Acute Myeloid Leukemia Intergroup. *J Clin Oncol.* 2004;**22**:3741–50.

10 Reiffers J, Gaspard MH, Maraninchi D, et al. Comparison of allogeneic or autologous bone marrow transplantation and chemotherapy in patients with acute myeloid leukemia in first remission: a prospective controlled trial. *Br J Haematol.* 1989;**72**:57–63.

11 Cassileth P, Harrington D, Appelbaum F, et al. Chemotherapy compared with autologous or allogeneic bone marrow transplantation in the management of acute myeloid leukemia in first remission. *N Engl J Med.* 1998;**339**:1649–56.

12 Keating S, de Witte T, Suciu S, et al. The influence of the HLA-matched sibling donor availability on treatment outcome for patients with AML: an analysis of the AML 8A study of the EORTC Leukaemia Cooperative Group and GIMEMA. *Br J Haematol.* 1998;**102**:1344–53.

13 Suciu S, Mandelli F, de Witte T, et al. Allogeneic compared with autologous stem cell transplantation in the treatment of patients younger than 46 years with acute myeloid leukemia (AML) in first complete remission (CR1): an intention-to-treat analysis of the EORTC/GIMEMA AML-10 trial. *Blood.* 2003;**102**:1232–40.

14 Breems DA, Lowenberg B. Autologous stem cell transplantation in the treatment of adults with acute myeloid leukaemia. *Br J Hematol.* 2005;**130**:825–33.

15 Tsimberidou AM, Stavroyianni N, Viniou N, et al. Comparison of allogeneic stem cell transplantation, high-dose cytarabine, and autologous peripheral stem cell transplantation as postremission treatment in patients with de novo acute myelogenous leukemia. *Cancer.* 2003;**97**:1721–31.

16 Harousseau JL, Cahn Jy, Pignon B, et al. Comparison of autologous bone marrow transplantation and intensive chemotherapy as postremission therapy in adult acute myeloid leukemia. *Blood.* 1997;**90**:2978–86.

17 Zittoun R, Mandelli F, Willemze R, et al. Autologous or allogeneic bone marrow transplantation compared with intensive chemotherapy in acute myelogenous leukemia. *N Engl J Med.* 1995;**332**:217–23.

18 Reiffers J, Stoppa AM, Attal M, et al. Allogeneic vs autologous stem cell transplantation vs chemotherapy in patients with acute myeloid leukemia in first remission: the BGMT 87 study. *Leukemia.* 1996;**10**:1874–82.

19 Bellido M, Tobias A, Brunet S, et al. Bone marrow and peripheral blood stem cell transplantation in adult patients in first remission. *Cochrane Database Syst Rev.* 2006;**2**.

20 Slovak ML, Kopecky KJ, Cassileth PA, et al. Karyotypic analysis predicts outcome of preremission and postremission therapy in adult acute myeloid leukemia: a Southwest Oncology Group/Eastern Cooperative Oncology Group Study. *Blood.* 2000;**96**:4075–83.

21 Burnett AK, Wheatley K, Goldstone AH, et al. The value of allogenic bone marrow transplant in patients with acute myeloid leukaemia at differing risk of relapse: results of the UK MRC AML 10 trial. *Br J Haematol.* 2002;**118**:385–400.

22 Ganser A, Krauter J, Hoelzer D, et al. Late consolidation for patients with standard risk AML up to 60 years: results of a prospective randomized comparison of high dose AraC and autologous PBSCT [abstract]. *Blood.* 2004;**104**:145.

23 Jourdan E, Boiron JM, Dastugue N, et al. Early allogeneic stem-cell transplantation for young adults with acute myeloblastic leukemia in first complete remission: an intent-to-treat long-term analysis of the BGMT experience. *J Clin Oncol.* 2005;**23**:7676–84.

24 Yanada M, Matsuo K, Emi N, et al. Efficacy of allogeneic hematopoietic stem cell transplantation depends on cytogenetic risk for acute myeloid leukemia in first disease remission. *Cancer.* 2005;**103**:1652–58.

25 Kottaridis PD, Gale RE, Frew ME, et al. The presence of a FLT3 internal tandem duplication in patients with acute myeloid leukemia (AML) adds important prognostic information to cytogenetic risk group and response to the first cycle of chemotherapy; analysis of 854 patients from the United Kingdom Medical Research Council AML 10 and 12 trials. *Blood.* 2001;**98**:1752–59.

26 Gale RE, Hills R, Kottaridis PD, et al. No evidence that FLT3 status should be considered as an indicator for transplantation in acute myeloid leukemia (AML): an analysis of 1135 patients, excluding acute promyelocytic leukemia, from the UK MRC AML 10 and 12 trials. *Blood.* 2005;**106**:3658–65.

27 Burnett AK, Goldstone AH, Stevens RM, et al. Randomised comparison of addition of autologous bone-marrow transplantation to intensive chemotherapy for acute myeloid leukemia in first remission: results of MRC AML 10 trial. *Lancet.* 1998;**351**:700–708.

28 Breems DA, Boogaerts MA, Dekker AW, et al. Autologous bone marrow transplantation as consolidation therapy in the treatment of adult patients under 60 years with acute myeloid leukemia in first complete remission: a prospective randomized Dutch-Belgian Haemato-Oncology Co-operative Group (HOVON) and Swiss Group for Clinical Cancer Research (SAKK) trial. *Br J Hematol.* 2004;**128**:59–65.

29 Nathan PC, Sung L, Crump M, et al. Consolidation therapy with autologous bone marrow transplantation in adults with acute myeloid leukemia: a meta-analysis. *J Natl Cancer Inst.* 2004;**96**:38–45.

30 Levi I, Grotto I, Yerushalmi R, et al. Meta-analysis of autologous bone marrow transplantation versus chemotherapy in adult patients with acute myeloid leukemia in first remission. *Leuk Res.* 2004;**28**:605–12.

31 Farag S, Ruppert A, Mrozek K, et al. Outcome of induction and postremission therapy in younger adults with acute myeloid leukemia with normal karyotype: a Cancer and Leukemia Group B Study. *J Clin Oncol.* 2005;**23**:482–93.

32 Tallman M, Rowlings P, Milone G, et al. Effect of postremission chemotherapy before human leukocyte antigen-identical sibling transplantation for acute myelogenous leukemia in first complete remission. *Blood.* 2000;**96**:1254–58.

33 Tallman MS, Perez WS, Lazarus HM, et al. Pretransplantation consolidation chemotherapy decreases leukemia relapse after autologous blood and bone marrow transplants for acute myelogenous leukemia in first remission. *Biol Blood Bone Marrow Transplantation.* 2006;**12**: 204–16.

34 Buchner T, Urbanitz D, Hiddemann W, et al. Intensified induction and consolidation with or without maintenance chemotherapy for acute myeloid leukemia (AML): two multicenter studies of the German AML Cooperative Group. *J Clin Oncol.* 1985;**3**:1583–89.

35 Hewlett J, Kopecky KJ, Head D, et al. A prospective evaluation of the roles of allogeneic marrow transplantation and low-dose monthly maintenance chemotherapy in the treatment of adult acute myelogenous leukemia (AML): a Southwest Oncology Group study. *Leukemia.* 1995;**9**:562–69.

36 Johnson SA, Prentice AG, Phillips MJ. Treatment of acute myeloid leukaemia with early intensive induction therapy. *Acta Oncol.* 1988;**27**:527–29.

37 Miyawaki S, Sakamaki H, Ohtake S, et al. A randomized, post-remission comparison of four courses of standard-dose consolidation therapy without maintenance therapy versus three courses of standard-dose consolidation with maintenance therapy in adults with acute myeloid leukemia. The Japan Adult Leukemia Study Group AML97 Study. *Cancer.* 2005;**104**:2726–34.

38 Jacobs P, Dubovsky DW, Wood L. In adult acute nonlymphoblastic leukaemia extended maintenance chemotherapy has no benefit. *Am J Hematol.* 1984;**16**:255–65.

39 Ohno R, Kobayashi T, Tanimoto M, et al. Randomized study of individualized induction therapy with or without vincristine, and of maintenance-intensification therapy between 4 or 12 courses in adult

acute myeloid leukemia: AML-87 Study of the Japan Adult Leukemia Study Group. *Cancer.* 1993;**71**:3888–95.

40 Buchner T, Hiddemann W, Berdel WE, et al. 6-thioguanine, cytarabine, and daunorubicin (TAD) and high-dose cytarabine and mitoxantrone (HAM) for induction, TAD for consolidation, and either prolonged maintenance by reduced monthly TAD or TAD-HAM-TAD and one course of intensive consolidation by sequential HAM in adult patients at all ages with de novo acute myeloid leukemia (AML): a randomized trial of the German AML Cooperative Group. *J Clin Oncol.* 2003;**21**:4496–504.

41 Buchner T, Berdel WE, Schoch C, et al. Double induction containing either two courses or one course of high-dose cytarabine plus mitoxantrone and postremission therapy by either autologous stem-cell transplantation or by prolonged maintenance for acute myeloid leukemia. *J Clin Oncol.* 2006;**24**:2480–89.

35 Current Areas of Controversy in the Treatment of Patients With Newly Diagnosed Acute Promyelocytic Leukemia

Martin S. Tallman, Syed A. Abutalib

Introduction

Acute promyelocytic leukemia (APL) was first described as a distinct and uncommon subtype of acute myeloid leukemia (AML) in 1957 (1). Features distinguishing APL from all other subtypes of AML include unusual sensitivity of the leukemia cells to anthracyclines, resulting in a high complete remission (CR) rate with this single agent (2), frequent presentation with leukopenia (3), a life-threatening coagulopathy (2,3), the PML-RAR alpha fusion transcript resulting from the t(15;17) translocation (4,5), and properties of the leukemia cells to differentiate with the vitamin A derivative all-trans retinoic acid (ATRA) [Vesanoid, Roche] (6) and undergo apoptosis with arsenic trioxide (ATO) [Trisenox, Cephalon Oncology] (7). Until the introduction ATRA in the 1990s, APL was treated in the same way as all other subtypes of AML. With conventional cytotoxic chemotherapy (dauorubicin and ara-C), APL was highly fatal, primarily due to a characteristic, early, severe, complex, and life-threatening bleeding disorder (2,3,8). With current practices to combine ATRA with anthracycline-based chemotherapy for induction and consolidation and to administer ATRA alone or with low-dose chemotherapy as maintenance (8) APL has become highly curable (8). Effective treatment strategies for patients with APL have evolved rapidly. After initial phase II trials demonstrated dramatic effectiveness of ATRA as a single agent (9–14), a number of clinical trials compared ATRA to conventional cytotoxic chemotherapy (15–18). These trials showed: (1) although ATRA does not significantly improve the CR rate, the relapse rate is reduced (15–18); (2) combining ATRA with chemotherapy results in a lower relapse rate than when ATRA is given until the achievement of CR and then followed sequentially by chemotherapy consolidation (17); and (3) maintenance ATRA alone or with low-dose chemotherapy, including 6-mercaptopurine and methotrexate, is more effective than no maintenance therapy (16,18). In phase II studies (LPA96 and LPA99), the Spanish cooperative group PETHEMA investigated omitting ara-C from induction and consolidation therapy to exploit the peculiar sensitivity of leukemic promyelocytes to anthracyclines, and reported favorable results with use of idarubicin and ATRA (19,20). Recent studies have explored therapy with single-agent ATO or a combination of ATO and ATRA, with or without chemotherapy (21–23).

Several studies have demonstrated that the most important factor predicting outcome in patients with APL is the white blood cell (WBC) count at initial presentation (24,25). The GIMEMA and PETHEMA cooperative groups classified patients as low, intermediate, and high risk for relapse based on the presenting WBC and platelet counts (26). Older age is another important unfavorable prognostic factor (24). The presence of the FLT3 internal tandem duplication mutation appears to confer an unfavorable prognosis (27–30), although there are conflicting data (31) and presence of the bcr3 (short) isoform of the PML-RAR-alpha fusion transcript may also confer an unfavorable prognosis (32). The identification of important prognostic factors has facilitated testing risk-adapted therapies. Despite excellent outcomes with contemporary strategies, several questions remain in treating newly diagnosed patients.

Questions

1. Is ara-C required in induction and consolidation in patients with newly diagnosed APL?
2. Can newly diagnosed patients with APL be treated with ATRA and ATO?
3. What is the best treatment for patients with high-risk APL?
4. Is maintenance therapy needed for all patients with APL?

Literature search and inclusion

In 1988, ATRA rapidly became incorporated into routine practice following the first major publication reporting its benefit in APL. For this reason, the search conducted in April 2007, included publications from January 1, 1987, to April 20, 2007, from MEDLINE using PubMed. The search terms included "acute promyelocytic

Evidence-based Hematology. Edited by Mark A. Crowther, Jeff Ginsberg, Holger J. Schünemann, Ralph M. Meyer, and Richard Lottenberg.

Table 35.1 *

Group	No. patients	CR (%)	Molecular CR (%)	DFS/EFS (%)	CIR (%)
JALSG (51,52)	283	94	98	69.2	NA
European APL (34)	340	96.5	98	93.3 (ara-C) 77.2 (w/o ara-C)	4.7 (ara-C) 15.9 (w/o ara-C)
GIMEMA (45)	298	94	99	90	5
PETHEMA (20)	426	90	98	81 90 risk-adapted	9.5 3.1
North American Intergroup (16,18)	50	70	NA	74	NA
GAMLCG (46)	51	92	91	88	NA

* CIR, CR, complete remission; DFS/EFS, disease-free survival/event-free survival; GAMLCG, German Acute Myeloid Leukemia Cooperative Group; JALSG, Japanese Adult Leukemia Study Group.

leukemia," "drug therapy," and "therapy," restricted to English language. Limitations included clinical trials, meta-analyses, practice guidelines, randomized controlled trial (RCT), clinical trial phase I, clinical trial phase II, clinical trial phase III, and clinical trial phase IV, comparative study, controlled clinical trial, corrected and republished article, guideline, multicenter study, humans, and cancer; MEDLINE and PubMed Central were imposed. Seventy-seven publications were retrieved. Computerized searches were also performed for abstracts from the annual meetings of the American Society of Hematology (ASH) and the American Society of Clinical Oncology (ASCO) taking place in the past five years. Abstracts were obtained by using the search engines associated with these Web sites and through review of relevant session agendas. The results of important citations are summarized in Table 35.1.

Grading of the quality of evidence and strengths of recommendations in this chapter are based on the guidelines proposed by the international Grading of Recommendations Assessment, Development, and Evaluation Working Group (GRADE) adopting the modification used by the American College of Chest Physicians that merges the very low and low categories of quality of evidence (see chapter 1).

Is ara-C required in induction and/or consolidation in patients with newly diagnosed APL?

Given the unusual sensitivity of leukemic promyelocytes to anthracyclines, it became reasonable to hypothesize that patients with newly diagnosed APL do not need ara-C during induction or consolidation. In the first of three studies, Estey and colleagues retrospectively compared outcomes of a contemporary cohort of patients treated with ATRA and idarubicin, but without ara-C, with a historical control group treated with ara-C combined with either doxorubicin, amsacrine (AMSA), or daunorubicin but without ATRA (33). In comparison with the historical cohort, no difference was observed in the CR rate (77%), but superior one-year disease-free survival of 87% was seen. Phase II studies from two cooperative groups (the Spanish group PETHEMA: LPA99, and the Italian group GIMEMA) have reported that combining ATRA with idarubicin alone (four doses of 12 mg/m^2 each) for induction (without ara-C) may be as effective in inducing CR as the combination of ara-C, ATRA, and an anthracycline (14,19,20). In the PETHEMA study, ara-C was not given in any treatment phase. In the GIMENA study, ara-C was given in consolidation as 1 gm/m^2/d for four days during cycle 1 and ara-C 150 mg/m^2 every eight hours subcutaneously days 1–5 during cycle 3 of consolidation. In the PETHEMA trial, ATRA was given in consolidation, and these investigators suggested that this addition may be beneficial for patients with intermediate and high-risk disease (20). In the LPA99 study, these patients received standard-dose ATRA, 45 mg/m^2/d on days 1–15, in combination with three courses of single-agent consolidation chemotherapy without ara-C. Evaluation of adding ATRA in consolidation was confounded by use of greater total doses of idarubicin in the first and third courses of consolidation, as compared with their previous LPA96 study (19). Nevertheless, these investigators were able to suggest that with these maneuvers the relapse and survival rates may be improved compared with those achieved in the LPA96 trial. Importantly, a beneficial effect on relapse rate appeared to be less in patients with high-risk disease.

In the only RCT testing the omission of ara-C in patients who receive ATRA, the European APL group observed a higher relapse rate among patients treated with ATRA plus daunorubicin without ara-C than among patients treated with ATRA plus daunorubicin and ara-C (daunorubicin cumulative dose, 495 mg/m^2) (34). This study was discontinued prematurely because 22 relapses occurred in the non–ara-C arm, of which three were molecular relapses, compared with only eight relapses, of which one was molecular relapses, in the ara-C arm. The two-year cumulative incidence of

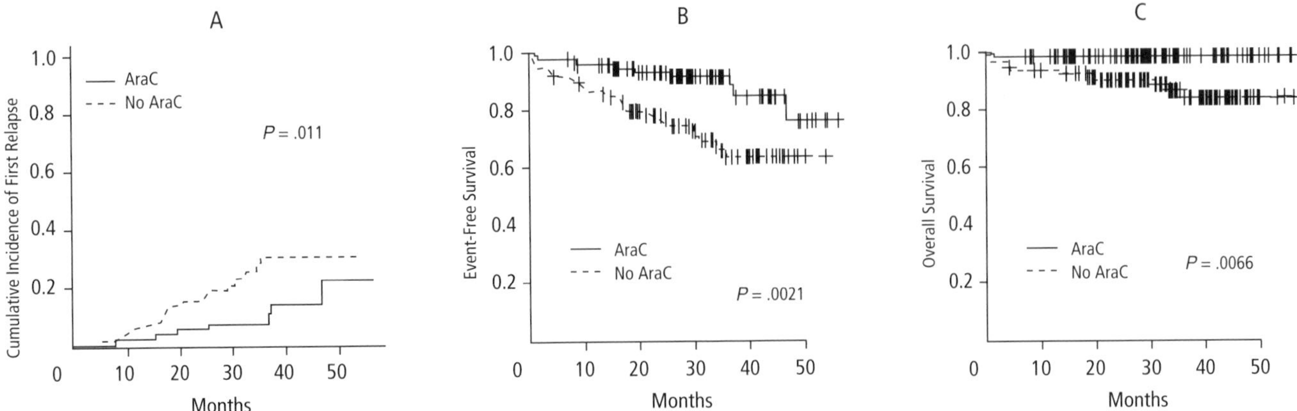

Figure 35.1 Cumulative incidence of (A) relapse, (B) event-free survival, and (C) overall survival of patients randomly assigned to cytarabine (AraC) or no AraC. From (34).

relapse (4.7% vs. 15.9%; $p = 0.001$) and two-year overall survival (97.9% vs. 89.6%; $p = 0.0066$) were both superior in the ara-C group (Figure 35.1). It is not clear whether these results, which differ from those reported by the PETHEMA group, can be explained by differences between idarubicin and daunorubicin, differences in the total cumulative doses of the anthracyclines, or because ATRA was used during consolidation in PETHEMA, but not by European APL Group. Of note is the discordance of these results with those of an RCT carried out during the pre-ATRA era; a GIMENA study demonstrated superior event-free survival with single-agent idarubicin as induction therapy as compared with idarubicin plus ara-C. In this study, no differences in CR rate or overall survival were detected (35).

Recommendations

1. Newly diagnosed patients with APL should be treated with ATRA in combination with either idarubicin or with daunorubicin and ara-C (Grade 1A).

2. At present, evidence suggests that the combination of ATRA and daunorubicin is not as effective as when these agents are administered with ara-C and cannot be recommended as initial therapy, at least in the doses of daunorubicin administered in the RCT testing this question (Grade 1B).

3. Higher-dose daunorubicin plus ATRA for induction may be as effective as when ATRA is given with daunorubicin and ara-C or when ATRA is given with idarubicin alone (Grade 2C). These speculations require confirmation with additional studies.

Can newly diagnosed patients be treated with ATRA and ATO?

Treatment with arsenic trioxide as a single agent in patients with relapsed and refractory APL leads to CR by conventional peripheral blood and bone marrow criteria in the majority of patients (36–42). In a U.S. multicenter trial of 40 patients with relapsed and refractory APL, all of whom had been previously exposed to ATRA, 85% of patients achieved morphologic CR after induction with single-agent ATO (40). Furthermore, of 29 evaluable patients who achieved CR using conventional criteria, 86% achieved molecular CR after induction or consolidation with ATO. These data encouraged the studies of ATO as part of initial induction (21–23,43).

Studies evaluating previously untreated high-risk patients, or those who developed leukocytosis during therapy, have explored the combination of ATO and ATRA with or without an anthracycline or the immunoconjugate gemtuzumab ozogamicin (GO), which is an anti-CD33 humanized monoclonal antibody chemically linked to the potent antibiotic calicheamicin. Investigators at the Shanghai Institute of Hematology evaluated 61 patients with newly diagnosed APL who were randomized to induction therapy with either ATRA as a single agent, ATO as a single agent, or the combination of ATRA (at half the conventional dose to avoid potential synergistic hepatotoxicity) plus ATO (23). All patients subsequently received intensive consolidation chemotherapy and maintenance therapy. Patients randomized to the combination arm achieved complete hematologic remission in a shorter median time period (25.5 days) than did those who received ATRA alone (40.5 days) or ATO alone (31 days). Furthermore, there was a significant reduction in the number of PML-RAR-alpha fusion transcript copies among patients in the combination arm. At a median follow-up of 18 months, no relapses were observed in 20 patients who achieved CR with combination therapy, compared with 7 of 37 patients who received monotherapy. Estey and colleagues treated 44 patients with ATRA and ATO (43). ATO began on day 10; high-risk patients (WBC $\geq$ 10,000 cells/μL) also received either GO or idarubicin. The overall CR rate of all patients was 87%, including 96% among low-risk and 79% among high-risk patients. The median follow-up of the 39 patients alive and in first CR was 16 months and all were molecularly negative at the last follow-up. The relapse-free survival at eight years was 90%.

Recent studies have suggested that single-agent ATO (21–22) is active therapy for some patients with newly diagnosed APL. Investigators in Iran treated patients with only two courses of ATO

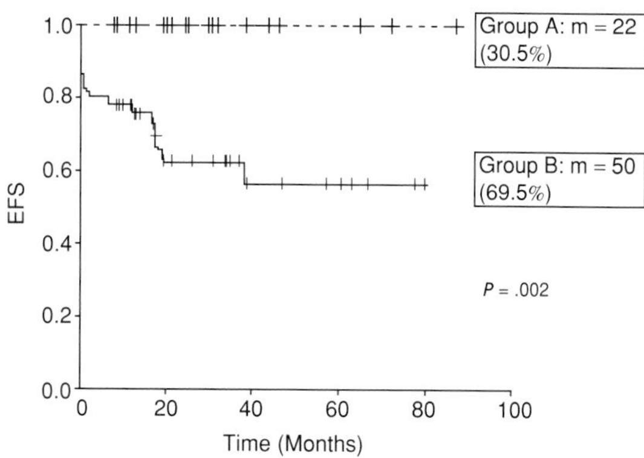

Figure 35.2 Comparison of Kaplan-Meier product limit estimate of event-free survival (EFS) between the good-risk group (group A: WBC count, $<5 \times 10^9$/L; platelet count, $>20 \times 10^9$/L) and the rest (group B).

and observed an 86% CR rate and a 92% molecular remission rate (21). However, a high relapse rate was observed suggesting undertreatment. In a phase II study conducted in India, 72 patients received one course of ATO for induction, one course for consolidation, and up to six courses of ATO (10 days per course) for consolidation (22); the CR rate was 86% and the three-year event-free, disease-free, and overall survival rates were 75%, 87%, and 86%, respectively. The molecular remission rate was 76%. Patients with a WBC count <5,000 cells/μL and a platelet count >20,000/μL had a three-year event-free, disease-free, and overall survival rates of 100%, while the others had rates of 63%, 80%, and 79%, respectively (Figure 35.2).

Although a small RCT suggested that the addition of ATRA to ATO in patients with relapsed and refractory APL does not improve the outcome compared with ATO alone (44) in patients with untreated APL, the combination appears to induce a more rapid CR and a more profound degree of molecular remission, with apparently no added toxicity compared with each agent alone. Among patients with very low-risk disease (WBC <5,000 cells/μL and platelets >20,000/μL), ATO as a single agent may be an effective therapeutic approach.

Recommendation

1. ATRA combined with anthracycline-based chemotherapy for induction and consolidation remains the standard treatment for newly diagnosed patients with APL. However, for patients who cannot be treated with anthracyclines (e.g., older adults, abnormal cardiac function), it is reasonable to consider treatment with a combination of ATRA plus ATO with or without an anthracycline or GO (Grade 1C).

What is the best treatment for patients with high-risk APL?

Treatment of high-risk APL is currently a major focus of research. Even with contemporary strategies, the three-year cumulative incidence of relapse for these patients is approximately 20% (20). Adding increased doses of idarubicin (in the PETHEMA LPA99 trial) and ATRA in consolidation may improve outcomes. More recent data suggest that ara-C or ATO may provide further benefits.

Ara-C has been evaluated in high-risk patients in three nonrandomized studies, with results suggesting a beneficial effect (34,45,46). The GIMEMA group (45) tested a consolidation treatment strategy consisting of ara-C 1 g/m^2/d for four days plus idarubicin for the first cycle; mitoxantrone and etoposide for the second cycle; and idarubicin, ara-C 150 mg/m^2 every eight hours subcutaneously for five days, and 6-thioguanine for the third cycle. Patients also received ATRA in conventional doses for 15 days during each consolidation course. With a median follow-up of two years, the cumulative incidence of relapse in high-risk patients was only 2%. The European APL Group also observed a low relapse rate among patients with a WBC count >10,000 cells/μL who received consolidation with ara-C 1–2 g/m^2 given every 12 hours (34). Two trials have been conducted by the German AML cooperative group. In the first trial, all patients received high-dose ara-C in induction, which resulted in a low relapse rate (46). In the second trial, patients were given ATRA plus idarubicin for induction followed by one cycle of ICE (idarubicin, ara-C, and etoposide) and then two cycles of HAM (high-dose ara-C and mitoxantrone) (47). Among 82 patients, 72 (88%) achieved CR and the relapse-free and overall survivals at 46 months were 83% and 82%, respectively.

The addition of ATO was tested in the recently completed phase III North American Intergroup Protocol C9710 (32,48,49). Patients received conventional ATRA, daunorubicin, and ara-C induction therapy and were then randomized to receive two 25-day courses of ATO followed by two courses of daunorubicin with one week of ATRA or two courses of daunorubicin and ATRA without prior ATO. Among 481 adults, the three-year event-free (77% vs. 59%; $p = 0.0013$) and overall (86% vs. 77%; $p = 0.029$) survivals were superior in patients allocated to ATO (48). The relapse rates at one-year among low- intermediate- and high-risk patients were 2%, 3%, and 7%, respectively (49). These results demonstrate superior outcomes with ATO, but it is important to note that the outcomes of the control arm were inferior to those expected and that results of the ATO arm were similar to those achieved without ATO in other studies. Therefore, it is not yet clear whether the addition of ATO to consolidation therapy should be standard.

Recommendations

1. High-risk patients appear to benefit from increased doses of idarubicin and ATRA in the consolidation phase (Grade 1B).
2. Intermediate or high doses of ara-C in combination with ATRA and idarubicin either in induction or in consolidation are effective therapies for high-risk patients (Grade 2C).
3. ATO in consolidation for all patients, including high-risk patients, is recommended (Grade 2A).

4. Gemtuzumab ozogamicin is effective when combined with ATRA, but the definitive role of GO in induction, consolidation, and or maintenance will require testing in RCTs (Grade 1C).

Is maintenance therapy needed for all patients with APL?

Two previous RCTs (the first North American Intergroup study and the European APL93 trial) suggested that maintenance therapy is beneficial. However, in these trials, the molecular status was not reported and the doses of anthracyclines were less than that used in the subsequent trials. Recent studies have suggested that maintenance therapy does not improve outcome for patients who are in molecular remission after intensive consolidation (50–52). In a trial carried out by the GIMEMA, 318 patients were randomized between 1993 and 1997 to 1 of 4 maintenance arms: oral 6-mercaptopurine (6-MP) and methotrexate, ATRA alone, ATRA alternating with 6-MP and methotrexate, or no further therapy after consolidation (50). Beginning in 1998, 268 patients in molecular remission after consolidation were randomized to only two of the arms, ATRA alone, or to ATRA plus 6-MP and methotrexate. There were 78 PML-RAR-alpha–negative patients randomized to 6-MP plus methotrexate, 83 to ATRA alone, 81 to ATRA plus 6-MP methotrexate, and 76 to no further therapy. No differences in molecular disease-free survivals were detected among the randomized arms. An RCT conducted by the Japanese Adult Leukemia Study Group (JALSG) (APL97), compared six courses of intensive maintenance chemotherapy without ATRA to observation in patients achieving a molecular remission after consolidation therapy and also found no benefit to maintenance therapy (51,52). Phase II data suggest that a state of molecular negativity can be achieved in more than 95% of patients who receive two to three courses of intensive anthracycline-based consolidation (20,25,45). Investigators at the Princess Margaret Hospital reported excellent outcomes with ATRA and chemotherapy induction and consolidation, without maintenance therapy; the five-year overall and leukemia-free survivals were 82% and 78%, respectively (53).

These studies suggest that patients with low- or intermediate-risk disease who achieve molecular remission after consolidation therapy may not require maintenance therapy. This issue is relevant because recent reports have suggested a small, but potentially important, incidence of secondary myelodysplastic syndrome and AML among patients treated with contemporary strategies, including maintenance chemotherapy (54,55). Given recent data demonstrating excellent outcomes in low-risk patients (WBC <20,000 cells/μL) receiving ATRA plus ATO or ATO alone, it may be possible to minimize not only maintenance therapy but also induction and consolidation chemotherapy, if future studies confirm these data. A new North American Intergroup trial will randomize low- and intermediate-risk patients in molecular remission after consolidation to either maintenance therapy with ATRA and low-dose chemotherapy or observation.

Recommendation

1. There are conflicting data regarding the benefits of maintenance therapy in patients with APL in CR after consolidation. Two previous RCTs have demonstrated a benefit, and several phase II trials, in which all patients received maintenance therapy, report excellent results. However, with the addition of new molecular techniques to monitor remission, preliminary publications of two other RCTs challenge whether there is a true benefit; these studies suggest that patients in molecular remission after intensive anthracycline-based chemotherapy do not benefit from postremission therapy with ATRA, ATRA plus low-dose chemotherapy or intensive cytotoxic chemotherapy. At the present time, it is recommended that most patients receive maintenance therapy with ATRA and low-dose chemotherapy with methotrexate and 6-mercaptopurine until further studies are completed (Grade 1B).

References

1 Hillestad LK. Acute promyelocytic leukemia. *Acta Med Scand.* 1957;**159**:189–94.
2 Bernard J, Mathe G, Boulay J, et al. Acute promyelocytic leukemia: a study made on 20 cases. *Schweiz Med Wochenschr.* 1959;**89**:604–8.
3 Bernard J, Weil M, Boiron M, et al. Acute promyelocytic leukemia: results of treatment by daunorubicin. *Blood.* 1973;**41**:489–96.
4 Grignani F, Ferrucci PF, Testa U, et al. The acute promyelocytic leukemia-specific PML-RAR alpha fusion protein inhibits differentiation and promotes survival of myeloid precursor cells. *Cell.* 1993;**74**:423–31.
5 Rowley JD, Golomb HM, Dougherty C. 15/17 translocation, a consistent chromosomal change in acute promyelocytic leukaemia. *Lancet.* 1977;**1**:549–50.
6 Breitman TR, Collins SJ, Keene BR. Terminal differentiation of human promyelocytic leukemic cells in primary culture in response to retinoic acid. *Blood.* 1981;**57**:1000–1004.
7 Chen GQ, Zhu J, Shi XG, et al. In vitro studies on cellular and molecular mechanisms of arsenic trioxide (As2O3) in the treatment of acute promyelocytic leukemia: As2O3 induces NB4 cell apoptosis with downregulation of Bcl-2 expression and modulation of PML-RAR alpha/PML proteins. *Blood.* 1996;**88**:1052–61.
8 Tallman MS, Nabhan C, Feusner JH, et al. Acute promyelocytic leukemia: evolving therapeutic strategies. *Blood.* 2002;**99**:759–67.
9 Huang ME, Ye YC, Chen SR, et al. Use of all-trans retinoic acid in the treatment of acute promyelocytic leukemia. *Blood.* 1988;**72**:567–72.
10 Warrell RP Jr, Frankel SR, Miller WH Jr, et al. Differentiation therapy of acute promyelocytic leukemia with tretinoin (all-trans-retinoic acid). *N Engl J Med.* 1991;**324**:1385–93.
11 Castaigne S, Chomienne C, Daniel MT, et al. All-trans retinoic acid as a differentiation therapy for acute promyelocytic leukemia. I. Clinical results. *Blood.* 1990;**76**:1704–9.
12 Chen ZX, Xue YQ, Zhang R, et al. A clinical and experimental study on all-trans retinoic acid-treated acute promyelocytic leukemia patients. *Blood.* 1991;**78**:1413–19.
13 Fenaux P, Castaigne S, Dombret H, et al. All-transretinoic acid followed by intensive chemotherapy gives a high complete remission rate and may

prolong remissions in newly diagnosed acute promyelocytic leukemia: a pilot study on 26 cases. *Blood.* 1992;**80**:2176–81.

14 Mandelli F, Diverio D, Avvisati G, et al. Molecular remission in PML/RAR alpha-positive acute promyelocytic leukemia by combined all-trans retinoic acid and idarubicin (AIDA) therapy. Gruppo Italiano-Malattie Ematologiche Maligne dell'Adulto and Associazione Italiana di Ematologia ed Oncologia Pediatrica Cooperative Groups. *Blood.* 1997;**90**:1014–21.

15 Fenaux P, Le Deley MC, Castaigne S, et al. Effect of all transretinoic acid in newly diagnosed acute promyelocytic leukemia. Results of a multicenter randomized trial. European APL 91 Group. *Blood.* 1993;**82**:3241–49.

16 Tallman MS, Andersen JW, Schiffer CA, et al. All-trans-retinoic acid in acute promyelocytic leukemia. *N Engl J Med.* 1997;**337**:1021–28.

17 Fenaux P, Chastang C, Chevret S, et al. A randomized comparison of all transretinoic acid (ATRA) followed by chemotherapy and ATRA plus chemotherapy and the role of maintenance therapy in newly diagnosed acute promyelocytic leukemia. The European APL Group. *Blood.* 1999;**94**:1192–200.

18 Tallman MS, Andersen JW, Schiffer CA, et al. All-trans retinoic acid in acute promyelocytic leukemia: long-term outcome and prognostic factor analysis from the North American Intergroup protocol. *Blood.* 2002;**100**:4298–302.

19 Sanz MA, Martin G, Rayon C, et al. A modified AIDA protocol with anthracycline-based consolidation results in high antileukemic efficacy and reduced toxicity in newly diagnosed PML/RARalpha-positive acute promyelocytic leukemia. PETHEMA group. *Blood.* 1999;**94**:3015–21.

20 Sanz MA, Martin G, Gonzalez M, et al. Risk-adapted treatment of acute promyelocytic leukemia with all-trans-retinoic acid and anthracycline monochemotherapy: a multicenter study by the PETHEMA group. *Blood.* 2004;**103**:1237–43.

21 Ghavamzadeh A, Alimoghaddam K, Ghaffari SH, et al. Treatment of acute promyelocytic leukemia with arsenic trioxide without ATRA and/or chemotherapy. *Ann Oncol.* 2006;**17**:131–34.

22 Mathews V, George B, Lakshmi KM, et al. Single-agent arsenic trioxide in the treatment of newly diagnosed acute promyelocytic leukemia: durable remissions with minimal toxicity. *Blood.* 2006;**107**:2627–32.

23 Shen ZX, Shi ZZ, Fang J, et al. All-trans retinoic acid/As2O3 combination yields a high quality remission and survival in newly diagnosed acute promyelocytic leukemia. *Proc Natl Acad Sci USA.* 2004;**101**:5328–35.

24 Asou N, Adachi K, Tamura J, et al. Analysis of prognostic factors in newly diagnosed acute promyelocytic leukemia treated with all-trans retinoic acid and chemotherapy. Japan Adult Leukemia Study Group. *J Clin Oncol.* 1998;**16**:78–85.

25 Burnett AK, Grimwade D, Solomon E et al. Presenting white blood cell count and kinetics of molecular remission predict prognosis in acute promyelocytic leukemia treated with all-trans retinoic acid: results of the randomized MRC trial. *Blood.* 1999;**93**:4131–43.

26 Sanz MA, Lo Coco F, Martin G, et al. Definition of relapse risk and role of nonanthracycline drugs for consolidation in patients with acute promyelocytic leukemia: a joint study of the PETHEMA and GIMEMA cooperative groups. *Blood.* 2000;**96**:1247–53.

27 Grimwade D, Gale RE, Hills R, et al. The relationship between FLT3 mutation status, biological characteristics and outcome in patients with acute promyelocytic leukemia [abstract]. *Blood.* 2003;**102**:334.

28 Kiyoi H, Naoe T, Yokota S, et al. Internal tandem duplication of FLT3 associated with leukocytosis in acute promyelocytic leukemia. Leukemia Study Group of the Ministry of Health and Welfare (Kohseisho). *Leukemia.* 1997;**11**:1447–52.

29 Kainz B, Heintel D, Marculescu R, et al. Variable prognostic value of FLT3 internal tandem duplications in patients with de novo AML and a normal karyotype, t(15;17), t(8;21) or inv(16). *Hematol J.* 2002;**3**:283–89.

30 Callens C, Chevret S, Cayuela JM, et al. Prognostic implication of FLT3 and Ras gene mutations in patients with acute promyelocytic leukemia (APL): a retrospective study from the European APL Group. *Leukemia.* 2005;**19**:1153–60.

31 Shih LY, Kuo MC, Liang DC, et al. Internal tandem duplication and Asp835 mutations of the FMS-like tyrosine kinase 3 (FLT3) gene in acute promyelocytic leukemia. *Cancer.* 2003;**98**:1206–16.

32 Stock W, Moser B, Sher DA, et al. PML-RAR alpha isoform at diagnosis is associated with disease-free survival (DFS) in patients enrolled in the intergroup trial (C-9710) for treatment of acute promyelocytic leukemia (APL) [abstract]. *Proc Am Soc Clin Oncol.* 2006;**24**:6504.

33 Estey E, Thall PF, Pierce S, et al. Treatment of newly diagnosed acute promyelocytic leukemia without cytarabine. *J Clin Oncol.* 1997;**15**:484–90.

34 Ades L, Raffoux, E, Chevret S, et al. Is ARAC useful in the treatment of APL? Results of a randomised trial from the European Acute Promyelocytic Leukemia Group. *J Clin Oncol.* 2006;**24**:5703–10.

35 Avvisati G, Petti MC, Lo Coco F, et al. Induction therapy with idarubicin alone significantly influences event-free survival duration in patients with newly diagnosed hypergranular acute promyelocytic leukemia: final results of the GIMEMA randomized study LAP 0389 with 7 years of minimal follow-up. *Blood.* 2002;**100**:3141–46.

36 Chen GQ, Shi XG, Tang W, et al. Use of arsenic trioxide (As2O3) in the treatment of acute promyelocytic leukemia (APL): I. As2O3 exerts dose-dependent dual effects on APL cells. *Blood.* 1997;**89**:3345–53.

37 Shen ZX, Chen GQ, Ni JH, et al. Use of arsenic trioxide (As2O3) in the treatment of acute promyelocytic leukemia (APL): II. Clinical efficacy and pharmacokinetics in relapsed patients. *Blood.* 1997;**89**:3354–60.

38 Soignet SL, Maslak P, Wang ZG, et al. Complete remission after treatment of acute promyelocytic leukemia with arsenic trioxide. *N Engl J Med.* 1998;**339**:1341–48.

39 Niu C, Yan H, Yu T, et al. Studies on treatment of acute promyelocytic leukemia with arsenic trioxide: remission induction, follow-up, and molecular monitoring in 11 newly diagnosed and 47 relapsed acute promyelocytic leukemia patients. *Blood.* 1999;**94**:3315–24.

40 Soignet SL, Frankel SR, Douer D, et al. United States multicenter study of arsenic trioxide in relapsed acute promyelocytic leukemia. *J Clin Oncol.* 2001;**19**:3852–60.

41 Lazo G, Kantarjian H, Estey E, et al. Use of arsenic trioxide (As2O3) in the treatment of patients with acute promyelocytic leukemia: the M. D. Anderson experience. *Cancer.* 2003;**97**:2218–24.

42 Liu YF, Shen ZX, Hu J, et al. Clinical observation on the efficacy of all-trans retinoic acid (ATRA) combined with arsenic trioxide (As2O3) in newly diagnosed acute promyelocytic leukemia (APL) [abstract 888]. *Blood.* 2004;**104**:253a.

43 Estey E, Garcia-Manero G, Ferrajoli A, et al. Use of all-trans retinoic acid plus arsenic trioxide as an alternative to chemotherapy in untreated acute promyelocytic leukemia. *Blood.* 2006;**107**:3469–73.

44 Raffoux E, Rousselot P, Poupon J, et al. Combined treatment with arsenic trioxide and all-trans-retinoic acid in patients with relapsed acute promyelocytic leukemia. *J Clin Oncol.* 2003;**21**:2326–34.

45 Lo Coco FA, Avvisati G, Vignetti M, et al. Front-line treatment of acute promyelocytic leukemia with AIDA induction followed by risk-adapted consolidation: results of the AIDA-2000 trial of the Italian GIMEMA group [abstract]. *Blood.* 2004;**104**: 392.

46 Lengfelder E, Reichert A, Schoch C, et al. Double induction strategy including high dose cytarabine in combination with all-trans retinoic acid: effects in patients with newly diagnosed acute promyelocytic leukemia. German AML Cooperative Group. *Leukemia.* 2000;**14**:1362–70.

47 Schlenk RF, Germing U, Hartmann F et al. High-dose cytarabine and mitoxantrone in consolidation therapy for acute promyelocytic leukemia. *Leukemia.* 2005;**19**:978–83.

48 Powell BL, Moser B, Stock W, et al. Consolidation with arsenic trioxide (As2O3) significantly improves event-free survival (EFS) and overall survival (OS) among patients with newly diagnosed acute promyelocytic leukemia (APL): North American Intergroup Protocol C9710 [cited 21 Mar 2007]. Available at: http://www.asco.org.

49 Powell BL, Moser B, Stock W, et al. Preliminary results from the North American Acute Promyelocytic Leukemia (APL) Study C9710. *Blood.* 2006;171a.

50 Avvisati G, Petti MC, Lo Coco F, et al. AIDA: the Italian way of treating acute promyelocytic leukemia (APL), final act [abstract 487]. *Blood.* 2003;**102**:142a.

51 Ohno R, Asou N. The recent JALSG study for newly diagnosed patients with acute promyelocytic leukemia (APL). *Ann Hematol.* 2004;**83** Suppl 1:S77–S78.

52 Asou N, Kishimoto Y, Kiyoi H, et al. A randomized study with or without maintenance chemotherapy in patients with acute promyelocytic leukemia who had become negative for PML-RAR-alpha transcript after consolidation therapy: the Japan Adult Leukemia Study Group (JALSG) APL97 study. *Blood.* **2006**;569a.

53 Gupta V, Yi QL, Brandwein J, et al. Role of all-trans-retinoic acid (ATRA) in the consolidation therapy of acute promyelocytic leukaemia (APL). *Leuk Res.* 2005;**29**:113–14.

54 Latagliata R, Petti MC, Fenu S, et al. Therapy-related myelodysplastic syndrome-acute myelogenous leukemia in patients treated for acute promyelocytic leukemia: an emerging problem. *Blood.* 2002;**99**: 822–24.

55 Zompi S, Viguie F. Therapy-related acute myeloid leukemia and myelodysplasia after successful treatment of acute promyelocytic leukemia. *Leuk Lymphoma.* 2002;**43**:275–80.

36 Chronic Lymphocytic Leukemia

Bruce D. Cheson

Introduction

Chronic lymphocytic leukemia (CLL) is the most common leukemia in Western countries with over 12,000 new cases projected in the United States in 2007 (1). Because it tends to be an indolent disease, it also has the greatest prevalence. There are no clear etiologic factors, although 10%–15% of patients have a family history of a hematologic malignancy (2). The median age at presentation is greater than 60 years, with 20% under 55 years and 10%–15% of patients younger than 50 years of age. Younger patients are more likely to die from CLL-related events, while older patients more often die from secondary malignancies and non-CLL causes (3).

A number of complications may occur in patients with CLL. These include an increased risk for cancers of the skin, gastrointestinal tract, and other common sites; transformation to aggressive lymphoid malignancies, including prolymphocytic leukemia or Richter's syndrome (a diffuse large B-cell lymphoma particularly resistant to therapy); and development of other hematologic malignancies, including acute myelogenous leukemia. In addition, at least 20% of patients will develop an autoimmune disorder, including immune-mediated thrombocytopenia, and these patients have an increased susceptibility to infections in part due to hypogammaglobulinemia, an inability to produce specific antibodies and abnormal activation of complement (4). The use of immunosuppressive therapies has markedly increased the number of opportunistic infections (5–7).

Questions

1. How is the diagnosis of CLL made?
2. What is the clinical relevance of newly identified prognostic factors?
3. What is the optimal approach to the initial treatment of patients with CLL?
4. How should patients with relapsed or refractory disease be managed?

Evidence-based Hematology. Edited by Mark A. Crowther, Jeff Ginsberg, Holger J. Schünemann, Ralph M. Meyer, and Richard Lottenberg.

Literature-search strategy and inclusions

Published manuscripts and abstracts were identified through PubMed and through the abstract books from recent American Society of Hematology and American Society of Clinical Oncology meetings. Selection of papers for inclusion was based on their importance as judged by the author. Review articles were not considered, and of those papers included, priority was given to large randomized trials followed by those phase II studies with adequately stated objectives and statistical considerations, and an adequate sample size.

Where graded recommendations are made in the text the grading system examining the quality of evidence and strengths of recommendations in this chapter are based on the guidelines proposed by the international Grading of Recommendations Assessment, Development, and Evaluation Working Group (GRADE) adopting the modification used by the American College of Chest Physicians that merges the "very low" and "low" categories of quality of evidence (see chapter 1).

How is the diagnosis of CLL made?

The diagnosis of CLL requires at least 5,000 clonal B cells/mm^3 in the peripheral blood (8). Examination of a blood smear should reveal a relatively homogeneous population of mature-appearing lymphocytes, with occasional smudge cells, often with some prolymphocytes that are larger with prominent nucleoli. The latter must be <55% to be CLL rather than prolymphocytic leukemia (9). Other lymphoid malignancies in a leukemic phase can be confused with CLL, such as hairy cell leukemia, marginal zone or follicular lymphoma, or T cell leukemias. The characteristic immunophenotype of CLL B cells helps distinguish among these entities: These B cells exhibit CD19 and CD20 (generally dim), CD23, and CD5, with monoclonality of light chains. Small numbers of CD5/CD20+ B cells can be detected in the blood of up to 5% of normal persons, referred to as benign lymphocytosis of unknown significance. Whether such patients will eventually progress to CLL is unknown.

A bone marrow aspiration is not needed for the diagnosis of CLL as adequate information can be obtained from the peripheral blood; however, the procedure is useful prior to therapy for an assessment of the normal bone marrow elements and to provide a baseline against which to compare the results of treatment. A lymph node biopsy is rarely indicated in CLL unless there is a concern of Richter's syndrome.

As a consequence of automated cell counting and a heightened awareness of the disorder, patients are diagnosed earlier in the course of their disease, with about half of the cases being asymptomatic at presentation.

Conclusion

The diagnosis of B-cell CLL can be made from routinely available evaluations of the peripheral blood, including cell counts, morphology, and flow cytometric analysis.

What is the clinical relevance of newly identified prognostic factors?

CLL patients are staged according to the clinical schemes of Rai in the United States and Binet in much of Europe (10,11). Both use physical examination and peripheral blood counts to separate patients into risk groups and are comparably prognostic. Rai stage 0 includes patients with only lymphocytosis (median survival >12.5 years); stage I, with lymphadenopathy (8.5 years); stage II, splenomegaly, with or without hepatomegaly (6 years); stage III, anemia (2–3 years); and stage IV, thrombocytopenia (2–3 years). This system was subsequently simplified to three stages (12); "low risk" (stage 0), "intermediate risk" (stages I–II), and "high risk" (stages III–IV). The Binet system designates stage A as fewer than three node-bearing areas (median survival >10 years); stage B, three or more node-bearing areas (5 years); stage C, anemia and thrombocytopenia (2 years) (13). The Binet system fails to identify Rai stage 0 patients. To complete this staging and to facilitate patient management of potential disease-related complications, required tests include a complete blood count with differential, reticulocyte count, direct antiglobulin test, quantitative immunoglobulins, complete metabolic panel with renal and liver function tests, serum LDH, and uric acid. A chest radiograph should be performed. However, CT scans are not yet part of standard care outside of a clinical trial, and CLL nodes are often not FDG-avid on positron emission tomography scans; therefore, this test should not be performed unless there is suspicion of Richter's transformation (14).

Fluorescent in situ hybridization demonstrates that 80% of patients have acquired chromosomal abnormalities, most often a 13q deletion, which occurs in about half of cases either alone or in combination with another abnormality (15). Normal karyotypes and trisomy 12 are the next in frequency followed by 17p-deletion (p53 mutation), and 11q-. There is a strong correlation between cytogenetics and outcome; 13q- being the most favorable, normal and trisomy 12 with an intermediate outcome, and the others and complex abnormalities with a poor survival. Newer studies suggest that expression of CD38, unmutated immunoglobulin heavy chain gene mutations, and expression of ZAP-70 are associated with an unfavorable outcome (16). There is currently no defined role for these new prognostic factors in the clinical management of patients with CLL and they should be reserved for clinical trials (17).

Conclusions

1. Standard laboratory tests (as described above) are sufficient for diagnosing and planning management of patients with CLL.
2. While several new biomarkers have been suggested as important for prognosis, these have not yet been prospectively validated to have predictive properties for determination of therapy, others are either not routinely available or reproducible among laboratories, and, thus, these studies are not required as part of standard clinical care.

What is the optimal approach to the initial treatment of patients with CLL?

Prospective randomized trials in early stage, asymptomatic patients in which early intervention with alkylating agents was compared with observation and later treatment upon progression failed to demonstrate any detrimental effect on patient survival by delaying treatment. Therefore, a current approach to such patients is to watch and wait until therapy is indicated by disease-related symptoms (fevers, sweats, unexplained weight loss, severe fatigue), massive or progressive lymphadenopathy or hepatosplenomegaly, autoimmune hemolytic anemia or thrombocytopenia unresponsive to corticosteroids, recurrent infections (8). Although the absolute lymphocyte count is not generally used as a criterion for initiating therapy, a rapid doubling of the peripheral blood lymphocyte count (<6 months) supports the decision to treat. Whether certain early stage, high-risk patients would benefit from early intervention has not yet been demonstrated.

Randomized trials comparing fludarabine with alkylating agent-based regimens show higher complete and overall response rates, a longer time to progression, but no survival advantage from the nucleoside analog (18–21). Despite the lack of a demonstrated survival benefit, based on the significant increase in time to progression that is not associated with high rates of severe toxicity, fludarabine-based therapy has replaced alkylating agent regimens as the standard initial treatment of CLL. This conclusion is supported by the Cochrane Report meta-analysis of five randomized trials that evaluated a total of 1,838 patients (22). The authors concluded that purine analogs induced a higher complete and overall response rate than alkylating-agent-based therapy and a longer progression-free survival. There was a suggestion of an overall survival advantage, but toxicity risks, including infections and hemolytic anemia, were greater. When only the studies evaluating fludarabine were included (i.e., the single study assessing cladribine was excluded), a survival benefit became apparent. The combination of fludarabine and cyclophosphamide improves response rate and time to progression compared with single agent fludarabine, but again, no survival advantage was detected; considerably more myelosuppression without an obvious increase in infections was noted (23,24).

Single-agent rituximab as initial treatment achieves a 51% response rate, with a median progression-free survival of only 18.6 months (25). Byrd et al. studied the combination of fludarabine and rituximab in a randomized phase II trial looking at concurrent versus sequential administration (26). They reported an overall and complete response rate of 90% and 47%, respectively, when the two agents were used concurrently, which was somewhat higher than when they were used sequentially (77% and 28%, respectively). Nevertheless, this difference did not translate into superior progression-free or overall survival and more myelotoxicity was seen. In a historical cohort comparison with another CALGB study evaluating fludarabine alone, superior survival was suggested for the antibody-containing combination (27).

Single-agent alemtuzumab has been compared in a randomized study with chlorambucil and has demonstrated prolonged progression-free survival, with particular efficacy in the particularly poor-risk patients with del17p (28). Asymptomatic cytomegalovirus viremia was documented in half the patients treated with alemtuzumab but was considered manageable. No survival advantage was detected.

Keating et al. treated 224 patients with the combination of fludarabine, cyclophosphamide, and rituximab and reported an overall response rate of 95% with 70% complete remissions (29). Major and minor infections occurred in 2.6% and 10% of cycles, respectively. Responses in the latter population of 177 patients included CR in 25%, nodular PR (nPR) in 16%, and PR in 32%; response correlated with type of and response to prior therapy (30). Nevertheless, most patients were unable to tolerate the full six cycles of therapy. Although the results with FCR superficially appear better than FR, the FCR patients were a median of eight years younger and had less advanced disease, which may explain the apparently superior rates. A randomized comparison between FR and FCR is needed to determine the standard therapy of untreated CLL (26,29).

High complete and overall response rates have also been reported with the combination of pentostatin, cyclophosphamide, and rituximab as initial therapy of CLL, with more than 90% of patients experiencing a response, including 41% complete remissions (31). How the safety and efficacy of this regimen compares with fludarabine-based therapy will require a randomized comparison.

Recommendations

1. Asymptomatic patients may be safely managed with observation and do not require initial therapy (Grade 1A). Indications for therapy include fevers, sweats, unexplained weight loss, severe fatigue, massive or progressive lymphadenopathy or hepatosplenomegaly, autoimmune hemolytic anemia or thrombocytopenia unresponsive to corticosteroids, and recurrent infections.
2. In patients requiring initial therapy, fludarabine is the treatment of choice based on the balance of disease control (time to progression) and avoidance of severe treatment-related toxicity associated with this therapy (Grade 1A).

How should patients with relapsed or refractory disease be managed?

Treatment options for patients who have progressed after initial therapy are determined, in part, by the initial treatment regimen, the quality, and duration of response to that regimen, and patient-related factors such as age, the size of lymph nodes, infection history, and performance status. More than half of patients initially treated with an alkylating agent will respond to fludarabine (18). In contrast, few meaningful responses can be achieved with chlorambucil in patients with progressive disease following initial therapy with fludarabine (18). Data evaluating treatment options in patients with relapsed disease principally come from phases I and II cohort studies or from small randomized trials that predominantly evaluate response rate. A number of options for patients with progressive disease are under evaluation, but randomized trials associated with mature results of disease control or overall survival have not yet been reported. Several of these options are summarized next.

Pentostatin. Responses with pentostatin are observed in 25%–30% of previously treated or untreated patients, although few are complete or durable (32–37). Toxicities include myelosuppression, immunosuppression, nausea, vomiting, fever, rash, and renal, neurotoxicity but without an apparent increase in secondary tumors (36–43). The combination of pentostatin, rituximab, and cyclophosphamide has generated promising results in patients who progress after or are refractory to fludarabine therapy (44).

Alemtuzumab. Alemtuzumab is a humanized monoclonal antibody that targets CD52 on the surface of B cells and T cells (7). Alemtuzumab is associated with responses in about 30% of patients with CLL failing alkylating agents and fludarabine but with rare complete remissions (45–47). The median time to response in an international trial was 1.5 months, the median duration of response 8.7 months, and the median survival 16 months, 32 months in responders (7). Patients with bulky lymphadenopathy appear unlikely to respond (48). The most frequent adverse events are infusion-related rigors (90%), fever (85%), nausea (53%), vomiting (38%), and mild-to-moderate rash in a third of patients. Because of an increased risk of *Pneumocystis carinii* and herpes viruses infections, antimicrobial prophylaxis is essential. Reactivation of cytomegalovirus occurs in a quarter of patients requiring weekly monitoring by polymerase chain reaction testing (7). The subcutaneous mode of administration appears to preserve activity while minimizing infusional toxicity (49).

Rituximab. Rituximab as a single agent induces partial responses in only 10%–15% of patients with relapsed or refractory CLL/SLL not previously exposed to this agent (50–55).

Fludarabine, cyclophosphamide, rituximab (FCR). The FCR regimen has been studied in previously treated patients (30). In 127 patients treated with a median of two prior regimens, the CR, nPR, and PR rates were 25%, 16%, and 32%, respectively. However, most patients were unable to tolerate the six planned cycles of therapy because the treatment was associated with significant myelosuppression and infections. The time to progression was about three years in those with a CR or nPR, but only 15 months in those with a partial response.

Other antibody therapies. Luxiliximab is a macaque-human chimeric monoclonal antibody with a strong similarity to the human antibody. It binds complement and mediates antibody-dependent cellular cytotoxicity by binding FcgammaRI and RII receptors. Although limited single-agent activity has been observed (56), in vitro data suggest synergy with fludarabine and rituximab and a phase I/II study of lumiliximab combined with fludarabine, cyclophosphamide, and rituximab has been completed (57). A randomized trial comparing FCR-luxiliximab with FCR alone is ongoing. Ofatumumab is a fully human monoclonal antibody targeting a novel epitope of the CD20 molecule. A phase I/II trial demonstrated significant depletion of CD19+CD5+ B cells and similar toxicity to rituximab with a high response rate in patients relapsing after fludarabine therapy (58).

Other new agents. Other drugs showing promise in CLL include lenalidomide, which is a second-generation immunomodulatory agent approved for patients with myelodysplastic syndrome and the 5q- chromosome abnormality, and for those with relapsed/refractory multiple myeloma. In a single-center study of patients with relapsed and refractory CLL, the response rate to lenalidomide was about 50% (59). Oblimersen sodium is an antisense molecule with modest single agent activity in CLL (60). A phase III trial comparing fludarabine plus cyclophosphamide with or without oblimersen in patients who with progressive disease after fludarabine therapy demonstrated a higher CR and nPR rate with the three-drug combination (61). Oblimersen has been combined with fludarabine and rituximab in preliminary testing with encouraging results (62). Related agents being tested in clinical trials include obatoclax and AT101 (63). Bendamustine is an alkylating agent-purine analogue hybrid that may be superior to chlorambucil in untreated CLL and is currently undergoing extensive study (64).

Stem cell transplantation. Allogeneic BMT data are limited in CLL, primarily because of the older age of the patients. In general, half the patients remain disease free for prolonged periods of time but treatment-related mortality is 25%–50% (58). Submyeloablative regimens may achieve successful engraftment without substantial acute GVHD and long-term responses; however, chronic GVHD is a serious complication (69,70). The published data for autologous stem cell transplantation for patients with CLL are limited and not encouraging (65,66,71–73).

Recommendations

1. Patients who relapse after single-agent fludarabine who do not have bulky lymphadenopathy ($\geq$5 cm) can be considered for alemtuzumab therapy (Grade 2C).
2. Younger patients and those with bulky disease may be treated with fludarabine and rituximab with or without cyclophosphamide (Grade 2C).
3. Patients who relapse after fludarabine and rituximab may respond to fludarabine-rituximab and cyclophosphamide (Grade 2C) or R-CHOP (Grade 2C).

References

1 Jemal A, Siegel R, Ward E, et al. Cancer statistics, 2007. *CA Cancer J Clin.* 2007;**57**:43–66.
2 Mauro FR, Giammartini E, Gentile M, et al. Clinical features and outcome of familial chronic lymphocytic leukemia. *Haematologica.* 2006;**91**:1117–20.
3 Mauro FR, Foa R, Cerretti R, et al. Autoimmune hemolytic anemia in chronic lymphocytic leukemia: clinical, therapeutic, and prognostic features. *Blood.* 2000;**95**:2786–92.
4 Heath ME, Cheson BD. Defective complement activity in chronic lymphocytic leukemia. *Am J Hematol.* 1985;**19**:63–73.
5 Cheson BD. Immunologic and immunosuppressive complications of purine analogue therapy. *J Clin Oncol.* 1995;**13**:2431–48.
6 Anaissie EJ, Kontoyiannis DP, O'Brien S, et al. Infections in patients with chronic lymphocytic leukemia treated with fludarabine. *Ann Intern Med.* 1998:**129**:559–66.
7 Keating MJ, Flinn I, Jain V, et al. Therapeutic role of alemtuzumab (CAMPATH-1H) in patients who have failed fludarabine: results of a large international study. *Blood.* 2002;**99**:3554–61.
8 Cheson BD, Bennett JM, Grever M, et al. National Cancer Institute-Sponsored Working Group guidelines for chronic lymphocytic leukemia: revised guidelines for diagnosis and treatment. *Blood.* 1996;**87**:4990–97.
9 Melo JV, Catovsky D, Galton DAG. The relationship between chronic lymphocytic leukaemia and prolymphocytic leukaemia. I. Clinical and laboratory features of 300 patients and characterization of an intermediate group. *Br J Haematol.* 1986;**63**:377–87.
10 Rai KR, Sawitsky A, Cronkite EP, et al. Clinical staging of chronic lymphocytic leukemia. *Blood.* 1975;**46**:219–34.

11 Binet JL, Catovsky D, Chandra P, et al. Chronic lymphocytic leukaemia: proposals for a revised prognostic staging system. *Br J Haematol.* 1981;**48**:365–67.

12 Rai KR. A critical analysis of staging in CLL. In: Gale RP, Rai KR, editors. Chronic *lymphocytic leukemia: recent progress and future direction.* New York: Alan R. Liss; 1987. p. 253.

13 Binet JL, Auquier A, Dighiero G, et al. A new prognostic classification of chronic lymphocytic leukemia derived from a multivariate survival analysis. *Cancer.* 1981;**48**:198–206.

14 Jerusalem G, Beguin Y, Najjar F, et al. Positron emission tomography (PET) with 18F-fluorodeoxyglucose (18F-FDG) for the staging of low-grade non-Hodgkin's lymphoma (NHL). *Ann Oncol.* 2001;**12**:825–30.

15 Döhner H, Stilgenbauer S, Benner A, et al. Genomic aberrations and survival in chronic lymphocytic leukemia. *N Engl J Med.* 2000;**343**:1910–16.

16 Rassenti LZ, Huynh L, Toy TL, et al. ZAP-70 compared with immunoglobulin heavy-chain gene mutation status as a predictor of disease progression in chronic lymphocytic leukemia. *N Engl J Med.* 2004;**351**:893–901.

17 Binet JL, Caligaris-Capio F, Catovsky D, et al. Perspectives on the use of new diagnostic tools in the treatment of chronic lymphocytic leukemia. *Blood.* 2006;**107**:859–61.

18 Rai KR, Peterson BL, Kolitz J, et al. Fludarabine compared with chlorambucil as primary therapy for chronic lymphocytic leukemia. *New Engl J Med.* 2000;**343**:1750–57.

19 Morrison VA, Rai KR, Peterson BL, et al. Therapy-related myeloid leukemias are observed in patients with chronic lymphocytic leukemia after treatment with fludarabine and chlorambucil: results of an intergroup study, Cancer and Leukemia Group B 9011. *J Clin Oncol.* 2002;**20**:3878–84.

20 French Cooperative Group on CLL, Johnson S, Smith AG, et al. Multicentre prospective randomised trial of fludarabine versus cyclophosphamide, doxorubicin, and prednisone (CAP) for treatment of advanced-stage chronic lymphocytic leukemia. *Lancet.* 1996;**347**:1432–38.

21 Leporrier M, Chevret S, Cazin B, et al. Randomized comparison of fludarabine, CAP, and ChOP, in 938 previously treated stage B and C-chronic lymphocytic leukemia. *Blood.* 2001;**98**:2319–25.

22 Steurer M, Pall G, Richards S, et al. Purine antagonists for chronic lymphocytic leukaemia (Review). *Cochrane Database Syst Rev.* 2007;3:CD004270.

23 Eichhorst B, Busch R, Hopfinger G, et al. Fludarabine plus cyclophosphamide versus fludarabine alone in first-line therapy of younger patients with chronic lymphocytic leukemia. *Blood.* 2006;**107**:885–91.

24 Flinn IW, Neuberg DS, Grever MR, et al. Phase III trial of fludarabine plus cyclophosphamide compared with fludarabine for patients with previously untreated chronic lymphocytic leukemia: US Intergroup Trial E2997. *J Clin Oncol.* 2007;**25**:793–98.

25 Hainsworth JD, Litchy S, Barton JH, et al. Single-agent rituximab as first-line and maintenance treatment for patients with chronic lymphocytic leukemia or small lymphocytic lymphoma: a phase II trial of the Minnie Pearl Cancer Research Network. *J Clin Oncol.* 2003;**21**:1746–51.

26 Byrd JC, Peterson B, Morrison VA, et al. Randomized phase 2 study of fludarabine with concurrent versus sequential treatment with rituximab in symptomatic, untreated patients with B-cell chronic lymphocytic leukemia: results from Cancer and Leukemia Group B 9712 (CALGB 9712). *Blood.* 2003;**101**:6–14.

27 Byrd JC, Rai K, Peterson BL, et al. The addition of rituximab to fludarabine may prolong progression-free survival and overall survival in patients with previously untreated chronic lymphocytic leukemia: an updated retrospective comparative analysis of CALGB 9712 and CALGB 9011. *Blood.* 2005;**105**:49–53.

28 Hillmen P, Skotnicki A, Robak T, et al. Alemtuzumab (Campath; MAB-CAMPATH) has superior progression-free survival vs chlorambucil as front-line therapy for patients with progressive B-cell chronic lymphocytic leukemia (BCLL) [abstract 301]. *Blood.* 2006;**108**:93a.

29 Keating MJ, O'Brien S, Albitar M, et al. Early results of a chemoimmunotherapy regimen of fludarfabine, cyclophosphamide, and rituximab (FCR) as initial therapy for chronic lymphocytic leukemia. *J Clin Oncol* 2005;**23**:4079–88.

30 Wierda W, O'Brien S, Wen S, et al. Chemoimmunotherapy with fludarabine, cyclophosphamide and rituximab for relapsed and refractory chronic lymphocytic leukemia. *J Clin Oncol.* 2005;**23**:4070–78.

31 Kay NE, Geyer SM, Call TG, et al. Combination chemoimmunotherapy with pentostatin, cyclophosphamide, and rituximab shows significant clinical activity with low accompanying toxicity in previously untreated B chronic lymphocytic leukemia. *Blood.* 2007;**109**:405–11.

32 Dearden C, Catovsky D. Deoxycoformycin in the treatment of mature B-cell malignancies. *Br J Cancer.* 1990;**62**:4–5.

33 Dillman RO, Mick R, McIntyre OR. Pentostatin in chronic lymphocytic leukemia: a phase II trial of Cancer and Leukemia Group B. *J Clin Oncol.* 1989;**7**:433–38.

34 Grever MR, Siaw MFE, Jacob WF, et al. The biochemical and clinical consequences of 2'-deoxycoformycin in refractory lymphoproliferative malignancy. *Blood.* 1981;**57**:406–17.

35 Ho AD, Ganeshaguru K, Knauf WU, et al. Clinical response to deoxycoformycin in chronic lymphoid neoplasms and biochemical changes in circulating malignant cells in vivo. *Blood.* 1988;**72**:1884–90.

36 Grever MR, Leiby JM, Kraut EH, et al. Low-dose deoxycoformycin in lymphoid malignancy. *J Clin Oncol.* 1985;**3**:1196–201.

37 Ho AD, Thaler J, Strykmans P, et al. Pentostatin in refractory chronic lymphocytic leukemia: a phase II trial of the European Organization for Research and Treatment of Cancer. *J Natl Cancer Inst.* 1990;**82**: 1416–20.

38 Grever MR, Coleman MS, Gray DP, et al. Definition of safe, effective, dosing regimen of 2'-deoxycoformycin with biochemical investigation. *Cancer Treat Symp.* 1984;**2**:43–49.

39 O'Dwyer PJ, Spiers ASD, Marsoni S. Association of severe and fatal infections and treatment with pentostatin. *Cancer Treat Rep.* 1986;**70**:1117–20.

40 O'Dwyer PJ, Wagner B, Leyland-Jones B, et al. 2'-deoxycoformycin (pentostatin) for lymphoid malignancies. *Ann Intern Med.* 1988;**108**:733–43.

41 Daeninck PJ, Johnston JB, Eisenhauer E, et al. Treatment of hairy cell leukemia with low-dose 2'deoxycoformycin: results of long-term follow-up [abstract 60]. *Proc ASCO.* 1997;**16**:17a.

42 Flinn IW, Kopecky KJ, Foucar MK, et al. Long-term results in hairy cell leukemia (HCL) treated with pentostatin [abstract 2575]. *Blood.* 1997:**90**:578a.

43 Cheson BD, Vena D, Barrett J, et al. Second malignancies as a consequence of nucleoside analog therapy of chronic lymphoid leukemias. *J Clin Oncol.* 1999;**17**:2454–60.

44 Lamanna N, Kalaycio M, Maslak P, et al. Pentostatin, cyclophosphamide, and rituximab is an active, well-tolerated regimen for patients with previously treated chronic lymphocytic leukemia. *J Clin Oncol* 2006;**24**:1575–81.

45 Österborg A, Dyer MJS, Bunjes D, et al. Phase II multicenter study of human CD52 antibody in previously treated chronic lymphocytic leukemia. *J Clin Oncol.* 1997;**15**:1567–74.

46 Keating MJ, Byrd J, Rai K, et al. Multicenter study of CAMPATH-1H in patients with chronic lymphocytic leukemia refractory to fludarabine [abstract 3118]. *Blood.* 1999;**94**:705a.

47 Rai KR, Coutré S, Rizzieri D, et al. Efficacy and safety of alemtuzumab (CAMPATH-1H) in refractory B-CLL patients treated on a compassionate basis [abstract 1538]. *Blood.* 2001;**98**:365a.

48 Moreton P, Kennedy B, Lucas G, et al. Eradication of minimal residual disease in B-cell chronic lymphocytic leukemia after alemtuzumab therapy is associated with prolonged survival. *J Clin Oncol.* 2005;**23**: 2971–79.

49 Lundin J, Kimby E, Björkholm M, et al. Phase II trial of subcutaneous anti-CD52 monoclonal antibody alemtuzumab (CAMPATH-1H) as first-line treatment for patients with B-cell chronic lymphocytic leukemia (B-CLL). *Blood.* 2002;**100**:768–73.

50 Nguyen DT, Amess JA, Doughty H, et al. IDEC-C2B8 anti-CD20 (rituximab) immunotherapy in patients with low-grade non-Hodgkin's lymphoma and lymphoproliferative disorders: evaluation of response on 48 patients. *Eur J Haematol.* 1999;**62**:76–82.

51 Maloney DG, Grillo-López AJ, White CA, et al. IDEC-C2B8 (Rituximab) anti-CD20- monoclonal antibody therapy in patients with relapsed low-grade non-Hodgkin's lymphoma. *Blood.* 1997;**90**:2188–95.

52 Piro LD, White CA, Grillo-Lopez AJ, et al. Extended rituximab (anti-CD20 monoclonal antibody) therapy for relapsed or refractory low-grade or follicular non-Hodgkin's lymphoma. *Ann Oncol.* 1999;**10**:655–61.

53 Winkler U, Jensen M, Manzke O, et al. Cytokine-release syndrome in patients with B-cell chronic lymphocytic leukemia and high lymphocyte counts after treatment with an anti-CD20 monoclonal antibody (Rituximab, IDEC-C2B8). *Blood.* 1999;**94**:2217–24.

54 Huhn D, von Schilling C, Wilhelm M, et al. Rituximab therapy of patients with B-cell chronic lymphocytic leukemia. *Blood.* 2001;**98**:1326–31.

55 Foran JM, Rohatiner AZ, Cunningham D, et al. European phase II study of rituximab (Chimeric anti-CD20 monoclonal antibody) for patients with newly diagnosed mantle-cell lymphoma and previously treated mantle-cell lymphoma, immunocytoma, and small B-cell lymphocytic lymphoma. *J Clin Oncol.* 2000;**18**:317–24.

56 Byrd J, O'Brien S, Flinn I, et al. Interim results from a phase I study of lumiliximab (IDEC-152, anti-CD23 antibody) therapy for relapsed or refractory CLL [abstract]. *Blood.* 2003;**102**:248.

57 Byrd JC, O'Brien S, Flinn IW, et al. Preliminary results from a phase I/II study of lumiliximab in combination with FCR for previously treated patients with chronic lymphocytic leukemia [abstract 113]. *Leuk Lymphoma.* 2005;**46**:S96.

58 Coiffier B, Tilly H, Pedersen LM, et al. HuMax CD20 fully human monoclonal antibody in chronic lymphocytic leukemia. Early results from an ongoing phase I/II clinical trial [abstract 448]. *Blood.* 2005;**106**:135a.

59 Chanan-Khan A, Miller KC, Musialo L, et al. Clinical efficacy of lenalidomide in patients with relapsed or refractory chronic lymphocytic leukemia: results of a phase II study. *J Clin Oncol.* 2006;**24**:5343–49.

60 O'Brien SM, Cunningham CC, Golenkov AK, et al. Phase I to II multicenter study of oblimersen sodium, a Bcl-2 antisense oligonucleotide, in patients with advanced chronic lymphocytic leukemia. *J Clin Oncol.* 2005;**23**:7697–702.

61 O'Brien S, Moore JO, Boyd TE, et al. Randomized phase 3 trial of fludarabine plus cyclophosphamide with or without oblimersen sodium (Bcl-2 antisense) in patients with relapsed or refractory chronic lymphocytic leukemia. *J Clin Oncol.* 2007;**25**:1114–20.

62 Mavromatis B, Rai KR, Wallace PK, et al. Efficacy and safety of the combination of Genasense (Oblimersen sodium, Bcl-2 antisense oligonucleotide), fludarabine and rituximab in previously treated and untreated subjects with chronic lymphocytic leukemia [abstract 2129]. *Blood.* 2005;**106**:602a.

63 O'Brien S, Kipps T, Faderl S, et al. A phase I trial of the small molecule pan-Bcl-2 family inhibitor GX15-070 administered intravenously (IV) every 3 233ks to patients with previously treated chronic lymphocytic leukemia (CLL). *Blood.* 2005;in press.

64 Knauf WU, Lissichkov T, Aldaoud A, et al. Bendamustine versus chlorambucil in treatment-naive patients with B-cell chronic lymphocytic leukemia: Results of an international study. *Blood.* 2007;**110**:609a (abstr).

65 Rabinowe SN, Soiffer RJ, Gribben JG, et al. Autologous and allogeneic bone marrow transplantation for poor prognosis patients with B-cell chronic lymphocytic leukemia. *Blood.* 1993;**82**:1366–76.

66 Khouri IF, Keating MJ, Vriesendorp HM, et al. Autologous and allogeneic bone marrow transplantation for chronic lymphocytic leukemia: preliminary results. *J Clin Oncol.* 1994;**12**:748–58.

67 Michallet M, Archimbaud E, Bandini G, et al. HLA-identical sibling bone marrow transplantation in younger patients with chronic lymphocytic leukemia. *Ann Intern Med.* 1996;**124**:311–15.

68 Khouri IF, Przepiorka D, van Besien K, et al. Allogeneic blood or marrow transplantation for chronic lymphocytic leukaemia: timing of transplantation and potential effect of fludarabine on acute graft-versus-host disease. *Br J Haematol.* 1997;**97**:466–73.

69 Slavin S, Nagler A, Naparstek E, et al. Nonmyeloablative stem cell transplantation and cell therapy as an alternative to conventional bone marrow transplantation with lethal cytoreduction for the treatment of malignant and nonmalignant hematologic diseases. *Blood.* 1998;**91**:756–63.

70 Khouri IF, Keating M, Körbling M, et al. Transplant-lite: induction of graft-versus malignancy using fludarabine-based nonablative chemotherapy and allogeneic blood progenitor-cell transplantation as treatment for lymphoid malignancies. *J Clin Oncol.* 1998;**16**:2817–24.

71 Khouri I, Keating MJ, Przepiorka D, et al. Stem cell transplantation (SCT) for chronic lymphocytic leukemia (CLL). Graft-versus-leukemia (GVL) without acute graft-versus-host disease (GVHD) [abstract 1814]. *Blood.* 1995;**86**:457.

72 Pavletic ZS, Bierman PJ, Vose JM, et al. High incidence of relapse after autologous stem-cell transplantation for B-cell chronic lymphocytic leukemia or small lymphocytic lymphoma. *Ann Oncol.* 1998;**9**:1023–26.

73 Sutton L, Maloum K, Gonzalez H, et al. Autologous hematopoietic stem cell transplantation as salvage treatment for advanced B cell chronic lymphocytic leukemia. *Leukemia.* 1998;**12**:1699–707.

37 Chronic Myeloid Leukemia

Irwin Walker

Introduction

Chronic myeloid leukemia (CML), with its classical Philadelphia chromosome marker, is caused by a fusion protein, BCR-ABL, the product of an abnormal chimeric gene formed by translocation of a portion of the ABL gene on chromosome 9 to the region adjacent to the BCR region on chromosome 22 (1). CML progresses through chronic, accelerated, and blastic phases, with consequent worsening prognosis, the median survival of patients with minimal or no treatment being four to five years (2).

Randomized trials conducted over 30 years have demonstrated improved survivals with successive new therapies (2–9). This evidence-based review uses combined cytarabine/interferon therapy as the historical starting point.

Questions

1. What is the recommended treatment for patients with CML at diagnosis?
2. What is the place of bone marrow transplantation at diagnosis?
3. What is the recommended treatment where first line treatment has failed?

Grading of the quality of evidence and strengths of recommendations in this chapter are based on the guidelines proposed by the international Grading of Recommendations Assessment, Development, and Evaluation Working Group (GRADE) adopting the modification used by the American College of Chest Physicians that merges the very low and low categories of quality of evidence (see chapter 1).

Evidence-based Hematology. Edited by Mark A. Crowther, Jeff Ginsberg, Holger J. Schünemann, Ralph M. Meyer, and Richard Lottenberg.
 ISBN: 978-1-4051-5747-6.

Literature-search strategy and inclusions

In keeping with the protocol for this publication, the weight of evidence was given, in order, to systematic reviews and meta-analyses, to randomized controlled trials, and then to other clinical trials. The literature search was conducted using MEDLINE, EMBASE, *Cochrane Database of Systematic Reviews* (DSR), TRIP database (www.tripdatabase.com), National Guideline Clearing House (www.guideline.gov), U.S. National Institutes of Health (clinicaltrials.gov), and the National Institutes of Health (www.cancer.gov/cancertopics/pdq).

What is the recommended treatment for patients with CML at the time of diagnosis?

Three systematic reviews were selected as being of high quality, and current to the period following the introduction of imatinib, from the National Institute for Clinical Excellence (NICE) (10), European LeukemiaNet (11), and Cancer Care Ontario Program in Evidenced Based Care (12). MEDLINE and EMBASE were searched for randomized trials published in the period (2004–2006) following the above reviews. No randomized trials were found.

Findings in Systematic Reviews

Data from the International Randomized Interferon versus STI571 (IRIS) trial (13) dominated the assessments of all three reviews. The IRIS trial compared imatinib (553 subjects) with the existing standard of combined interferon/cytarabine (553 subjects). The primary endpoint was freedom from progression, defined as the occurrence of either accelerated phase, blast phase, loss of either complete hematologic response or major cytogenetic response, or death. The estimated rate of freedom from progression to accelerated-phase or blast-crisis, at 18 months, was 96.7% in the imatinib group and 91.5% in the combination-therapy group ($p < 0.001$). After a median follow-up of 19 months, the estimated rate of a major cytogenetic response was 87.1% in the imatinib group and 34.7% in the combination-therapy group ($p < 0.001$). The estimated rates of complete cytogenetic response were 76.2% and 14.5%, respectively ($p < 0.001$). Finally, imatinib was better tolerated than the combination therapy, frequencies of grade 3 or 4 toxicities, withdrawals due to intolerability, and crossovers all being higher in the combined therapy group. A total of 79 patients (14.3%) in the imatinib group and 493 patients (89.2%) in the combination-therapy group either discontinued treatment or crossed over to the alternative treatment group.

The conclusions of all three reviews were that imatinib was superior to combined interferon/cytarabine therapy, and was the first choice of therapy, at a starting dose of 400 mg daily. However, the reviews also concluded that the optimal dose had not been determined.

Long-term follow-up of the IRIS trial

The IRIS trial was published with a median follow up of 19 months and a 60-month follow-up has also been published (14). Of the 553 patients randomized to imatinib, 69% have remained on therapy, and overall survival is 89% (92% when censored at bone marrow transplantation). Ninety-three percent of patients have been free of progression to accelerated phase or blast crisis. There were two important additional observations: (1) the rate of progression to accelerated phase or blast crisis was lower in the fourth and fifth years (0.9% and 0.6%, respectively) than in each of the first three years (1.5%, 2.8%, and 1.6% respectively), indicating that initial responses have been durable; (2) failure to achieve a major cytogenetic response (either complete or partial) at one year was a predictor for subsequent progression to accelerated phase or blast crisis (3% and 7% for complete and partial responders, 19% for the remainder). The difference between complete and partial responders was not statistically significant, but the difference between either of these responders and those remaining was highly statistically significant ($p < 0.001$).

Survival is the most important endpoint in CML; however, a survival advantage of imatinib could not be demonstrated in the IRIS trial. The trial design did not include survival as an endpoint, and, further, 65% of interferon-treated patients had crossed over to imatinib by 60 months, and only 3% of patients remained on this therapy. In the absence of information on survival from randomized trials, two retrospective cohort comparison studies have been performed, both finding improved survival with imatinib compared with interferon/cytarabine (15,16). These two studies are important in providing the only information ever likely to become available on the impact on survival of imatinib compared with interferon-based therapy. Though these studies were not randomized, the findings are consistent. Further, the cohorts used by Roy et al. for their comparison had previously been well defined, having been arms of previous randomized trials.

Recommendation

Imatinib, 400 mg/d, is the recommended treatment for newly diagnosed patients with Philadelphia-positive (or BCR:ABL positive) CML. (Grade 1A).

Predictors for progression to accelerated phase or blast crisis include failure to achieve a hematological remission at 3 months, a major cytogenetic remission at 12 months, and a major molecular remission at 12 months.

What is the place of bone marrow transplantation at the time of diagnosis?

Findings in searches for reviews and randomized trials in transplantation

Two systematic reviews of transplantation in CML were identified, one reviewing the results of full allogeneic transplantation as part of an overall review of therapy of CML (6), the other, more recently, reviewing nonmyeloablative transplantation in general (17). These reviews failed to identify randomized trials comparing transplantation with other modes of therapy in CML, either of the classic randomized design or the method of biological randomization used most often in transplant studies (18,19). A subsequent search for randomized trials undertaken for this review likewise failed to find any randomized trials. The only systematic, though not randomized, study comparing transplantation with other therapies was conducted in the pre-imatinib era; this was a systematic and matched comparison of the results of transplantation from the International Bone Marrow Transplant Registry with the results of hydroxyurea or interferon therapy from the German CML Study Group (20). This study showed a survival advantage for chemotherapy in the first 4–5.5 years after diagnosis then with a crossover in the survival curves; transplanted patients subsequently survived better than chemotherapy-treated patients with the time of crossover varying according to the Sokal risk group. There have been two uncontrolled series reported recently of patients with CML undergoing transplantation, using non-myeloablative and ablative conditioning, respectively. The European Group for Blood and Marrow Transplantation (EBMT) has reported on 118 patients undergoing nonmyeloablative transplantation a median of 11.7 months since diagnosis and with median age 48 years; three-year disease-free and overall survivals were 44.9% and 69%, respectively (21). EBMT has reported also the results of patients undergoing transplantation with ablative conditioning (22); of 1,828 patients transplanted in first chronic phase from 1980 to 1990, survival at 5, 10, 15, and 20 years has been 51%, 46%, 40%, and 38%, respectively. Of 1,621 patients transplanted using only sibling donors, survival at 15 years has been 41%. Two-year survivals of three cohorts transplanted from 1980 to 1990, 1991 to 1999, and 2000 to 2003 have improved by 50% (relative risk of 0.5 for most recent cohort) due to a decrease in transplant mortality. Multivariate analysis showed a low EBMT risk score (23–25) and use of a sibling donor as significant for prediction of survival, 49% of patients with a score of 0–1 being expected to live 20 years.

The positive qualities of data from EBMT are the high level of reporting and the large numbers of patients; however, the data suffer from a lack of prospective criteria for transplantation, and, ultimately, by lacking a matched comparison group the data fall down in not being able to address the question of most appropriate therapy.

Other information regarding bone marrow transplantation

Three systematic studies, while not comparing transplantation with other modes of therapy, are relevant to decisions about performing transplantation and to the way of performing the procedure itself. First, the well-validated EBMT risk score (23–25) provides a prediction of transplant-related mortality; second, a long-term follow-up of four randomized trials showed similar rates of survival for the two most commonly used preparative regimens of BuCy (busulfan/cyclophosphamide) and CyTBI (cyclophosphamide/total body irradiation); third, addition of antithymocyte globulin may decrease the rate of chronic graft versus host disease and improve survival of patients receiving grafts from unrelated donors (26).

In conclusion, there is no high-level scientific evidence on which to compare transplantation over other therapies in the imatinib era. Furthermore, while transplantation is the only modality known to produce a cure in a substantial number of patients, the high early mortality (26% at two years for patients transplanted in first chronic phase) stands in contrast to the 93% five-year survival of patients treated with imatinib in the IRIS trial.

Recommendation

Transplantation should be recommended only for patients for whom newer drugs have failed or have resulted in unacceptable toxicity (Grade 1C).

What is the recommended treatment for patients with CML where first line treatment has failed?

How is "failure" defined?

Absolute failure of imatinib therapy is defined as either failure to attain a complete hematological response, progression to either accelerated phase or blast crisis, excessive toxicity, or intolerance. Other definitions, based on laboratory criteria, of failure to attain either a major cytogenetic remission (<35% Ph+ cells) or a major molecular response (>3 log reduction in BCR:ABL transcripts), as well as their timing, are more controversial. Recognizing this, the European LeukemiaNet (11) has classified endpoints at various time points as either "failure," "suboptimal response," or "warnings." The authors designated their classification as "operational"; however, longer follow-up from the IRIS trial continues to support and even strengthens this classification. The specific treatment recommendations assigned to each designation must however be considered tentative given the extensive clinical research results rapidly becoming available, on dosage of imatinib, combination with other agents, and introduction of new agents.

Table 37.1 Percentage of subjects randomized to imatinib (IRIS trial) having long-term event-free survival (EFS), according to degree of cytogenetic and molecular responses.

Endpoints		Time points of observation*		
Type	**Response**	**6 months %**	**12 months %**	**18 months %**
Cytogenetic response	Complete	95[†]	97[‡]	99[‡]
	Partial		93[‡]	90[‡,§]
	Minimal or none	75[†,§,‖]	81[‡,§]	83[‡]
Molecular response	Complete		100[¶]	100[‡]
	Major			98[‡]
	Minor		93[§,¶]	87[‡,§]

*%, percent of subjects with long-term EFS.
[†] At 24 months.
[¶] At 30 months.
[‡] At 60 months.
[§] Statistically significantly inferior to best result.
[‖] Significant only for "no response" (Ph = cells >95%); molecular responses are those in subjects having "Complete" or "Partial" cytogenetic responses.

The overall survival of patients on imatinib in the IRIS trial after five years was 89%, and all patients achieving both a complete cytogenetic response (0% Ph+ cells) and a major molecular response (>3 log suppression) at 18 months continued in chronic phase without AP or BC thereafter; this then indicates total success, and any lesser result could be regarded as relative or absolute failure. However, even those who achieved a complete cytogenetic response at 18 months but lacked a major molecular response had only a 2% likelihood of AP or BC, and this difference was not significant. Overall, 99% of all patients achieving a major cytogenetic remission at 12 months continued without AP/BC regardless of molecular response, while if only a partial response was achieved (<35% Ph+ cells) 10% of patients progressed to AP or BC.

Table 37.1 summarizes the likelihood of long-term event-free survival of the 553 patients randomized to imatinib on the IRIS study as predicted by the attainment of various endpoints at different time periods. The data are taken from three follow-up reports of this study (14,27,28).

What options are available to treat patients that have failed imatinib therapy?

There is a lack of randomized trials to guide either the choice or the timing of therapy for those who have failed imatinib, and the risks and benefits of each option may in turn differ for each definition of "failure," for example, bone marrow transplantation for patients in accelerated phase compared with those lacking only a major molecular response. This review will be confined to describing agents that are available for clinical use, either licensed or in advanced stage of clinical trials.

Two newly developed drugs, dasatinib and nilotinib, have dramatically changed the considerations for patients failing imatinib therapy being, like imatinib, relatively specific inhibitors of BCR:ABL and low in toxicity. In mid-2006, the U.S. National Cancer Institute announced their availability for clinical use following the completion of phase I trials (29,30) in patients with imatinib resistance or intolerance (31).

Dasatinib. Dasatinib (BMS-354825, Bristol-Myers Squibb) is an orally available ABL kinase inhibitor that differs from imatinib in that it can bind to both the active and inactive conformations of the ABL kinase domain. Dasatinib also inhibits a distinct spectrum of kinases that overlaps with the array of kinases that imatinib inhibits (29). Eighty-four subjects (74 CML, 10 with ALL) who were resistant (86%) or intolerant (14%) to imatinib took part in a phase I dose-escalation trial to determine tolerance. Subjects were treated with doses up to 180 mg/d (single dose) or 70 mg twice daily. Sixty percent of patients required dose interruptions, and 25% required dose reductions, but apparently, no patients withdrew from the study as a result of toxic effects, which seemed to be transient in many instances. The commonest nonhematological toxicities were pleural effusions in 18% and transient disturbances of liver function in 8.3%. Patients previously experiencing toxicities with imatinib did not experience the same toxicities with dasatinib. For patients in chronic phase ($n = 40$), complete hematologic and major cytogenetic responses were 92% and 45%, respectively. Of those in accelerated phase ($n = 11$), complete hematologic response was achieved in 45%. Of those in blast crisis ($n = 23$), complete hematologic responses were seen in 35%, but these responses were uniformly short-lived.

Nilotinib. Nilotinib (AMN107, Novartis) is a new, orally active, aminopyrimidine-derivative tyrosine kinase inhibitor that is more potent against CML cells in vitro than is imatinib and was active in 32 of 33 imatinib-resistant cell lines with mutant ABL kinases (30). One hundred and nineteen subjects (106 CML, 13 ALL) with resistance to imatinib took part in a phase I dose-escalation trial. The maximum tolerated dose was 600 mg bid, but there was no discernable difference in response rate with the lower dose of 400 mg bid, and the side-effect profile was better. Grade 4 hematologic toxicities were common, but nonhematologic toxicities were uncommon, consisting mostly of abnormalities in laboratory changes in liver function or lipase, or in skin changes. Complete hematologic responses were seen in 11 of 17 (65%) of patients in chronic phase, in 26 of 56 (46%) of patients in accelerated phase, and in 2 of 24 patients with myeloid blast crisis. Complete cytogenetic responses were seen in 35%, 27%, and 21% of these groups. In October 2007, on the evidence from phase II studies (32, 33), the U.S. Federal Drug Authority (FDA) gave accelerated approval for the use of nilotinib in patients failing or intolerant of other therapies.

Comparison of dasatinib and imatinib in patients resistant to imatinib. The START-R study (34) compared dasatinib 70 mg bid to imatinib 800 mg daily in patients resistant to imatinib 400–600 mg daily. The major endpoint was complete cytogenetic response. One hundred and fifty patients were randomized in a 2:1 ratio, 101 to dasatinib and 49 to imatinib. The duration of follow-up was 15 months. Dasatinib was found to be superior to imatinib with respect to complete hematologic responses (93% versus 82%, $p = .034$), major cytogenetic response rates (52% versus 33%, $p = .023$), complete cytogenetic response (40% versus 16%, $p = .004$), and attainment of major molecular responses (16% versus 4%, $p = .038$). Treatment failure (hazard ratio 0.16, $p < .001$) and progression-free survival (hazard ratio 0.16, $p < .001$) also favoured dasatinib. Superficial edema and fluid retention were more common with imatinib, while pleural effusions and cytopenias were more frequent and severe with dasatinib.

In June 2006, the FDA gave accelerated approval for dasatinib use in patients failing prior therapies, the recommended dose being 70 mg bid. Subsequently, a four-arm study (34) was conducted comparing doses of 140 mg daily with 100 mg daily, both as single daily doses, and divided doses twice daily. A dose of 100 mg taken once daily resulted in fewer side effects with no diminution in effectiveness.

Bone marrow transplantation

There is a complete lack of comparative trials involving transplantation with which to guide a choice toward bone marrow transplantation in patients failing imatinib. Survival after transplantation in accelerated phase or blast crisis is poor; EBMT experience being 29% and 18% at five years, respectively (22).

Recommendation

For patients failing imatinib therapy at 400-600 mg daily, dasatinib at a dose of 100 mg once daily is highly effective (Grade 1A). Alternatively, nilotinib at a dose of 400 mg twice daily can also be recommended.

References

1 Goldman J. M, Melo J. V. Chronic myeloid leukemia—advances in biology and new approaches to treatment. *N Engl J Med.* 2003;**349**(15):1451–64.

2 Anonymous. Interferon alfa versus chemotherapy for chronic myeloid leukemia: A meta-analysis of seven randomized trials. Chronic myeloid leukemia trialists' collaborative group. *J Natl Cancer Inst.* 1997;**89**(21):1616–20.

3 Anonymous. Chronic granulocytic leukaemia: Comparison of radiotherapy and busulphan therapy. Report of the medical research council's working party for therapeutic trials in leukaemia. *Br Med J.* 1968;**1**(5586):201–8.

4 Hehlmann R, Heimpel H, Hasford J, et al. Randomized comparison of busulfan and hydroxyurea in chronic myelogenous leukemia: Prolongation of survival by hydroxyurea: the German CML study group. *Blood.* 1993;**82**(2):398–407.

5 Chronic Myeloid Leukemia Trialists' Collaborative Group. Hydroxyurea versus busulphan for chronic myeloid leukaemia: an individual patient data meta-analysis of three randomized trials. *Br J Haematol.* 2000;**110**(3):573–76.

6 Silver RT, Woolf SH, Hehlmann R, et al. An evidence-based analysis of the effect of busulfan, hydroxyurea, interferon, and allogeneic bone marrow transplantation in treating the chronic phase of chronic myeloid leukemia: developed for the American Society of Hematology. *Blood.* 1999;**94**(5):1517–36.

7 Guilhot F, Chastang C, Michallet M, et al. Interferon alfa-2b combined with cytarabine versus interferon alone in chronic myelogenous leukemia. *N Engl J Med.* 1997;**337**(4):223–29.

8 Walker I, Benger A, Browman G, et al. Drug therapy for chronic myeloid leukaemia. *Curr Oncol.* 2000;**7**(4):229–41.

9 Randomized trial of splenectomy in Ph1-positive chronic granulocytic leukaemia, including an analysis of prognostic features. *Br J Haematol.* 1983;**54**(3):415–30.

10 Dalziel K, Round A, Stein K, et al. Effectiveness and cost-effectiveness of imatinib for first-line treatment of chronic myeloid leukaemia in chronic phase: a systematic review and economic analysis. *Health Technol Assess.* 2004;**8**(28):1–120.

11 Baccarani M, Saglio G, Goldman J, et al. Evolving concepts in the management of chronic myeloid leukemia: Recommendations from an expert panel on behalf of the European Leukemia Net. *Blood.* 2006;**108**(6):1809–20.

12 Treatment of chronic myeloid leukemia with imatinib [homepage on the Internet]. Toronto (ON): Cancer Care Ontario (CCO) Hematology Disease Site Group. 16 Jul 2004 [cited 12 Nov 2006]. Available from: www.guideline.gov.

13 O'Brien SG, Guilhot F, Larson RA, et al. Imatinib compared with interferon and low-dose cytarabine for newly diagnosed chronic-phase chronic myeloid leukemia. *N Engl J Med.* 2003;**348**(11):994–1004.

14 Druker BJ, Guilhot F, O'Brien SG, et al. Five-year follow-up of patients receiving imatinib for chronic myeloid leukemia. *N Engl J Med.* 2006;**355**(23):2408–17.

15 Kantarjian HM, Talpaz M, O'Brien S, et al. Survival benefit with imatinib mesylate versus interferon-alpha-based regimens in newly diagnosed chronic-phase chronic myelogenous leukemia. *Blood.* 2006;**108**(6):1835–40.

16 Roy L, Guilhot J, Krahnke T, et al. Survival advantage from imatinib compared with the combination interferon-alpha plus cytarabine in chronic-phase chronic myelogenous leukemia: historical comparison between two phase 3 trials. *Blood.* 2006;**108**(5):1478–84.

17 Djulbegovic B, Seidenfeld J, Bonnell C, et al. Nonmyeloablative allogeneic stem-cell transplantation for hematologic malignancies: a systematic review. *Cancer Control.* 2003;**10**(1):17–41.

18 Burnett AK, Wheatley K, Goldstone AH, et al. The value of allogeneic bone marrow transplant in patients with acute myeloid leukaemia at differing risk of relapse: results of the UK MRC AML 10 trial. *Br J Haematol.* 2002;**118**(2):385–400.

19 Cassileth PA, Harrington DP, Appelbaum FR, et al. Chemotherapy compared with autologous or allogeneic bone marrow transplantation in the management of acute myeloid leukemia in first remission. *N Engl J Med.* 1998;**339**(23):1649–56.

20 Gale RP, Hehlmann R, Zhang MJ, et al. Survival with bone marrow transplantation versus hydroxyurea or interferon for chronic myelogenous leukemia: the German CML study group. *Blood.* 1998;**91**(5):1810–19.

21 Crawley C, Szydlo R, Lalancette M, et al. Outcomes of reduced-intensity transplantation for chronic myeloid leukemia: an analysis of prognostic factors from the chronic leukemia working party of the EBMT. *Blood.* 2005;**106**(9):2969–76.

22 Gratwohl A, Brand R, Apperley J, et al. Allogeneic hematopoietic stem cell transplantation for chronic myeloid leukemia in Europe 2006: transplant activity, long-term data and current results. An analysis by the chronic leukemia working party of the European group for blood and marrow transplantation (EBMT). *Haematologica.* 2006;**91**(4):513–21.

23 Gratwohl A, Hermans J, Goldman J, et al. Risk assessment for patients with chronic myeloid leukaemia before allogeneic blood or marrow transplantation. *Lancet.* 1998;**352**(9134):1087–92.

24 Passweg JR, Walker I, Sobocinski KA, et al. Validation and extension of the EBMT risk score for patients with chronic myeloid leukaemia (CML) receiving allogeneic haematopoietic stem cell transplants. *Br J Haematol.* 2004;**125**(5):613–20.

25 De Souza CA, Vigorito AC, Ruiz MA, et al. Validation of the EBMT risk score in chronic myeloid leukemia in brazil and allogeneic transplant outcome. *Haematologica.* 2005;**90**(2):232–37.

26 Bacigalupo A, Lamparelli T, Barisione G, et al. Thymoglobulin prevents chronic graft-versus-host disease, chronic lung dysfunction, and late transplant-related mortality: long-term follow-up of a randomized trial in patients undergoing unrelated donor transplantation. *Biol Blood Marrow Transplantation.* 2006;**12**(5):560–65.

27 Druker B, Gathmann I, Bolton AE. Probability and impact of obtaining acytogenetic response to imatinib as initial therapy for chronic myeloid leukemiain chronic phase. *Blood.* 2003;**102**:182a (abstr).

28 Guilhot F. Sustained durability of responses plus high rates of cytogenetic responses result in long term benefit for newly diagnosedchronic phase chronic myeloid leukemia treated with imatinib therapy: update from the IRIS study. *Blood.* 2004;**104**:10a (abstr).

29 Talpaz M, Shah NP, Kantarjian H, et al. Dasatinib in imatinib-resistant philadelphia chromosome-positive leukemias. *N Engl J Med.* 2006;**354**(24):2531–41.

30 Kantarjian H, Giles F, Wunderle L, et al. Nilotinib in imatinib-resistant CML and philadelphia chromosome-positive ALL. *N Engl J Med.* 2006;**354**(24):2542–51.

31 National Cancer Institute. Nilotinib and dasatinib are safe, potentially effective treatment for pH-positive leukemias. Available from: http://www.cancer.gov.libaccess.lib.mcmaster.ca/clinicaltrials/results/nilotinib-and-dasatinib0706.

32 Le Coutre P, Bhalla K, Giles F, *et al.*, A phase II study of nilotinib, a novel tyrosine kinase inhibitor administered to imatinib-resistant and -intolerant patients with chronic myelogenous leukemia (CML) in chronic phase (CP), *Blood* **108** (2006), p. 53A (abstr 165).

33 Hochhaus A, Erben P, Branford S, *et al.*, Hematologic and cytogenetic response dynamics to nilotinib (AMN107) depend on the type of BCR-ABL mutations in patients with chronic myelogeneous leukemia (CML) after imatinib failure, *Blood* **108** (2006), p. 225A (abstr 749).

34 Kantarjian H, Pasquini R, Hamerschlak N, et al. Dasatinib or high-dose imatinib for chronic-phase chronic myeloid leukemia after failure of first-line imatinib: a randomized phase 2 trial. *Blood.* 2007;**109**:5143–5150.

35 Shah NP, Kim DW, Kantarjian HM, Rousselot P, Dorlhiac-Llacer PE, Milone JH, et al. Dasatinib 50 mg or 70 mg BID compared to 100 mg or 140 mg QD in patients with CML in chronic phase (CP) who are resistant or intolerant to imatinib: one-year results of CA180034. *J Clin Oncol.* 2007;25(18S): (abstr).

38 Selected Management of Patients with Myelodysplastic Syndromes

John M. Storring, Karen W. L. Yee

Introduction

An estimated 10,268 new cases of myelodysplastic syndromes (MDS) were diagnosed in the United States in 2003 with an overall incidence rate of 3.1 per 100,000 (1,2). However, disease incidence increases with age, with an approximate fivefold difference in estimates for those diagnosed at ages 60–69 years compared with those at ages 80 years and older (7.8 per 100,000 versus 39.3 per 100,000) (2). The myelodysplastic syndromes comprise a heterogenous group of clonal hematopoietic stem cell disorders characterized by ineffective hematopoiesis and peripheral cytopenias in the presence of a normo- or hypercellular bone marrow (3). Recently, the World Health Organization (WHO) classification (4) has superseded the French-American-British (FAB) classification (5) of the MDS subgroups. Although the FAB and WHO classifications have prognostic significance, the International Prognostic Scoring System (IPSS), which was derived from multivariate analysis of predominantly untreated patients with de novo MDS (6) has been used more frequently in treatment decision making and clinical trials. The IPSS score employs objective parameters and thus allows for improved reproducibility. Furthermore, the development and employment of a standardized criteria for assessing response in patients with MDS has ensured comparability between studies and permitted evaluation of the clinical significance of new therapeutic agents (7,8).

Treatment has generally been limited to observation and supportive measures as the patients are usually older with frequent comorbidities and clinically efficacious interventions were lacking. Therefore, the patients usually succumb to complications arising from their cytopenias with a proportion dying from leukemic transformation (6). Recently, data have been published to support the idea that disease-modifying treatment with novel agents is efficacious in selected patients.

Questions

1. What is the role of lenalidomide in patients with previously untreated or treated MDS?
2. What is the role of the hypomethylating agents, azacitidine, and decitabine, in patients with MDS?
3. What constitutes a reasonable management approach to using drug therapy for patients with MDS?

Literature search and inclusion

A computer search of the following databases was performed: MEDLINE (1966 through to May 2007) and PubMed (http://www4.ncbi.nlm.nih.gov/PubMed/, as of May 14, 2007) with restriction to the English language. Both medical subject heading and text word-search terms for myelodysplasia and myelodysplastic syndrome were combined with those terms for azacitidine, decitabine, and lenalidomide. These terms were than combined with the search terms for the following study designs: practice guidelines, systematic reviews, or meta-analyses, reviews, clinical trials, randomized controlled trials (RCTs) and controlled clinical trials. Conference proceedings of the American Society of Hematology (2000–2006) and the American Society of Clinical Oncology (2000–2007) were searched. Only randomized controlled trials or phase II trials involving at least 20 patients were included.

Where possible, the grading of the quality of evidence and strengths of recommendations in this chapter are based on the guidelines proposed by the International Grading of Recommendations Assessment, Development, and Evaluation Working Group (GRADE) adopting the modification used by the

Evidence-based Hematology. Edited by Mark A. Crowther, Jeff Ginsberg, Holger J. Schünemann, Ralph M. Meyer, and Richard Lottenberg.

American College of Chest Physicians that merges the "very low" and "low" categories of quality of evidence (see chapter 1).

What is the role of lenalidomide in patients with previously untreated or treated MDS?

The tumor microenvironment and cytokine milieu, secreted by the malignant cells or marrow stromal cells, are important for survival, growth, and resistance of a variety of hematological malignancies, including MDS (9–11). The precise mechanism of action of immunomodulating drugs, such as thalidomide and its derivatives (e.g., lenalidomide), are unclear and may be mediated by antiangiogenesis, immunomodulation, or direct cytotoxic effects (12). Lenalidomide is more potent and effective, with fewer toxicities, than thalidomide (12).

In a single-center phase II trial (MDS-001), 43 patients with de novo MDS and transfusion-dependent or symptomatic anemia received single-agent lenalidomide at doses of 10 or 25 mg orally per day continuously or 10 mg orally per day for 21 days every 28 days (13). All patients had either failed therapy with recombinant erythropoietin or had an endogenous serum level of more than 500 U/L. No patients had received prior cytotoxic therapy. Eighty-eight percent of patients had a low- or intermediate-1 (INT-1) risk IPSS score (6). Neutropenia and thrombocytopenia occurred in 65% and 74% of patients, respectively, and necessitated treatment interruption or dose reductions in 58% of patients. Other common toxicities were pruritus, diarrhea, and urticaria. The overall response rate (ORR) was 56% [major hematological improvement-erythroid (HI-E) 49%; minor HI-E 7%] (7). Responses were observed at all dose levels; median time to response increased from 9 weeks to 11.5 weeks for patients treated with the 25 mg dose and those treated with 10 mg daily for 21 out of 28 days, respectively. The response rate was highest among those patients with a clonal interstitial deletion involving chromosome 5q31.1 compared with those with a normal karyotype or other abnormal karyotypes (83% vs. 57% vs. 12%, respectively; $p = 0.007$). However, the pharmacological target in the chromosome 5q31 region remains to be defined. Disease duration, FAB classification, IPSS risk category, and number of prior therapies did not correlate with response. Of the 20 patients with clonal cytogenetic abnormalities, 10 had a complete cytogenetic remission (CCyR). After a median follow-up of 81 weeks, the median response duration for major HI-E had not been reached (after >48 weeks) and the median hemoglobin level was 132 g/L compared with baseline hemoglobin levels of 80–83 g/L.

A confirmatory phase II multicenter study (MDS-003) evaluated the clinical efficacy of lenalidomide in 148 patients with low- or INT-1 risk de novo MDS, clonal interstitial deletion involving chromosome 5q31, and transfusion-dependent anemia (14). Lenalidomide was initially administered at a dose/schedule of either 10 mg orally daily for 21 days every 28 days (n = 46) and then amended to 10 mg orally daily continuously (n = 102) because of the shorter time to response observed in the pilot study (13). Although 74% of patients had an isolated 5q deletion, only 27% of patients fulfilled the criteria for del5q syndrome. Twenty-five percent had one or more cytogenetic abnormalities in addition to del(5q). Eighty-one percent of patients had low- or INT-1 risk MDS; unclassified in 14% of patients. Thirty-nine percent had received prior cytotoxic therapy. The most frequently reported toxicities were grade 3 or 4 neutropenia (55%) and thrombocytopenia (44%); neutropenic fever occurred in only 4.1% of patients. Other common adverse events were pruritus, rash, diarrhea, and fatigue. Eighty percent of patients required dose reductions. Twenty-four percent of patients were removed prior to evaluation of response at 24 weeks (due to a lack of benefit in 5%, adverse event 11%, and other 7%). In total, 11 deaths occurred, three of which were due to neutropenic infection and suspected to be drug related. In an intent-to-treat analysis, the ORR was 76%; transfusion independence was achieved in 67% of patients. A minor HI-E was observed in 9% of patients. Thirty-eight (45%) of 85 evaluable patients achieved a CCyR. There was no significant difference in response rate between the two treatment schedules ($p = 0.26$). Median time to response was 4.6 weeks. Probability of hematologic and cytogenetic response was independent of karyotype complexity and chromosomal deletion breakpoint. Hematologic and cytogenetic responses were significantly higher in patients with preserved thrombopoiesis ($p = 0.003$) and lower transfusion requirements ($p = 0.01$). Disease progression may be associated with the inability of lenalidomide to inhibit angiogenesis in the bone marrow ($p = 0.0005$) (15). After a median follow-up of 104 weeks, the median response duration for transfusion independence had not been reached. The impact of lenalidomide on overall survival and quality of life is unclear. At the current time, there are only anecdotal reports describing activity of lenalidomide in patients with therapy-related MDS (16). Limited data on the cost-effectiveness of lenalidomide in transfusion-dependent patients with low- or INT-1 risk MDS and an associated deletion 5q31 abnormality have been presented (17). A randomized, double-blinded, European trial (MDS-004) is currently evaluating these two daily doses of lenalidomide (5 mg and 10 mg) compared with placebo in low- or INT-1 risk MDS patients with transfusion-dependent anemia and a deletion 5q31 abnormality.

A phase II study (MDS-002) is evaluating the effect of lenalidomide in patients with MDS and transfusion-dependent anemia without del(5)(q31) aberrations (18–20). Lenalidomide was administered at 10 mg orally daily for 21 days every 28 days or 10 mg orally daily continuously. Of 215 patients enrolled in the study, 169 had confirmed low- or INT-1 risk MDS. Grade 3 or 4 neutropenia and thrombocytopenia occurred in 19% and 15% of patients, respectively, and necessitated dose interruption or dose reduction. In an intent-to-treat analysis, ORR was 44% (transfusion independence 27%). Of the 169 patients with low- or INT-1 risk, the ORR was 51% (transfusion independence 33%). Median time to response was 4.5 weeks. With a median follow-up of 58 weeks, the median duration of transfusion independence was 41 weeks with a median increase in hemoglobin of 33 g/L.

Recommendations

1. Three phase II studies have demonstrated that lenalidomide has clinically important activity in treating patients with *de novo* MDS. This activity includes resolution of a transfusion-dependent state. Recognizing the limitations of evidence that is based on phase II studies, treatment with lenalidomide may be a reasonable option for patients. Preliminary evidence suggests that this option may be most helpful for patients with low or INT-1 risk MDS that is associated with del(5)(q31), and a trial of therapy is therefore recommended (Grade 1C).

As only a small number of patients with INT-2 or high-risk MDS and del(5)(q31) abnormalities have received lenalidomide, treating these patients with lenalidomide is therefore associated with greater uncertainty of benefit. Despite this uncertainty, treatment of selected patients may be considered after full discussions of the limitations of the data and the potential risks of therapy (Grade 2C).

At the current time, preliminary results of the trial of lenalidomide in patients without del(5)(q31) abnormalities have only been published in abstract form; therefore, there is insufficient evidence to permit definite recommendations regarding lenalidomide in patients with transfusion-dependent anemia due to low- and INT-1 risk MDS with alternate [not del(5)(q31)] cytogenetic abnormalities (including normal karyotype) (Grade 2C).

2. There is insufficient evidence evaluating lenalidomide in patients with treatment-related MDS; therefore, treatment of these patients cannot be recommended at this time (Grade 2C).

3. When providing treatment with lenalidomide, an initial dose of 10 mg/d is recommended as this was the dose that has been most studied (Grade 1C). The optimum duration of therapy is unclear. In responding patients who are tolerating therapy, treatment may continue indefinitely (Grade 2C).

What is the role of the hypomethylating agents, azacitidine and decitabine, in patients with MDS?

Recent evidence demonstrates that epigenetic silencing of genes is associated with myelodysplasia and that a worse prognosis may be correlated with hypermethylation of certain genes (21–26). Azacitidine and decitabine, nucleoside analogues, act as hypomethylating agents. Decitabine (5-aza-deoxycytidine) is the deoxy derivative of azacitidine, which is a more potent in vitro inhibitor of DNA methyltransferase (27).

Azacitidine

Only one RCT was identified; the Cancer and Leukemia Group B (CALGB) compared azacitidine with supportive care in 191 patients with MDS categorized by FAB classification (28). Patients were randomized to azacitidine 75 mg/m^2/d administered subcutaneously for seven consecutive days every four weeks or supportive care. Patients on the supportive-care-only arm were permitted to cross over to receive azacitidine treatment, if there was disease progression after four months of supportive care; 53% of patients crossed over from supportive care to azacitidine. Complete cytogenetic data to determine IPSS score was available only for 81 patients (low 9%; INT-1 45%; INT-2 27%; high 19%) (6). Twenty percent of patients had secondary MDS and 17% had received prior therapy. The most common toxicity with azacitidine was myelosuppression. However, therapy with azacitidine did not increase the rate of infection or bleeding (29).

Therapy with azacitidine resulted in a higher response rates [23% (complete remission, CR 7%; partial remission, PR 16%) vs. 0%, $p < 0.0001$], which is comparable to what had been observed in the phase II trials (29–33). Significant hematologic improvement (HI) was observed in patients receiving azacitidine (37% vs. 5%). Response to azacitidine was independent of MDS classification. Median time to best response was 3.1 months. Median duration of response (CR, PR, or HI) was 15 months. Therapy with azacitidine was associated with a prolonged median time to event (i.e., AML or death) (21 months vs. 12 months; $p = 0.007$), but no difference in median survival was detected (20 vs. 14 months; $p = 0.10$). However, the analysis of survival was confounded as 53% of patients receiving supportive care crossed over to receive azacitidine. Therefore, a secondary six-month landmark analysis was performed that included 155 patients; median survival for the azacitidine group was significantly improved compared with patients receiving supportive care who crossed over late or never (18 vs. 11 months, $p = 0.03$). There was a significant improvement in quality of life (i.e., general well-being, psychosocial distress, physical functioning, fatigue, and dyspnea), as assessed by the Mental Health Inventory and the European Organization for Research and Treatment of Cancer (EORTC) Quality of Life Questionnaire, in patients receiving azacitidine ($p < 0.05$) (28,34).

Decitabine

Again, only one RCT was identified; low-dose decitabine was compared with supportive care in 170 patients with MDS categorized by FAB classification (IPSS score INT-1 31%; INT-2 44%; high 26%) (6,35). Patients were randomized to 15 mg/m^2 decitabine administered intravenously over three hours every eight hours for three consecutive days every six weeks for up to 10 cycles (for a total dose of 135 mg/m^2 per cycle) or supportive care. Fourteen percent of patients had secondary MDS, and 21% had received prior therapy. The groups were comparable for numerous risk factors, including median time from diagnosis (29 weeks for the decitabine arm vs. 35 weeks for the supportive care). Primary toxicity was myelosuppression. More grade 3 or 4 toxicities, including febrile neutropenia and hematologic toxicity, occurred in the decitabine arm compared to the supportive care arm.

Therapy with decitabine resulted in a higher response rates [17% (CR 9%; PR 8%) vs. 0%, $p < 0.001$]. There was also a significant HI after decitabine therapy compared to supportive care (13% vs. 7%, $p < 0.001$). Responses were observed across all IPSS groups. Median duration of response was 10.3 months. Median time to response (CR or PR) was 3.3 months or after two cycles of decitabine therapy. Differences in median time to event (i.e., AML or death) (12.1 vs. 7.8 months; $p = 0.16$) and median survival (14 vs. 14.9 months; $p = 0.636$) were not detected between the decitabine and control groups. However, subgroup analyses suggested prolonged median times to AML progression or death in patients with INT-2 or high-risk MDS (12.0 vs. 6.8 months; $p = 0.03$) or *de novo* MDS (12.6 vs. 9.4 months; $p = 0.04$) in those receiving decitabine compared with supportive care. There was a significant improvement in quality of life (i.e., global health status, physical functioning, fatigue, and dyspnea), as assessed by the EORTC Quality of Life Questionnaire, in patients receiving decitabine ($p < 0.05$). Confirmation of these findings is awaited by the completion of a phase III multicenter trial comparing the same dose/schedule of decitabine to supportive care in elderly patients (age ≥60 years old) with MDS that is currently being performed by the EORTC.

A cross-trial comparison of the overall response rates (i.e., CR+PR+HI) obtained after therapy with decitabine is less than that reported for the CALGB RCT comparing azacitidine to supportive care (28), even after reanalysis of the results using the International Working Group response criteria (30% vs. 47%) (29). This may be due to differences between the patient population treated, as a higher proportion of patients enrolled in the decitabine trial had INT-2 or high-risk IPSS scores compared to those enrolled in the CALGB study [69% vs. 37 of 81 (46%) patients, respectively], and fewer cycles of decitabine were administered compared with azacitidine (median 3 cycles vs. 9 cycles). Similarly, the response rates reported in the RCCT are lower than that obtained with similar (36–38) and alternative dosing schedules (39); however, this may be due to differences in dose intensity (36–39) or patient selection with more INT-2 and high-risk patients treated in the RCCT (70% vs. 39%) (35,39). There are no randomized trials comparing azacitidine to decitabine.

Recommendations

1. Azacitidine is indicated for the treatment of patients with the following treatment-related or de novo MDS FAB subtypes: refractory anemia (RA) or refractory anemia with ringed sideroblasts (RARS) (if accompanied by neutropenia or thrombocytopenia or requiring transfusions), refractory anemia with excess blasts (RAEB), refractory anaemia with excess blasts in transformation (RAEB-t), and chronic myelomonocytic leukemia (CMML) (Grade 1B). The duration of therapy is unclear. In the absence of disease progression, patients should receive at least four cycles of therapy before evaluating for a response (Grade 1B).

2. Decitabine is indicated for the treatment of patients with MDS, including previously treated and untreated, de novo and secondary MDS of all FAB subtypes (RA, RARS, RAEB, RAEB-t, and CMML), and INT-1, INT-2, and high-risk IPSS groups (Grade 1B). The duration of therapy is unclear. In the absence of disease progression, patients should receive at least four cycles of therapy before evaluating for a response (Grade 1C).

What constitutes a reasonable management approach to using drug therapy for patients with MDS?

This chapter has discussed three agents that are currently licensed for the treatment of MDS. However, there is considerable overlap between the patients who would be candidates for each of these agents. There are no RCTs comparing these agents to one another nor is there much information on response rates to the alternative drugs in patients who have failed to respond to one agent (40). Nonetheless, a treatment approach, based on cross-trial comparisons of the phase II and III studies with these agents, is warranted to optimize management strategies in patients with MDS. The recommendations that follow must, however, be interpreted with caution as high-quality evidence does not exist.

Treatment decisions should be made based on the patient's IPSS score, overall clinical picture, and treatment-related toxicities. For patients with low- or INT-1 risk MDS, significant mortality arises from complications of marrow failure, including iron overload from red cell transfusions, and comorbid conditions (6). Therefore, criteria for initiation of therapy include evidence of progressive marrow failure, as manifested by the development of, or worsening of, anemia requiring transfusions, neutropenia with or without infections, or thrombocytopenia in the presence or absence of bleeding. As patients with INT-2 or high-risk MDS have a poorer overall survival and higher likelihood of transformation to acute myeloid leukemia (6), appropriate patients should receive therapy at the time of diagnosis. Choice of therapy should be guided by not only the IPSS score (i.e., low/INT-1 vs. INT-2/high risk) and comorbidities but also the presence of specific karyotype abnormalities [e.g., del(5)(q31)] and candidacy for intensive therapy.

A reasonable plan for integrating these agents into an overall management plan is shown in Figure 38.1. As above, these recommendations should be interpreted with caution because of the lack of direct comparative data from phase III trials. In addition, included is a recommendation to consider use of an erythropoietin stimulating agent (ESA). A full review of data for use of ESAs in myelodysplasia (± a granulocyte colony stimulating factor) is beyond the scope of this review. While there are recommendations that support use of ESAs as a standard practice (41), other data have suggested that such a practice may not be cost-effective (42).

Recommendation

In patients with clinically significant cytopenias for whom therapy with these agents appears to provide benefit, reasonable approaches for patients with low/INT-1 and INT-2/high-risk are described in Figures 38.1A and 38.B, respectively (Grade 2C).

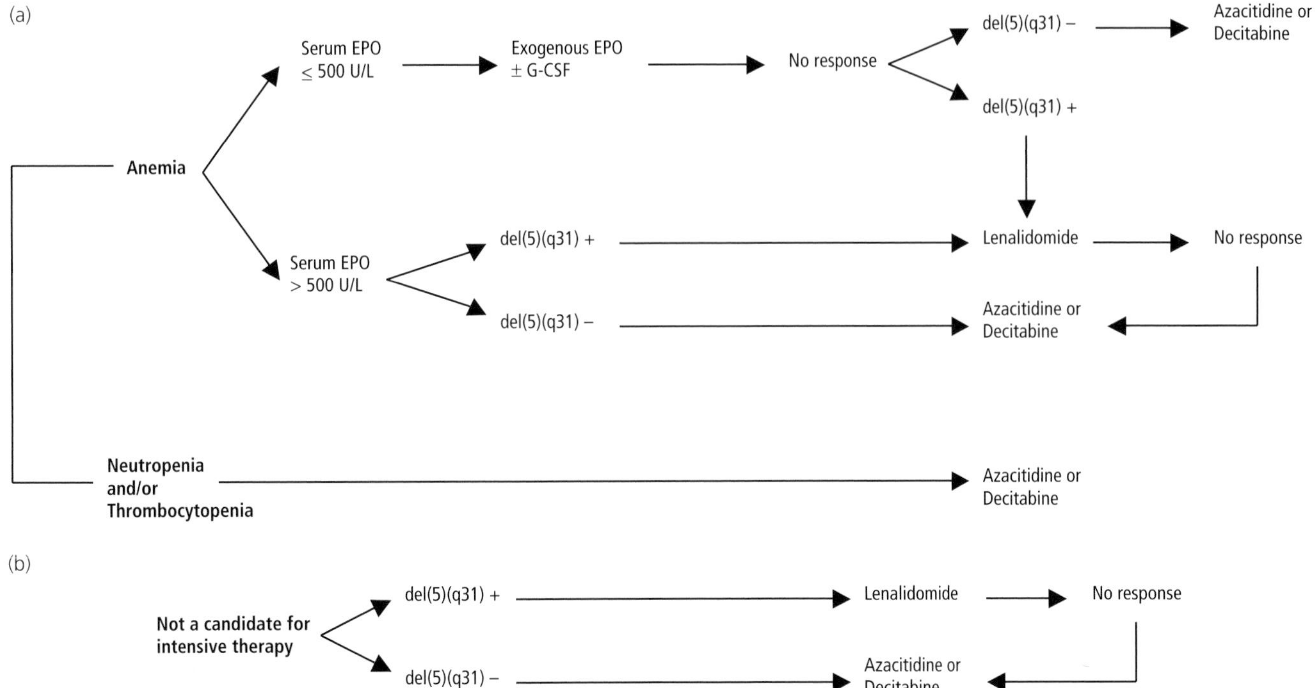

Figure 38.1 Treatment approach that incorporates agents available for patients with myelodysplastic syndromes. (a) Patients with low- or INT-1 risk MDS, (b) Patients with INT-2 or High-risk MDS.

These recommendations are based on cross-trial comparisons of trials testing lenalidomide, azacitidine, and decitibine. No direct comparative data from randomized controlled trials are available; therefore, recommendations should be interpreted with caution (Grade 2C). As indicated in the text, data evaluating therapy with erythropoietic stimulating agents and granulocyte colony stimulating factors have not been included within the scope of this chapter.

References

1 Rollison DE, Hayat M, Smith M, et al. First report of national estimates of the incidence of myelodysplastic syndromes and chronic myeloproliferative disorders from the U.S. SEER Program *Blood.* 108; 2006.

2 Ries LAG, Melbert D, Krapcho M, et al. SEER Cancer Statistics Review, 1975–2004, National Cancer Institute. Bethesda, MD. https://seer.cancer.gov/csr/1975_2004/, based on November 2006 SEER data submission, posted to the SEER Web site, 2007.

3 Corey SJ, Minden MD, Barber DL, et al. Myelodysplastic syndromes: the complexity of stem-cell diseases. *Nat Rev Cancer.* 2007;**7**:118–29.

4 Harris NL, Jaffe ES, Diebold J, et al. World Health Organization classification of neoplastic diseases of the hematopoietic and lymphoid tissues: report of the Clinical Advisory Committee meeting-Airlie House, Virginia, November 1997. *J Clin Oncol.* 1999;**17**:3835–49.

5 Bennett JM, Catovsky D, Daniel MT, et al. Proposals for the classification of the myelodysplastic syndromes. *Br J Haematol.* 1982;**51**:189–99.

6 Greenberg P, Cox C, LeBeau MM, et al. International scoring system for evaluating prognosis in myelodysplastic syndromes. *Blood.* 1997;**89**:2079–88.

7 Cheson BD, Bennett JM, Kantarjian H, et al. Report of an international working group to standardize response criteria for myelodysplastic syndromes. *Blood.* 2000;**96**:3671–74.

8 Cheson BD, Greenberg PL, Bennett JM, et al. Clinical application and proposal for modification of the International Working Group (IWG) response criteria in myelodysplasia. *Blood.* 2006;**108**:419–25.

9 Flores-Figueroa E, Gutierrez-Espindola G, Montesinos JJ, et al. In vitro characterization of hematopoietic microenvironment cells from patients with myelodysplastic syndrome. *Leuk Res.* 2002;**26**:677–86.

10 Aguayo A, Kantarjian H, Manshouri T, et al. Angiogenesis in acute and chronic leukemias and myelodysplastic syndromes. *Blood.* 2000;**96**:2240–45.

11 Sawanobori M, Yamaguchi S, Hasegawa M, et al. Expression of TNF receptors and related signaling molecules in the bone marrow from patients with myelodysplastic syndromes. *Leuk Res.* 2003;**27**:583–91.

12 Bartlett JB, Dredge K, Dalgleish AG. The evolution of thalidomide and its IMiD derivatives as anticancer agents. *Nat Rev Cancer.* 2004;**4**:314–22.

13 List A, Kurtin S, Roe DJ, et al. Efficacy of lenalidomide in myelodysplastic syndromes. *N Engl J Med.* 2005;**352**:549–57.

14 List A, Dewald G, Bennett J, et al. Lenalidomide in the myelodysplastic syndrome with chromosome 5q deletion. *N Engl J Med.* 2006;**355**:1456–65.

15 Buesche G, Dieck S, Giagounidis A, et al. Anti-angiogenic in vivo effect of lenalidomide (CC-5013) in myelodysplastic syndrome with del(5q) chromosome abnormality and its relation to the course of the disease. *Blood.* 2005;**106**:113a.

16 Melchert M, Williams C, List A. Remitting activity of lenalidomide in treatment-induced myelodysplastic syndrome. *Leukemia.* 2007;**21**:1576–78.

17 Goss TF, Szende A, Schaefer C, et al. Cost-effectiveness of lenalidomide in treating patients with transfusion-dependent myelodysplastic syndromes (MDS) in the United States. *J Clin Oncol.* 2006;**24**:332s.

18 Bartlett JB, Tozer A, Stirling D, et al. Recent clinical studies of the immunomodulatory drug (IMiD) lenalidomide. *Br J Cancer.* 2005;**93**:613–19.

19 List AF, Gewald G, Bennett J, et al. Results of the MDS-002 and -003 international phase II studies evaluating lenalidomide (CC-5013; Revlimida) in the treatment of transfusion-dependent (TD) patients with myelodysplastic syndrome (MDS). *Haematologica.* 2005;**90**:307–8.

20 List AF, Baker AF, Green S, et al. Lenalidomide: targeted anemia therapy for myelodysplastic syndromes. *Cancer Control.* 2006;**13** Suppl:4–11.

21 Wu SJ, Yao M, Chou WC, et al. Clinical implications of SOCS1 methylation in myelodysplastic syndrome. *Br J Haematol.* 2006;**135**:317–23.

22 Aggerholm A, Holm MS, Guldberg P, et al. Promoter hypermethylation of p15INK4B, HIC1, CDH1, and ER is frequent in myelodysplastic syndrome and predicts poor prognosis in early-stage patients. *Eur J Haematol.* 2006;**76**:23–32.

23 Christiansen DH, Andersen MK, Pedersen-Bjergaard J. Methylation of p15INK4B is common, is associated with deletion of genes on chromosome arm 7q and predicts a poor prognosis in therapy-related myelodysplasia and acute myeloid leukemia. *Leukemia.* 2003;**17**:1813–19.

24 Quesnel B, Guillerm G, Vereecque R, et al. Methylation of the p15(INK4b) gene in myelodysplastic syndromes is frequent and acquired during disease progression. *Blood.* 1998;**91**:2985–90.

25 Tien HF, Tang JH, Tsay W, et al. Methylation of the p15(INK4B) gene in myelodysplastic syndrome: it can be detected early at diagnosis or during disease progression and is highly associated with leukaemic transformation. *Br J Haematol.* 2001;**112**:148–54.

26 Uchida T, Kinoshita T, Nagai H, et al. Hypermethylation of the p15INK4B gene in myelodysplastic syndromes. *Blood.* 1997;**90**:1403–9.

27 Creusot F, Acs G, Christman JK. Inhibition of DNA methyltransferase and induction of Friend erythroleukemia cell differentiation by 5-azacytidine and 5-aza-2'-deoxycytidine. *J Biol Chem.* 1982;**257**:2041–48.

28 Silverman LR, Demakos EP, Peterson BL, et al. Randomized controlled trial of azacitidine in patients with the myelodysplastic syndrome: a study of the cancer and leukemia group B. *J Clin Oncol.* 2002;**20**:2429–40.

29 Silverman LR, McKenzie DR, Peterson BL, et al. Further analysis of trials with azacitidine in patients with myelodysplastic syndrome: studies 8421, 8921, and 9221 by the Cancer and Leukemia Group B. *J Clin Oncol.* 2006;**24**:3895–903.

30 Gryn J, Zeigler ZR, Shadduck RK, et al. Treatment of myelodysplastic syndromes with 5-azacytidine. *Leuk Res.* 2002;**26**:893–97.

31 Anthony S, Lyons R, Cosgriff T, et al. Transfusion independence assessed using three alternative dosing schedules of azacitidine in patients with myelodysplastic syndromes. *J Clin Oncol.* 2006;**24**:355s.

32 Silverman L, Holland JF, Demakos EP. Azacytidine (azaC) in myelodysplastic syndromes (MDS) CALGB 8421 and 8921. *Ann Hematol.* 1994;**68**:12.

33 Silverman LR, Holland JF, Weinberg RS, et al. Effects of treatment with 5-azacytidine on the in vivo and in vitro hematopoiesis in patients with myelodysplastic syndromes. *Leukemia.* 1993;**7** Suppl 1:21–29.

34 Kornblith AB, Herndon JE II, Silverman LR, et al. Impact of azacytidine on the quality of life of patients with myelodysplastic syndrome treated in a randomized phase III trial: a Cancer and Leukemia Group B Study. *J Clin Oncol.* 2002;**20**:2441–52.

35 Kantarjian H, Issa JP, Rosenfeld CS, et al. Decitabine improves patient outcomes in myelodysplastic syndromes: results of a phase III randomized study. *Cancer.* 2006;**106**:1794–803.

36 Wijermans P, Lubbert M, Verhoef G, et al. Low-dose 5-aza-2'-deoxycytidine, a DNA hypomethylating agent, for the treatment of high-risk myelodysplastic syndrome: a multicenter phase II study in elderly patients. *J Clin Oncol.* 2000;**18**:956–62.

37 Wijermans PW, Krulder JW, Huijgens PC, et al. Continuous infusion of low-dose 5-Aza-2'-deoxycytidine in elderly patients with high-risk myelodysplastic syndrome. *Leukemia.* 1997;**11** Suppl 1:S19–S23.

38 Wijermans PW, Lubbert M, Verhoef G. Low dose decitabine for elderly high risk MDS patients: who will respond? *Blood.* 2002;**100**:96a.

39 Kantarjian H, Oki Y, Garcia-Manero G, et al. Results of a randomized study of 3 schedules of low-dose decitabine in higher-risk myelodysplastic syndrome and chronic myelomonocytic leukemia. *Blood.* 2007;**109**:52–57.

40 Borthakur G, Ravandi-Kashani F, Cortes J, et al. Decitabine induces responses in patients with myelodysplastic syndrome (MDS) after failure of azacitidine therapy. *Blood.* 2006;**108**:157a.

41 Bowen D, Culligan D, Jowitt S, et al. Guidelines for the diagnosis and therapy of adult myelodysplastic syndromes. *Br J Haematol.* 2003;**120**:187–200.

42 Casadevall N, Durieux P, Dubois S, et al. Health, economic, and quality-of-life effects of erythropoietin and granulocyte colony-stimulating factor for the treatment of myelodysplastic syndromes: a randomized, controlled trial. *Blood.* 2004;**104**:321–27.

39 Evidence-based Treatment of Burkitt Lymphoma in Adults

John Gerecitano, David J. Straus

Introduction

Denis Burkitt initially described an aggressive and rapidly fatal sarcoma (later reclassified as lymphoma) in 1958 (1). Since then, our understanding of the pathophysiology and optimal treatment of Burkitt lymphoma (BL) has advanced so that adult patients with this diagnosis may be cured with well-defined chemotherapeutic regimens. Since this disease is rare, representing less than 2% of non-Hodgkin lymphoma in adults (2), large randomized phase III trials have not been possible. Treatment recommendations are based on small phase II trials and anecdotal experience. Despite the lack of "high-quality" evidence, data from the trials presented in this chapter provide a convincing argument for the use of short, intense courses of chemotherapeutic cocktails with intrathecal prophylaxis. There are currently three recognized forms of this aggressive lymphoma: (1) the endemic form originally described by Burkitt, which is largely confined to equatorial Africa, (2) sporadic BL, which is seen in immunocompetent patients both within and outside of this region, and (3) HIV-associated BL. The hallmark of all BL is the overexpression of the *c-myc* gene, which results from a translocation event that brings this gene (located on the short arm of chromosome 8) into juxtaposition with the strong enhancer elements of immunoglobulin coding regions (either the heavy-chain coding region on the short arm of chromosome 14, the kappa light-chain region on the long arm of chromosome 2, or the lambda light-chain region on the short arm of chromosome 22). In 1999, the World Health Organization/Revised European American Lymphoma (WHO/REAL) classification system required that the diagnosis of BL be based on the typical histologic appearance of monotonous medium-sized lymphoid cells with a proliferative index (most commonly measured using the Ki-67 stain) of greater than 99% and, when available, cytogenetic analysis confirming a *c-myc* translocation (3). Although the WHO recognizes the Ann Arbor staging system as the standard for this and other lymphomas, many investigators have used other systems to describe the extent of disease and extranodal involvement in patients with BL. The major determinants of survival reflected in these staging systems include tumor burden (usually represented by the size of the predominant mass and serum lactate dehydrogenase (LDH) levels) and involvement of the central nervous system (CNS) or bone marrow.

Questions

1. Is there a role for surgical "debulking" in Burkitt lymphoma?
2. What is the optimal therapy for adult patients?
3. Is the outcome of treatment worse for patients with Burkitt lymphoma associated with HIV infection than those without HIV infection?
4. What is the role of recombinant urate oxidase as tumor lysis syndrome prophylaxis/treatment in Burkitt lymphoma?

Literature-search strategy and inclusion

A search of PubMed was conducted using the terms "Burkitt lymphoma," "Burkitt's lymphoma," or "small noncleaved cell lymphoma," and "treatment," "trial," or "therapy." Publications dealing primarily with pediatric patients and case reports were excluded. Those publications that did not include a sufficient number of patients with Burkitt lymphoma (less than three), or that included BL patients but did not report results for this subcategory were excluded. Articles and abstracts that do not meet these criteria have been included, at the authors' discretion, to illustrate historical or clinical aspects of the disease and its treatment.

Grading of the quality of evidence and strengths of recommendations in this chapter are based on the guidelines proposed by the international Grading of Recommendations Assessment, Development, and Evaluation Working Group (GRADE) adopting the

Evidence-based Hematology. Edited by Mark A. Crowther, Jeff Ginsberg, Holger J. Schünemann, Ralph M. Meyer, and Richard Lottenberg.

modification used by the American College of Chest Physicians that merges the "very low" and "low" categories of quality of evidence (see chapter 1).

Is there a role for surgical "Debulking" in Burkitt lymphoma?

Since BL was initially thought of as a sarcoma, it is not surprising that surgery remained a mainstay of treatment for a long time (4,5). Even after effective chemotherapeutic modalities were developed, surgery was considered the standard of care in order to debulk the disease and decrease the tumor lysis caused by subsequent chemotherapy (6,7). This recommendation was based mainly on retrospective analyses with small numbers of patients. However, there is a strong potential for selection bias because only those patients with relatively limited disease and therefore good prognosis were surgical candidates. More recent retrospective analyses in children highlight the fact that those patients who undergo surgery are more likely to have smaller disease burdens, which would predict a better outcome regardless of local interventions (8). Surgery has been shown to increase complications, delay effective chemotherapy and decrease survival (9). This, coupled with the fact that most recurrences involve the CNS and other areas outside the initial area of presentation, argue strongly against surgery as a routine part of care in BL patients unless indicated for other reasons.

Recommendation

Surgical debulking is not recommended for patients with Burkitt lymphoma, even if bulky disease is present (Grade 1C).

What is the optimal therapy for adult patients?

The rapid rate of growth and relapse in BL has led to the speedy accrual of clinical data because disease-free survival and cure rate ascertainment requires relatively short-term follow-up. However, evaluation and comparison of clinical trials is difficult because (1) the rarity of the disease leads to limited accrual at individual centers, (2) disease classification has changed as our understanding of the pathophysiology of the disease has advanced and new diagnostic techniques have become available, (3) the staging and prognostic factors used in different trials vary, and (4) early awareness of poor responses has led to mid-trial treatment changes during many of these studies. Treatment for BL has historically followed three patterns that include treatment as per other aggressive histology lymphomas, such as diffuse large B-cell lymphoma (DLBCL), use of the same regimens as for treatment of acute lymphoblastic leukemia (ALL), and short, intensive therapy. Combinations and schedules successfully used in other aggressive lymphomas with relatively high growth rates have not shown promise in BL, reflecting the close to 100% proliferation rate in this lymphoma (10). Retrospective studies of patients treated with cyclophosphamide, doxorubicin, vincristine, and prednisone (CHOP) (11) (the standard of care in other aggressive lymphomas) and CHOP-like (12) regimens have demonstrated complete response rates between 61% and 72% and disappointing long-term survivals of 45%–55%.

Since early classification schemes categorized some presentations of BL as a form of ALL, the first drug combinations resembled regimens that were commonly used in both diseases. Since the CNS was frequently the site of relapse in early trials (13,14), two main strategies developed to prevent CNS recurrences: (1) treatment with high doses of methotrexate and cytarabine (15), which could cross the blood–brain barrier and (2) direct intrathecal administration of these drugs (16,17). Further attempts to prevent relapse included prolonged maintenance therapies extrapolated from ALL treatment regimens (18–20). Eventually, it became apparent that initial treatment with more intense courses, employing multiple active drugs over a short period of time with adequate CNS prophylaxis, led to equivalent if not superior results. Many adult induction regimens have been modeled after pediatric treatments, especially those used in ALL (21,22). In general, these regimens incorporate combinations of anthracyclines, alkylators, and vinca alkaloids, alternating with high doses of CNS-penetrating treatments (methotrexate or cytarabine), and include intrathecal prophylaxis (5,23–29).

Although many of the above studies illustrate successful and viable treatment options for BL, most of the regimens are complex and have not been validated. The two most promising and widely studied modern regimens for the treatment of BL have been developed at MD Anderson Cancer Center (MDACC) (30) and the U.S. National Cancer Institute (NCI) (23) and could be described as short, intensive therapies. Hyperfractionated cyclophosphamide, vincristine, doxorubicin, and dexamethasone (hyper-CVAD) was originally developed at MDACC for the treatment of pediatric ALL. HyperCVAD in alternation with cycles of high-dose methotrexate and cytarabine in 26 patients with leukemic BL was first reported in 1999 (30). Complete responses were obtained in 81% of patients, with a three-year survival rate of 49%. Addition of rituximab to this regimen has been reported recently in adult patients with BL (31). In 28 assessable patients with a median follow-up of 22 months, complete remissions were achieved in 86% (with one additional CR after salvage transplant), and, with a median follow-up time of 22 months, the estimated three-year overall survival was 89%. These results are especially impressive given that the median age of this population was 46 years, and 29% of patients were over age 60 years (31). Thus, the addition of rituximab to intensive chemotherapy may provide results in adults with BL similar to those that have been reported in the past with children. The most widely independently validated chemotherapeutic regimen used in BL is the CODOX-M-IVAC regimen (cyclophosphamide, doxorubicin, vincristine, high-dose methotrexate-ifosfamide, etoposide, high-dose cytarabine) developed at the NCI (32). Building on their experience using 15 cycles of the CODOX-M regimen, Magrath et al. (32) used an alternating regimen with nonoverlapping agents, combined with an intervening infusion of high-dose methotrexate and interspersed intrathecal therapy. The authors treated "low-risk" patients with three cycles of CODOX-M alone, whereas patients with more advanced disease received a full four cycles of alternating therapy. The initial trial of this regimen in a group of 72 adult and pediatric patients achieved an extremely impressive 92% two-year event-free survival. These data were obtained in a select group of young patients (median age 25) and therefore required validation in other patients populations. An international experience with CODOX-M/IVAC was reported in 2002 (33). Although the two-year EFS of 64.6% was not as high in this study, the median age of patients was 35, with 40 of the 52 patients presenting with high-risk disease (note that risk categorization was defined in a slightly different way in the two publications). Of note, the international study also required central pathology review to confirm the diagnosis of BL, whereas the Magrath paper included all small, noncleaved non-Hodgkin lymphoma (NHL) as diagnosed by the various referral centers. A retrospective analysis of 13 HIV-negative patients with a median age of 37 supported the efficacy of this regimen, with a two-year event-free survival of 92% (34). Validation of the CODOX-M/IVAC regimen was recently reported in an even older patient population (median age 47) (35). Toxicity of this regimen was decreased by lowering the dose of methotrexate infusions (to prevent the 58% rate of mucositis seen by Magrath (32), capping the dose of vincristine and decreasing intrathecal cytarabine (to prevent the 27% rate of neurotoxicity). A decreased cyclophosphamide dose was balanced by an increased dose of doxorubicin. This study achieved a response rate similar to that seen in the international evaluation (two-year progression-free survival of 64%) in an even older patient population.

Recommendation

Short, intensive therapy such as with CODOX-M/IVAC is recommended for adult patients with Burkitt lymphoma when the goal of therapy is prolonged disease control and maximum duration of overall survival. This therapy is recommended over alternative options such as CHOP or regimens that are used to treat ALL (Grade 1C).

Is the outcome of treatment worse for patients with Burkitt lymphoma associated with HIV infection than those without HIV infection?

When compared with the general population, patients infected with the human immunodeficiency virus (HIV) are at a higher risk of developing aggressive lymphomas and presenting with more advanced disease. Early studies sought to reduce the risk of opportunistic infections by decreasing the intensity of treatment regimens in HIV-positive populations. Two studies evaluated a reduced-dose m-BACOD regimen (methotrexate, bleomycin, doxorubicin, cyclophosphamide, vincristine, and dexamethasone) in HIV-associated NHL patients (36–38). Both regimens led to a two-year survival rate of less than 30% in this group with both large and small cell lymphomas. In these and other studies, a low CD4 count was a major factor associated with a short survival (38,39). However, the dramatic reductions in HIV viral load achieved with highly active antiretroviral therapy (HAART) (40) has also been shown to raise CD4 counts, thereby improving immune and hematopoietic cellular functions. A retrospective study of HIV-positive patients at one institution showed a dramatic improvement in survival for patients with DLBCL using HAART (41). Since these patients were treated with similar chemotherapeutic regimens before and after the institution of HAART, the increased survival probably indicates a better tolerance for chemotherapy. These benefits did not, however, extend to patients with HIV and BL, who fared equally poorly both before and after HAART when treated with m-BACOD and CHOP-like regimens. Unlike other HIV-associated illnesses (including DLBCL), BL commonly occurs in patients with CD4 counts above 200/dL (42). It was clear that low- or standard-dose chemotherapy regimens like the two versions of m-BACOD were inadequate treatment for Burkitt lymphoma regardless of the presence or absence of HIV infection. In 2003, two small studies, one retrospective and one prospective, demonstrated the ability of HIV-infected patients to tolerate the CODOX-M-IVAC regimen with rates of myelosuppression and infectious complications similar to a comparison group of HIV-negative patients, regardless of prior or concurrent HAART therapy (34,43). A German retrospective study showed the tolerability of a seven-drug dose-intense regimen in HIV-positive BL and BLL patients (44), and an MDACC trial did the same for Hyper-CVAD (45). All four trials have shown the feasibility of concomitant treatment with dose-dense chemotherapy and HAART, with survival rates ranging from 48% (45) to 72% (44).

Recommendation

Patients with HIV-related BL should be treated as aggressively as immunocompetent patients, since they often have well-preserved CD4 counts that can be maintained with HAART (Grade 1C).

What is the role of recombinant urate oxidase as tumor lysis syndrome prophylaxis/treatment in Burkitt lymphoma?

The combination of large tumor burden at presentation and the high sensitivity of BL to cytotoxic agents present a high risk of tumor lysis syndrome, which can manifest as toxicity to a number of organs, with particularly lethal risks involving the nervous system, heart, and kidneys. Characteristic metabolic consequences include hyperkalemia, hypocalcemia, hyperphosphatemia, and the development of a metabolic acidosis. In addition, high levels of uric acid in the bloodstream can also overwhelm the renal clearance system, resulting in renal failure secondary to the precipitation of urate crystals in the renal tubule (46). Standard components of management include brisk intravenous hydration with a simple isotonic solution (such as normal saline) aimed at maintaining a renal output of at least 2.5 L/d and judicious use of diuretics such as mannitol or furosemide, sodium polystyrene sulphonate for treatment of hyperkalemia, and oral phosphate binders such as aluminum hydroxide. Severe electrolyte disturbances may require dialysis.

Hyperuricemia can be prevented with the use of xanthine oxidase inhibitors and institution of an alkaline diuresis. It is therefore standard practice to begin treatment with allopurinol in patients with BL at the time of diagnosis. One published dose recommendation for allopurinol is 100 mg/m^2 orally every eight hours with at least a 50% reduction in dose for patients in renal failure (46). Unfortunately, urine alkalinization can increase precipitation of calcium phosphate (47). Furthermore, allopurinol can lead to an increase in serum xanthine, which is insoluble (especially in alkaline urine) and can itself precipitate in the renal tubules leading to obstructive uropathy (48,49). Urate oxidase is an enzyme that converts uric acid into allantoin, a highly soluble metabolic product. Rasburicase is a recombinant form of urate oxidase. A randomized multicenter trial comparing rasburicase with allopurinol was conducted in 52 pediatric patients undergoing treatment for leukemia or lymphoma (50). Patients in the rasburicase arm had an 86% reduction in plasma uric acid within the first four hours of intravenous administration, compared with a 12% reduction in the allopurinol arm. During the first 96 hours, patients in the rasburicase arm had a 2.6-fold reduction in exposure to hyperuricemia compared with those treated with allopurinol, an effect which was even more pronounced in the nine patients with BL, who experienced a fourfold reduction in uric acid exposure during this period. Although this study was not powered to detect differences in acute renal failure, trends toward improved creatinine values were also seen in the rasburicase group. Because a breakdown product of uric acid metabolism is hydrogen peroxide, oxidative damage to red blood cells can occur in patients with glucose-6-phosphate dehydrogenase deficiency, and hemolysis has been observed in at least one such patient (47). Rasburicase has been approved by the U.S. Food and Drug Administration for the treatment of hyperuricemia caused by cancer therapy in children. Two large compassionate use trials demonstrate close to 100% efficacy in decreasing serum uric acid levels to normal values in adults and children with a variety of malignancies, with consequent lower-than-expected rises in creatinine and use of hemodialysis (51,52). A more targeted group of 100 adult patients with aggressive lymphoma has also been studied, with similar results (53).

Although highly effective, rasburicase can be quite expensive; the manufacturer recommends a five-day course in pediatric patients that costs upward of $4,000 (54). To contain expenses, several authors have used modified approaches to rasburicase use. Hummel et al. reported on four patients treated with lower doses and/or shorter duration of rasburicase in whom serum uric acid decreased and renal function improved without further treatment (55). Three other authors have reported on small groups of patients treated with a single dose of rasburicase to lower uric acid levels, followed by the prophylactic use of allopurinol during chemotherapeutic treatment of leukemia or lymphoma (56,57). In all cases, this strategy resulted in renal improvement and maintenance of safe levels of serum uric acid. Since urate oxidase will quickly lower uricemia without preventing further buildup and allopurinol will prevent the production of uric acid without treating existing hyperuricemia, this combination approach provides a cost-effective alternative that is already in use at other institutions (58).

Recommendation

For patients with features of established tumor lysis syndrome, treatment with rasburicase is recommended (Grade 1B).

References

1 Burkitt D. A sarcoma involving the jaws in African children. *Br J Surg.* 1958;**46**(197):218–23.

2 The Non-Hodgkin's Lymphoma Classification P. A Clinical evaluation of the International Lymphoma Study Group classification of non-Hodgkin's lymphoma. *Blood.* 1997;**89**:3909–18.

3 Harris NL, Jaffe ES, Diebold J, et al. The World Health Organization classification of neoplastic diseases of the hematopoietic and lymphoid tissues: report of the Clinical Advisory Committee meeting, Airlie House, Virginia, November, 1997. *Ann Oncol.* 1999;**10**(12):1419–32.

4 Kemeny MM, Magrath IT, Brennan MF. The role of surgery in the management of American Burkitt's lymphoma and its treatment. *Ann Surg.* 1982;**196**(1):82–86.

5 Janus C, Edwards BK, Sariban E, et al. Surgical resection and limited chemotherapy for abdominal undifferentiated lymphomas. *Cancer Treat Rep.* 1984;**68**(4):599–605.

6 Magrath IT, Lwanga S, Carswell W, et al. Surgical reduction of tumour bulk in management of abdominal Burkitt's lymphoma. British medical journal. 1974;**2**(5914):308–12.

7 Ziegler JL. Treatment results of 54 American patients with Burkitt's lymphoma are similar to the African experience. *N Engl J Med.* 1977;**297**(2):75–80.

8 Shamberger RC, Weinstein HJ. The role of surgery in abdominal Burkitt's lymphoma. *J Pediatr Surg.* 1992;**27**(2):236–40.

9 Frappaz D, Miron I, Brunat-Mentigny M, et al. Is there still a place for initial surgery in advanced Burkitt's lymphomas (BL) [abstract 1295]? *Proc Am Soc Clin Oncol.*

10 Hagemeister FB. Results of treatment of small non-cleaved cell lymphoma in patients without positive HIV serology. *Leuk Lymphoma.* 1993;**10** Suppl:21–27.

11 Kaiser U, Uebelacker I, Havemann K. Non-Hodgkin's lymphoma protocols in the treatment of patients with Burkitt's lymphoma and lymphoblastic lymphoma: a report on 58 patients. *Leuk Lymphoma.* 1999;**36**(1–2):101–8.

12 Economopoulos T, Dimopoulos MA, Foudoulakis A, et al. Burkitt's lymphoma in Greek adults: a study of the Hellenic co-operative oncology group. *Leuk Res.* 2000;**24**(12):993–98.

13 Ziegler JL, Magrath IT, Nkrumah FK, et al. Evaluation of CCNU (NSC-79037) used for the prevention of CNS involvement in Burkitt's lymphoma. *Cancer Chemother Rep.* 1975;**59**(6):1155–56.

14 Williams CK, Folami AO, Seriki O. Patterns of treatment failure in Burkitt's lymphoma. *Eur J Cancer Clin Oncol.* 1983;**19**(6):741–46.

15 Todeschini G, Tecchio C, Degani D, et al. Eighty-one percent event-free survival in advanced Burkitt's lymphoma/leukemia: no differences

in outcome between pediatric and adult patients treated with the same intensive pediatric protocol. *Ann Oncol.* 1997;**8** Suppl 1:77–81.

16 Ziegler JL, Bluming AZ. Intrathecal chemotherapy in Burkitt's lymphoma. *Br Med J.* 1971;**3**(5773):508–12.

17 Nkrumah FK, Perkins IV. Burkitt's lymphoma: a clinical study of 110 patients. *Cancer.* 1976;**37**(2):671–76.

18 Patte C, Philip T, Rodary C, et al. Improved survival rate in children with stage III and IV B cell non-Hodgkin's lymphoma and leukemia using multi-agent chemotherapy: results of a study of 114 children from the French Pediatric Oncology Society. *J Clin Oncol.* 1986;**4**(8):1219–26.

19 Straus DJ, Wong GY, Liu J, et al. Small non-cleaved-cell lymphoma (undifferentiated lymphoma, Burkitt's type) in American adults: results with treatment designed for acute lymphoblastic leukemia. *Am J Med.* 1991;**90**(3):328–37.

20 Hoelzer D, Ludwig WD, Thiel E, et al. Improved outcome in adult B-cell acute lymphoblastic leukemia. *Blood.* 1996;**87**(2):495–508.

21 Di Nicola M, Carlo-Stella C, Mariotti J, et al. High response rate and manageable toxicity with an intensive, short-term chemotherapy programme for Burkitt's lymphoma in adults. *Br J Haematol.* 2004;**126**(6): 815–20.

22 Divine M, Casassus P, Koscielny S, et al. Burkitt lymphoma in adults: a prospective study of 72 patients treated with an adapted pediatric LMB protocol. *Ann Oncol.* 2005;**16**(12):1928–35.

23 Magrath IT, Janus C, Edwards BK, et al. An effective therapy for both undifferentiated (including Burkitt's) lymphomas and lymphoblastic lymphomas in children and young adults. *Blood.* 1984;**63**(5):1102–11.

24 Murphy SB, Bowman WP, Abromowitch M, et al. Results of treatment of advanced-stage Burkitt's lymphoma and B cell (SIg+) acute lymphoblastic leukemia with high-dose fractionated cyclophosphamide and coordinated high-dose methotrexate and cytarabine. *J Clin Oncol.* 1986;**4**(12):1732–39.

25 Bernstein JI, Coleman CN, Strickler JG. Combined modality therapy for adults with small noncleaved cell lymphoma (Burkitt's and non-Burkitt's types). *J Clin Oncol.* 1986;**4**(6):847–58.

26 McMaster ML, Greer JP, Greco FA, et al. Effective treatment of small-noncleaved-cell lymphoma with high-intensity, brief-duration chemotherapy. *J Clin Oncol.* 1991;**9**(6):941–46.

27 Waits TM, Greco FA, Greer JP, et al. Effective therapy for poor-prognosis non-Hodgkin's lymphoma with 8 weeks of high-dose-intensity combination chemotherapy. *J Clin Oncol.* 1993;**11**(5):943–49.

28 Philip T, Biron P, Philip I, et al. Massive therapy and autologous bone marrow transplantation in pediatric and young adults Burkitt's lymphoma (30 courses on 28 patients: a 5-year experience). *Eur J Cancer Clin Oncol.* 1986;**22**(8):1015–27.

29 Soussain C, Patte C, Ostronoff M, et al. Small noncleaved cell lymphoma and leukemia in adults: a retrospective study of 65 adults treated with the LMB pediatric protocols. *Blood.* 1995;**85**(3):664–74.

30 Thomas DA, Cortes J, O'Brien S, et al. Hyper-CVAD program in Burkitt's-type adult acute lymphoblastic leukemia. *J Clin Oncol.* 1999;**17**(8):2461–70.

31 Thomas DA, Faderl S, O'Brien S, et al. Chemoimmunotherapy with hyper-CVAD plus rituximab for the treatment of adult Burkitt and Burkitt-type lymphoma or acute lymphoblastic leukemia. *Cancer.* 2006;**106**(7):1569–80.

32 Magrath I, Adde M, Shad A, et al. Adults and children with small non-cleaved-cell lymphoma have a similar excellent outcome when treated with the same chemotherapy regimen. *J Clin Oncol.* 1996;**14**(3): 925–34.

33 Mead GM, Sydes MR, Walewski J, et al. An international evaluation of CODOX-M and CODOX-M alternating with IVAC in adult Burkitt's lymphoma: results of United Kingdom Lymphoma Group LY06 study. *Ann Oncol.* 2002;**13**(8):1264–74.

34 Wang ES, Straus DJ, Teruya-Feldstein J, et al. Intensive chemotherapy with cyclophosphamide, doxorubicin, high-dose methotrexate/ifosfamide, etoposide, and high-dose cytarabine (CODOX-M/IVAC) for human immunodeficiency virus-associated Burkitt lymphoma. *Cancer.* 2003;**98**(6):1196–205.

35 Lacasce A, Howard O, Lib S, et al. Modified magrath regimens for adults with Burkitt and Burkitt-like lymphomas: preserved efficacy with decreased toxicity. *Leuk Lymphoma.* 2004;**45**(4):761–67.

36 Levine AM, Wernz JC, Kaplan L, et al. Low-dose chemotherapy with central nervous system prophylaxis and zidovudine maintenance in AIDS-related lymphoma: a prospective multi-institutional trial. *JAMA*; 1991;**266**(1):84–8.

37 Kaplan LD, Straus DJ, Testa MA, et al. Low-dose compared with standard-dose m-BACOD chemotherapy for non-Hodgkin's lymphoma associated with human immunodeficiency virus infection. National Institute of Allergy and Infectious Diseases AIDS Clinical Trials Group. *N Engl J Med.* 1997;**336**(23):1641–48.

38 Straus DJ, Huang J, Testa MA, et al. Prognostic factors in the treatment of human immunodeficiency virus-associated non-Hodgkin's lymphoma: analysis of AIDS Clinical Trials Group protocol 142—low-dose versus standard-dose m-BACOD plus granulocyte-macrophage colony-stimulating factor. National Institute of Allergy and Infectious Diseases. *J Clin Oncol.* 1998;**16**(11):3601–6.

39 Knowles DM, Chamulak GA, Subar M, et al. Lymphoid neoplasia associated with the acquired immunodeficiency syndrome (AIDS). The New York University Medical Center experience with 105 patients (1981–1986). *Ann Intern Med.* 1988;**108**(5):744–53.

40 Palella FJ Jr, Delaney KM, Moorman AC, et al. Declining morbidity and mortality among patients with advanced human immunodeficiency virus infection. HIV Outpatient Study investigators. *N Engl J Med.* 1998;**338**(13):853–60.

41 Lim ST, Karim R, Nathwani BN, et al. AIDS-related Burkitt's lymphoma versus diffuse large-cell lymphoma in the pre-highly active antiretroviral therapy (HAART) and HAART eras: significant differences in survival with standard chemotherapy. *J Clin Oncol.* 2005;**23**(19):4430–38.

42 Davi F, Delecluse HJ, Guiet P, et al. Burkitt-like lymphomas in AIDS patients: characterization within a series of 103 human immunodeficiency virus-associated non-Hodgkin's lymphomas. Burkitt's Lymphoma Study Group. *J Clin Oncol.* 1998;**16**(12):3788–95.

43 Lichtman SM, Calderon N. Alternating CODOX-M and IVAC in HIV positive patients with Burkitt's lymphoma [abstract 2471]. *Proc Am Soc Clin Oncol.* 2003;**22**:614.

44 Horst H-A, Faetkenheuer G, Wyen C, et al. AIDS-associated Burkitt- or Burkitt-like lymphoma—the short-term, multiagent and dose intensive B-ALL protocol is feasible and effective [abstract 1001]. *Blood.* 2003;**102**(11).

45 Cortes J, Thomas D, Rios A, et al. Hyperfractionated cyclophosphamide, vincristine, doxorubicin, and dexamethasone and highly active antiretroviral therapy for patients with acquired immunodeficiency syndrome-related Burkitt lymphoma/leukemia. *Cancer.* 2002;**94**(5):1492–99.

46 Cairo MS, Bishop M. Tumour lysis syndrome: new therapeutic strategies and classification. *Br J Haematol.* 2004;**127**(1):3–11.

47 Pui CH. Rasburicase: a potent uricolytic agent. *Expert Opin Pharmacother.* 2002;**3**(4):433–42.

48 Band PR, Silverberg DS, Henderson JF, et al. Xanthine nephropathy in a patient with lymphosarcoma treated with allopurinol. *N Engl J Med.* 1970;**283**(7):354–57.

49 Landgrebe AR, Nyhan WL, Coleman M. Urinary-tract stones resulting from the excretion of oxypurinol. *N Engl J Med.* 1975;**292**(12): 626–27.

50 Goldman SC, Holcenberg JS, Finklestein JZ, et al. A randomized comparison between rasburicase and allopurinol in children with lymphoma or leukemia at high risk for tumor lysis. *Blood.* 2001;**97**(10):2998–3003.

51 Jeha S, Kantarjian H, Irwin D, et al. Efficacy and safety of rasburicase, a recombinant urate oxidase (Elitektrade]), in the management of malignancy-associated hyperuricemia in pediatric and adult patients: final results of a multicenter compassionate use trial. *Leukemia.* 2004;**19**(1):34–38.

52 Bosly A, Sonet A, Pinkerton CR, et al. Rasburicase (recombinant urate oxidase) for the management of hyperuricemia in patients with cancer: report of an international compassionate use study. *Cancer.* 2003;**98**(5):1048–54.

53 Coiffier B, Mounier N, Bologna S, et al. Efficacy and safety of rasburicase (recombinant urate oxidase) for the prevention and treatment of hyperuricemia during induction chemotherapy of aggressive non-Hodgkin's lymphoma: results of the GRAAL1 (Groupe d'Etude des Lymphomes de l'Adulte Trial on Rasburicase Activity in Adult Lymphoma) study. *J Clin Oncol.* 2003;**21**(23):4402–6.

54 Cheson BD, Dutcher BS. Managing malignancy-associated hyperuricemia with rasburicase. *J Support Oncol.* 2005;**3**(2):117–24.

55 Hummel M, Buchheidt D, Reiter S, et al. Successful treatment of hyperuricemia with low doses of recombinant urate oxidase in four patients with hematologic malignancy and tumor lysis syndrome. *Leukemia.* 2003;**17**(12):2542–44.

56 Lee AC, Li CH, So KT, et al. Treatment of impending tumor lysis with single-dose rasburicase. *Ann Pharmacother.* 2003;**37**(11):1614–17.

57 Liu CY, Sims-McCallum RP, Schiffer CA. A single dose of rasburicase is sufficient for the treatment of hyperuricemia in patients receiving chemotherapy. *Leuk Res.* 2005;**29**(4):463–65.

58 Cruz JM, Chauvenet AR. Optimizing care with rasburicase. *J Support Oncol.* 2005;**3**(2):127–28.

40 Primary Central Nervous System Lymphoma

Tamara Shenkier

Introduction

Primary central nervous system lymphoma (PCNSL) is a rare type of extranodal non-Hodgkin's lymphoma (NHL) confined to the craniospinal axis without evidence of systemic spread. It should be distinguished from nodal or extranodal NHL that has disseminated to the CNS, which is a different clinical entity. The incidence of PCNSL in the immunocompetent population has been rising over the past three decades for reasons that are unclear (1). Whole-brain irradiation (WBXRT) was the mainstay of care for years. A Radiation Therapy Oncology Group (RTOG) study of WBXRT at 40 Gray (Gy) plus a 20 Gy boost to the involved area demonstrated an overall response of 90%. However, responses were not durable with the vast majority of relapses occurring in the brain. The median survival was 12 months and fewer than 5% of patients survived five years (2). In addition, a significant proportion of survivors developed leukoencephalopathy, a debilitating neurotoxicity which presents as a decline in cognitive or physical function (3). Given the low efficacy of irradiation as monotherapy, combined modality treatment (CMT) with chemotherapy and WBXRT was subsequently employed. Only one reported randomized trial has been conducted looking at CMT (4). It is of historical interest only because it used CHOP chemotherapy, a regimen that does not penetrate well across the intact blood-brain barrier (BBB). The trial closed earlier than planned through poor accrual and there was no clear benefit seen.

Successful inroads were subsequently made by employing methotrexate, an antimetabolite that can penetrate the intact BBB. Methotrexate has a modest role to play in the treatment of systemic lymphoma but has become the most important single agent in the treatment of PCNSL. High-dose methotrexate (MTX) refers to systemically administered MTX, infused over four to six hours, at doses higher than 1 g/m^2 and usually over 3.5 g/m^2, followed by folinic acid rescue (5). There is consensus that the use MTX-based chemotherapy with or without the addition of whole-brain radiotherapy (WBXRT) seems to be the most effective approach in the treatment of PCNSL. Survival is still inferior to that seen when aggressive non-Hodgkin's lymphoma involves other extranodal sites suggesting an intrinsic biological resistance (6,7) or a limitation imposed by the presence of the BBB despite the favorable profile of single agent MTX (8,9). Furthermore, combined modality therapy is still associated with an unacceptably high risk of neurotoxicity particularly in patients over age 60 years at diagnosis (10). In view of the drawbacks of CMT and the high initial response rate of PCNSL to chemotherapy, the strategy of using systemic therapy alone, with WBXRT reserved only for patients with disease progression, has been increasingly employed (11–13). No direct comparison of CMT and chemotherapy is available; therefore, no firm conclusions can be made regarding the relative efficacy of these two strategies. However, it is clear that the risk of leukoencephalopathy is much lower when systemic therapy is administered as a single modality (12,14,15).

Since there are no published randomized controlled trials using MTX based therapy, the optimal treatment of PCNSL remains undefined. Our current treatment policies are derived from phase II trials and population based cohorts. In these types of studies, prognostic variables such as age ($\leq$60 versus $>$60 years) and performance status (PS) are often more important determinants of outcome than treatment (16). The selection and enrollment criteria in phase II trials must be carefully scrutinized when comparing treatment approaches between studies and these results should be interpreted with caution. Although results compiled from clinical trials suggest progress in the treatment of PCNSL, survival improvements are not reflected in population-based cohorts. Two single-center population-based studies (17,18) and a surveillance, epidemiology, and end results (SEER) cancer registry study of 1,565 immunocompetent patients with PCNSL (19) describe overall median survivals ranging from 9 to 17 months. These data are sobering and are more generalizable than results from phase II trials, but they also include uninformative cases of

Evidence-based Hematology. Edited by Mark A. Crowther, Jeff Ginsberg, Holger J. Schünemann, Ralph M. Meyer, and Richard Lottenberg.

patients not suitable for any treatment apart from symptom palliation.

Questions

1. In patients less than age 60 years at presentation:
   a. Is combined modality therapy with chemotherapy and whole brain irradiation the standard of care?
   b. Which chemotherapy regimen should be used?
   c. Can the dose of whole brain irradiation be reduced or omitted in patients who achieve a complete response with chemotherapy?
2. In patients older than age 60 at presentation what treatment approach optimizes the balance between achieving cure and minimizing neurotoxicity?
3. What is the optimal treatment at relapse?

The evaluation of these questions will be predominantly based on case series data. As the results of some case series may be applicable to more than one question, this chapter will have a different format than used in other chapters. The results of the overall database will be described and answers to all questions will be provided in a summary section.

Literature-search strategy and inclusions

All literature searches employed PubMed MEDLINE at the National Library of Medicine. First a search for randomized controlled trials and primary CNS lymphoma (PCNSL) was performed. Only one ongoing German trial was described the results of which are not yet published (20). A search for "systematic review" and "primary CNS lymphoma" yielded only two articles neither of which was relevant. Next, a search using the parameters "primary CNS lymphoma" or "PCNSL" combined with "treatment" or "therapy" was performed limited to "English" and the dates 1999–2006, the past seven years being most pertinent to current practice. Two hundred fifty-eight articles were retrieved. Articles were manually reviewed and excluded as irrelevant for the following reasons: PCNSL in immunosuppressed hosts (e.g., AIDS or HIV-related lymphomas, posttransplant lymphoproliferative disorders); secondary CNS dissemination; other extranodal lymphomas (e.g., breast, testicular, sinus); pediatric age group; focus other than treatment (e.g., imaging or pathology); unusual histology (e.g., low grade lymphomas); reports containing fewer than 15 patients; and overviews of previously published data. Seventy-four articles were retained. A separate search was conducted which combined "central nervous system" or "brain" or "primary" and "lymphoma" with terminology specific to study type: "retrospective," "cohort study," "population based," "phase II," and "clinical trials." One hundred and forty papers were retrieved. The results were then limited to "English" and the dates 1999–2006 and articles were excluded for the same reasons outlined above. Sixty-eight articles remained. The results of the first and second searches were combined and duplicates were discarded. These 114 papers were again manually reviewed for relevance. Sixty-four English language articles and abstracts published from 1999 to 2006 remained and were directly applicable to this review.

Grading of the quality of evidence and strengths of recommendations in this chapter are based on the guidelines proposed by the international Grading of Recommendations Assessment, Development, and Evaluation Working Group (GRADE) adopting the modification used by the American College of Chest Physicians that merges the very low and low categories of quality of evidence (see chapter 1).

Summary of literature extraction

Only one randomized trial in PCNSL has been conducted. In this multicenter German study, complete responders to carmustine, methotrexate(MTX) 1.5 g/m2, procarbazine, and dexamethasone (BMPD) chemotherapy were randomized to either whole-brain irradiation (WBXRT) or observation (20). The final results have not yet been reported, but a preliminary publication reported that the median survival was significantly longer at centers accruing at least four patients than at those with fewer patients (31.5 vs. 9.5 months, $p = 0.03$), indicating that institutional experience treating PCNSL is another possible prognostic factor (21). Therefore, trials providing lesser levels of evidence will be reviewed. Table 40.1 shows large retrospective series, which include both treatment and outcome data in patients which PCNSL and Table 40.2 tabulates the phase II trials of combined modality therapy (CMT). The largest and potentially most useful studies for the purposes of treatment recommendations will be summarized.

A retrospective Japanese study of 132 patients with PCNSL treated with irradiation alone between 1990 and 1999 demonstrated a median overall survival (OS) of 18 months and an OS at five years of 18% (22). Among the patients aged 16–65 years with good performance status (a subset of patients who would have been eligible for the EORTC combined modality treatment trial) (23) the median survival was 26 months. These are the best-possible results using single modality irradiation and should now be the standard against which phase II trials of CMT are compared. Neurotoxicity data was not reported.

The median OS of 226 patients with PCNSL treated in the French Federation of Cancer Centres between 1980 and 1995 was 16 months (24,25). Treatment with any MTX and cytarabine based chemotherapy (compared to WBXRT alone) correlated with better survival in univariate analysis but after adjustment for known prognostic variables administration of MTX remained the only treatment-related factor independently correlated with survival. Survivors experienced significant neurotoxicity especially patients over age 60 who received >50 Gy.

Reni assembled data from 19 prospective series of 288 patients treated with MTX based therapy: either CMT or chemotherapy alone (26). Median OS was 40 months, which reflects the highly selective nature of the individual studies. A dose of at least 3 g/m^2

Table 40.1 Series of >100 patients in PCNSL reporting both treatment and outcome data.*

Reference	Study type	No. of patients	Median age (y)	Treatment Regimens	Total No.	No. Containing MTX	Median OS (mo)	OS at 5 y (%)	Neuro toxicity	Comments
(22)	3 multicenter studies 1990 onward	132	63	Only WBXRT 40 Gy + 10 Gy boost	 132		18 (26 if <65 y)	18 (24 if <65 y)	NA	
(26)	Review of published prospective studies using MTX-based Rx	288	NA	Any WBXRT (immediate or delayed) MTX only ± WBXRT MTX + other Cx ± WBXRT	100	 102 186	40	40	NA	(1) Individual studies had fewer than 35 pts. (2) not a formal meta-analysis
(27)	Multicenter compilation of individual data ITT analysis	370	61	Cx alone Cx → WBXRT(45 Gy) WBXRT(45 Gy) → Cx	32 197 36	25 135 9	20 24 (if MTX used)	24	21%	ara-c associated with improved survival
(24,25)	French retrospective data from studies 1978–1995	226	61	WBXRT alone Some Cx→WBXRT	59 162	 94	16 30 (if MTX used)	19 36 (if MTX used)	19% 69% if >50 Gy	MTX beneficial in all ages
(17)	Population-based British Columbia	122	60	WBXRT alone (≥35 Gy/20) MTX alone MTX→WBXRT palliative	37 34	 23 28	18 39 (if any MTX ≥ 1 g/m^2 used)	19 23	4% (MTX alone) 16% severe (WBXRT)	(1) Median OS 17 mo for entire cohort (2) Analysis by treatment administered
(18)	Single center 1989–2001	164	62	WBXRT CMT Palliative HDC	47 40 8	 65	10 14 1 28	26 (2 y) 36 (2 y)		Median OS 7.5 mo for entire cohort
(55)	Multicenter	248	61	WBXRT alone Cx → WBXRT Cx alone Cx palliative	60 129 35 24	 108	12 overall		NA	
(56)	Nationwide Japan 1985–1994	466 (380 had WBXRT)	60	WBXRT alone Any Cx→WBXRT	181 189	 31	18 (22 if <60 y)	15		(1) 8% T cell phenotype (2) 30–39.9 Gy has median OS 24 mo

*WBXRT, whole-brain irradiation; OS, overall survival; ara-c, cytarabine; Gy, Gray; Rx, treatment; HDC, high dose chemotherapy; Cx, chemotherapy; MTX, methotrexate; NA, data not available.

Table 40.2 Results of combined modality therapy (CMT) for PCNSL using MTX-Based regimens followed by WBXRT.*

References	Chemotherapy: Pre-XRT (MTX g/m²)	Chemotherapy: Post-XRT	Institution	No. of patients	WBXRT Median age (y)	dose Gy (boost)	Median PFS (mo)	Median OS (mo)	5 y OS (%)	Neurotoxicity	Comments
(10,28)	MTX **3.5** VCR procarbazine	ara-c	single	57	65	45	129	51 overall NR if <60 y 29 if >60 y	43	30% overall 26% <60 y and WBXRT 74% >60 y and WBXRT 4% chemo only	Cause of death: PCNSL 61% neurotoxicity 25%; no primary WBXRT given to 26 pts (22 >60 y and 4 <60 y)
(28,30)	MTX **2.5** VCR procarbazine	ara-c	Multi RTOG	102	57	45 36 HFX if CR	24	37 50 if <60 y 22 if >60 y	32	15% HFX only delayed its onset	No difference in OS between standard and HFX WBXRT
(31,32)	MTX**1**		Multi	46	58	45 (5.4)	40	33	37	30% at 5 y 58% if >60 y	
(23,59)	MTX **3** teniposide carmustine		Multi EORTC	52	51	40		46	58 (3 y)	63% overall in survivors but severe in 21%	10% acute toxic death
(33)	MTX **0.5** pirarubicin cyclo etoposide VCR procarbazine	same q4mo × 2 y	Multi	32	61	20–30	39	68	56 (wide CI)	10% death due to neurotoxicity; 7/18 long-term survivors had dementia	10% acute toxic death
(60)	MTX **3.5** bleomycin cyclo VCR procarbazine ara-c		Single	38	56	45 deferred if CR with chemo	28 if CR with chemo	42	60	None reported based on MMSE	25/36 CR to Cx; 16 relapses in 25
(61)	MTX **1** thiotepa procarbazine		Single	17	53	41 (+14)	18	32	25	29% grade 5	
(34)	MTX **3.5** ara-c idarubicin thiotepa		Multi	41	57	30 if CR 36 if PR 45 if <PR (9)	3 y FFS 43%	15	41	NR	10% acute toxic death
(35,36)	CHOD → MTX **1.5** ara-c VCR carmustine		Multi	77	60	1986–1995 45 (10) 1996–2001 30.6 if CR		40	37	0 if XRT 30.6 Gy; 8% (mild) if <60 y and 45 Gy 60% if >60 y and 45 Gy	9% acute toxic deaths; more relapses if 30.6 Gy especially if <60 y

*MTX, methotrexate; HFX, hyperfractionated; WBXRT or XRT, whole-brain irradiation; FFS, failure-free survival; ara-c, cytarabine; MMSE, mini-mental status exam; VCR, vincristine; CI, confidence interval; No., number; cyclo, cyclophosphamide; PFS, progression-free survival; CHOD, cyclophosphamide, doxorubicin, vincristine, dexamethasone; OS, overall survival; Gy, Gray; Cx, chemotherapy.

of MTX correlated with better survival in univariate analysis. In the 118 patients who received this dose of MTX, age $\leq$60 years, Karnofsky performance status $\geq$70 and the addition of cytarabine remained significantly associated with OS in multivariate analysis. If a complete response (CR) was obtained with chemotherapy, patients who received WBXRT at relapse appeared to do equally well as those who were immediately irradiated. Finally, those who received $\geq$40 Gy fared no better than those treated with lower doses.

In another large report, 23 centers submitted data to the International Extranodal Lymphoma Study Group (IELSG) on 378 immunocompetent patients with PCNSL diagnosed between 1980 and 1999, 135 of whom were treated with MTX based CMT (27). Median OS for the entire cohort was 20 months and 24 months when MTX based chemotherapy was used. The latter group had a significantly improved survival with respect to those treated with 45 Gy of WBXRT alone. This was independent of age and performance status. Similar to the Reni paper, those treated with MTX plus high-dose cytarabine exhibited improved survival compared with those treated with MTX alone. In contrast, there was no correlation between MTX dose (1 to 2.9 g/m^2 vs. $\geq$3 g/m^2) and survival.

The data in Table 40.2 show the results of phase II trials of CMT several of which warrant more detailed description. The long-term results from the Memorial Sloan Kettering Cancer Center (MSKCC) and subsequent multicenter RTOG study using a modification of that protocol have recently been published (10,28–30). The protocol included procarbazine and vincristine in combination with MTX, followed by 45 Gy WBXRT (modified later to 36 Gy with hyperfractionation for complete responders in the RTOG study) and finally cytarabine. The median OS was 51 months for the single center trial and 37 months in the RTOG trial with patients younger than 60 years faring extremely well (median OS not reached and 50 months, respectively). With hyperfractionation, lower total doses of WBXRT were administered and OS was not compromised compared with those who received 45 Gy. Thirty percent of survivors developed leukoencephalopathy with an incidence of 74% in irradiated patients older than 60 years. This complication was delayed but not eliminated in those who received the hyperfractionated dose schedule. Finally, a subgroup of patients who refused WBXRT following complete response to chemotherapy only had a 4% incidence of neurotoxicity.

In comparison, long-term results using single-agent MTX at a dose of 1 g/m^2 followed by a higher dose of total dose of irradiation achieved a median OS of 33 months with 30% of survivors demonstrating significant neurotoxicity (58% of those over 60 years) (31,32). A multicenter EORTC trial enrolled 52 patients up to age 65 years to a multiagent MTX based regimen followed by 40 Gy of WBXRT. The median survival of 46 months is similar to that of younger patients in the RTOG trial but the 10% incidence of acute toxic deaths and the 21% rate of severe neurotoxicity (63% all grades) preclude the widespread adoption of this regimen.

Three of the trials in Table 40.2 used a tailored approach to WBXRT, with the administered dose reduced according to response or age (33–36). The median OS for these trials ranged from 15 to 68 months with 10% of patients experiencing an acute toxic death from the multiagent chemotherapy regimens. The results on neurotoxicity are conflicting, with the Japanese trial reporting significant rates of dementia despite using a maximum WBXRT dose of 30 Gy and the Bessel data showing no clinically significant neurotoxicity for those who received <30.6 Gy. In the Bessel trial, long-term disease control was inferior for patients younger than 60 years who received 30.6 Gy of WBXRT compared to those who received 45 Gy.

The studies using chemotherapy alone as planned initial treatment for patients with PCNSL are shown in Table 40.3. Several important points can be made. First progression-free survival (PFS) for chemotherapy alone is inferior to that achieved with CMT. In contrast, the OS results are comparable underscoring the efficacy of salvage therapy, usually WBXRT, for those who experience progression. Second, two separate multicenter trials (12,37) have tested methotrexate as a single agent at a dose of 8 g/m^2 and have reported very different outcomes with median survivals of 25 and 55 months, respectively. There is no obvious reason for this discrepancy. Third, when multiagent chemotherapy is employed a lower dose of MTX (1 to 5 g/m^2) is generally administered (13,38,39) and the more intense the initial chemotherapy regimen the greater the acute treatment related mortality. OS is still superior to the PFS in these trials reflecting the efficacy of salvage therapy. Fourth, intra-arterial chemotherapy with blood–brain barrier disruption is effective but is complicated to administer, associated with acute adverse events and therefore not widely applicable (40,41). Finally, long-term neurotoxicity is lower for those patients with sustained remissions after chemotherapy alone but serious neurotoxicity is seen in those patients who receive salvage WBXRT in doses greater than 36Gy.

Several small studies have used high dose chemotherapy and stem cell rescue (either with or without WBXRT) (42–44) as first-line treatment of PCNSL. These have not been shown to be sufficiently superior to standard approaches to warrant their use outside of the clinical trial setting.

Most patients with PCNSL will experience a relapse. There is no Grade 1 evidence available to establish a standard of care for relapsed PCNSL. Table 40.4 outlines the published data (45–54). WBXRT is generally employed following progression after chemotherapy alone. MTX can be administered again if the disease-free interval is long. Other agents that cross the BBB, including those given at high dose with stem cell support, have also been employed.

Recommendations

A trade-off exists that includes potentially superior disease control associated with combined modality therapy and reduced risks of neurotoxicity/leukencephalopathy associated with chemotherapy alone. Based on the limited data available, the following are recommended:

1. For patients less than age 60 years at presentation:
   a. Is combined modality therapy with chemotherapy and whole brain irradiation the standard of care?

Table 40.3 Results of trials of initial MTX-based chemotherapy in PCNSL.*

References	Chemotherapy (Systemic)		Setting	No. of Patients	Median age (y)	ORR (%) CR/PR	PFS mo median	OS mo median	2 y OS%	Neuro toxicity	Acute toxic deaths	Comments
	MTX Dose g/m^2	Other Drugs										
(11)	8	None	Single	31	63	100 65/35	17	30	63	None		
(37,57)	8	None if < CR, WBXRT 45 Gy or PCV	Multi	37	60	NA 30/NA	10	25	51	58% if WBXRT salvage; 10% if no WBXRT		Trial aborted early due to low ORR
(12,54,58)	8	None	Multi	25	59	74 52/22	13	55	68	15% if WBXRT at relapse but 0% if dose <36 Gy/20		
(40,41)	2.5 with BBB disruption & IA administration	(a) Cyclo procarbazine (b) Cyclo etoposide	Single	74	60	84 65/19	NA	41	NA	None	5% (+7% stroke)	<60 y median OS 86 mo >60 y median OS 16 mo
(38)	1	Lomustine procarbazine steroids	Multi	50	72 (all pts >60 y)	48 42/6 (after 1 cycle)	7	14	50	7% in long-term responder	4%	
(13)	5 "Bonn Protocol"	ara-c ifosphamide vincristine cyclo vindesine steroids	Multi	65	62	71 61/10	21	50	69	3%	9%	<61 y median OS not reached >61 y median OS 34 mo
(39)	3	Lomustine procarbazine steroids;5 mo of maintenance Cx and deferred WBXRT if CR	3 sites	64	47 (all pts <60 y)	90 52/38	13	Not reached at 54 mo f/u	NA	9% (none in chemo alone group)	3%	Consolidation or salvage XRT n = 27 HDC n = 23
(7)	8	Temozolomide rituximab; if CR then ara-c etoposide	Single	21	59	NA 52/NA	11.5	Not reached at 27 mo f/u	NA			

*MTX, methotrexate; PFS, progression-free survival; Gy, Gray; ORR, overall response rate; OS, overall survival; IA, intra-arterial; CR, complete response; ara-c, cytarabine; NA, not available; PR, partial response; WBXRT or XRT, whole-brain irradiation; cyclo, cyclophosphamide; BBB, blood–brain barrier; f/u, follow–up; Cx, chemotherapy; PCV, procarbazine; CCNU, vincristine.

Table 40.4 Studies of $\geq$15 patients of salvage therapy for relapsed or refractory PCNSL.*

Reference	Type	No.	Median age (y)	Treatment	ORR%	Median (months) PFS	OS	Long term	Comments
(45)	Retrospective review 24 papers	173	57% <60 y 43% >60 y	Various including WBXRT	NA	NA	NA		2 mo vs. 14 mo OS for no Rx vs. any Rx
(46)	Phase II	22	53	(a) Cytarabine etoposide (b) HDC in responders	71 after (a)	NA	64% (3 y)	14 in CR median f/u 41 mo	5/7 pts >60 y died acutely
(47)	Retrospective review previously treated with CHOD/BVAM	16	54	Etoposide cytarabine ifosfamide	37	5	6	80% of responders alive at 12 mo	1 episode encephalopathy 50% febrile neutropenia
(48)	Multicenter retrospective MTX Rx (median TTR 24 mo)	22	58	MTX	91	NA	62		Only included patients previously in CR 2° first-line MTX
(48)	Phase II	23	60	Temozolomide	26	2	4	3 of 8 in CR median f/u 16 mo	
(50)	Retrospective review single institution	15	69	Temozolomide rituximab (IT MTX if CSF +)	53	2.2	14	3 of 6 in CR at 9, 11, 22 mo	Low platelets
(51,52)	Phase II	24	53	Topotecan	37	2.5	7	3 of 4 in CR at 12, 15, 24 mo	11 patients received Rx after topotecan (WBXRT in 9)
(62)	Retrospective review of German studies n = 143	44	59	33/44 14 Cx 12 WBXRT 7 CMT		NA	4.5	9 alive >10 mo	
(54)	Relapsed or refractory post- MTX	27	67	WBXRT Median 36 Gy	74	10	11	40% alive at 24 mo	15% neurotoxicity if dose > 36 Gy

*PFS, progression-free survival; HDC, high-dose chemotherapy; WBXRT, whole-brain irradiation; IT MTX, intrathecal methotrexate; Cx, chemotherapy; OS, overall survival; TTR, time to relapse; CHOD/BVAM, Reference (63); Gy, Gray; CMT, combined modality therapy.

Methotrexate-based CMT, using a minimum dose of 1 g/m^2 is recommended over use of WBXRT as a single modality (Grade 1C).

Use of chemotherapy alone, may be appropriate in order to reduce neurotoxicity. When given as a single modality, the chemotherapy should follow the principles described below with respect to optimum chemotherapy and omission of radiation (Grade 2C).

b. Which chemotherapy regimen should be used?

Proper testing of chemotherapy regimens in randomized trials has not been performed. Thus, no one regimen has been proven superior to another.

When used as a single agent, the dose of methotrexate should be 8 g/m^2, prorated to creatinine clearance (Grade 2C).

The MSKCC/RTOG regimen of methotrexate, procarbazine, vincristine (with cytarabine administered following WBXRT) has been the most widely tested in phase II trials, and its efficacy appears to be at least comparable to other options and it is associated with the least acute toxicity of the multiagent chemotherapy protocols. Use of this regimen is a reasonable option when combined modality therapy is chosen (Grade 2C).

While cytarabine has been used in most multiagent protocols, multivariate analyses of retrospective studies have not consistently supported its additive role. Therefore, there are insufficient data to recommend routine inclusion of this agent (Grade 2C).

c. Can the dose of whole brain irradiation be reduced or omitted in patients who achieve a complete response with chemotherapy?

When combined with chemotherapy, the dose of WBXRT should be kept to less than 40 Gy (Grade 1C).

Progression-free survival is superior when combined modality therapy is used. However, a strategy of delayed WBXRT for patients who achieve a complete response with chemotherapy does not appear to adversely influence overall survival compared with immediate irradiation. Radiation treatment can be deferred until relapse so that the risk of neurotoxicity can be minimized. If WBXRT is used as part of primary therapy a dose range of 31–40 Gy appears to best balance efficacy with toxicity (Grade 2C).

2. In patients older than age 60 at presentation what treatment approach optimizes the balance between achieving cure and minimizing neurotoxicity?

CMT is associated with an unacceptable risk of severe neurotoxicity in patients older than 60 years. Therefore, unless treatment is directed at short-term palliation only, these patients should be treated with chemotherapy alone (Grade 1C).

3. What is the optimal treatment at relapse?

There is no standard of care for treatment of PCNSL at relapse.

Whole-brain radiation therapy is generally employed following progression after chemotherapy alone (Grade 2C).

Methotrexate can be readministered if the durable disease control was achieved with initial therapy (Grade 2C).

References

1 Olson JE, Janney CA, Rao RD, et al. The continuing increase in the incidence of primary central nervous system non-Hodgkin lymphoma: a surveillance, epidemiology, and end results analysis. *Cancer.* 2002;**95**(7):1504–10.

2 Nelson DF. Radiotherapy in the treatment of primary central nervous system lymphoma (PCNSL). *J Neurooncol.* 1999;**43**(3):241–47.

3 O'Neill BP, Wang CH, O'Fallon JR, et al. The consequences of treatment and disease in patients with primary CNS non-Hodgkin's lymphoma: cognitive function and performance status. North Central Cancer Treatment Group. *Neuro Oncol.* 1999;**1**(3):196–203.

4 Mead GM, Bleehen NM, Gregor A, et al. A medical research council randomized trial in patients with primary cerebral non-Hodgkin lymphoma: cerebral radiotherapy with and without cyclophosphamide, doxorubicin, vincristine, and prednisone chemotherapy. *Cancer.* 2000;**89**(6):1359–70.

5 Green MR, Chowdhary S, Lombardi KM, et al. Clinical utility and pharmacology of high-dose methotrexate in the treatment of primary CNS lymphoma. *Expert Rev Neurother.* 2006;**6**(5):635–52.

6 Camilleri-Broet S, Criniere E, Broet P, et al. A uniform activated B-cell-like immunophenotype might explain the poor prognosis of primary central nervous system lymphomas: analysis of 83 cases. *Blood.* 2006;**107**(1):190–96.

7 Issa S, Hwang J, Karch J, et al. Treatment of primary CNS lymphoma with induction high-dose methotrexate, temozolomide, rituximab followed by consolidation cytarabine/etoposide: a pilot study with biomarker analysis. *Proc Annu Meeting ASCO.* 2006;**24**(Pt 1 Suppl 18):7595.

8 Doolittle ND, Miner ME, Hall WA, et al. Safety and efficacy of a multicenter study using intraarterial chemotherapy in conjunction with osmotic opening of the blood-brain barrier for the treatment of patients with malignant brain tumors. *Cancer.* 2000;**88**(3):637–47.

9 Hiraga S, Arita N, Ohnishi T, et al. Rapid infusion of high-dose methotrexate resulting in enhanced penetration into cerebrospinal fluid and intensified tumor response in primary central nervous system lymphomas. *J Neurosurg.* 1999;**91**(2):221–30.

10 Abrey LE, Yahalom J, DeAngelis LM. Treatment for primary CNS lymphoma: the next step. *J Clin Oncol.* 2000;**18**(17):3144–50.

11 Guha-Thakurta N, Damek D, Pollack C, Hochberg FH. Intravenous methotrexate as initial treatment for primary central nervous system lymphoma: response to therapy and quality of life of patients. *J Neurooncol.* 1999;**43**(3):259–68.

12 Batchelor T, Carson K, O'Neill A, et al. Treatment of primary CNS lymphoma with methotrexate and deferred radiotherapy: a report of NABTT 96-07. *J Clin Oncol.* 2003;**21**(6):1044–49.

13 Pels H, Schmidt-Wolf IGH, Glasmacher A, et al. Primary central nervous system lymphoma: results of a pilot and phase II study of systemic and intraventricular chemotherapy with deferred radiotherapy [see comment]. *J Clin Oncol.* 2003;**21**(24):4489–95.

14 Correa DD, DeAngelis LM, Shi W, et al. Cognitive functions in survivors of primary central nervous system lymphoma. *Neurology.* 2004;**62**(4):548–55.

15 Fliessbach K, Helmstaedter C, Urbach H, et al. Neuropsychological outcome after chemotherapy for primary CNS lymphoma: a prospective study. *Neurology.* 2005;**64**(7):1184–88.

16 Ferreri AJM, Blay J-Y, Reni M, et al. Prognostic scoring system for primary CNS lymphomas: the International Extranodal Lymphoma Study Group experience. *J Clin Oncol.* 2003;**21**(2):266–72.

17 Shenkier TN, Voss N, Chhanabhai M, et al. The treatment of primary central nervous system lymphoma in 122 immunocompetent patients: a population-based study of successively treated cohorts from the British Colombia Cancer Agency. *Cancer.* 2005;**103**(5):1008–17.

18 Feuerhake F, Baumer C, Cyron D, et al. Primary CNS lymphoma in immunocompetent patients from 1989 to 2001: a retrospective analysis of 164 cases uniformly diagnosed by stereotactic biopsy. *Acta Neurochir (Wien).* 2006;**148**(8):831–38; discussion 8.

19 Omuro AMP, Ben-Porat LS, Panageas KS, et al. Delayed neurotoxicity in primary central nervous system lymphoma. *Arch Neurol.* 2005;**62**(10):1595–600.

20 Thiel E, Nowrousian M, Hossfeld D, et al. The BMPD study with randomized whole-brain-irradiation (WBI) for primary CNS lymphoma (PCNSL). *J Cancer Res Clin Oncol.* 2002;**128**(Suppl 1).

21 Korfel A, Martus P, Nowrousian MR, et al. Response to chemotherapy and treating institution predict survival in primary central nervous system lymphoma. *Br J Haematol.* 2005;**128**(2):177–83.

22 Shibamoto Y, Ogino H, Hasegawa M, et al. Results of radiation monotherapy for primary central nervous system lymphoma in the 1990s. *Int J Radiat Oncol Biol Phys.* 2005;**62**(3):809–13.

23 Poortmans PM, Kluin-Nelemans HC, Haaxma-Reiche H, et al. High-dose methotrexate-based chemotherapy followed by consolidating radiotherapy in non-AIDS-related primary central nervous system lymphoma: European Organization for Research and Treatment of Cancer Lymphoma Group Phase II Trial 20962. *J Clin Oncol.* 2003;**21**(24):4483–88.

24 Blay JY, Conroy T, Chevreau C, et al. High-dose methotrexate for the treatment of primary cerebral lymphomas: analysis of survival and late neurologic toxicity in a retrospective series. *J Clin Oncol.* 1998;**16**(3):864–71.

25 Blay JY, Ongolo-Zogo P, Sebban C, et al. Primary cerebral lymphomas: unsolved issues regarding first-line treatment, follow-up, late neurological toxicity and treatment of relapses. The FNCLCC. French Federation Nationale des Centres de Lutte contre le Cancer. *Ann Oncol.* 2000;**11** Suppl 1:39–44.

26 Reni M, Ferreri AJ, Guha-Thakurta N, et al. Clinical relevance of consolidation radiotherapy and other main therapeutic issues in primary central nervous system lymphomas treated with upfront high-dose methotrexate. *Int J Radiat Oncol Biol Phys.* 2001;**51**(2):419–25.

27 Ferreri AJM, Reni M, Pasini F, Calderoni A, et al. A multicenter study of treatment of primary CNS lymphoma. *Neurology.* 2002;**58**(10):1513–20.

28 Gavrilovic IT, Hormigo A, Yahalom J, et al. Long-term follow-up of high-dose methotrexate-based therapy with and without whole brain irradiation for newly diagnosed primary CNS lymphoma. *J Clin Oncol.* 2006;**24**(28):4570–74.

29 DeAngelis LM, Seiferheld W, Schold SC, et al. Combination chemotherapy and radiotherapy for primary central nervous system lymphoma: Radiation Therapy Oncology Group Study 93-10 [see comment]. *J Clin Oncol.* 2002;**20**(24):4643–48.

30 Fisher B, Seiferheld W, Schultz C, et al. Secondary analysis of Radiation Therapy Oncology Group study (RTOG) 9310: an intergroup phase II combined modality treatment of primary central nervous system lymphoma. *J Neurooncol.* 2005;**74**(2):201–5.

31 O'Brien P, Roos D, Pratt G, et al. Phase II multicenter study of brief single-agent methotrexate followed by irradiation in primary CNS lymphoma. *J Clin Oncol.* 2000;**18**(3):519–26.

32 O'Brien PC, Roos DE, Pratt G, et al. Combined-modality therapy for primary central nervous system lymphoma: long-term data from a Phase II multicenter study (Trans-Tasman Radiation Oncology Group). *Int J Radiat Oncol Biol Phys.* 2006;**64**(2):408–13.

33 Yamanaka R, Morii K, Shinbo Y, et al. Modified ProMACE-MOPP hybrid regimen with moderate-dose methotrexate for patients with primary CNS lymphoma. *Ann Hematol.* 2005;**84**(7):447–55.

34 Ferreri AJM, Dell'Oro S, Foppoli M, et al. MATILDE regimen followed by radiotherapy is an active strategy against primary CNS lymphomas. *Neurology.* 2006;**66**(9):1435–38.

35 Bessell EM, Lopez-Guillermo A, Villa S, et al. Importance of radiotherapy in the outcome of patients with primary CNS lymphoma: an analysis of the CHOD/BVAM regimen followed by two different radiotherapy treatments. *J Clin Oncol.* 2002;**20**(1):231–36.

36 Bessell EM, Graus F, Lopez-Guillermo A, et al. Primary non-Hodgkin's lymphoma of the CNS treated with CHOD/BVAM or BVAM chemotherapy before radiotherapy: long-term survival and prognostic factors. *Int J Radiat Oncol Biol Phys.* 2004;**59**(2):501–8.

37 Herrlinger U, Kuker W, Uhl M, et al. NOA-03 trial of high-dose methotrexate in primary central nervous system lymphoma: final report. *Ann Neurol.* 2005;**57**(6):843–47.

38 Hoang-Xuan K, Taillandier L, Chinot O, et al. Chemotherapy alone as initial treatment for primary CNS lymphoma in patients older than 60 years: a multicenter phase II study (26952) of the European Organization for Research and Treatment of Cancer Brain Tumor Group [see comment]. *J Clin Oncol.* 2003;**21**(14):2726–31.

39 Omuro AM, Taillandier L, Chinot O, et al. Methotrexate (MTX), procarbazine and CCNU for primary central nervous system lymphoma (PCNSL) in patients younger than 60: can radiotherapy (RT) be deferred? *J Clin Oncol (Suppl).* 2006;**24**:70s (abstr).

40 McAllister LD, Doolittle ND, Guastadisegni PE, et al. Cognitive outcomes and long-term follow-up results after enhanced chemotherapy delivery for primary central nervous system lymphoma. *Neurosurgery.* 2000;**46**(1):51–60.

41 Kraemer DF, Fortin D, Doolittle ND, et al. Association of total dose intensity of chemotherapy in primary central nervous system lymphoma (human non-acquired immunodeficiency syndrome) and survival. *Neurosurgery.* 2001;**48**:1033–41.

42 Abrey LE, Moskowitz CH, Mason WP, et al. Intensive methotrexate and cytarabine followed by high-dose chemotherapy with autologous stem-cell rescue in patients with newly diagnosed primary CNS lymphoma: an intent-to-treat analysis. *J Clin Oncol.* 2003;**21**(22):4151–56.

43 Illerhaus G, Marks R, Ihorst G, et al. High-dose chemotherapy with autologous stem-cell transplantation and hyperfractionated radiotherapy as first-line treatment of primary CNS lymphoma. *J Clin Oncol.* 2006;**24**(24):3865–70.

44 Colombat P, Lemevel A, Bertrand P, et al. High-dose chemotherapy with autologous stem cell transplantation as first-line therapy for primary CNS lymphoma in patients younger than 60 years: a multicenter phase II study of the GOELAMS group. *Bone Marrow Transplant.* 2006;**38**(6):417–20.

45 Reni M, Ferreri AJ, Villa E. Second-line treatment for primary central nervous system lymphoma. *Br J Cancer.* 1999;**79**(3–4):530–34.

46 Soussain C, Suzan F, Hoang-Xuan K, et al. Results of intensive chemotherapy followed by hematopoietic stem-cell rescue in 22 patients with refractory or recurrent primary CNS lymphoma or intraocular lymphoma. *J Clin Oncol.* 2001;**19**(3):742–49.

47 Arellano-Rodrigo E, Lopez-Guillermo A, Bessell EM, et al. Salvage treatment with etoposide (VP-16), ifosfamide and cytarabine (Ara-C) for

patients with recurrent primary central nervous system lymphoma. *Eur J Haematol.* 2003;**70**(4):219–24.

48 Plotkin SR, Betensky RA, Hochberg FH, et al. Treatment of relapsed central nervous system lymphoma with high-dose methotrexate. *Clin Cancer Res.* 2004;**10**(17):5643–46.

49 Reni M, Mason W, Zaja F, et al. Salvage chemotherapy with temozolomide in primary CNS lymphomas: preliminary results of a phase II trial. *Eur J Cancer.* 2004;**40**(11):1682–88.

50 Enting RH, Demopoulos A, DeAngelis LM, et al. Salvage therapy for primary CNS lymphoma with a combination of rituximab and temozolomide [see comment]. *Neurology.* 2004;**63**(5):901–3.

51 Fischer L, Thiel E, Klasen HA, et al. Response of relapsed or refractory primary central nervous system lymphoma (PCNSL) to topotecan. *Neurology.* 2004;**62**(10):1885–87.

52 Fischer L, Thiel E, Klasen HA, et al. Long-term remissions in relapsed/refractory primary central nervous system lymphoma (PCNSL) after topotecan chemotherapy. *J Clin Oncol (Meeting Abstracts).* 2005;**23**(16 Suppl):1528–.

53 Jahnke K, Thiel E, Martus P, et al. Relapse of primary central nervous system lymphoma: clinical features, outcome and prognostic factors. 2006;**80**(2):159–65.

54 Nguyen PL, Chakravarti A, Finkelstein DM, et al. Results of whole-brain radiation as salvage of methotrexate failure for immunocompetent patients with primary CNS lymphoma. *J Clin Oncol.* 2005;**23**(7):1507–13.

55 Bataille B, Delwail V, Menet E, et al. Primary intracerebral malignant lymphoma: report of 248 cases. *J Neurosurg.* 2000;**92**(2):261–66.

56 Hayabuchi N, Shibamoto Y, Onizuka Y. Primary central nervous system lymphoma in Japan: a nationwide survey. *Int J Radiat Oncol Biol Phys.* 1999;**44**(2):265–72.

57 Herrlinger U, Schabet M, Brugger W, et al. German Cancer Society Neuro-Oncology Working Group NOA-03 multicenter trial of single-agent high-dose methotrexate for primary central nervous system lymphoma. *Ann Neurol.* 2002;**51**(2):247–52.

58 Batchelor T, Grossman S, Carson K, et al. Updated results from NABTT CNS consortium studies in primary CNS lymphoma. Annual Meeting Proceedings. *Am Soc Clin Oncol.* 2004;**23**:111 (abstr).

59 Harder H, Holtel H, Bromberg JE, et al. Cognitive status and quality of life after treatment for primary CNS lymphoma. *Neurology.* 2004;**62**(4):544–47.

60 Silvani A, Salmaggi A, Eoli M, et al. Methotrexate based chemotherapy and deferred radiotherapy for primary central nervous system lymphoma (PCNSL): single institution experience. *J Neuro-Oncol.* 2007;**82**:273–9.

61 Omuro AMP, DeAngelis LM, Yahalom J, et al. Chemoradiotherapy for primary CNS lymphoma: an intent-to-treat analysis with complete follow-up. *Neurology.* 2005;**64**(1):69–74.

62 Jahnke K, Korfel A, Martus P, et al. High-dose methotrexate toxicity in elderly patients with primary central nervous system lymphoma. *Proc Ann Meeting ASCO.* 2005;**16**(3):445–49.

63 Bessell EM, Graus F, Lopez-Guillermo A, et al. CHOD/BVAM regimen plus radiotherapy in patients with primary CNS non-Hodgkin's lymphoma. *Int J Radiat Oncol Biol Phys.* 2001;**50**(2):457–64.

41 Diffuse Large B-cell Lymphoma

Michael Crump

Introduction

Diffuse large B-cell lymphoma (DLBCL) is the most common aggressive histology lymphoma diagnosed in North America and Europe. Recent data from the SEER (surveillance, epidemiology, and end results) program described an incidence of DLBCL in the United States of 7.1 per 100,000 persons per year (1). Approximately one-third of patients present with localized disease, defined as Ann Arbor Stage I or II, with 50% of these patients having disease involving extranodal sites. Therapy for extranodal disease and specific histologic subtypes such as T-cell–rich B-cell lymphoma and primary mediastinal large B cell lymphoma tends to mirror that studied in nodal DLBCL. Therefore, these patients will be included in this overview.

Patients with localized or advanced stage DLBCL and good performance status and organ function are treated with curative intent. During the 1990s, various multiagent combination chemotherapy regimens were compared in order to evaluate the concepts of dose intensity and the strategy of using alternating, non-cross-resistant regimens to improve outcomes in patients with aggressive non-Hodgkin's lymphoma (NHL) (2–6). These trials, and a systematic review of randomized trials comparing standard cyclophosphamide, doxorubicin, vincristine, and prednisone (CHOP) to "third-generation" regimens (7), showed no advantage to these regimens and established CHOP as the accepted standard to which future regimens should be compared. Currently, patients with DLBCL are treated with anthracycline-based chemotherapy regimens, mainly employing doxorubicin, and more recently, in combination with the anti-CD20 antibody rituximab (8–10). With the exception of HIV-related non-Hodgkin's lymphoma (11), the addition of rituximab has improved response rate, time to progression, and overall survival in all prospective, randomized studies reported to date and has become the standard of care for patients with this histology. However, despite the therapeutic advance provided by chemoimmunotherapy, a number of important questions remain with regard to the management of DLBCL and its variants.

The incidence of DLBCL rises sharply in persons over the age of 50, and the majority of cases in North America are diagnosed in patients over the age of 60 (1). Because elderly patients may tolerate aggressive chemotherapy poorly, and frequently have one or more significant comorbidities, alternative chemotherapy regimens have been explored in this patient population in an attempt to reduce toxicity while maintaining treatment efficacy and the possibility of cure.

Questions

1. Should patients with DLBCL receive involved-field radiation as part of primary therapy?
2. Should young patients with a good response to chemotherapy who are at high risk for recurrence receive consolidation with autologous stem cell transplantation?
3. Should rituximab be added to second-line therapy for patients with relapsed disease?
4. Should patients with advanced DLBCL receive dose-dense CHOP chemotherapy supported by filgrastim (G-CSF)?
5. Should older patients with DLBCL receive CHOP chemotherapy with curative intent?

Literature-search strategy and inclusion

MEDLINE (Ovid) (1950 to January 2007, week 3) and the Cochrane Library (2006, Issue 4) databases were searched. In MEDLINE the following Medical Subject Heading (MeSH) terms were used: "lymphoma, b-cell"; "exp lymphoma, diffuse"; "exp lymphoma, high-grade"; "exp lymphoma, intermediate-grade"; "exp lymphoma, large-cell"; and "exp lymphoma, undifferentiated." In addition, variations of the following text words were

Evidence-based Hematology. Edited by Mark A. Crowther, Jeff Ginsberg, Holger J. Schünemann, Ralph M. Meyer, and Richard Lottenberg.

also used: "diffuse large cell lymphoma," "aggressive lymphoma," "high grade non-Hodgkin lymphoma (NHL)," and "intermediate grade NHL." Those terms were combined with search terms for the following publication types and study designs: systematic reviews, meta-analyses, and randomized controlled trials (RCTs). The Cochrane Library search was similar. The proceedings of the annual meetings of the American Society of Hematology (ASH) and American Society of Clinical Oncology were searched electronically for trial results available in abstract form. The trials were reviewed by a research methodologist and the author to exclude duplications and reports describing nonrandomized trials. Seventy-nine trials were found that met inclusion criteria.

Grading of the quality of evidence and strengths of recommendations in this chapter are based on the guidelines proposed by the international Grading of Recommendations Assessment, Development, and Evaluation Working Group (GRADE) adopting the modification used by the American College of Chest Physicians that merges the very low and low categories of quality of evidence (see chapter 1).

Should patients with DLBCL receive involved-field radiation as part of primary therapy?

Although aggressive histology lymphomas such as DLBCL are very radiosensitive, distant relapse occurs frequently even with the extended-field radiotherapy. Combined modality treatment has allowed for a decrease in radiation field size and improved systemic disease control in stages I and II aggressive histology lymphoma (12).

The literature search identified five RCTs (13–17) and one systematic review (18) evaluating the benefit of the addition of involved-field radiation therapy (RT) to chemotherapy. The systematic review evaluated RT for all histologies and did not include trials published after 2003.

An RCT conducted by the Southwest Oncology Group (SWOG) demonstrated that three cycles of CHOP chemotherapy followed by involved-field radiation produced superior event-free and overall survival compared with eight cycles of CHOP alone (13). However, after additional follow-up, although the observed differences at five years remain, there have been more subsequent relapses in the radiation arm of the trial, and event-free and overall survival at ten years are the same in the two arms (19). The Eastern Cooperative Oncology Group (ECOG) performed a trial in stages I and II aggressive lymphoma utilizing eight cycles of CHOP chemotherapy, with patients achieving a complete response subsequently randomized to receive involved-field radiation (30 Gray [Gy]) or no further therapy; those with a partial response were assigned to local radiation (40 Gy) (14). In that study, involved-field radiation improved the six-year disease-free survival (73% vs. 56%), but no difference in overall survival was detected. Patients with a partial response, who were assigned to receive RT 40 Gy, had six-year failure-free survival of 63%.

Two recent trials by the Groupe d'Etude de Lymphomes de l'Adulte (GELA) tested the use of chemotherapy alone compared to chemotherapy followed by radiation in patients with low-risk aggressive lymphoma. In the first, patients age 60 years old or less with stages I and II lymphoma (DLBCL in 80% of cases) and no adverse International Prognostic Index (IPI) factors were randomized to three cycles of CHOP plus involved-field radiation, or chemotherapy alone with the intensive doxorubicin (Adriamycin®), cyclophosphamide, vindesine, bleomycin, and prednisone (ACVBP) induction and sequential consolidation (16). After a median follow-up of nearly eight years, event-free and overall survivals were significantly better in patients receiving chemotherapy alone, despite a slightly higher rate of local recurrence. The second study enrolled 576 patients older than age 60 with no IPI risk factors and compared four cycles of CHOP plus involved-field radiation (40 Gy in 22 fractions over five weeks) to CHOP alone (17). The median patient age was 68, and only 8% of patients had bulky disease at presentation. After a median follow up of seven years, event-free survival at five years is 61% in the chemotherapy alone group and 64% in the combined modality treatment group (p = NS).

A recent meta-analysis of five RCTs testing RT in localized aggressive lymphoma concluded that. although these studies are heterogeneous, there is no clear indication of benefit from the addition of involved-field RT following chemotherapy, or in place of a longer course of chemotherapy (20). As systemic chemotherapy becomes more effective, the role of involved-field RT may decrease. Notably, disease stage and bulk of disease remain important predictors of outcome in these trials regardless of therapy received.

Recommendation

Patients with localized stages I and II DLBCL should not routinely receive involved-field RT as consolidation of a complete response. Patients with a partial response may derive benefit from involved field radiation (Grade 2A).

Should patients with a good response to chemotherapy who are at high risk for recurrence receive consolidation with autologous stem cell transplantation?

The search strategy yielded 12 RCTs (21–32) and one meta-analysis (33). The majority of these trials compared standard durations of therapy (six to eight cycles of CHOP-like chemotherapy) to the same chemotherapy for a shorter number of cycles plus autologous stem cell transplantation (ASCT), or added ASCT as consolidation following a full course of chemotherapy. Two trials tested the concept of high-dose sequential therapy, without standard induction treatment, compared with CHOP or equivalent treatment (23,32). Although most studies enrolled "high-risk" patients, only two trials (27,31) specifically targeted patients who were at high-risk by the IPI, and the percentage of patients with high-intermediate or high-risk disease ranged from 31% to 100%. Though not all studies provided information on immunophenotyping, enrollment of patients with T cell lymphoma ranged from 2% to 10%, and anaplastic large cell lymphoma from 6% to 12%.

The intention-to-treat analyses of these trials consistently has shown a lack of improvement in disease-free or overall survival. The fraction of patients assigned high-dose therapy who did not complete protocol treatment (i.e., who did not receive high-dose therapy) varied but was as high as 40% (26,31).

Two RCTs did report an improvement in overall survival, but these were based on unplanned subset analyses. A reanalysis of the LNH-87 trial demonstrated benefit from high-dose therapy in patients considered high-risk according to the IPI (34,35), and an unplanned subset analysis of the GOELEMS trial similarly showed an improvement for patients with high-intermediate risk IPI scores (30). However, taken together, these trials have not shown an improvement in overall survival compared with conventional dose chemotherapy (33). A meta-analysis of 15 RCTs, including 2,728 patients, showed no evidence of improvement in survival following ASCT (36). A retrospective analysis of patients entered on two RCTs testing high-dose therapy and ASCT did not suggest any benefit from ASCT for patients with peripheral T-cell lymphoma, a group of patients with a particularly poor outcome with standard therapy (37).

Currently, a North American Intergroup RCT led by SWOG compares eight cycles of R-CHOP to six cycles R-CHOP followed by ASCT. This is the only ongoing RCT testing the utility of ASCT in patients receiving optimal chemoimmunotherapy.

Recommendation

For patients responding to primary chemotherapy, high-dose therapy with stem cell support does not improve progression-free or overall survival and is not recommended (Grade 1A).

Should rituximab be added to second-line therapy for patients with relapsed disease?

Only one RCT was identified; this was published as an ASH abstract (38).

There have been difficulties in conducting RCTs testing the role of rituximab as a part of second-line therapy for patients with DLBCL. At least two large cooperative group trials, one in Europe and the second in the United States, were initiated but closed prematurely because of poor accrual. Phase II or cohort studies have reported improved outcomes when rituximab is included compared with historical controls. For example, superior complete response rates have been suggested by a comparison of second-line chemotherapy prior to stem cell transplantation with R-ICE (rituximab, ifosfamide, carboplatin, and etoposide) as opposed to ICE (39). Improvement in disease control posttransplant could not be determined because of the retrospective nature of this analysis.

Recently, the Dutch-Belgium Group, HOVON, presented the results of an RCT testing the addition of rituximab to DHAP-VIM chemotherapy for patients with relapsed aggressive histology B-cell lymphoma (38). Patients with at least a partial response to two cycles received an additional cycle for stem cell mobilization, followed by high-dose BEAM chemotherapy and ASCT. This study randomized over 200 patients; less than 5% had received prior rituximab. The addition of rituximab to second-line chemotherapy improved the complete and overall response rates (77% vs. 49%), as well as failure-free survival and overall survival post-transplant ($p < 0.001$). Although this study clearly demonstrates benefits, the impact adding rituximab for patients who have DLBCL that progresses during, or recurs after, completion of initial chemoimmunotherapy that included rituximab is unclear. There are currently no data regarding improvement in disease control by the addition of rituximab to the second-line treatment of patients who are not undergoing ASCT.

Recommendation

The inclusion of rituximab with second-line chemotherapy prior to autologous transplantation for patients who are rituximab-naïve is recommended (Grade 1B). The addition of rituximab to the second-line chemotherapy, of those who have previously received chemoimmunotherapy, cannot be supported by the available data (Grade 2C).

Should patients with advanced DLBCL receive dose-dense chemotherapy supported by growth factors?

The potential of hematopoietic growth factors such as filgrastim (G-CSF) to support a more dose-intensive chemotherapy or a shortened chemotherapy treatment schedule has facilitated the evaluation of chemotherapy dose intensity in aggressive histology lymphoma.

Two recent trials by the German High-Grade Lymphoma Study Group tested the addition of etoposide to CHOP chemotherapy (CHOEP) and the use of a two-week treatment cycle compared to three weeks, using a factorial design (40,41). Patients under the age of 60 with a favorable prognosis (normal LDH) were randomized to six cycles of CHOP on a 21- or 14-day schedule, the latter supported by G-CSF, or CHOEP-21 or -14. In this younger cohort with favorable prognosis lymphoma, CHOEP produced a higher complete remission rate and five-year event-free survival rate (69 vs. 58, $p = 0.004$) (40). Interval reduction improved overall survival in multivariate analysis but not in the direct comparison of the 14- versus 21-day schedules.

The same strategies were evaluated in as second trial in older patients: those aged 61–75 were randomized to the same treatment regimens as in the previous trial, CHOP-21 or CHOP-14, and CHOEP-21 or CHOEP-14 (41). Complete remission rate was inferior in the CHOP-21 arm, and five-year event-free survival, and overall survivals were superior for CHOP-14 (44% vs. 32% for event-free survival and 53% vs. 41% for overall survival). There was no improvement in disease control from the addition of etoposide to either the shortened or standard schedule, but the five-drug regimen produced greater toxicity. A second trial evaluating therapy intensification in patients age 18–65 years with aggressive NHL has recently been reported (42). Eligible patients had intermediate-risk lymphoma according to HOVON criteria (stage II and LDH >1.5 times normal or stages III–IV and LDH $<1.5\times$ normal). Patients were randomized to receive standard CHOP-21 or intensified CHOP (I-CHOP), consisting of increased doses of cyclophosphamide and doxorubicin, with treatment every 14 days for six cycles. The complete overall response rates were similar in the two arms, and the estimated six-year overall survival for CHOP 21 was 50% versus 61% for I-CHOP (hazard ratio 0.83, 0.62–1.11). Disease-free survival was also similar in the two groups. There are currently no data from trials evaluating the impact of intensifying treatment schedule in the setting of the addition of rituximab (14- vs. 21-day R-CHOP).

Recommendation

Intensification of therapy by using G-CSF allows treatment every 14 days and improves outcomes in patients with DLBCL; however, none of the trials reported to date have compared this strategy to R-CHOP on a 21-day schedule, and therefore, this strategy does not replace R-CHOP administered on a 21-day schedule as a treatment standard (Grade 2B). The GELA is currently comparing R-CHOP-21 to R-CHOP-14, but no results are available.

Should older patients with DLBCL receive CHOP chemotherapy with curative intent?

The literature search yielded 12 RCTs focusing on chemotherapy strategies for older patients, defined as those 60 or 70 years of age or older. Three trials investigated the addition of rituximab (9,43,63), while the others compared chemotherapy regimens, either with simple substitutions of another agent (including mitoxantrone) for doxorubicin, or more complex regimen comparisons (44–51). In addition, 12 other trials evaluating anthracycline substitutions were identified, although these trials did not specifically target an older patient population but included patients over the age of 65 (52–61). One systematic review on this topic, published in 2002, was also retrieved (62). Trials conducted specifically to evaluate supportive care (for example, prevention of febrile neutropenia) were not included (51).

In two studies, use of mitoxantrone (CNOP) produced inferior rates of complete response and overall survival compared to CHOP (44,48). Conversely, in a large trial, including more than 500 patients comparing an eight-week regimen of cyclophosphamide, etoposide, vincristine, bleomycin, prednisone, and either doxorubicin or mitoxantrone, the complete remission rate and overall survival at four years was significantly better for patients receiving mitoxantrone (50% vs. 28%, $p = 0.001$) (47). However, a subsequent trial, that included 784 patients, compared the six drug mitoxantrone-containing regimen, PMitCEBO, to CHOP in patients over the age of 60 and showed no difference in response rate, time to progression, or overall survival (46).The GELA attempted to improve on the results of the LNH-94 regimen (ACVBP followed by multidrug consolidation) in high-risk elderly patients. The strategy employed alternating cycles of ACVBP with VIMMM (VM26, ifosfamide, methotrexate, methyl-GAG, and methotrexate) and an alternating consolidation with VIM and ACVM (doxorubicin, cyclophosphamide, vindesine, and methotrexate) (48). There was no improvement in complete response rate or overall survival, but both regimens were associated with high-treatment-related mortality (19% and 26%). The ACVBP regimen was subsequently compared to standard CHOP chemotherapy in previously untreated patients aged 61–69 with at least one IPI risk factor (49). This regimen, which includes intensified chemotherapy with CNS prophylaxis followed by sequential consolidation, was superior in terms of complete response rate, five-year event-free survival, and overall survival. However, ACVBP chemotherapy was associated with an increased risk of early death compared with CHOP (13% vs. 7%, $p = 0.014$). Patients in the CHOP arm experienced more CNS progression but did not receive CNS prophylaxis.

An improvement in response rate and failure-free survival has been demonstrated in two trials adding rituximab to CHOP chemotherapy (9,43). Updated results from the GELA trial in over 400 patients shows an improvement in event-free and overall survival at five years, irrespective of the number of IPI risk factors at diagnosis (43). The second trial by the ECOG confirmed an improvement in response rate and disease control but no difference in overall survival (9). The latter study employed a maintenance rituximab strategy, with four weekly doses given every six months for two years. This study demonstrated that maintenance rituximab improved failure-free survival after CHOP but not after R-CHOP. In light of the fact that the majority of the patients now receive rituximab concurrently with each cycle of CHOP, there is currently no indication for the use of maintenance rituximab following a response to induction treatment.

The German High-Grade Lymphoma Study Group (GHGLSG) has demonstrated improvement in event-free and overall survival by shortening the treatment interval from 21 to 14 days, by the use of G-CSF support as described above (41). This improvement was not at the expense of a higher incidence of fever and neutropenia or other hematologic and nonhematologic toxicity. This shortened chemotherapy course, CHOP-14 was the standard arm for a second randomized trial by the GHGLSG (63). A factorial design was again used to evaluate the benefit from the addition of rituximab with each chemotherapy treatment and determine the optimum number of cycles of treatment (6 vs. 8). This study has been reported in abstract form and showed similar survival with six or eight cycles of chemotherapy, and confirmed the benefit of the addition of rituximab to CHOP even when given on a 14-day cycle. The superiority of R-CHOP-14 compared with CHOP-14 was recently confirmed in a trial by the HOVON and Nordic lymphoma groups in patients age 65–85 (median 72 years) (64). This study, reported in abstract form, demonstrated improvement in failure-free survival (hazard ratio $= 0.60$, $p = 0.007$) and overall survival ($p = 0.05$). Twenty-two percent of patients in that study discontinued treatment because of toxicity, and 14% experienced grade 3 or 4 infection.

Recommendation

The optimum chemotherapy regimen in elderly patients (over the age of 60) with DLBCL is R-CHOP-21 given for six cycles (Grade 1A). Data from randomized trials are not yet available to determine if R-CHOP-14 improves outcomes compared with R-CHOP-21. There is currently no advantage to the use of eight cycles of therapy in patients with a complete response after six cycles. Substitution of another agent for doxorubicin in this combination is not recommended as a strategy to improve toxicity or overall survival (Grade 1A). The choice of more intensive and prolonged regimens such as ACVBP, in the absence of rituximab, cannot be recommended at this time (Grade 2A).

References

1 Morton LM, Wang SS, Devesa SS, et al. Lymphoma incidence patterns by who subtype in the United States, 1992–2001. *Blood.* 2006;**107**:265–76.

2 Gordon LI, Andersen J, Colgan J, et al. Advanced diffuse non-Hodgkin's lymphoma: analysis of prognostic factors by the international index and by lactic dehydrogenase in an intergroup study. *Cancer.* 1995;**75**:865–73.

3 Fisher RI, Gaynor ER, Dahlberg S, et al. Comparison of a standard regimen (CHOP) with three intensive chemotherapy regimens for advanced non-Hodgkin's lymphoma. *N Engl J Med.* 1993;**328**:1002–6.

4 Wolf M, Matthews JP, Stone J, et al. Long-term survival advantage of MACOP-B over CHOP in intermediate-grade non-Hodgkin's lymphoma: the Australian and New Zealand Lymphoma Group. *Ann Oncol.* 1997;**8** Suppl 1:71–75.

5 Montserrat E, Garcia-Conde J, Vinolas N, et al. CHOP vs. Promace-Cytabom in the treatment of aggressive non-Hodgkin's lymphomas: long-term results of a multicenter randomized trial. (Pethema: Spanish Cooperative Group for the Study of Hematological Malignancies Treatment, Spanish Society Of Hematology). *Eur J Haematol.* 1996;**57**:377–83.

6 Jerkeman M, Anderson H, Cavallin-Stahl E, et al. Chop versus MACOP-B 01–A Nordic Lymphoma Group Randomized Trial. *Ann Oncol.* 1999;**10**:1079–86.

7 Messori A, Vaiani M, Trippoli S, et al. survival in patients with intermediate or high grade non-Hodgkin's lymphoma: meta-analysis of randomized studies comparing third generation regimens with CHOP. *Br J Cancer.* 2001;**84**:303–7.

8 Coiffier B, Lepage E, Briere J, et al. CHOP chemotherapy plus rituximab compared with CHOP alone in elderly patients with diffuse large-B-cell lymphoma. *N Engl J Med.* 2002;**346**:235–42.

9 Habermann TM, Weller EA, Morrison VA, et al. Rituximab-CHOP versus CHOP alone or with maintenance rituximab in older patients with diffuse large B-cell lymphoma. *J Clin Oncol.* 2006;**24**:3121–27.

10 Pfreundschuh M, Trumper L, Osterborg A, et al. CHOP-like chemotherapy plus rituximab versus CHOP-like chemotherapy alone in young patients with good-prognosis diffuse large-B-cell lymphoma: a randomised controlled trial by the Mabthera International Trial (MINT) Group. *Lancet Oncol.* 2006;**7**:379–91.

11 Kaplan LD, Lee JY, Ambinder RF, et al. Rituximab does not improve clinical outcome in a randomized phase 3 trial of CHOP with or without rituximab in patients with HIV-associated non-Hodgkin lymphoma: AIDS-Malignancies Consortium Trial 010. *Blood.* 2005;**106**:1538–43.

12 Yahalom J, Varsos G, Fuks Z, et al. Adjuvant cyclophosphamide, doxorubicin, vincristine, and prednisone chemotherapy after radiation therapy in stage I low-grade and intermediate-grade non-Hodgkin lymphoma: results of a prospective randomized study. *Cancer.* 1993;**71**:2342–50.

13 Miller TP, Dahlberg S, Cassady JR, et al. Chemotherapy alone compared with chemotherapy plus radiotherapy for localized intermediate- and high-grade non-Hodgkin's lymphoma. *N Engl J Med.* 1998;**339**:21–26.

14 Horning SJ, Weller E, Kim K, et al. Chemotherapy with or without radiotherapy in limited-stage diffuse aggressive non-Hodgkin's lymphoma: Eastern Cooperative Oncology Group Study 1484. *J Clin Oncol.* 2004;**22**:3032–38.

15 Aviles A, Fernandezb R, Perez F, et al. Adjuvant radiotherapy in stage IV diffuse large cell lymphoma improves outcome. *Leuk Lymphoma.* 2004;**45**:1385–89.

16 Reyes F, Lepage E, Ganem G, et al. ACVBP versus CHOP plus radiotherapy for localized aggressive lymphoma. *N Engl J Med.* 2005;**352**:1197–1205.

17 Bonnet C, Fillet G, Mounier N, et al. CHOP alone compared with CHOP plus radiotherapy for localized aggressive lymphoma in elderly patients: a study by the Groupe D'etude Des Lymphomes De L'adulte. *J Clin Oncol.* 2007;**25**:787–92.

18 Gustavsson A, Osterman B, Cavallin-Stahl E. A systematic overview of radiation therapy effects in non-Hodgkin's lymphoma. *Acta Oncol.* 2003;**42**:605–19.

19 Miller TP, Leblanc M, Spier CM, et al. CHOP alone compared to chop plus radiotherapy for early stage aggressive non-Hodgkin's lymphomas: update of the Southwest Oncology Group (SWOG) randomized trial. *Blood.* 2001;**98**:S742–S43.

20 Fried DB, Morris DE, Shea TC, et al. A systematic review evaluating the addition of radiation therapy to chemotherapy for localized aggressive non-Hodgkin's lymphoma: what is the role of radiotherapy? *Blood.* 2004;**104**:862a (abstr).

21 Haioun C, Lepage E, Gisselbrecht C, et al. Comparison of autologous bone marrow transplantation with sequential chemotherapy for intermediate-grade and high-grade non-Hodgkin's lymphoma in first complete remission: a study of 464 patients. Groupe D'etude Des Lymphomes De L'adulte. *J Clin Oncol.* 1994;**12**:2543–51.

22 Martelli M, Vignetti M, Zinzani Pl, et al. High-dose chemotherapy followed by autologous bone marrow transplantation versus dexamethasone, cisplatin, and cytarabine in aggressive non-Hodgkin's lymphoma with partial response to front-line chemotherapy: a prospective randomized Italian Multicenter Study. *J Clin Oncol.* 1996;**14**:534–42.

23 Gianni AM, Bregni M, Siena S, et al. High-dose chemotherapy and autologous bone marrow transplantation compared with MACOP-B in aggressive B-cell lymphoma. *N Engl J Med.* 1997;**336**:1290–97.

24 Santini G, Salvagno L, Leoni P, et al. VACOP-B versus VACOP-B plus autologous bone marrow transplantation for advanced diffuse non-Hodgkin's Lymphoma: results of a prospective randomized trial by the Non-Hodgkin's Lymphoma Cooperative Study Group. *J Clin Oncol.* 1998;**16**:2796–2802.

25 Kluin-Nelemans HC, Zagonel V, Anastasopoulou A, et al. Standard chemotherapy with or without high-dose chemotherapy for aggressive non-Hodgkin's lymphoma: randomized phase III EORTC study. *J Natl Cancer Inst.* 2001;**93**:22–30.

26 Kaiser U, Uebelacker I, Abel U, et al. Randomized study to evaluate the use of high-dose therapy as part of primary treatment for "aggressive" lymphoma. *J Clin Oncol.* 2002;**20**:4413–19.

27 Gisselbrecht C, Lepage E, Molina T, et al. Shortened first-line high-dose chemotherapy for patients with poor-prognosis aggressive lymphoma. *J Clin Oncol.* 2002;**20**:2472–79.

28 Vitolo U, Liberati AM, Cabras MG, et al. High dose sequential chemotherapy with autologous transplantation versus dose-dense chemotherapy MEGACEOP as first line treatment in poor-prognosis diffuse large cell lymphoma: an "Intergruppo Italiano Linfomi" randomized trial. *Haematologica.* 2005;**90**:793–801.

29 Olivieri A, Santini G, Patti C, et al. Upfront high-dose sequential therapy (HDS) versus VACOP-B with or without HDS in aggressive non-Hodgkin's lymphoma: long-term results by the NHLCSG. *Ann Oncol.* 2005;**16**:1941–48.

30 Milpied N, Deconinck E, Gaillard F, et al. Initial treatment of aggressive lymphoma With high-dose chemotherapy and autologous stem-cell support. *N Engl J Med.* 2004;**350**:1287–95.

31 Martelli M, Gherlinzoni F, De Renzo A, et al. Early autologous stem-cell transplantation versus conventional chemotherapy as front-line therapy in high-risk, aggressive non-Hodgkin's lymphoma: an Italian multicenter randomized trial. *J Clin Oncol.* 2003;**21**:1255–62.

32 Betticher DC, Martinelli G, Radford JA, et al. Sequential high dose chemotherapy as initial treatment for aggressive sub-types of non-Hodgkin lymphoma: results of the international randomized phase III trial (Mistral). *Ann Oncol.* 2006;**17**:1546–52.

33 Strehl J, Mey U, Glasmacher A, et al. High-dose chemotherapy followed by autologous stem cell transplantation as first-line therapy in aggressive non-Hodgkin's lymphoma: a meta-analysis. *Haematologica.* 2003;**88**:1304–15.

34 Haioun C, Lepage E, Gisselbrecht C, et al. Benefit of autologous bone marrow transplantation over sequential chemotherapy in poor-risk aggressive non-Hodgkin's lymphoma: updated results of the prospective study LNH87-2. Groupe D'etude Des Lymphomes De L'adulte. *J Clin Oncol.* 1997;**15**:1131–37.

35 Haioun C, Lepage E, Gisselbrecht C, et al. Survival benefit of high-dose therapy in poor-risk aggressive non-Hodgkin's lymphoma: final analysis of the prospective LNH87-2 protocol—a Groupe D'etude Des Lymphomes De L'adulte Study. *J Clin Oncol.* 2000;**18**:3025–30.

36 Greb A, Bohlius J, Trelle S, et al. High-dose chemotherapy with autologous stem cell support in first-line treatment of aggressive non-Hodgkin lymphoma—results of a comprehensive meta-analysis. *Cancer Treat Rev.* 2007;**33**:338–46.

37 Mounier N, Gisselbrecht C, Briere J, et al. All aggressive lymphoma subtypes do not share similar outcome after front-line autotransplantation: a matched-control analysis by the Groupe D'etude Des Lymphomes De L'adulte (GELA). *Ann Oncol.* 2004;**15**:1790–97.

38 Vellenga E, van Patten WLJ, van 'T Veer MB, et al. Rituximab (Mabthera) improves the treatment results of DHAP-VIM-DHAP and ASCT in relapsed/progressive aggressive $CD20^+$ NHL: a prospective randomized HOVON trial. *Blood.* 2008;**111**:537–43.

39 Kewalramani T, Zelenetz AD, Nimer SD, et al. Rituximab and ice as second-line therapy before autologous stem cell transplantation for relapsed or primary refractory diffuse large B-cell lymphoma. *Blood.* 2004;**103**:3684–88.

40 Pfreundschuh M, Trumper L, Kloess M, et al. Two-weekly or 3-weekly CHOP chemotherapy with or without etoposide for the treatment of young patients with good-prognosis (normal LDH) aggressive lymphomas: results of the NHL-B1 trial of the DSHNHL. *Blood.* 2004;**104**:626–33.

41 Pfreundschuh M, Trumper L, Kloess M, et al. Two-weekly or 3-weekly CHOP chemotherapy with or without etoposide for the treatment of elderly patients with aggressive lymphomas: results of the NHL-B2 trial of the DSHNHL. *Blood.* 2004;**104**:634–41.

42 Verdonck LF, Notenboom A, De Jong DD, et al. Intensified 12-week CHOP (I-CHOP) plus G-CSF compared with standard 24-week CHOP (CHOP-21) for patients with intermediate-risk aggressive non-Hodgkin lymphoma: a Phase 3 trial of the Dutch-Belgian Hemato-Oncology Cooperative Group (HOVON). *Blood.* 2007;**109**:2759–66.

43 Feugier P, Van Hoof A, Sebban C, et al. Long-term results of the R-CHOP study in the treatment of elderly patients with diffuse large B-cell lymphoma: a study by the Groupe D'etude Des Lymphomes De L'adulte. *J Clin Oncol.* 2005;**23**:4117–26.

44 Sonneveld P, De Ridder M, Van Der Lh, et al. Comparison Of doxorubicin and mitoxantrone in the treatment of elderly patients with advanced diffuse non-Hodgkin's lymphoma using CHOP versus CNOP chemotherapy. *J Clin Oncol.* 1995;**13**:2530–39

45 Bosly A, Lepage E, Coiffier B, et al. Outcome is not improved by the use of alternating chemotherapy in elderly patients with aggressive lymphoma. *Hematol J.* 2001;**2**:279–85.

46 Burton C, Linch D, Hoskin P, et al. A phase III trial comparing CHOP to PMITCEBO with or without G-CSF in patients aged 60 plus with aggressive non-Hodgkin's lymphoma. *Br J Cancer.* 2006;**94**:806–13.

47 Mainwaring PN, Cunningham D, Gregory W, et al. Mitoxantrone is superior to doxorubicin in a multiagent weekly regimen for patients older than 60 with high-grade lymphoma: results of a BNLI randomized trial of PADRIACEBO versus PMITCEBO. *Blood.* 2001;**97**:2991–97.

48 Osby E, Hagberg H, Kvaloy S, et al. CHOP is superior to CNOP in elderly patients with aggressive lymphoma while outcome is unaffected by filgrastim treatment: results of a Nordic Lymphoma Group randomized trial. *Blood.* 2003;**101**:3840–48.

49 Tilly H, Lepage E, Coiffier B, et al. Intensive conventional chemotherapy (ACVBP regimen) compared with standard CHOP for poor-prognosis aggressive non-Hodgkin lymphoma. *Blood.* 2003;**102**:4284–89.

50 Zinzani PL, Gherlinzoni F, Storti S, et al. Randomized trial of 8-week versus 12-week VNCOP-B plus G-CSF regimens as front-line treatment in elderly aggressive non-Hodgkin's lymphoma patients. *Ann Oncol.* 2002;**13**:1364–69.

51 Zinzani PL, Pavone E, Storti S, et al. Randomized trial with or without granulocyte colony-stimulating factor as adjunct to induction VNCOP-B treatment of elderly high-grade non-Hodgkin's lymphoma. *Blood.* 1997;**89**:3974–79.

52 Al Ismail SA, Whittaker JA, Gough J. Combination chemotherapy including epirubicin for the management of non-Hodgkin's lymphoma. *Eur J Cancer Clin Oncol.* 1987;**23**:1379–84.

53 Bertini M, Freilone R, Botto B, et al. Idarubicin in patients with diffuse large cell lymphomas: a randomized trial comparing VACOP-B (A = doxorubicin) vs VICOP-B (I = idarubicin). *Haematologica.* 1997;**82**:309–13.

54 Bezwoda W, Rastogi RB, Erazo VA, et al. Long-term results of a multicentre randomised, comparative phase III trial of CHOP versus CNOP regimens in patients with intermediate- and high-grade non-Hodgkin's lymphomas. Novantrone International Study Group. *Eur J Cancer.* 1995;**31a**:903–11.

55 Brugiatelli M, Federico M, Gobbi PG, et al. Epidoxorubicin vs idarubicin containing regimens in intermediate and high grade non-Hodgkin's lymphoma: preliminary results Of A Multicentric randomized trial. *Haematologica.* 1993;**78**:306–12.

56 Economopoulos T, Dimopoulos Ma, Mellou S, et al. Treatment of intermediate- and high-grade non-Hodgkin's lymphoma using CEOP versus CNOP. *Eur J Haematol.* 2002;**68**:135-43.

57 Federico M, Clo V, Brugiatelli M, et al. Efficacy of two different promacecytabom derived regimens in advanced aggressive non-Hodgkin's lymphoma: final report of a multicenter trial conducted by GISL. *Haematologica.* 1998;**83**:800–811.

58 Guglielmi C, Gherlinzoni F, Amadori S, et al. A phase III comparative trial of M-BACOD vs M-BNCOD in the treatment of stage II–IV diffuse non-Hodgkin's lymphomas. *Haematologica.* 1989;**74**:563–69.

59 Nair R, Ramakrishnan G, Nair NN, et al. A randomized comparison of the efficacy and toxicity of epirubicin and doxorubicin in the treatment of patients with non-Hodgkin's lymphoma. *Cancer.* 1998;**82**:2282–88.

60 Pavlovsky S, Santarelli MT, Erazo A, et al. Results of a randomized study of previously-untreated intermediate and high grade lymphoma using CHOP versus CNOP. *Ann Oncol.* 1992;**3**:205–9.

61 Zinzani Pl, Martelli M, Storti S, et al. Phase III comparative trial using CHOP vs CIOP in the treatment of advanced intermediate-grade non-Hodgkin's lymphoma. *Leuk Lymphoma.*1995;**19**:329–35.

62 Kouroukis CT, Browman GP, Esmail R, et al. Chemotherapy for older patients with newly diagnosed, advanced-stage, aggressive-histology non-Hodgkin Lymphoma: a systematic review. *Ann Intern Med.* 2002;**136**:144–52.

63 Pfreundschuh M, Schubert J, Ziepurt M, et al. Six versus eight cycles of bi-weekly CHOP-14 with or without rituximab in elderly patients with aggressive $CD20^+$ B-cell lymphomas: a randomised controlled trial (RICOVER-60). *Lancet Oncol.* 2008;**9**:105–116.

64 Sonneveld P, Van Putten W, Biesma DH, et al. Phase III trial of 2-weekly CHOP with rituximab for aggressive B-cell non-Hodgkin's lymphoma in elderly patients. *Blood.* 2006;**108**.

42 Follicular Lymphoma

Kevin Imrie, Matthew Cheung

Introduction

Follicular lymphoma (FL) is the second most common subtype of non-Hodgkin's lymphoma, accounting for approximately 35% of the 61,000 cases of NHL estimated to occur in 2006 in North America (1). It is the most common of the indolent lymphomas and represents the prototype of this group of histologies. One-third of patients with follicular lymphoma present with what appears to be localized disease and have historically been treated with local irradiation with the intent of long-term disease control. Patients with advanced disease, in contrast, do not appear to be have the potential for cure with currently available therapies. The lack of curative potential, combined with the increasing array of treatment options, has led to a wide variation in approach to therapy. Defining an optimal approach to treatment has been challenging given the long natural history of the disease and the tendency of patients to receive multiple lines of therapy over a number of years. Despite these limitations, increasing numbers of well-conducted randomized trials are emerging to help inform and define practice.

Literature-search strategy and inclusion

A search for randomized trials, systematic reviews, and published practice guidelines were completed in the Cochrane Library (2006, Issue 3) and MEDLINE (1966–August 2006, week 2). The full literature search strategy can be found at (http://web.mac.com/kimrie/iWeb/Site/Welcome.html). A primary author and a research methodologist independently reviewed search results. We included studies of follicular lymphoma as well as those dealing with patients with "low-grade" or "indolent" lymphoma in which a large proportion of patients had follicular lymphoma. If no randomized trials could be identified to address an identified question, lesser evidence was considered.

Evidence-based Hematology. Edited by Mark A. Crowther, Jeff Ginsberg, Holger J. Schünemann, Ralph M. Meyer, and Richard Lottenberg.

Search results

A total of 2,064 citations were recovered (MEDLINE 1,929, Cochrane 135). Eighteen meta-analyses or systematic reviews citations were recovered. Many of the citations retrieved were not in fact randomized trials, systematic reviews, or meta-analyses or were duplicate citations or updates of previously published trials; 41 randomized trials, two systematic reviews, and two meta-analyses met inclusion. Because no randomized trials addressing prognostic factors could be identified, lesser evidence was used to address this question (question 8). Lesser-quality evidence was also considered to evaluate the role of radioimmunoconjugate therapy, as only one randomized trial that did not address the question fully was identified.

Systematic reviews and meta-analyses

Two published systematic reviews were identified. A systematic overview of chemotherapy effects in indolent non-Hodgkin's lymphoma published by the Swedish Council of Technology Assessment in *Acta Oncologica* in 2001 (2,3) was well-conducted, but its publication prior to 18 of 41 randomized trials included in this review limits its utility. A second review published by the Italian Society of Hematology took the form of a consensus panel rather than a systematic review and was not included (4). Two meta-analyses addressing the role of interferon-alpha were identified and are addressed in question 4 (5,6).

Grading of the quality of evidence and strengths of recommendations in this chapter are based on the guidelines proposed by the international Grading of Recommendations Assessment, Development, and Evaluation Working Group (GRADE) adopting the modification used by the American College of Chest Physicians that merges the very low and low categories of quality of evidence (see chapter 1).

1. Should patients with limited stage follicular lymphoma receive systemic therapy in combination with local radiotherapy?

Six randomized trials compare the combination of chemotherapy with radiotherapy to radiotherapy alone in indolent non-Hodgkin's lymphoma (7–11). Most of these trials antedate modern lymphoma classification systems and were relatively underpowered to exclude a meaningful benefit. Only one trial restricted inclusion to indolent lymphomas. This study randomized 148 patients with localized indolent lymphoma to receive radiotherapy or radiotherapy plus chlorambucil. There was no difference in relapse rate, and relapse-free survival and survival were comparable at 10 and 15 years in the two arms. The remaining trials included patients with aggressive histologies and did not demonstrate improvement in survival with the addition of chemotherapy to radiation. No published trials addressing the benefit of adding chemoimmunotherapy to radiation have been published.

Recommendation

Patients with limited-stage follicular lymphoma should be treated with radiation therapy as a single modality (Grade 1B).

2. Do all patients with advanced stage follicular lymphoma require therapy at the time of diagnosis?

Treatment at the time of diagnosis has been compared to observation in asymptomatic patients with advanced-stage follicular lymphoma in three randomized trials (12–15). The largest of these was a trial comparing treatment with oral chlorambucil at diagnosis to a "watch-and-wait" policy in newly diagnosed asymptomatic patients with advanced stage indolent lymphoma (13). Three hundred and nine patients were enrolled, 65% of whom had follicular lymphoma. At a median follow-up of 16 years, actuarial 10-year survival was comparable in the two arms (45% vs. 34%, $p = \text{NS}$). The chance of remaining free of any treatment at 10 years if observed from the time of diagnosis was 19% and was 40% for those over the age of 70 at enrollment. Two smaller trials confirmed also failed to find improved outcome with treatment at diagnosis (12,15). All three trials compared observation to relatively "gentle" chemotherapy. One small trial comparing aggressive chemotherapy with ProMACE-MOPP and total nodal irradiation to "watchful waiting" was presented in preliminary form in 1988; however, no conclusions could be drawn at the time of the analysis presented (12). No other trials comparing more intensive (anthracycline or purine-based) regimens or immunochemotherapy to a "watch-and-wait" strategy have been published.

Recommendation

Asymptomatic patients with newly diagnosed advanced stage follicular lymphoma should be initially managed with observation (Grade 1A).

3. Has any one chemotherapy regimen been demonstrated to be superior?

Numerous randomized trials have compared one regimen to another in follicular and indolent lymphomas (12–25). These trials are summarized in Table 42.1. The studies compare a wide array of regimens including alkylating agent, purine analogue, and anthracycline-based combinations. Many of these trials were conducted prior to modern lymphoma classification systems, and many were underpowered to exclude small but important differences in survival. Only one trial reported a survival difference (17). This study, conducted by the Groupe d'Étude des Lymphomes de l'Adulte (GELA), compared a relatively intensive regimen of cyclophosphamide, doxorubicin, teniposide, and prednisone (CHVP) with 18 months of interferon alpha to fludarabine. Patients were permitted entry into the study regardless of the percentage of large cell involvement (as long as <50% of the infiltration was of a diffuse pattern) and one-fourth of participants had a significant (>15%) large cell component. Five-year overall survival was 77% in the CHVP-interferon arm compared with 62% in the fludarabine arm ($p < 0.05$). However, some of this improvement may be attributable to the use of interferon maintenance following induction (see question 4) and the inclusion of some patients with transformed lymphoma. No other randomized trials have provided comparative evidence with this particular regimen. Four of the 10 remaining trials report differences in disease control between the arms studied. In some series, purine-analogue or anthracycline-based regimens appear to result in superior disease control than in alkylator-based regimens. This observation was not consistent, with two recently published large well conducted studies reporting no better disease control with purine analogues (17) or anthracyclines (21) when compared with alkylator-based regimens.

Recommendation

As long-term outcomes appear comparable with alkylating agent, purine analogue, or anthracycline-based regimens, no definitive conclusions can be reached regarding a treatment of choice among these options (Grade 2B).

4. What is the role of interferon?

Before the advent of rituximab, the role of interferon had been the most closely scrutinized question in the management of follicular lymphoma. Ten randomized trials have been published as well as two meta-analyses (5,6,23,26–35). The meta-analysis conducted

Table 42.1 Randomized trials comparing chemotherapy regimens in follicular lymphoma.*

References	Author	N	Arms	RR	Disease-control	Survival
					Median	5-y OS
(15)	Brice	193	Observation	NA (p = NS)	24 mo (p = NS)	78 (p = NS)
			Prednimustine	78%	40 mo	70
			Interferon	70%	35 mo	84
					2-y FFP	2-y OS
(16)	Coiffier	131	CHVP Interferon		63% ($p < 0.05$)	77% ($p < 0.05$)
			Fludarabine		49%	62%
					5-y PFS	5-y OS
(17)	Hagenbeek	381	Fludarabine	70% ($p < 0.001$)	8% (p = NS)	65% (p = NS)
			CVP	52%	25%	56%
						5-y OS
(18)	Kimby	132	ChP	36% ($p = 0.01$)	NR	41% (p = NS)
			CHOP	60%	NR	44%
					Median PFS	Median OS
(19)	Klasa	91	Fludarabine	64% (p = NS)	11 mo ($p = 0.03$)	57 mo (p = NS)
			CVP	52%	9 mo	44 mo
(20)	Lister	66	Chlorambucil	74% (p = NS)	NR	NR
			CVP	83%	NR	NR
					10-y PFS	10-y OS
(21)	Peterson	228	Cyclophosphamide	89% (p = NS)	25% (p = NS)	44% (p= NS)
			CHOP-B	93%	33%	46%
					5-yr PFS	5-yr OS
(22)	Tsimberidou	142	FND	97% (p = NS)	41% ($p = 0.02$)	44% (p = NS)
			ATT	97%	50%	46%
					Median PFS	
(23)	Unterhalt	246	PmM	83% (p = NS)	31 mo ($p = 0.04$)	NR
			COP	83%	14 mo	NR
					19 mo PFS	42 mo OS
(24)	Zinzani	199	Fludarabine	85% (p = NS)	62% ($p = 0.02$)	73% (p = NS)
			Fludarabine-Idarubicin	81%	84%	72%
(25)	Zinzani		Fludarabine-mitoxantrone	96% (p = NS)	71% (p = NS)†	NR
			CHOP	98%	54%	NR

*ATT, alternating triple therapy; CHOP, cyclophosphamide, adriamycin, vincristine, prednisone; CHOP-B, cyclophosphamide, adriamycin, vincristine, prednisone, bleomycin; ChP-chlorambucil, prednisone; CHVP, cyclophosphamide, adriamycin, teniposide, prednisone; COP, cyclophosphamide, vincristine, prednisone; CVP, cyclophosphamide, vincristine, prednisone; FND, fludarabine, mitoxantrone, dexamethasone; NR, not reported; PmM, prednimustine mitoxantrone.

by Rohatiner et al. was well conducted and included all of the important randomized trials (6). This analysis reports that the addition of interferon did not significantly influence response rate but that the use of interferon was associated with an absolute 8% difference in survival at 10 years. The benefit in survival was seen when interferon was given with relatively intensive initial chemotherapy, at a cumulative dose of $\geq$36 million units per month and when it was given with chemotherapy rather than as maintenance. Despite this demonstrated benefit, the use of interferon has been limited by the perceived toxicity of long-term use as well as the need to use this agent in combination with relatively intensive chemotherapy regimens. Trials evaluating the role of interferon given in combination with rituximab-containing regimens are ongoing.

Recommendation

The use of interferon is associated with improved survival particularly when given in high doses and along with relatively intensive chemotherapy. However, the potential benefit must be carefully balanced with the potential for long-term toxicity and impact on quality of life for the individual patient. The benefit of adding interferon to rituximab in induction and maintenance therapy (see question 5) has not been evaluated. Therefore, the routine use of interferon is not recommended (Grade 2A).

5. What is the role of rituximab in?

a. First-line therapy
b. Beyond first line
c. Maintenance

Rituximab (Mabthera/Rituxan, Roche, Basel, Switzerland) is a chimeric IgG1 monoclonal antibody directed against the CD20 surface antigen found on most normal and neoplastic B lymphocytes(36). Since an initial demonstration of benefit with rituximab monotherapy in relapsed FL, there have been multiple large randomized studies detailing the use of rituximab in combination with initial combination chemotherapy, in the relapsed setting, and most recently, as maintenance therapy to sustain patients in remission. Six randomized trials evaluating the role of rituximab in these setting were identified. These trials are summarized in Table 42.2.

a. First-line therapy

Two randomized trials have studied the use of rituximab in combination with chemotherapy in patients with previously untreated advanced-stage follicular lymphoma. Marcus et al. compared cyclophosphamide, vincristine, and prednisone (CVP) plus rituximab (CVP-R) with CVP alone in 321 patients (37). Patients randomized to receive rituximab in combination with chemotherapy had a significantly improve response rate (81% vs. 57%; $p < 0.0001$) and median time to progression (32 months vs. 15 months; $p < 0.0001$). Survival was not reported to be different between the two arms, however, this trial was recently updated in abstract form and authors now report improved survival (hazard ratio [HR] 0.6, 95% confidence interval [CI] 0.38–0.96; $p = 0.03$) (38).

In a German Low-Grade Study Group (GLSG) trial, Hiddemann et al. reported a comparison of CHOP-R with cyclophosphamide, doxorubicin, vincristine, and prednisone (CHOP) alone in 428 patients with previously untreated advanced-stage follicular lymphoma (39). Although follow-up has been brief in this report (median 18 months), superior response rates and disease control (time-to-treatment failure) have so far translated into a survival benefit for patients who received R-CHOP (estimated probability of survival at 2 years 95% vs. 90%, $p = 0.016$).

Recommendation

Rituximab should be used in combination with chemotherapy regimens such as CVP and CHOP as initial therapy for patients with previously untreated follicular lymphoma (Grade 1A).

b. Beyond first line

Two trials studied anthracycline/anthracenedione-based chemotherapy with or without rituximab in patients with resistant or relapsed indolent lymphoma (40,41). Both trials included only patients who were rituximab-naïve. Interpretation of the results of both trials is complicated by the fact that both studies included a second randomization to rituximab maintenance or observation (see question 5c). Both reports documented superior progression-free survival in patients who received rituximab. The GLSG reported that the addition of rituximab to a chemotherapy regimen consisting of fludarabine, cyclophosphamide, and mitoxantrone was associated with improved progression-free survival (median 16 months vs. 10 months; $p = 0.0381$) and survival overall survival (40). The second trial led by the European Organization for Research and Treatment of Cancer reported that the addition of rituximab to CHOP chemotherapy was associated with improved progression-free survival (median 33 months vs. 20 months; HR 0.65, $p = 0.0003$) and a trend towards improved three-year survival (83% vs. 72%; HR 0.74, $p = 0.096$) (41). Responding patients in both studies underwent a second randomization comparing rituximab maintenance with observation (described below).

None of the randomized trials evaluating the role of rituximab in combination with chemotherapy beyond first-line included patients who had previously received rituximab.

Recommendations

1. Previously treated patients who are appropriate candidates for further chemotherapy and who have not previously received rituximab should receive treatment in combination with rituximab (Grade 1A).
2. Insufficient evidence exists to allow for definitive recommendations regarding retreatment with rituximab in combination with chemotherapy for patients who have previously received rituximab (grade 2C).

c. Maintenance

The role of rituximab as maintenance therapy for patients with indolent B-cell lymphomas has been tested in four published randomized trials (40–43).

Two randomized trials studied the role of maintenance rituximab (MR) following induction treatment with rituximab monotherapy (42,43). The MR strategy resulted in extended disease control (event- or progression-free survival) compared with observation alone in both studies. Neither report detailed a benefit in overall survival.

Two trials studied the use of MR following response to combination chemotherapy (with or without rituximab) for relapsed FL. Both trials incorporated initial randomizations to chemotherapy with or without rituximab before second randomizations comparing MR with observation (40,41). In one report (40) that included patients with relapsed follicular and mantle cell lymphoma, MR was associated with a prolonged response duration (median not reported vs. 17 months; $p < 0.001$) and a trend toward improved three-year overall survival (82% vs. 55%; $p = 0.056$). In a study (41) exclusively in patients with relapsed or refractory disease,

Table 42.2 Randomized controlled trials evaluating chemotherapy plus rituximab versus non-rituximab regimens in follicular lymphoma.*

Author, study	N rand	Patients	Treatment	RR	Disease control	OS
First-line therapy						
Marcus (37,38)	321	First-line follicular	CVP-R vs. CVP	81% vs. 57%; $p < 0.0001$	Median TTP, 34 vs. 15 mo; $p < 0.0001$	3-y OS: 89% vs. 81%; $p = 0.07$
Hiddemann (39)	428	First-line follicular	CHOP-R vs. CHOP	96% vs. 90%; $p = 0.011$	Median TTF, not reached in either group; TTF superior in R-CHOP group (relative risk 0.40); $p < 0.0001$	Median OS not reached in either group; estimated probability of survival at 2 years, 95% vs. 90%; $p = 0.016$
Beyond first-line therapy						
Forstpointner (40)	147	Relapsed follicular and mantle	FCM-R vs. FCM	79% vs. 58%; $p =$ 0.01	Median PFS, 16 vs. 10 mo; $p = 0.0381$	Median, not reached vs. 24 mo ($p = 0.0030$)
Van Oers (41)	465	Relapsed/ resistant follicular NHL	CHOP-R vs. CHOP	CR after induction: 30% vs. 16%; $p < 0.0001$	Median PFS 33 vs. 20 mo (HR 0.65; $p = 0.0003$)	3-y OS, 83% vs. 72% (HR 0.74; $p = 0.096$)

Author, study	N rand	Patients	Induction Treatment	Maintenance Treatment	Disease control	OS
Maintenance therapy						
Ghielmini (42)	202	**Untreated and relapsed**[†] follicular lymphoma	Rituximab	R maint vs. Obs	Median EFS 23 vs. 12 mo ($p = 0.024$)	NR
Hainsworth (43)	90	**Relapsed**[†] indolent NHL (follicular or SLL)	Rituximab	R maint vs. Obs[‡]	Median PFS, 32 vs. 7 mo ($p = 0.007$)	3 y, 72% vs. 68%, $p =$ NS
Forstpointner (40)	NR[§]	**Relapsed** follicular or mantle cell lymphoma	FCM or R-FCM[‖]	R maint vs. Obs	Median response duration, not reached vs. 17 mo; $p = 0.001$	3 y, 82% vs. 55%; $p = 0.056$
Van Oers (41)	334	**Relapsed/ resistant** follicular NHL	CHOP-R vs. CHOP	R maint vs. Obs	Median PFS 52 vs. 15 mo (HR 0.40; $p < 0.0001$)	3 y, 85% vs. 77% (HR 0.52; $p = 0.011$)

*abst, abstract; CHOP, cyclophosphamide, doxorubicin, vincristine, prednisone; CR, complete response; CVP, cyclophosphamide, vincristine, prednisone; EFS, event-free survival; est, estimated; eval, evaluable; FCM, fludarabine, cyclophosphamide, mitoxantrone; maint, maintenance; max, maximum; mo, month; N, number; NHL, non-Hodgkin's lymphoma; NR, not reported; NS, not significant; obs, observation; OS, overall survival; PFS, progression-free survival; PR, partial response; pts, patients; rand, randomized; R, rituximab; RR, response rate; SD, stable disease; SLL, small lymphocytic lymphoma; TTF, time-to-treatment failure; vs., versus; y, year.

[†] No previous treatment with rituximab.

[‡] Obs, retreatment at progression.

[§] Number of patients in each group not given.

[‖] First randomization stopped after 147 patients; all subsequent patients received induction R-FCM (136 of 174 evaluable patients for the second randomization received R-FCM).

MR was associated with an improvement in progression-free survival (median 52 months vs. 15 months; HR 0.40 $p < 0.0001$) and three-year overall survival (85% vs. 77%; HR 0.52 $p = 0.011$) compared with observation. In the subgroup of patients who had received rituximab with initial induction chemotherapy, MR continued to demonstrate an improvement in progression-free survival and a statistically insignificant improvement in overall survival ($p = 0.059$).

No published randomized studies have addressed the use of MR following initial combination chemotherapy (with or without rituximab).

Recommendation

For patients with follicular lymphoma who respond to treatment with combination chemotherapy or rituximab, this treatment should be followed by the use of maintenance rituximab (Grade: first line 1B; second line 1A).

6. What is the role of radioimmunoconjugate therapy?

Radioimmunoconjugates are radioisotope-bound monoclonal antibodies that target radiation specifically to sites of lymphoma involvement. Initial studies of early examples of these agents, including yttrium (^{90}Y)-ibritumomab tiuxetan and iodine (^{131}I)-tositumomab, have suggested benefit in patients with relapsed or refractory FL, with activity demonstrated even in patients with rituximab-refractory disease (44,45). A single randomized trial has subsequently been completed in which ^{90}Y-ibritumomab tiuxetan was compared with rituximab monotherapy in 143 patients with relapsed or refractory low-grade, follicular, or transformed lymphoma (46) ^{90}Y-ibritumomab tiuxetan was associated with a higher overall response rate (80% vs. 56%; $p = 0.002$) but similar time-to-progression (11.2 vs. 10.1 months; $p = 0.173$). No evidence of improvement in quality of life or overall survival was reported. Severe hematologic toxicity occurred commonly (approximately 60% of patients) and in a delayed fashion (with count nadirs seven to nine weeks after therapy). Although limited non-randomized data suggest a lower rate of toxicity in less heavily pretreated patients, no randomized data is available for use of radioimmunoconjugates in this context.

Recommendation

Radioimmunoconjugates are active agents in relapsed and refractory CD20+ indolent lymphoma. However, as there is insufficient evidence that they are superior to other existing treatment options, routine use of radioimmunoconjugates is recommended only when other options are not appropriate (Grade 2C).

7. What is the role of stem cell transplantation?

Autologous stem cell transplantation (ASCT) following myeloablative therapy therapy has been studied in FL for patients with relapsed disease and following initial induction therapy. A single phase III study is available in younger patients (age ≤65) in the relapsed setting (47). In this three-arm trial, patients responding to chemotherapy were randomized to further chemotherapy, myeloablative therapy and ASCT, or myeloablative therapy followed by re-infusion of an autologous graft first treated with ex vivo purging. Patients who proceeded with either ASCT arm (purged or unpurged) sustained improvements in progression-free and overall survival (HR 0.40, 95% CI 0.18–0.89) compared with patients treated with chemotherapy alone. Accrual to this study was incomplete, and the limited sample size may have resulted in important baseline differences between treatment arms.

Three randomized trials have also documented the role of ASCT following the initial induction remission in FL. Two studies have reported improvements in event-free or progression-free survival with the use of ASCT (48,49). In one study by the GLSG, ASCT was compared with interferon maintenance in patients <60 who first responded to CHOP-like chemotherapy (48). In another study from the French GOELAMS (Groupe Ouest-Est des Leucemies et des Autres Maladies du Sang), ASCT was compared with a standard chemotherapy regimen combined with interferon in patients ≤60 with a high-burden disease (49). Despite improved disease control in these studies, no improvements in overall survival were detected in either trial. Of concern, both studies documented increased rates of secondary malignancies, including myelodysplasia and acute leukemia, in patients proceeding with ASCT. A third report from the GELA similarly compared a standard chemotherapy regimen plus interferon with chemotherapy followed by ASCT in patients ≤60 (50). No differences in event-free or overall survival have been attained with ASCT in this report. The report from GELA did not find excessive rates of secondary tumors in patients randomized to ASCT.

Recommendations

1. For patients with follicular lymphoma in first remission, there is no consistent evidence that outcomes are superior with ASCT; therefore, this treatment is not recommended for these patients (Grade 2A).

2. For patients with relapsed disease, a single study suggests that ASCT is superior to chemotherapy alone; this level of evidence is felt to be insufficient to warrant transplantation as a standard treatment (Grade 2B).

8. Can treatment be tailored to prognosis?

No randomized trials of risk factor adapted therapy strategies were identified in our search. Two prognostic scoring systems are in common use in follicular lymphoma. The first is the International Prognostic Index (IPI) developed for use in aggressive histology lymphoma and published in 1993, which has been reported to be predictive of outcome in follicular lymphoma as well (51). More recently in 2004, a prognostic index developed specifically for use in follicular lymphoma, the Follicular Lymphoma Prognostic Factor Index (FLIPI) has been published (52). This index uses age, stage, LDH, hemoglobin level, and number of nodal sites to categorize patients into three risk groups (low risk, intermediate risk, and high risk). Results were analyzed according to at least one of these indexes in four of the randomized trials included in the review (37,39,49,50). In no case was a differential treatment effect reported according to risk group. In one report, the GOELAMS trial that demonstrated improved event-free survival with ASCT compared to standard therapy, the benefit in disease control with ASCT reached statistical significance in the subgroup of patients with high-risk FLIPI scores but did not in intermediate or low-risk disease. This likely reflects limited power to detect differences in the subgroup analysis rather than a differential effect in the high-risk subgroup. Prospective randomized trials examining risk-adapted therapy will be required to definitively answer this question.

Recommendation

There is insufficient evidence to allow for definitive recommendations to treat subgroups differently according to prognostic factors (Grade 2C).

Acknowledgment

We would like to thank Adam Haynes for his assistance in developing and conducting the structured search of the literature.

References

1 Jaffe E. Harris, N, Stein, H, et al. *Pathology and genetics of tumors of haematopietic and lymphoid tissues.* Lyon: IARC; 2001.

2 Brandt L, Kimby, E, Nygren, P, et al. A systematic overview of chemotherapy effects in indolent non-Hodgkin's lymphoma. *Acta Oncol.* 2001;**40**(2–3):213–23.

3 Nygren P, and Glimelius, B. The Swedish Council on Technology Assessment in Health Care (SBU) report on Cancer Chemotherapy—project objectives, the working process, key definitions and general aspects on cancer trial methodology and interpretation. *Acta Oncol.* 2001;**40**(2–3):155–65.

4 Barosi G, Carella, A, Lazzarino, M, et al. Management of nodal indolent (non marginal-zone) non-Hodgkin's lymphomas: practice guidelines from the Italian Society of Hematology, Italian Society of Experimental Hematology and Italian Group for Bone Marrow Transplantation. *Haematologica.* 2005;**90**(9):1236–57.

5 Allen IE, Ross, SD, Borden, SP, et al. Meta-analysis to assess the efficacy of interferon-alpha in patients with follicular non-Hodgkin's lymphoma. *J Immunother.* 2001;**24**(1):58–65.

6 Rohatiner AZ, Gregory, WM, Peterson, B, et al. Meta-analysis to evaluate the role of interferon in follicular lymphoma. *J Clin Oncol.* 2005;**23**(10):2215–23.

7 Carde P, Burgers, JM, van Glabbeke, M, et al. Combined radiotherapy-chemotherapy for early stages non-Hodgkin's lymphoma: the 1975–1980 EORTC controlled lymphoma trial. *Radiother Oncol.* 1984;**2**(4):301–12.

8 Kelsey SM, Newland, AC, Hudson, GV, et al. A British National Lymphoma Investigation randomised trial of single agent chlorambucil plus radiotherapy versus radiotherapy alone in low grade, localised non-Hodgkins lymphoma. *Med Oncol.* 1994;**11**(1):19–25.

9 Landberg TG, Hakansson, LG, Moller, TR, et al. CVP-remission-maintenance in stage I or II non-Hodgkin's lymphomas: preliminary results of a randomized study. *Cancer.* 1979;**44**(3):831–38.

10 Monfardini S, Banfi, A, Bonadonna, G, et al. Improved five-year survival after combined radiotherapy-chemotherapy for stage I-II non-Hodgkin's lymphoma. *Int J Radiat Oncol Biol Phys.* 1980;**6**(2):125–34.

11 Nissen NI, Ersboll, J, Hansen, HS, et al. A randomized study of radiotherapy versus radiotherapy plus chemotherapy in stage I-II non-Hodgkin's lymphomas. *Cancer.* 1983;**52**(1):1–7.

12 Young RC, Longo, DL, Glatstein, E, et al. The treatment of indolent lymphomas: watchful waiting v aggressive combined modality treatment. *Semin Hematol.* 1988;**25**(2 Suppl 2):11–16.

13 Ardeshna KM, Smith, P, Norton, A, et al. Long-term effect of a watch and wait policy versus immediate systemic treatment for asymptomatic advanced-stage non-Hodgkin lymphoma: a randomised controlled trial. *Lancet.* 2003;**362**(9383):516–22.

14 Young RC, Longo, D.L, Glatstein, E, et al. Watchful waiting vs aggressive combined modality therapy in the treatment of stage III-IV indolent non-Hodgkin's lymphoma. *Proc Am Soc Clin Oncol.* 1987;**6:**200a.

15 Brice P, Bastion, Y, Lepage, E, et al. Comparison in low-tumor-burden follicular lymphomas between an initial no-treatment policy, prednimustine, or interferon alfa: a randomized study from the Groupe d'Etude des Lymphomes Folliculaires. Groupe d'Etude des Lymphomes de l'Adulte. *J Clin Oncol.* 1997;**15**(3):1110–17.

16 Coiffier B, Neidhardt-Berard, EM, Tilly, H, et al. Fludarabine alone compared to CHVP plus interferon in elderly patients with follicular lymphoma and adverse prognostic parameters: a GELA study. Groupe d'Etudes des Lymphomes de l'Adulte. *Ann Oncol.* 1999;**10**(10):1191–97.

17 Hagenbeek A, Eghbali, H, Monfardini, S, et al. Phase III intergroup study of fludarabine phosphate compared with cyclophosphamide, vincristine, and prednisone chemotherapy in newly diagnosed patients with stage III and IV low-grade malignant non-Hodgkin's lymphoma. *J Clin Oncol.* 2006;**24**(10):1590–96.

18 Kimby E, Bjorkholm, M, Gahrton, G, et al. Chlorambucil/prednisone vs. CHOP in symptomatic low-grade non-Hodgkin's lymphomas: a randomized trial from the Lymphoma Group of Central Sweden. Ann Oncol 1994;**5** Suppl 2:S67–S71.

19 Klasa RJ, Meyer, RM, Shustik, C, et al. Randomized phase III study of fludarabine phosphate versus cyclophosphamide, vincristine, and prednisone in patients with recurrent low-grade non-Hodgkin's lymphoma previously treated with an alkylating agent or alkylator-containing regimen [see comment]. *J Clin Oncol.* 2002;**20**(24):4649–54.

20 Lister TA, Cullen, MH, Beard, M.E, et al. Comparison of combined and single-agent chemotherapy in non-Hodgkin's lymphoma of favourable histological type. *Br Med J.* 1978;**1**(6112):533–37.

21 Peterson BA, Petroni, GR, Frizzera, G, et al. Prolonged single-agent versus combination chemotherapy in indolent follicular lymphomas: a study of the cancer and leukemia group B. *J Clin Oncol.* 2003;**21**(1):5–15.

22 Tsimberidou AM. McLaughlin, P, Younes, A, et al. Fludarabine, mitoxantrone, dexamethasone (FND) compared with an alternating triple therapy (ATT) regimen in patients with stage IV indolent lymphoma. *Blood.* 2002;**100**(13):4351–57.

23 Unterhalt M, Herrmann, R, Tiemann, M, et al. Prednimustine, mitoxantrone (PmM) vs cyclophosphamide, vincristine, prednisone (COP) for the treatment of advanced low-grade non-Hodgkin's lymphoma. German Low-Grade Lymphoma Study Group. *Leukemia.* 1996;**10**(5):836–43.

24 Zinzani PL, Magagnoli, M, Moretti, L, et al. Randomized trial of fludarabine versus fludarabine and idarubicin as frontline treatment in patients with indolent or mantle-cell lymphoma. *J Clin Oncol.* 2000;**18**(4):773–79.

25 Zinzani PL, Pulsoni, A, Perrotti, A, et al. Fludarabine plus mitoxantrone with and without rituximab versus CHOP with and without rituximab as

front-line treatment for patients with follicular lymphoma. *J Clin Oncol.* 2004;**22**(13):2654–61.

26 Chisesi T, Congiu, M, Contu, A, et al. Randomized study of chlorambucil (CB) compared to interferon (alfa-2b) combined with CB in low-grade non-Hodgkin's lymphoma: an interim report of a randomized study. Non-Hodgkin's Lymphoma Cooperative Study Group. *Eur J Cancer.* 1991;**27** Suppl 3:S31–S33.

27 Solal-Celigny P. Lepage, E, Brousse, N, et al. Recombinant interferon alfa-2b combined with a regimen containing doxorubicin in patients with advanced follicular lymphoma. Groupe d'Etude des Lymphomes de l'Adulte. *N Engl J Med.* 1993;**329**(22):1608–14.

28 Solal-Celigny P, Lepage, E, Brousse, N, et al. Doxorubicin-containing regimen with or without interferon alfa-2b for advanced follicular lymphomas: final analysis of survival and toxicity in the Groupe d'Etude des Lymphomes Folliculaires 86 Trial. *J Clin Oncol.* 1998;**16**(7):2332–38.

29 Smalley RV, Andersen, JW, Hawkins, MJ, et al. Interferon alfa combined with cytotoxic chemotherapy for patients with non-Hodgkin's lymphoma. *N Engl J Med.* 1992;**327**(19):1336–41.

30 Andersen JW, and Smalley, RV. Interferon alfa plus chemotherapy for non-Hodgkin's lymphoma: five-year follow-up. *N Engl J Med.* 1993;**329**(24):1821–22.

31 Smalley RV, Weller, E, Hawkins, MJ, et al. Final analysis of the ECOG I-COPA trial (E6484) in patients with non-Hodgkin's lymphoma treated with interferon alfa (IFN-alpha2a) plus an anthracycline-based induction regimen. *Leukemia.* 2001;**15**(7):1118–22.

32 Arranz R, Garcia-Alfonso, P, Sobrino, P, et al. Role of interferon alfa-2b in the induction and maintenance treatment of low-grade non-Hodgkin's lymphoma: results from a prospective, multicenter trial with double randomization. *J Clin Oncol.* 1998;**16**(4):1538–46.

33 Hagenbeek A, Carde, P, Meerwaldt, JH, et al. Maintenance of remission with human recombinant interferon alfa-2a in patients with stages III and IV low-grade malignant non-Hodgkin's lymphoma. European Organization for Research and Treatment of Cancer Lymphoma Cooperative Group. *J Clin Oncol.* 1998;**16**(1):41–47.

34 Aviles A. Duque, G, Talavera, A, et al. Interferon alpha 2b as maintenance therapy in low grade malignant lymphoma improves duration of remission and survival. *Leuk Lymphoma.* 1996;**20**(5–6):495–99.

35 Fisher RI, Dana, BW, LeBlanc, M, et al. Interferon alpha consolidation after intensive chemotherapy does not prolong the progression-free survival of patients with low-grade non-Hodgkin's lymphoma: results of the Southwest Oncology Group randomized phase III study 8809. *J Clin Oncol.* 2000;**18**(10):2010–16.

36 McLaughlin P, Grillo-Lopez, AJ, Link, BK, et al. Rituximab chimeric anti-CD20 monoclonal antibody therapy for relapsed indolent lymphoma: half of patients respond to a four-dose treatment program. *J Clin Oncol.* 1998;**16**(8):2825–33.

37 Marcus R, Imrie, K, Belch, A, et al. CVP chemotherapy plus rituximab compared with CVP as first-line treatment for advanced follicular lymphoma. *Blood.* 2005;**105**(4):1417–23.

38 Marcus R, Solal-Celigny, P, Imrie, K, et al. MabThera (Rituximab) plus cyclophosphamide, vincristine and prednisone (CVP) chemotherapy improves survival in previously untreated patients with advanced follicular non-Hodgkins lymphoma (NHL). *Blood.* 2006;**108**(11):481.

39 Hiddemann W, Kneba, M, Dreyling, M, et al. Frontline therapy with rituximab added to the combination of cyclophosphamide, doxorubicin, vincristine, and prednisone (CHOP) significantly improves the outcome for patients with advanced-stage follicular lymphoma compared with therapy with CHOP alone: results of a prospective randomized study of the German Low-Grade Lymphoma Study Group. *Blood.* 2005;**106**(12):3725–32.

40 Forstpointner R, Dreyling, M, Repp, R, et al. The addition of rituximab to a combination of fludarabine, cyclophosphamide, mitoxantrone (FCM) significantly increases the response rate and prolongs survival as compared with FCM alone in patients with relapsed and refractory follicular and mantle cell lymphomas: results of a prospective randomized study of the German Low-Grade Lymphoma Study Group. *Blood.* 2004;**104**(10):3064–71.

41 van Oers MH, Klasa, R, Marcus, RE, et al. Rituximab maintenance improves clinical outcome of relapsed/resistant follicular non-Hodgkin lymphoma in patients both with and without rituximab during induction: results of a prospective randomized phase 3 intergroup trial. *Blood.* 2006;**108**(10):3295–301.

42 Ghielmini M, Schmitz, SF, Cogliatti, SB, et al. Prolonged treatment with rituximab in patients with follicular lymphoma significantly increases event-free survival and response duration compared with the standard weekly × 4 schedule. *Blood.* 2004;**103**(12):4416–23.

43 Hainsworth JD, Litchy, S, Shaffer, DW, et al. Maximizing therapeutic benefit of rituximab: maintenance therapy versus re-treatment at progression in patients with indolent non-Hodgkin's lymphoma—a randomized phase II trial of the Minnie Pearl Cancer Research Network [see comment]. *J Clin Oncol.* 2005;**23**(6):1088–95.

44 Witzig TE, Flinn, IW, Gordon, LI, et al. Treatment with ibritumomab tiuxetan radioimmunotherapy in patients with rituximab-refractory follicular non-Hodgkin's lymphoma. *J Clin Oncol.* 2002;**20**(15):3262–69.

45 Horning SJ, Younes, A, Jain, V, et al. Efficacy and safety of tositumomab and iodine-131 tositumomab (Bexxar) in B-cell lymphoma, progressive after rituximab. *J Clin Oncol.* 2005;**23**(4):712–19.

46 Witzig TE, Gordon, L.I, Cabanillas, F, et al. Randomized controlled trial of yttrium-90-labeled ibritumomab tiuxetan radioimmunotherapy versus rituximab immunotherapy for patients with relapsed or refractory low-grade, follicular, or transformed B-cell non-Hodgkin's lymphoma. *J Clin Oncol.* 2002;**20**(10):2453–63.

47 Schouten HC, Kvaloy, S, Sydes, M, et al. The CUP trial: a randomized study analyzing the efficacy of high dose therapy and purging in low-grade non-Hodgkin's lymphoma (NHL). *Ann Oncol.* 2000;**11** Suppl 1:S91–S94.

48 Lenz G. Drelying, M, Schiegnitz, E, et al. Myeloablative radiochemotherapy followed by autologous stem cell transplantation in first remission prolongs progression-free survival in follicular lymphoma: results of a prospective, randomized trial of the German Low-Grade Lymphoma Study Group. *Blood.* 2004;**104**(9):2667–74.

49 Deconinck EF, Foussard, C, Milpied, N, et al. High-dose therapy followed by autologous purged stem-cell transplantation and doxorubicin-based chemotherapy in patients with advanced follicular lymphoma: a randomized multicenter study by GOELAMS. *Blood.* 2005;**105**(10):3817–23.

50 Sebban C, Mounier, N, Brousse, N, et al. Standard chemotherapy with interferon compared with CHOP followed by high-dose therapy with autologous stem cell transplantation in untreated patients with advanced follicular lymphoma: the GELF-94 randomized study from the Groupe d'Etude des Lymphomes de l'Adulte (GELA). *Blood.* 2006;**108**(8):2540–44.

51 A predictive model for aggressive non-Hodgkin's lymphoma: the International Non-Hodgkin's Lymphoma Prognostic Factors Project. *N Engl J Med.* 1993;**329**(14): 987–94.

52 Solal-Celigny P, Roy, P, Colombat, P, et al. Follicular lymphoma international prognostic index. *Blood.* 2004;**104**(5):1258–65.

43 Lymphoblastic Lymphoma

Tyler Y. Kang, John W. Sweetenham

Introduction

Lymphoblastic lymphoma (LBL) is a rare and highly aggressive type of non-Hodgkin lymphoma (NHL) that accounts for less than 2% of all lymphomas (1). The disease can be composed of either precursor T- or B-lymphocytes, with 85%–90% being of T-cell origin and occurs mostly in young adult men, with a median age of twenty (2,3). Frequently, patients present with rapidly developing bulky mediastinal disease and are at risk of bone marrow and central nervous system (CNS) involvement.

The morphologic, immunophenotypic, and genetic features of LBL are indistinguishable from acute lymphoblastic leukemia (ALL). Therefore, the World Health Organization classification has unified these diagnoses into "precursor T or B cell lymphoblastic lymphoma/leukemia," underlining the highly aggressive nature of the disease. The immunophenotypic features that characterize T-cell lymphoblastic lymphomas include expression of the T-cell markers CD7, CD5, and CD2 and markers of primitive cells, including terminal deoxynucleotidyl transferase (TdT), CD99, and CD 34 (4,5). Surface CD3 is typically negative, but cytoplasmic CD3 is positive. The B-cell types express the above primitive markers plus pan-B-cell markers such as CD19 and CD79a. Rearrangements of the T-cell receptor gene can occur in both T- and B-cell LBLs; presence is thus not useful for diagnosis. Gene expression profiling in precursor T-cell disease can be used as a prognostic tool, as it characterizes various stages of thymocyte maturation that may be associated with different clinical outcomes (6). Future treatment paradigms are likely to be based on the molecular pathogenesis of the disease and exploitation of targets such as HOX 1+ cluster, FLT3, TEL-AML1, and MLL genes (7).

Evidence-based Hematology. Edited by Mark A. Crowther, Jeff Ginsberg, Holger J. Schünemann, Ralph M. Meyer, and Richard Lottenberg.

Questions

1. Do aggressive ALL-type regimens improve outcome?
2. Does CNS prophylaxis improve outcome, including survival?
3. Does stem cell transplantation after first remission improve outcome?
4. Does the type of transplantation (autologous vs. allogeneic) influence outcome?
5. Does mediastinal radiation improve outcome?

Literature-search strategy and inclusion

A literature search was performed using the PubMed and Ovid databases using the term "lymphoblastic lymphoma." In addition to use of terms relevant to each clinical question, further search terms include "clinical trials," "systematic reviews," "meta-analysis," and "randomized controlled studies." Because of the paucity of available randomized controlled trials (RCTs) and meta-analyses, further cross-referencing of journal articles were done to locate other pertinent papers, including relevant reports of trials assessing adult ALL and pediatric ALL/LBL.

Grading of the quality of evidence and strengths of recommendations in this chapter are based on the guidelines proposed by the international Grading of Recommendations Assessment, Development, and Evaluation Working Group (GRADE) adopting the modification used by the American College of Chest Physicians that merges the "very low" and "low" categories of quality of evidence (see chapter 1).

Do aggressive ALL-type regimens improve outcome?

Early treatment approaches of LBL utilized conventional-dose lymphoma protocols such as cyclophosphamide, doxorubicin,

Table 43.1 Comparison of treatment regimens and outcome.*

References	Therapy	No. of patients	Disease-free survival	Overall survival
Conventional therapy				
Anderson (1983) (12)	COMP	40 (pediatric)	34% (5 y)	45% (5 y)
Colgan (1994) (8)	CHOP-like	39	49% (6 y)	51% (6 y)
Kaiser (1999) (9)	CHOP-like	29	38% ($3^1/_2$y)	41% ($3^1/_2$ y)
Conventional therapy and transplantation				
Le Gouill (2003) (11)	ACVBP type	92	22% (34 mo)	32% (34 mo)
Intensive induction				
Anderson (1983) (12)	LSA_2L_2	124 (pediatric)	64% (5 y)	67% (5 y)
Sweetenham (2001) (23)	LSA_2L_2 type	34	24% (3 y)	45% (3 y)
Hoelzer (2002) (13)	ALL-type	45	62% (7 y)	51% (7 y)
Thomas (2004) (14)	HyperCVAD	33	66% (3 y)	70% (3 y)
First remission transplantation after intensive induction				
Sweetenham (1994) (21)	High dose ctx + Auto	105	63% (6 y)	64% (6 y)
Jost (1995) (10)	MACOP-B + Auto	20	31% (3 y)	48% (3 y)
Sweetenham (2001) (23)	Induction + Auto	31	55% (3 y)	56% (3 y)

*ACVBP; Adriamycin® (doxorubicin), cyclophosphamide, Oncouin® (vincristine), bleomycin and prednisone. ALL, acute lymphoblastic leukemia; COMP, cyclophosphamide, vincristine, doxorubicin, methotrexate, prednisone.

vincristine, prednisone (CHOP), cyclophosphamide, vincristine, doxorubicin, methotrexate, prednisone (COMP); and methotrexate, doxorubicin, cyclophosphamide, vincristine, prednisone, bleomycin (MACOP-B) with or without CNS prophylaxis (8,9). These regimens were associated with complete response (CR) rates of 50%–70%, but long-term disease-free survival (DFS) was observed in less than 50% of patients. The use of high-dose therapy and autologous stem cell transplantation for patients achieving a CR with these regimens did not appear to improve outcomes (10). In a recent French Groupe d'Etudes des Lymphomes del l'Adulte (GELA) study of 92 patients treated with LNH 87 and 93 protocols, consisting of ACVBP and intrathecal methotrexate, 71% entered CR but the median relapse-free survival (RFS) was 10 months and overall survival was 32% at 5 years (11).

Regimens similar to those used to treat ALL have therefore been tested. An RCT comparing COMP with an intensive 10-drug regimen called LSA_2L_2 in children with LBL showed that the two-year failure-free survival was significantly better with LSA_2L_2 (76% vs. 26%, $p = 0.0002$) (12). More recent studies using ALL regimens such as that conducted by the German Multicenter Study Group protocol for adult ALL and the testing of the HyperCVAD regimen have demonstrated CR rates of 93% and 91% and long-term DFS of 65% at seven years and 66% at three years, respectively (13,14).

While cross-trial comparisons suggest substantial improvements in outcomes with use of ALL regimens, these are small cohort studies; RCTs involving large patient numbers are difficult to conduct because of the rarity of LBL (Table 43.1).

Therefore, while these data support the use of intensive ALL-like regimens for the treatment of LBL, the level of evidence providing this support must be considered modest.

Recommendation

In adult patients with LBL, treatment with the same regimens that are used to treat adults with ALL is recommended (Grade 1C).

Does CNS prophylaxis improve outcome, including survival?

Involvement of the CNS at presentation occurs in 7%–20% of patients with LBL (14,15). Without appropriate prophylaxis, CNS relapse may occur in as many as 50% of these patients. Even with prophylaxis, if therapy is given in later phases of treatment, CNS recurrences may be observed in up to 30% of cases (16). However, when combined with CNS radiation, earlier administration of intrathecal methotrexate has been shown in uncontrolled studies to reduce the CNS relapse rate to 3%, but an effect on survival was not obvious (17). No RCTs have directly tested CNS prophylaxis, and such trials are unlikely to ever be conducted. Drawing from parallels in childhood ALL and using historical cohort comparisons, studies in which some form of CNS prophylaxis was provided suggest important improvements in outcome (18).

Thus, CNS prophylaxis is an accepted requirement of therapy; however, the optimum form of prophylaxis is uncertain. Benefits of cranial irradiation have been suggested in many studies, but concerns of neuropsychologic sequelae and the potential of second malignancies have limited its use (19). Trials that incorporate high-dose systemic plus intrathecal chemotherapy (e.g., methotrexate) without cranial radiation have shown very low rates of CNS relapse (14), suggesting that such a strategy may obviate the need for radiation. To address this question further, a multicenter historical cohort comparison of the NHL-BFM95 and NHL BFM

90/86 trials, evaluating patients who had responded well to systemic chemotherapy, was conducted in the pediatric population in Austria, Germany, and Switzerland (20). This comparison showed that five-year DFS was 88% in 156 patients treated with intrathecal chemotherapy alone versus 91% in the 163 patients who received additional cranial radiation ($p = 0.35$); the five-year overall survivals were 85% versus 89% ($p = 0.32$), respectively. These results suggest that when patients have a good response to chemotherapy, use of intrathecal chemotherapy alone is as effective as treatment which includes cranial irradiation.

Recommendations

1. Adult patients with LBL should receive prophylactic CNS therapy (Grade 1C).

2. The optimum form of CNS prophylactic therapy is uncertain. Treatment with high-dose intravenous plus intrathecal methotrexate appears to provide comparable disease control as compared with cranial radiation, reduces the risk of neurologic sequelae, and is thus the preferred form of therapy (Grade 2C).

Does stem cell transplantation after first remission improve outcome?

While intensive, ALL-like regimens have improved response rates of LBL, relapse rates continue to be relatively high. Strategies using high-dose (myeloablative) therapy and stem cell transplantation have therefore been tested; many studies include small patient numbers and are from single institutions and are thus confounded by selection bias. In a large registry series, the European Group for Blood and Marrow Transplantation (EBMT) reported that outcomes of 214 patients who had received a variety of prior therapies, including conventional lymphoma chemotherapy or intensive ALL-like regimens, and then underwent autologous transplantation (21). Of 105 patients undergoing transplantation in first complete remission (CR1), long-term overall survival was 63% as compared with only 31% in those undergoing transplantation after initial disease progression. The Dutch-Belgian Hemato-Oncology Cooperative Group subsequently reported a phase II study in which 15 patients with LBL underwent two courses of high-dose induction chemotherapy followed by autologous transplantation (22); 13 of 15 patients responded to initial chemotherapy and completed the entire treatment protocol. At 5 years, the estimated overall survival was 46% and event-free survival was 40%, suggesting that early transplantation might improve outcomes.

This hypothesis was tested in an RCT conducted by the EBMT and the United Kingdom Lymphoma Group. In this study, 98 patients who achieved CR1 were initially entered and 65 were randomized to receive conventional chemotherapy, which included ALL-type maintenance therapy or high-dose therapy and autologous transplantation (23). Main reasons for failure to randomize included patient choice, morbidity and mortality from induction therapy, or progressive disease. The three-year RFS was 55% with autologous transplantation versus 22% with maintenance chemotherapy ($p = 0.065$). A difference in overall survival at three years was not detected (56% vs. 45%; $p = 0.71$). Potential reasons for lack of difference in overall survival included insufficient power given the small number of randomized patients. Although the trial was terminated early due to slow accrual, a post hoc power calculation indicated that a different conclusion would have been unlikely. Also, the superior RFS together with the lack of detectable difference in overall survival may have been contributed by successful second-line therapy with autologous transplantation in subsequent relapses.

These data therefore do not lead to definitive conclusions. At present, autologous transplantation remains a reasonable treatment strategy. Improvements in both maintenance therapies and transplantation technology will require ongoing comparisons of these options. However, it is clear that the intensity of initial chemotherapy is important in determining the outcome of this disease (Table 43.1).

Recommendation

Although differences in overall survival have not been demonstrated, treatment with autologous transplantation improves long-term disease control in adult patients with lymphoblastic lymphoma and is thus a preferred option (Grade 2B).

Does the type of transplantation (autologous vs. allogeneic) influence outcome?

Allogeneic transplantation has theoretical advantages over autologous transplantation as the risk of tumor contamination of the reinfused stem cell product is avoided and allogeneic transplantation provides immunologic therapy through a "graft versus lymphoma" effect. An early study from the Netherlands in which adult patients with LBL/ALL underwent allogeneic transplantation in CR1 showed a five-year actuarial overall survival of 48% (24). Studies comparing allogeneic and autologous transplantation have been reported, but sample sizes are small and results variable. With the establishment of large transplantation databases, several studies have attempted to address whether allogeneic transplantation might be a superior option.

The International Bone Marrow Transplant and the Autologous Blood and Marrow Transplant Registries have been evaluated to compare outcomes of 76 HLA-identical sibling matched allogeneic and 128 autologous transplantations (25). Treatment-related mortality (TRM) was significantly higher in those undergoing allogeneic transplantation (25% vs. 5%, $p < 0.001$), but a lower relapse rate was observed (34% vs. 56%, $p = 0.004$). As disease-free and overall survivals were similar, the authors concluded that any advantage gained from improved disease control associated with the allogeneic procedure was offset by the increased morbidity of the procedure. A second evaluation of the EBMT's database compared 1,332 patients undergoing autologous transplantation with 314 who underwent allogeneic transplantation (26). While the relapse rate was again higher with autologous transplantation, overall survival was superior because of the higher TRM associated with allogeneic transplantation.

Recommendation

Given the low incidence of treatment-related mortality, therapy with autologous transplantation is preferred over allogeneic transplantation, even allowing for the higher relapse rate associated with the autologous procedure (Grade 1C).

Does mediastinal radiation improve outcome?

Patients with LBL may present with bulky mediastinal disease; the utility of adjuvant mediastinal radiotherapy has therefore been investigated. In the pediatric population, radiation therapy has not been demonstrated to improve survival (27,28), and as sequelae of mediastinal radiation may include secondary malignancies and cardiac toxicities, use of radiation is not considered a standard practice. Although many of these studies were randomized studies, mediastinal radiotherapy was usually not given in a randomized fashion, and the results with respect to mediastinal irradiation cannot be interpreted as such. Outcomes of chemotherapy in adult patients have been inferior to those observed in children, principally due to poorer disease control. Therefore, augmented means of achieving disease control, including use of mediastinal radiation, continue to be debated.

A small retrospective review performed at MD Anderson involving 47 adult patients with LBL attempted to address this question (29); 43 patient who achieved CR with a variety of chemotherapies were assessed. None of the 19 patients who received mediastinal radiotherapy experienced mediastinal recurrence, whereas 8 of 24 patients who did not get radiation had mediastinal relapse. However, a major confounding factor was that 16 of 19 patients who received mediastinal radiotherapy had Hyper-CVAD, while most of the patients without radiation (18 of 24) had other forms of chemotherapy. Overall survival and freedom-from-progression were not significantly different. This small study suggests that there may be an improvement in local control with the use of adjuvant mediastinal radiation but the results are far from conclusive.

Recommendation

Currently, available data are insufficient to recommend that patients with bulky mediastinal disease who achieve a CR with an intensive ALL regimen and who will continue to receive maintenance therapy with that regimen or will proceed to undergo autologous transplantation also require mediastinal radiation (Grade 2C).

References

1 A clinical evaluation of the International Lymphoma Study Group classification of non-Hodgkin's lymphoma. The Non-Hodgkin's Lymphoma Classification Project. *Blood.* 1997;**89**(11):3909–18.

2 Rosen PJ, Feinstein DI, Pattengale PK, et al. Convoluted lymphocytic lymphoma in adults: a clinicopathologic entity. *Ann Intern Med.* 1978;**89**(3):319–24.

3 Nathwani BN, Diamond LW, Winberg CD, et al. Lymphoblastic lymphoma: a clinicopathologic study of 95 patients. *Cancer.* 1981;**48**(11):2347–57.

4 Sheibani K, Nathwani BN, Winberg CD, et al. Antigenically defined subgroups of lymphoblastic lymphoma. Relationship to clinical presentation and biologic behavior. *Cancer.* 1987;**60**(2):183–90.

5 Link MP, Stewart SJ, Warnke RA, et al. Discordance between surface and cytoplasmic expression of the Leu-4 (T3) antigen in thymocytes and in blast cells from childhood T lymphoblastic malignancies. *J Clin Invest.* 1985;**76**(1):248–53.

6 Griffith RC, Kelly DR, Nathwani BN et al. A morphologic study of childhood lymphoma of the lymphoblastic type: the pediatric Oncology Group experience. *Cancer.* 1987;**59**(6):1126–31.

7 Pui CH, Evans WE. Treatment of acute lymphoblastic leukemia. *N Engl J Med.* 2006;**354**(2):166–78.

8 Colgan JP, Andersen J, Habermann TM, et al. Long-term follow-up of a CHOP-based regimen with maintenance therapy and central nervous system prophylaxis in lymphoblastic non-Hodgkin's lymphoma. *Leuk Lymphoma.* 1994;**15**(3–4):291–96.

9 Kaiser U, Uebelacker I, Havemann K. Non-Hodgkin's lymphoma protocols in the treatment of patients with Burkitt's lymphoma and lymphoblastic lymphoma: a report on 58 patients. *Leuk Lymphoma.* 1999;**36**(1–2):101–8.

10 Jost LM, Jacky E, Dommann-Scherrer C, et al. Short-term weekly chemotherapy followed by high-dose therapy with autologous bone marrow transplantation for lymphoblastic and Burkitt's lymphomas in adult patients. *Ann Oncol.* 1995;**6**(5):445–51.

11 Le Gouill S, Lepretre S, Briere J, et al. Adult lymphoblastic lymphoma: a retrospective analysis of 92 patients under 61 years included in the LNH87/93 trials. *Leukemia.* 2003;**17**(11):2220–24.

12 Anderson JR, Wilson JF, Jenkin DT, et al. Childhood non-Hodgkin's lymphoma: the results of a randomized therapeutic trial comparing a 4-drug regimen (COMP) with a 10-drug regimen (LSA2-L2). *N Engl J Med.* 1983;**308**(10):559–65.

13 Hoelzer D, Gokbuget N, Digel W, et al. Outcome of adult patients with T-lymphoblastic lymphoma treated according to protocols for acute lymphoblastic leukemia. *Blood.* 2002;**99**(12):4379–85.

14 Thomas DA, O'Brien S, Cortes J, et al. Outcome with the hyper-CVAD regimens in lymphoblastic lymphoma. *Blood.* 2004;**104**(6):1624–30.

15 Aljurf M, Zaidi SZ. Chemotherapy and hematopoietic stem cell transplantation for adult T-cell lymphoblastic lymphoma: current status and controversies. *Biol Blood Marrow Transplant.* 2005;**11**(10):739–54.

16 Coleman CN, Cohen JR, Burke JS, et al. Lymphoblastic lymphoma in adults: results of a pilot protocol. *Blood.* 1981;**57**(4):679–84.

17 Coleman CN, Picozzi VJ Jr, Cox RS, et al. Treatment of lymphoblastic lymphoma in adults. *J Clin Oncol.* 1986;**4**(11):1628–37.

18 Thomas DA, Kantarjian HM. Lymphoblastic lymphoma. *Hematol Oncol Clin North Am.* 2001;**15**(1):51–95, vi.

19 Pui CH, Cheng C, Leung W, et al. Extended follow-up of long-term survivors of childhood acute lymphoblastic leukemia. *N Engl J Med.* 2003;**349**(7):640–49.

20 Burkhardt B, Woessmann W, Zimmermann M, et al. Impact of cranial radiotherapy on central nervous system prophylaxis in children and adolescents with central nervous system-negative stage III or IV lymphoblastic lymphoma. *J Clin Oncol.* 2006;**24**(3):491–99.

21 Sweetenham JW, Liberti G, Pearce R, et al. High-dose therapy and autologous bone marrow transplantation for adult patients with lymphoblastic lymphoma: results of the European Group for Bone Marrow Transplantation. *J Clin Oncol.* 1994;**12**(7):1358–65.

22 van Imhoff GW, van der Holt B, MacKenzie MA, et al. Short intensive sequential therapy followed by autologous stem cell transplantation in adult Burkitt, Burkitt-like and lymphoblastic lymphoma. *Leukemia.* 2005;**19**(6):945–52.

23 Sweetenham JW, Santini G, Qian W, et al. High-dose therapy and autologous stem-cell transplantation versus conventional-dose consolidation/maintenance therapy as postremission therapy for adult patients with lymphoblastic lymphoma: results of a randomized trial of the European Group for Blood and Marrow Transplantation and the United Kingdom Lymphoma Group. *J Clin Oncol.* 2001;**19**(11):2927–36.

24 De Witte T, Awwad B, Boezeman J, et al. Role of allogenic bone marrow transplantation in adolescent or adult patients with acute lymphoblastic leukaemia or lymphoblastic lymphoma in first remission. *Bone Marrow Transplant.* 1994;**14**(5):767–74.

25 Levine JE, Harris RE, Loberiza FR Jr, et al. A comparison of allogeneic and autologous bone marrow transplantation for lymphoblastic lymphoma. *Blood.* 2003;**101**(7):2476–82.

26 Peniket AJ, Ruiz de Elvira MC, Taghipour G, et al. An EBMT registry matched study of allogeneic stem cell transplants for lymphoma: allogeneic transplantation is associated with a lower relapse rate but a higher procedure-related mortality rate than autologous transplantation. *Bone Marrow Transplant.* 2003;**31**(8):667–78.

27 Eden OB, Hann I, Imeson J, et al. Treatment of advanced stage T cell lymphoblastic lymphoma: results of the United Kingdom Children's Cancer Study Group (UKCCSG) protocol 8503. *Br J Haematol.* 1992;**82**(2):310–16.

28 Tubergen DG, Krailo MD, Meadows AT, et al. Comparison of treatment regimens for pediatric lymphoblastic non-Hodgkin's lymphoma: a Childrens Cancer Group study. *J Clin Oncol.* 1995;**13**(6):1368–76.

29 Dabaja BS, Ha CS, Thomas DA, et al. The role of local radiation therapy for mediastinal disease in adults with T-cell lymphoblastic lymphoma. *Cancer.* 2002;**94**(10):2738–44.

44 Mantle Cell Lymphoma

C. Tom Kouroukis

Introduction

What is currently known as mantle cell lymphoma (MCL) has previously been classified as centrocytic lymphoma (1), intermediate lymphocytic lymphoma (2), and intermediately differentiated lymphoma (3). In 1992, a unified description of this entity was made using morphology and immunohistochemistry and the term "mantle cell lymphoma" was coined (4). This entity is notable for being intensely CD20 positive, CD5 positive and CD23 negative. The t(11;14)(q13;q32) translocation, which approximates the immunoglobulin heavy chain locus at 14q32 and the bcl-1 oncogene at 11q13 results in the overexpression of cyclin D1, which regulates transition from G1 to S phase of the cell cycle. This translocation is detectable by cytogenetics in up to 50% of cases of MCL as diagnosed by morphology and immunohistochemistry (3) and overexpression of cyclin D1 has been detectable in almost all cases of MCL in some series (5).

Mantle cell lymphoma makes up approximately 6%–8% of all cases of non-Hodgkin lymphoma (6). In previous series, it appeared that patients with MCL treated with aggressive chemotherapy experienced shorter response durations and progression-free survivals compared with patients with intermediate grade lymphoma (7). Also, when treated with less toxic regimens, patients with MCL experienced a shorter survival compared with patients with indolent lymphoma (7). These findings suggested that MCL has the worst features of both indolent and aggressive histology lymphoma; that is, it has the incurability of the indolent lymphomas and the aggressiveness of the intermediate grade lymphomas. Median survival times range from three to four years (7–10).

Evidence-based Hematology. Edited by Mark A. Crowther, Jeff Ginsberg, Holger J. Schünemann, Ralph M. Meyer, and Richard Lottenberg.

Questions

1. What is the role of anthracycline or anthracenedione-based chemotherapy in adults with newly diagnosed or relapsed MCL?
2. What is the role of rituximab (as a single agent, in combination with chemotherapy) in adults with newly diagnosed or relapsed MCL?
3. What is the role of high dose chemotherapy and stem cell transplantation in patients with newly diagnosed or relapsed MCL?

Literature-search strategy and results

Two search strategies used: one for the electronic databases listed below and a second strategy to search the abstracts of the American Society of Hematology (ASH) and the American Society of Clinical Oncology (ASCO) meetings. Regarding the electronic databases, the following were searched:

- *Cochrane Database of Systematic Reviews* (first quarter 2007)
- *ACP Journal Club* (1991 to March/April 2007)
- Database of Abstracts of Reviews of Effects (second quarter 2007)
- Cochrane Central Register of Controlled Trials (second quarter 2007)
- EMBASE (1980 to 2007, week 18)
- Ovid MEDLINE® In-Process and other non-indexed citations and Ovid MEDLINE® 1950 to present (May 7, 2007).

Separate search strategies were used for systematic reviews or meta-analyses and for randomized controlled trials (RCTs). Details are included in the Appendix. The search for systematic reviews and meta-analyses identified 16 citations with two addressing questions relevant to this chapter. The search for RCTs yielded 680 citations from which nine RCTs were identified. Some of the RCTs were published updates as abstracts or second papers (11–23): in five (13–15,17–22), the results of MCL patients were obtained by subgroup analysis and three studies (11,12,16) included MCL patients exclusively. One study compared two nonanthracycline chemotherapy regimens in patients with indolent and MCL, without rituximab, since no information on the MCL subgroup was available, the study was not discussed further (23).

Abstract searches were done from 2004 to 2006 inclusively from the ASH and ASCO meetings using the following words in the abstract title "mantle cell lymphoma." A total of 145 abstracts were found for American Society of Hematology and 30 abstracts for American Society of Clinical Oncology. The results of the abstracts are discussed in the individual sections that follow.

Grading of the quality of evidence and strengths of recommendations in this chapter are based on the guidelines proposed by the international Grading of Recommendations Assessment, Development, and Evaluation Working Group (GRADE) adopting the modification used by the American College of Chest Physicians that merges the very low and low categories of quality of evidence (see chapter 1).

What is the role of anthracycline or anthracenedione-based chemotherapy in adults with newly diagnosed or relapsed MCL?

Three studies (in four publications) (19–22) were found that address this question. None of the abstracts provided additional information. The studies tested chemotherapy, including an anthracycline or anthracenedione, against chemotherapy without anthracyclines or anthracenediones (19,20,22) or a regimen containing an anthracycline against a regimen containing an anthracenedione (21). One study published the treatment data (19) separately from data comparing responses between patients with follicular lymphoma and those with MCL (20). These studies extracted data from a subgroup of patients with previously untreated MCL.

In a study by Zinzani et al. (22), patients between 18 and 65 years of age with previously untreated indolent lymphoma or MCL were randomized to fludarabine alone versus fludarabine with idarubicin. Of the total of 199 eligible patients, 29 had MCL. There was no significant difference detected in the MCL subgroup in the complete response rate (27% vs. 33%) and in the partial response rate (45% vs. 28%) for those receiving fludarabine alone compared to fludarabine with idarubicin, respectively. In the entire group of patients, there were improvements in relapse-free and progression-free survivals favoring the anthracycline-containing treatment, but there was no detectable difference in relapse-free survival in the small number of patients with MCL. There were no differences in important toxicities detected between the two treatment groups.

Anthracenediones, like mitoxantrone, were developed as less toxic alternatives to anthracyclines (24). Combination chemotherapy with mitoxantrone, cyclophosphamide, and prednisone (MCP) was tested against cyclophosphamide, doxorubicin, vincristine, and prednisone (CHOP) by Nickenig et al. (21) in patients with follicular lymphoma and MCL. Eighty-six previously untreated patients with MCL were randomized to either MCP or CHOP for 6 to 8 cycles. In the subgroup of patients with MCL, the response rate appeared higher with CHOP but was not statistically significant (87% versus 73%, $p = 0.08$). There was no detectable difference in time-to-treatment failure in the MCL subgroup (median 21 vs. 15 months for CHOP and MCP, respectively, $p = 0.14$). In terms of overall survival in the MCL subgroup, the median measured 61 months after CHOP chemotherapy compared with 48 months after MCP ($p = 0.058$). Higher rates of hematological toxicity were observed following MCP compared with CHOP, and a greater difficulty in mobilizing stem cells in patients younger than 60 years.

In a study by the German Low Grade Lymphoma Study Group (19), patients with previously untreated, advanced stage indolent lymphoma, including MCL, were randomized to prednimustine and mitoxantrone (PmM) or to a combination of cyclophosphamide, vincristine, and prednisone (COP). There was a second randomization to interferon alpha or to observation alone after eight cycles of initial therapy. In the initial publication of this study (19), from a total of 246 patients, 46 were diagnosed with either centrocytic lymphoma or mantle cell lymphoma. The response rate in the evaluable subgroup of 39 patients with centrocytic lymphoma or MCL appeared higher in those patients treated with PmM compared with COP (27% vs. 5%, *p*, not provided). Event-free survival was only reported for the entire group of patients. In a subsequent publication of this study (20), MCL patients experience a slower response to chemotherapy and a shorter median event-free and overall survival of 8 months and 28 months, respectively, compared with follicular lymphoma patients (24 months and 7 years, respectively).

Recommendation

Anthracycline-containing therapy (e.g., CHOP) has evolved to become the most common initial treatment for patients with MCL. This standard has evolved without clear supporting data from RCTs. Without available data to refute this standard, it is reasonable to recommend that CHOP be considered the standard first line of therapy (Grade 2B). When comparing doxorubicin versus mitoxantrone-containing regimens, a subgroup analysis from one study that includes a small number of patients suggests that it is unlikely that therapy with mitoxantrone will be superior, and it may be inferior. Thus, there is insufficient evidence to recommend a mitoxantrone-containing regimen over CHOP (Grade 2B).

What is the role of rituximab (as a single agent, in combination with chemotherapy) in adults with newly diagnosed or relapsed MCL?

Two systematic reviews and four studies (11,13–18) evaluated rituximab in patients with either untreated or relapsed MCL.

Rituximab as single-agent therapy

In an RCT of the Swiss Group for Clinical Cancer Research (16), previously untreated and relapsed patients with MCL were given rituximab as a single agent, 375 mg/m^2 weekly for 4 weeks followed by randomization in those patients who lacked progression to either observation alone or intermittent rituximab, 375 mg/m^2 once every 8 weeks for four injections. Upon relapse or progression, treatment was left to the discretion of the patient's physician. At week 12 of treatment, 27% of 104 patients did not progress and proceeded to randomization. There were no differences detected in response rate, best response, or event-free survival (progression, relapse, second tumor, death from any cause) between the two groups (median 6 versus 12 months, observation versus rituximab treatment, respectively, $p = 0.45$ or $p = 0.1$, depending on the statistical test used). Patients treated with ongoing rituximab experienced more prolonged decreases in B lymphocyte subsets, but there were no differences in any serious adverse events.

Rituximab as a component of multiagent therapy

A systematic review and practice guideline from Cancer Care Ontario Program in Evidence-Based Care examined studies of rituximab in patients with lymphoma (25). A number of studies contained information regarding MCL patients, but these were already identified during the searches done for RCTs included in this section. A systematic review and meta-analysis done by the Cochrane Haematological Malignancies Group (26) looked at immunochemotherapy with rituximab in patients with indolent or MCL. The three RCTs (11,13,17,18) identified in the Cochrane Review reporting on outcomes in MCL patients are discussed in this section. The Cochrane Review pooled the three studies despite the differences in chemotherapy regimens and that the studies contained previously untreated and relapsed patients. The overall response rate favored rituximab with chemotherapy ($Z = 2.62$, $p = 0.009$), and these studies were not statistically heterogeneous (chi-square 0.64, df $= 2$, $p = 0.73$). The hazard ratio for overall survival in the pooled analysis for the MCL patients also favoured the chemotherapy and rituximab group ($Z = 2.04$, $p = 0.04$) but the heterogeneity statistic was borderline, suggesting the studies were statistically heterogeneous (chi-square 5.21, df $= 2$, $p = 0.07$).

In a study by the German Low Grade Lymphoma Study Group (11), patients with previously untreated MCL were randomized to six cycles of cyclophosphamide, doxorubicin, vincristine, and prednisone (CHOP), with or without rituximab (375 mg/m^2 on day 0). Responding patients up to the age of 65 years were offered participation in another randomized study of high-dose therapy and autologous stem cell transplantation versus maintenance interferon therapy. Patients treated with rituximab had a superior overall (94% vs. 75%, $p = 0.0054$), and complete response rate (34% vs. 7%, $p = 0.00024$), and time-to-treatment failure compared to patients receiving CHOP (median 21 vs. 14 months, $p = 0.013$). There were no differences detected in progression-free survival or in the two-year survival probability (76% in both treatment arms). Apart from infusion-related reactions to the rituximab, there were no differences in any adverse events between the two groups.

Another study by the German Low Grade Lymphoma Study Group included patients with relapsed or refractory follicular or MCL (13). Patients were randomized to fludarabine, cyclophosphamide, and mitoxantrone (FCM) with or without rituximab. Out of 128 evaluable patients, 48 patients had MCL. Patients in the R-FCM treatment group who experienced a response underwent a further randomization to rituximab maintenance 375 mg/m^2 intravenously weekly for 4 weeks at months 3 and 6. The authors did not indicate whether patients may have received previous rituximab-containing therapy. In the entire group of patients, the response rate was improved with R-FCM, but in the subgroup of MCL patients, there was no statistically significant difference in the response rate (46% vs. 58%) between patients receiving FCM versus R-FCM, respectively. After a median observation time of 18 months, overall survival in the MCL group was improved with R-FCM compared with FCM alone (median not reached versus 11 months, $p = 0.0042$). There were no major differences in any toxicities between the two groups of patients although there was more lymphopenia seen in the rituximab-containing group. In two follow-up abstract reports (14,15), it was noted that all patients who received rituximab maintenance experienced an improved duration of response (median not reached versus 17 months, $p = 0.0024$), although the results for the MCL subgroup are not known, only that the progression-free survival was significantly different ($p = 0.049$) between those patients that did or did not receive maintenance rituximab.

An interim analysis of a study in patients with indolent lymphoma comparing mitoxantrone, chlorambucil, prednisone with or without rituximab was prepared by the Ostdeutsche Studiengruppe Hämatologie und Onkologie (17). There is no breakdown in the interim results by disease subtype and disease control and survival data are not available. As of the date of the preparation of this chapter, despite the publication of an abstract report (18), the results of this study regarding the MCL patients are not yet available (M. Herold, personal communication).

Recommendations

1. In previously untreated patients with MCL, the addition of rituximab to CHOP results in superior overall and complete response rates and time-to-treatment failure. The one available study did not detect a difference in survival, but this study's design included subsequent co-interventions of autologous stem cell transplantation or interferon maintenance therapy, which may have influenced this outcome. By including rituximab with initial treatment, important benefits are observed and no associated important additional toxicities are noted. Therefore, inclusion of rituximab is recommended (Grade 1A).

2. In patients with relapsed MCL, the addition of rituximab to FCM was associated with a superior overall survival. This finding is one of statistical and clinical significance, but obtained through a subgroup analysis. Although details are not available, maintenance rituximab in the FCM-R study may also have conferred a benefit in progression-free survival. Rituximab is therefore recommended as part of multi-agent treatment for patients who have relapsed MCL (Grade 1B). As described by Imrie and Cheung in chapter 42 with respect to follicular lymphoma, there are insufficient data to evaluate the role of retreatment with rituximab-containing therapy for patients who have previously received this agent.

3. At present, there are insufficient data to justify use of rituximab maintenance following single-agent rituximab therapy for patients with MCL (Grade 1C).

What is the role of high dose chemotherapy and stem cell transplantation in patients with newly diagnosed or relapsed MCL?

An RCT done by the European MCL network (12) included adults less than age 65 years, with stage III or IV previously untreated MCL and an Eastern Cooperative Oncology Group performance status of 0–2. Patients were allocated to myeloablative radiochemotherapy followed by autologous transplantation or interferon alpha maintenance therapy. The majority of patients were received CHOP, with or without rituximab, and many had participated in a previous study of CHOP with or without rituximab (11). Patients received intensified mobilization chemotherapy with Dexa-BEAM (dexamethasone, BCNU, etoposide, cytarabine, and melphalan) followed by conditioning with total body irradiation (12 Gy) and high-dose cyclophosphamide; 122 evaluable patients with a median age of 55 years were followed. Of those treated with transplantation, 81% attained a CR and 17% a PR compared with 37% and 62%, respectively, for those patients treated with interferon alpha maintenance therapy. The median time-to-treatment failure was superior in the transplantation group (29 vs. 15 months, $p = 0.0023$), as was the median progression-free survival (39 vs. 17 months, $p = 0.011$). A subgroup analysis evaluating those patients who achieved a complete remission with CHOP (±rituximab) demonstrated an even longer progression-free survival (median 46 months) compared with interferon alpha maintenance therapy (24 months, $p = 0.0019$). No difference in overall survival at 3 years was detected between the two groups (83% and 77%, respectively, for transplantation and interferon maintenance therapy groups). No differences in overall survival were detected between patients who underwent transplantation in complete or partial remission. More frequent rates of hematological toxicities, infections due to cytopenia and infectious mortality, mucositis, and gastrointestinal, pulmonary, renal, and hepatic toxicities were seen in patients undergoing transplantation. Patients treated with interferon alpha more often experienced muscle and bone pain and depression. A Cox regression analysis could only identify transplantation and a low International Prognostic Index score to be independently associated with an improved progression-free survival.

Recommendation

In previously untreated patients with MCL, autologous stem cell transplantation is associated with a higher response rate, and an approximate doubling in the median time-to-treatment failure and progression-free survival compared with interferon maintenance therapy. Despite increased toxicities and the lack of a demonstrated survival advantage, autologous transplantation is therefore a reasonable option to include as initial therapy for MCL patients (Grade 2A). The decision to offer autologous transplantation to MCL patients is complex and should account for underlying comorbidities and be based on the measured benefits against patient preferences and toxicities.

References

1 Meusers P, Engelhard M, Bartels H, et al. Multicentre randomized therapeutic trial for advanced centrocytic lymphoma: anthracycline does not improve the prognosis. *Hematol Oncol.* 1989;**7**(5):365–80.

2 Weisenburger DD, Nathwani BN, Diamond LW, et al. Malignant lymphoma, intermediate lymphocytic type: a clinicopathologic study of 42 cases. *Cancer.* 1981;**48**(6):1415–25.

3 Bookman MA, Lardelli P, Jaffe ES, et al. Lymphocytic lymphoma of intermediate differentiation: morphologic, immunophenotypic, and prognostic factors. *J Natl Cancer Inst.* 1990;**82**(9):742–48.

4 Banks PM, Chan J, Cleary M, et al. Mantle cell lymphoma: a proposal for unification of morphologic, immunologic, and molecular data. *Am J Surg Pathol.* 1992;**16**:637–40.

5 de Boer CJ, Schuuring E, Dreef E, et al. Cyclin D1 protein analysis in the diagnosis of mantle cell lymphoma. *Blood.* 1995;**86**(7):2715–23.

6 The Non-Hodgkin's lymphoma classification project. A clinical evaluation of the International Lymphoma Study Group classification of non-Hodgkin's lymphoma. *Blood.* 1997;**89**(11):3909–18.

7 Teodorovic I, Pittaluga S, Kluin-Nelemans JC, et al. Efficacy of four different regimens in 64 mantle-cell lymphoma cases: Clinicopathologic comparison with 498 other non-Hodgkin's lymphoma subtypes. *J Clin Oncol.* 1995;**13**(11):2819–26.

8 Fisher RI, Dahlberg S, Nathwani B, et al. A clinical analysis of two indolent lymphoma entities: Mantle cell lymphoma and marginal zone lymphoma (including the mucosa-associated lymphoid tissue and monocytoid B-cell subcategories): a Southwest Oncology Group Study. *Blood.* 1995;85:1075–82.

9 Weisenburger D, Vose J, Greiner T, et al. Mantle cell lymphoma: a clinicopathologic study of 68 cases from the Nebraska Lymphoma Study Group. *Am J Hematol.* 2000;**64**:190–96.

10 Argatoff LH, Connors JM, Klasa RJ, et al. Mantle cell lymphoma: a clinicopathologic study of 80 cases. *Blood.* 1997;**89**(6):2067–78.

11 Lenz G, Dreyling M, Hoster E, et al. Immunochemotherapy with rituximab and cyclophosphamide, doxorubicin, vincristine, and prednisone significantly improves response and time to treatment failure, but not long-term outcome in patients with previously untreated mantle cell lymphoma: results of a prospective randomized trial of the German Low Grade Lymphoma Study Group (GLSG). *J Clin Oncol.* 2005;**23**(9):1984–92.

12 Dreyling M, Lenz G, Hoster E, et al. Early consolidation by myeloablative radiochemotherapy followed by autologous stem cell transplantation in first remission significantly prolongs progression-free survival in mantle-cell lymphoma: results of a prospective randomized trial of the European MCL Network. *Blood.* 2005;**105**(7):2677–84.

13 Forstpointner R, Dreyling M, Repp R, et al. The addition of rituximab to a combination of fludarabine, cyclophosphamide, mitoxantrone (FCM) significantly increases the response rate and prolongs survival as compared with FCM alone in patients with relapsed and refractory follicular and mantle cell lymphomas: results of a prospective

randomized study of the German Low-Grade Lymphoma Study Group. *Blood.* 2004;**104**(10):3064–71.

14 Dreyling M, Forstpointner R, Gramatzki M, et al. Rituximab maintenance improves progression-free and overall survival rates after combined immuno-chemotherapy (R-FCM) in patients with relapsed follicular and mantle cell lymphoma: final results of a prospective randomized trial of the German Low Grade Lymphoma Study Group (GLSG). *Am Soc Clin Oncol.* 2006;**24**:7502.

15 Hiddemann W, Forstpointner R, Dreyling M, et al. Rituximab maintenance prolongs response duration after salvage therapy with R-FCM in patients with relapsed follicular lymphomas and mantle cell lymphomas: results of a prospective randomized trial of the German Low Grade Lymphoma Study Group (GLSG). *ASH Ann Meeting Abstr.* 2005;**106**(11):920.

16 Ghielmini M, Schmitz SF, Cogliatti S, et al. Effect of single-agent rituximab given at the standard schedule or as prolonged treatment in patients with mantle cell lymphoma: a study of the Swiss Group for Clinical Cancer Research (SAKK). *J Clin Oncol.* 2005;**23**(4):705–11.

17 Herold M, Dolken G, Fiedler F, et al. Randomized phase III study for the treatment of advanced indolent non-Hodgkin's lymphomas (NHL) and mantle cell lymphoma: chemotherapy versus chemotherapy plus rituximab. *Ann Hematol.* 2003;**82**(2):77–79.

18 Herold M, Haas A, Srock S, et al. Addition of rituximab to first-line MCP (mitoxantrone, chlorambucil, prednisolone) chemotherapy prolongs survival in advanced follicular lymphoma—4-year follow-up results of a phase III trial of the East German Study Group Hematology and Oncology (OSHO#39). *ASH Ann Meeting Abstr.* 2006;**108**(11):484.

19 Unterhalt M, Herrmann R, Tiemann M, et al. Prednimustine, mitoxantrone (PmM) vs cyclophosphamide, vincristine, prednisone (COP) for the treatment of advanced low-grade non-Hodgkin's lymphoma. German Low-Grade Lymphoma Study Group. *Leukemia.* 1996;**10**(5):836–43.

20 Hiddemann W, Unterhalt M, Herrmann R, et al. Mantle-cell lymphomas have more widespread disease and a slower response to chemotherapy compared with follicle-center lymphomas: results of a prospective comparative analysis of the German low-grade lymphoma study group. *J Clin Oncol.* 1998;**16**(5)1922–30.

21 Nickenig C, Dreyling M, Hoster E, et al. Combined cyclophosphamide, vincristine, doxorubicin, and prednisone (CHOP) improves response rates but not survival and has lower hematologic toxicity compared with combined mitoxantrone, chlorambucil, and prednisone (MCP) in follicular and mantle cell lymphomas: results of a prospective randomized trial of the German Low-Grade Lymphoma Study Group. *Cancer.* 2006;**107**(5):1014–22.

22 Zinzani PL, Magagnoli M, Moretti L, et al. Randomized trial of fludarabine versus fludarabine and idarubicin as frontline treatment in patients with indolent or mantle-cell lymphoma. *J Clin Oncol.* 2000;**18**(4):773–79.

23 Herold M, Schulze A, Niederwieser D, et al. Bendamustine, vincristine and prednisone (BOP) versus cyclophosphamide, vincristine and prednisone (COP) in advanced indolent non-Hodgkin's lymphoma and mantle cell lymphoma: results of a randomised phase III trial (OSHO# 19). *J Cancer Res Clin Oncol.* 2006;**132**(2):105–12.

24 Faulds D, Balfour JA, Chrisp P, et al. Mitoxantrone: a review of its pharmacodynamic and pharmacokinetic properties, and therapeutic potential in the chemotherapy of cancer. *Drugs.* 1991;**41**(3):400–49.

25 Cheung MC, Haynes AE, Meyer RM, et al. Rituximab in lymphoma: a systematic review and consensus practice guideline from Cancer Care Ontario. *Cancer Treat Rev.* 2007;**33**(2):161–76.

26 Schulz H, Bohlius JF, Trelle S, et al. Immunochemotherapy with rituximab and overall survival in patients with indolent or mantle cell lymphoma: a systematic review and meta-analysis. *J Natl Cancer Inst.* 2007;**99**(9):706–14.

Appendix

Search strategies for reports evaluating therapies for patients with mantle cell lymphoma

1. Strategy for systematic reviews and meta-analyses (numbers indicate citations identified)

1.1 meta-analysis.mp. (68504)
1.2 systematic review.mp. (36779)
1.3 1 or 2 (88486)
1.4 mantle cell lymphoma.mp. (3163)
1.5 mantle cell lymphoma.sh. (1585)
1.6 4 or 5 (3163)
1.7 3 and 6 (16)

2. Strategy for Randomized Controlled Trials

2.1 mantle cell lymphoma.mp. [mp = ti, ot, ab, tx, kw, ct, sh, hw, tn, dm, mf, nm] (3163)
2.2 mantle cell lymphoma.sh. (1585)
2.3 1 or 2 (3163)
2.4 randomized controlled trial.pt. (461116)
2.5 controlled clinical trial.pt. (148014)
2.6 randomized controlled trials.sh. (53359)
2.7 random allocation.sh. (77953)
2.8 double-blind method.sh. (166725)
2.9 single-blind method.sh. (17717)
2.10 4 or 5 or 6 or 7 or 8 or 9 (692869)
2.11 limit 10 to humans [Limit not valid in: CDSR,ACP Journal Club,DARE,CCTR; records were retained] (666398)
2.12 clinical trial.pt. (709506)
2.13 exp clinical trials/ (661522)
2.14 (clin$ adj25 trial$).ti,ab. (296745)
2.15 ((singl$ or doubl$ or trebl$ or tripl$) adj25 (blind$ or mask$)).ti,ab. (279977)
2.16 placebos.sh. (43684)
2.17 placebo$.ti,ab. (296813)
2.18 random$.ti,ab. (939868)
2.19 research design.sh. (49193)
2.20 12 or 13 or 14 or 15 or 16 or 17 or 18 or 19 (1965570)
2.21 comparative study.sh. (91167)
2.22 exp evaluation studies/ (695990)
2.23 follow up studies.sh. (361831)
2.24 prospective studies.sh. (263550)
2.25 (control$ or prospectiv$ or volunteer$).ti,ab. (3578517)
2.26 21 or 22 or 23 or 24 or 25 (4513393)
2.27 11 or 20 or 26 (5454678)
2.28 3 and 27 (938)
2.29 remove duplicates from 28 (680)

45 Management of Patients with Peripheral T-cell Lymphoma

Kerry J. Savage

Introduction

Peripheral T-cell lymphomas (PTCLs) are a biologically diverse and uncommon group of diseases accounting for only 12%–15% of all cases in Western populations (1). By definition, they represent all TCLs of postthymic origin as opposed to the "precursor" lesion, lymphoblastic lymphoma. Compared to their B-cell counterparts, PTCLs remain largely unexplored and the optimal treatment ill-defined due to disease rarity and biological heterogeneity. The importance of the distinction between the mature B-cell and T-cell lymphomas and the impact on prognosis has only recently been fully appreciated. The Working Formulation did not yet incorporate immunophenotypic information and the updated Kiel Classification, although recognizing the T-cell phenotype, required subclassification of PTCLs based on morphologic subtypes and failed to recognize several clinicopathological entities (2). It wasn't until the REAL (Revised European–American Lymphoma) classification (Table 45.1) in 1994 which integrated morphologic, phenotypic, molecular and clinical information that the full spectrum of T-cell neoplasms was recognized and this provided the basis for the recently published WHO (World Health Organization) classification with some modifications (Table 45.1) (3). This review highlights the current state of the evidence related to the prognostic significance and some specifics of therapy related to peripheral T-cell lymphoma.

Questions

1. Is the prognosis of peripheral T-cell lymphoma inferior to patients with diffuse large B-cell lymphoma?
2. Are there any histologic subtypes of peripheral T-cell lymphoma with a more favorable prognosis?
3. Is cyclophosphamide, doxorubicin, vincristine, and prednisone (CHOP) the optimal therapy in PTCL? Should any of the PTCL subtypes be treated differently?
4. Should patients with PTCL be treated with primary autologous stem cell transplantation?
5. Is the outcome of patients with relapsed or refractory PTCL similar to diffuse large B-cell lymphoma (DLBCL) following autologous stem cell transplantation?

Evidence-based Hematology. Edited by Mark A. Crowther, Jeff Ginsberg, Holger J. Schünemann, Ralph M. Meyer, and Richard Lottenberg.

Literature-search strategy and inclusion

The PubMed database was searched to delineate all English, survival and treatment studies on adults with PTCLs from 1994 to 2006, to capture an era where PTCLs were recognized as a distinct group of diseases. Lymphoblastic lymphoma, mycosis fungoides, and leukemic-type PTCLs (LGL, HTLV1-associated T-cell lymphoma/leukemia and prolymphocytic leukemia) were excluded. Additional components of the search strategies specific to the questions addressed are indicated within the analyses of each question.

Grading of the quality of evidence and strengths of recommendations in this chapter are based on the guidelines proposed by the international Grading of Recommendations Assessment, Development, and Evaluation Working Group (GRADE) adopting the modification used by the American College of Chest Physicians that merges the "very low" and "low" categories of quality of evidence (see chapter 1).

Is the prognosis of peripheral T-cell lymphoma inferior to patients with diffuse large B-cell lymphoma?

The PubMed database was searched using the terms "peripheral t-cell lymphoma and survival" to identify all reports evaluating the prognosis of PTCLs, excluding for this purpose, studies evaluating primary transplant, specific novel treatment studies in relapsed patients, pediatric and HIV reports. Initially, 122 papers

Table 45.1 Revised European-American Lymphoma (REAL) and World Health Organization (WHO) classifications of T-cell and NK neoplasms.

REAL Classification	WHO Classification
Precursor T-cell neoplasm	**Precursor T-cell neoplasm**
Precursor T-lymphoblastic lymphoma/leukemia	Precursor T-lymphoblastic lymphoma/leukemia
Peripheral T-cell and NK-cell neoplasms	**Mature (peripheral) T-cell neoplasms**
T-cell chronic lymphocytic leukemia/	**Predominantly leukemic/disseminated**
Prolymphocytic leukemia	T-cell prolymphocytic leukemia
Large granular lymphocyte leukemia	T-cell granular lymphocytic leukemia
T-cell type and NK-cell type	NK-cell leukemia
Adult T-cell lymphoma/leukemia (HTLV1+)	Adult T-cell lymphoma/leukemia (HTLV1 +)
Angioimmunoblastic T-cell lymphoma	**Predominantly nodal**
Peripheral T-cell lymphoma, unspecified	Angioimmunoblastic T-cell lymphoma
Anaplastic large cell lymphoma, T/null-cell types	Peripheral T-cell lymphoma, unspecified
	Anaplastic large-cell lymphoma, T/null-cell, primary systemic type
Mycosis fungoides/Sezary syndrome	**Predominantly extranodal**
Angiocentric lymphoma	Mycosis fungoides/Sezary syndrome
Intestinal T-cell lymphoma	Anaplastic large-cell lymphoma, T/null-cell, primary cutaneous type
	Extranodal NK/T-cell lymphoma nasal and nasal type
	Enteropathy-type T-cell lymphoma
	Hepatosplenic $\gamma\delta$ T-cell lymphoma
	Subcutaneous panniculitis-like T-cell lymphoma

were retrieved. Manual exclusion of additional studies not directly pertaining to the question (including analyses of biological markers) reports of less than 25 cases for individual PTCL subtypes, non-T-cell lymphomas, and reviews resulted in 18 relevant papers (Table 45.2). The majority of these studies classified (or reclassified) PTCL according to the REAL classification and the most common subtype evaluated was PTCLU (unspecified). Only five of the reports reclassified patients according to the WHO. Three of these studies directly compared the prognosis of PTCL DLBCL (Table 45.2) (4–6).

There was heterogeneity in the reporting of outcome analyses with some studies combining all subtypes whereas others evaluated individual PTCL disease entities (Table 45.2). Some studies included a subset of pediatric patients and some did not specify the minimum age of inclusion. Further, since all series were retrospective in nature, treatments were variable, but the majority evaluated either CHOP or second- or third-generation CHOP-type regimens.

Overall, the survival of the PTCLs was poor with five-year estimates ranging from 26% to approximately 50%. Those studies that evaluated survival in specific histologic subtypes reported overall survival (OS) estimates for PTCLU from 20%–45% with similar results observed for angioimmunoblastic T-cell lymphoma (AILT) (7–12). Reports comparing the survival of PTCL to a cohort of similarly treated DLBCL patients, demonstrated an inferior event-free or overall survival in the PTCL subgroup (4–6). One analyses determined that this difference was confined to the nonanaplastic large cell lymphoma (ALCL) patients (4). A recent study specifically compared the survival of PTCLU with DLBCL, thus removing the heterogeneity generated when comparisons are made combining all PTCL subtypes. In this analysis, overall survival was inferior in the PTCLU group as anticipated; however, the disease-free survival (DFS), which only considers those patients who have achieved a complete remission, was similar in PTCLU and DLBCL suggesting that if a complete remission (CR) is achieved the duration of remission is also influenced by clinical prognostic factors rather than exclusively by disease immunophenotype.

Conclusion

Although the collective literature is based exclusively on retrospective analyses, the consistency of these reports supports that patients with PTCL have an inferior prognosis compared to DLBCL.

Are there any histologic subtypes of peripheral T-cell Lymphoma with a more favorable prognosis?

The prognostic importance of T- versus B-cell phenotype does not apply to all of the PTCL histologic subtypes. In the comprehensive PTCL survival analyses outlined in Table 45.2, several studies evaluated the prognostic significance of the ALCL histologic subtype and found that it had a more favorable prognosis (4,5,8,11–14). This is also consistent with findings from the non-Hodgkin's classification project where ALCL patients had a more favorable outcome than other PTCLs and also DLBCL (15). Some

Table 45.2 Studies of prognosis in peripheral T-cell lymphomas.*

Study	Country (n)	Classification	Treatment	PTCL Subtypes	EFS	OS	DLBCL EFS OS		Comment
Sonnen (2005) (8)	Europe (125)	WHO	Heterogeneous CHOP/CHOP-like ±XRT Palliative ASCT	All PTCLU (56%) AILT ALCL	—	43 45 28 61	—	–	Most patients were ALK-positive Histologic subtype did not impact overall survival in MVA IPI predictive of survival in PTCLs
Morabito (2004) (6)	Europe (297)	WHO	CHOP/CHOP-like (2nd or 3rd) (90%) ASCT	PTCLU	–	42	–	56	Overall survival of PTCLU inferior to DLBCL ($p = 0.0012$) but not in MVA If CR, DFS equivalent ($p = 0.1$) IPI predictive of survival in PTCLU
Savage (2004) (9)	North America (199)	WHO	CHOP/CHOP-like 75%–90%	PTCLU (64%) AILT ALCL ALK pos ALK neg CUTALCL NK/TCL	20 13 43 — — 56 15	35 36 43 58 34 78 24	—	—	Survival analyses on all patients (most treated with anthracycline-based CHT) ALK-pos ALCL trend to improved OS over ALK-neg ALCL (58% vs. 34%, $p = 0.35$) IPI predictive of survival in PTCLU and ALCL
Gallamini (2004) (43)	Europe (385)	WHO	CHOP/CHOP-like Non-anthracyline ASCT	PTCLU (100%)	—	43	—	—	Exclusively evaluated PTCLU IPI predictive of survival in PTCLU New T-cell prognostic index also developed
ten Berge (2003) (7)	Europe (133)	WHO	CHOP	PTCLU (35%) ALCL ALK pos ALK neg AILT		20 90 40 35 $p =$ 0.0001	—	—	Some pediatric cases included ALK-pos ALCL more favorable prognosis than ALK neg ALCL. ALK neg ALCL survival did not differ significantly than PTCLU IPI predictive of survival I n ALK neg ALCL
Arrowsmith (2003) (11)	North American (92)	REAL	CHOP-type Palliative or local therapy	All PTCLU (30%) ALCL (43%) AILT Other	22 17 40 0	49 42 58 26	—	—	Some pediatric cases included Survival more favorable with ALCL (ALK pos and ALK neg ALCL survival was not compared) IPI predictive of survival in grouped PTCL analysis
Rudiger (2002) (44)	International (96)	REAL	Combination CHT	All PTCLU AILT "Angiocentric"	20	26	—	—	Survival analyses only on patients treated with combination CHT No difference in survival among PTCL subtypes (ALK status unknown) IPI predictive of survival in grouped PTCL analysis

Musson (2003) (7,16)	Europe (104)	REAL	Chemotherapy or combined modality (60%) – type not specified	All PTCLU ALCL AILT Angiocentric Intestinal Cutaneous	— MS	52 34 mo 65.4 102	—	—	No difference in survival between PTCL subtypes ALK status unknown
Pellatt (2002) (10)	Europe (120)	REAL	Combination CHT (CHOP) (60%–70%) Single agent	All PTCLU AILT ALCL ETTL	39	36 40 30 60 25 $p =$ 0.035			Survival in ALCL more favorable
Kim (2002) (45)	Korea (78)	REAL	Combination CHT (86%)	All PTCLU (40%) Angiocentric ALCL AILT Other	— MS	36 (5 y) 12 (mo) 29 25 4 $p = 0.04$	 18 51 NR 4		Histologic subtype did not impact survival in MVA IPI predictive of survival in PTCLs
Weisenburger (2001) (13)	International	REAL (129)	Adriamycin-based (80%)	All PTCL ALCL	56	75			ALCL (70% ALK pos) more favorable survival than other PTCLs ($p < 0.001$) Survival estimates for PTCL reported in Rudiger et al.
Lee (1999) (46)	Korea (125)	REAL	Not stated	PTCLU (43%) Angiocentric	—	—	—	—	Overall survival of DLBCL superior to PTCLU ($p = 0.0043$) (Estimates not provided)
Isobe (1999) (47)	Japan (45)	REAL	Not stated	ALL PTCL (non-ALCL) PTCLU (15.5%) Angiocentric AILT ATLL ALCL	-	$<$30% $>$70%	-	-	Overall survival comparison to B-cell lymphomas included all B-cell histologic subtypes
Gisselbrecht (1998) (4)	Europe (288)	Kiel	Heterogeneous (4 trials) mBACOD ACVB or NCVB VIM3/ACVB CVP or CTVP	All PTCL PTCLU (56%) AILT ALCL "Non-ALCL"		41 64 35 $p =$ 0.0001		52 $p=$ 0.0004	PTCLs inferior survival compared to BCL (mostly DLBCL) ALCL more favorable prognosis c/w BCL and other non-ALCL

(cont.)

Table 45.2 (*Continued.*)

Study	Country (n)	Classification	Treatment	PTCL Subtypes	EFS	OS	DLBCL EFS OS		Comment
Lopez-Guillermo (1998) (12)	Europe (174)	REAL	CHOP or CHOP-like (89%)	All PTCL PTCLU (55%) ALCL AILT Angiocentric Intestinal	MS	38 22 mos 65 20 25 4			Survival more favourable with ALCL in MVA ($p = 0.03$) IPI predictive of survival in PTCLU
Melnyk (1997)	North America (68)	REAL	Heterogeneous (6 trials) CHOP/CHOP-like CHOPDBleo/DHAP ASHAP/MBACOS /MINE ASHAP or MBACOS + MINE	All PTCL PTCLU (66%) ALCL AILT Angiocentric	38	38	56 $p = 0.001$	63 $p = 0.001$	PTCL inferior survival compared to DLBCL No difference among PTCL subtypes (subgroups small)
Ansell (1997)	North America (78)	REAL	CHOP/CHOP like (2nd 3rd generation) Palliative/XRT alone	All PTCL PTCLU (68%) ALCL AILT Angiocentric Intestinal	—	22 mos (MS)	—	—	IPI predictive of survival in grouped PTCL analysis
Ascani (1997) (14)	Europe (168)	REAL	CHOP-like (2nd 3rd generation) Aggressive pediatric protocols	All PTCL PTCLU (46%) AILT ALCL Other		38 (8 y)			Included some pediatric cases ALCL superior survival compared to non-ALCL ($p = 0.0001$)

*MS, median survival; mos, months; OS, overall survival; EFS, event-free survival; IPI, International Prognostic Index; CHT, chemotherapy; PTCLU, peripheral T cell lymphoma, unspecified; AILT, angioimmunoblastic T-cell lymphoma; NK/TCL, Extranodal NK/T cell lymphoma nasal and nasal type; ALCL, anaplastic large cell lymphoma; ALK pos, ALK positive; ALK neg, ALK negative.

Table 45.3 Studies evaluating prognosis in ALK pos and ALK neg T- and null-cell ALCL.

Study	Classification	Treatment	Frequency	EFS		OS		Comment
			ALK pos	ALK pos	ALK neg	ALK pos	ALK neg	
ten Berge, 2000 Europe (85) (17)	REAL	Not stated	38%	—	—	90	35 $p = 0.0003$	Outcome of ALK neg ALCL poor in nodal and extranodal sites Some pediatric cases included
Gascoyne 1999 (57) (18,19)	REAL	CHOP	54%	88	37 $p < 0.0001$	93	37 $p < 0.00001$	Estimates only for T- and null-cell ALCL
Falini 1999 (78)	REAL	Combination chemotherapy Pediatric protocols	60%	82 (DFS)	28	71	15 $p < 0.0007$	Some pediatric cases included

*ALCL, anaplastic large cell lymphoma; ALK, pos ALK positive; ALK, neg ALK negative; OS, overall survival; EFS, event-free survival.

studies did not find outcome differences between ALCL and non-ALCL subtypes (Table 45.2) (5,16). The differences between these analyses likely reflects additional heterogeneity within systemic ALCL which is now believed to be comprised of two very biologically and clinically different subtypes, ALK positive (pos) and ALK negative (neg). ALK or anaplastic lymphoma kinase overexpression is most commonly due to t(2;5)(p23;35), which fuses the ALK gene on 2p23 to the nucleophosmin gene on 5q35, resulting in expression of the ALK protein which has constitutive tyrosine kinase activity. Other variant partner chromosomes have also been recognized, all resulting in ALK expression which can be identified by immunohistochemical methods (2).

A second PubMed review was undertaken specifically in ALCL where ALK status has been reported. Older analyses often include B-cell ALCL, which is now recognized as a subtype of DLBCL. The initial screen using the same criteria as above yielded 48 papers. Exclusion of reports on biologic prognostic factors, other marker studies, in vitro and animal analyses resulted in 22 relevant reports on ALCL. Of these eight, were duplicate studies (Table 45.2). A number of studies were excluded that contained cases of anaplastic-like Hodgkin's lymphoma or distinction between T- and null-cell ALCL and B-cell ALCL was not possible in the survival analyses. In total three papers were identified that exclusively evaluated the prognostic significance of ALK positive status in T-cell or null-cell ALCL (Table 45.3) (17–19). The frequency of ALK positivity was 40%–60% and all studies demonstrated a superior five-year OS in ALK-pos ALCL (71%–93%) than ALK-neg ALCL (15%–35%). This was also confirmed in multivariate analysis, adjusting for other prognostic factors. Of note, pediatric cases were also included in some of these analyses.

The WHO classification recognizes that ALCL should be divided into two subtypes, primary systemic type and primary cutaneous type due to differences in immunophenotype, genetics and clinical behavior. Meticulous staging is critical to rule out the presence of systemic ALCL with secondary cutaneous involvement. In contrast to systemic ALCL, cutaneous ALCL has an indolent course, lacks the t(2;5)(p23;35) and are ALK and EMA negative but usually express cutaneous lymphocyte antigen. It typically occurs in older men as solitary, asymptomatic cutaneous or subcutaneous reddish-violet nodules/tumors. Extracutaneous disease can occur in 10% of patients, mainly in regional lymph nodes, and most often in patients with multiple lesions. It wasn't until the revised WHO classification that it was distinguished as a separate entity from systemic ALCL. As such, some studies of ALCL prior to 1999 may have included both systemic and cutaneous types. A recent large review of 146 cases of primary cutaneous ALCL from the Dutch and Austrian cutaneous lymphoma registries demonstrated a 10-year disease-specific survival (DSS) of 95% (20). This is also consistent with other report which also summarized previous literature, where the DSS (95%–100%) and OS (83%–100%), is reflective of the indolent course with a propensity to relapse (9,21).

Conclusions

Expression of ALK in cases of T- and null-cell ALCL identifies populations with different prognoses. Those with ALK-pos ALCL have a more favorable prognosis.

Recommendation

Cutaneous ALCL should be considered a more indolent and should be separated from other PTCLs for treatment decisions (Grade 1C). ALK expression should be assessed in all cases of ALCL.

Is CHOP the optimal therapy in PTCL? Should any of the PTCL subtypes be treated differently?

CHOP-type chemotherapy is the standard treatment of PTCLs. The large Intergroup trial comparing CHOP to 2nd and 3rd generation regimens in diffuse large-cell lymphoma failed to reveal any benefit of the more intensive regimens and CHOP emerged as the standard therapy (22). However, this study was performed in an era when immunophenotyping was not universally available thus the impact of these specific treatment regimens in the subgroup of patients with T-cell lymphomas was not assessable. There have been no randomized phase III studies since this landmark analysis that have compared CHOP to an alternate treatment regimen exclusively in PTCLs, however, a number of studies have evaluated dose-intensive regimens in all aggressive lymphomas. A PubMed search was performed to identify all randomized controlled treatment studies published 1999 or later using the terms "aggressive lymphoma," excluding transplantation. Fifty-four studies were identified, 10 of which compared novel regimens to CHOP therapy. Three RCT studies evaluated treatment regimens in localized aggressive lymphomas, however, none these reported on separate results for those tumors with a T-cell phenotype. The largest and most recent study published was performed by the German Non-Hodgkin's Lymphoma Group (DSHNHL) evaluating whether the reduction of treatment intervals from three (CHOP-21) to two weeks (CHOP-14) or the addition of etoposide (CHOEP) would improve outcome in elderly patients or young "good prognosis" patients with aggressive lymphomas (23,24). In this pre-rituximab era, CHOP-14 and CHOEP improved EFS and OS in elderly patients (NHL-B2) and young patients (NHL-B 1), respectively. Although, a proportion of patients in each of these trials did have an aggressive lymphoma with a T-cell phenotype (5.8% NHL-B2; 13.7% NHL-B1), most of the patients had anaplastic large cell lymphoma (no ALK reporting) and further, insufficient numbers in each treatment group precluded analysis of the subset of patients with T-cell lymphoma in these two four-arm trials (23,24). The remainder of the studies was too small to evaluate the superiority (or inferiority) of a particular regimen in T-cell lymphomas and outcome analyses pertaining to the T-cell subgroup were not reported. As a result, CHOP has been widely utilized in PTCL but with the notable exception of ALK-pos ALCL, outcomes have been poor (Table 45.2). However, given the lack of evidence of a superior regimen, it remains the standard therapy in PTCL.

Generally, treatment approaches to date have been similar among the PTCL subtypes. One exception is extranodal NK/T-cell lymphoma (NK/TCL), a predominant PTCL subtype in Asian populations. Morphologically, these tumors demonstrate angiocentric invasion, vascular destruction, and necrosis. They are positive for Epstein-Barr virus (EBV), which is thought to play a role in tumor pathogenesis. NK/TCLs are typically very locally aggressive with five-year OS, ranging in the literature from 25% to 50% (25), the variability likely reflecting inconsistent reporting of immunophenotyping and EBV status. Nasal-type NK/TCL occur in the skin, gastrointestinal tract or testis often with advanced stage disease and appear to have an inferior survival to nasal NK/TCL with long term remissions achieved in only 10%–15% of cases (25).

The majority of patients present with localized disease receive combined modality therapy (CMT) with CHOP/CHOP-type chemotherapy followed by involved-field radiotherapy (RT) akin to the therapy recommendations for localized DLBCL (26). Frequently, disease progression occurs during anthracycline-based chemotherapy in patients with NK/TCLs suggesting an inherent chemoresistance that may be related to expression of P-glycoprotein resulting in multidrug resistance (27). With this, several centers have advocated that primary radiotherapy be utilized in the treatment of NK/TCL. Radiotherapy has not been formally compared with CMT or chemotherapy alone in a randomized phase III trial in this entity. A PubMed review was undertaken of all studies of "NK/T-cell lymphoma" or "angiocentric" lymphoma and treatment with radiotherapy, limited to the years 1999 to 2006 due to inconsistent reporting of immunophenotyping before this. Seventy-two studies were found and after exclusion of studies with less than 25 patients, studies that included B-cell lymphomas, case reports and studies of biological markers, 21 papers relevant to the study question, including 8 reviews, 1 editorial, and 12 primary treatment studies were reviewed; no randomized trials were identified. Further review eliminated three primary treatment reports due to insufficient reporting of immunophenotyping details required to exclude the possible inclusion of B-cell lymphomas, yielding nine studies to analyze the role of radiation therapy (Table 45.4). All but one study included only Asian populations.

Survival rates ranged from 15% to 83% and the single case series of Caucasian patients from an Italian group, showed a very poor prognosis (five-year OS 18%). A recent retrospective cohort study of 105 patients treated in China with localized NK/TCL demonstrated that patients treated with primary radiotherapy had an equivalent five-year OS (66% vs. 76%) and PFS (61% vs. 66%) to patients treated with CMT, suggesting that chemotherapy did not provide any additional benefit (28). Interestingly, the CR rate following RT was 83% compared with 20% after initial chemotherapy; however, the latter improved to 81% following the RT. The survival estimates in this study are high and this may reflect that not all patients had uniform CD56 and EBV analysis. In the retrospective cohort study by You and colleagues, seven patients received RT alone and had a significantly improved outcome compared with patients who received primary chemotherapy with the addition of radiation only in the event if a CR was not achieved (83% vs. 29%, $p = 0.03$) (27). Within this study, the authors compared the survival of patients who received any radiotherapy to those who did not and similarly found improved OS in the former group (50% vs. 23%, $p = 0.025$). Improved outcome using primary radiation therapy compared with CMT has been seen in other analyses (29,30). Other studies have noted equivalent results with primary radiation therapy or CMT but increased primary progression was observed with intended up-front chemotherapy than radiotherapy (31). Radiation therapy does appear to salvage some cases of primary chemotherapy failure (27).

Although there are limitations due to the retrospective nature of these analyses and biases introduced by the selection of patients for specific treatments, all of the studies demonstrated either equivalent or superior outcomes for radiotherapy alone compared to CMT. Collectively, these results support that radiation should be utilized the primary therapy in localized NK/T-cell lymphoma. Whether chemotherapy either during or after radiation impacts cure rates is unknown.

The other exception to the treatment paradigm for PTCLs is cutaneous ALCL. This subtype typically has an indolent natural history and propensity to relapse. The majority of patients can be treated with localized excision with or without radiotherapy and overly aggressive treatment should be avoided. Patients with

Table 45.4 Survival of nasal NK/T cell lymphoma treated with primary radiotherapy or combined modality therapy in the past 6 years. Adapted from Li et al (29).

Author	Classification	Country (n)	Location (%)	Pathology	Stage	Therapy (n)	5y OS %	Comment
Li (2006) (28)	REAL	China (105)	Nasal	Angiocentric morph All patients positive for at least 1 T- or NK-cell marker	I, II	RT (31) RT + CT or CT + RT (34) CT (3)	66 76 $p = 0.84$	CD56, CD57, and EBV not performed in all cases RT dose 45-60 Gy
Pagano (2006)	WHO	Italy (26)	Nasal (62)	Angiocentric CD3ε+, CD56+, TIA1, granzyme B, EBV+	I–IV	CHOP/CHOP-type + RT CHOP/CHOP-type	18	Non-anthracyline-based chemotherapy in 32%
Kim (2006) (48)	WHO	Korea (43)	Nasal (67)		I, II	CEOP-B +/- RT	No difference	
Kim (2005) (49)	WHO	Korea (114)	Nasal	CD3ε+, CD56+ (87%) EBV + (75%)	I, II	RT CHOP/CHOP-type + RT CHOP/CHOP-type	69 56 44 $p = 0.087$	
Li (2004) (28)	Not stated	Taiwan (77, stage I/II n = 56)	Nasal (56)	Angiocentric CD3+ and or TCR PCR, CD56 ±, EBV ±	I–IV	RT RT + CHOP/CHOP-like CHT	50 (I, II only) 59 15 $p = 0.01$	Included PTCL EBV and CD56 not performed on all cases RT dose 40–50 y
Chim (2004) (30)	WHO	Hong Kong (67)	Nasal	Angiocentric morp CD3ε+, CD56+ EBV+	I–IV	RT (7) CHOP/CHOP-like+ RT	83 32 $p = 0.03$	12 patients had non-anthracycline-based regimens
You (2004)	Not stated	Taiwan (46)	Nasal (46)	Angiocentric CD3 (surface) CD56+	I, II	RT (6) CHOP/CHOP-like +/-RT	50 (any RT) 23 p = 0.017	EBV not performed in all cases RT dose 54–60Gy Patients treated with CHT were given RT after 3 or 6 cycles if CR not achieved (83% vs. 29%) 5 y OS
Kim (2003) (50)	REAL	Korea (59, stage I/II n = 41)	Nasal (76)	Angiocentric CD3, CD56 ±, EBV	I–IV	CHOP ± RT	44 (2y) 53 (I, II 2y)	RT added at physicians discretion CR rate post CHT stage I, II 43%
Cheung (2002)	WHO	China (79)	Nasal	CD3ε+, CD56+	I, II	RT CHOP/CHOP-like + RT	30 40 $p = 0.87$	6 patients received HDT ASCT consolidation

*RT, radiotherapy; EBV, Epstein-Barr virus; OS, overall survival.

disseminated or extracutaneous disease may benefit from systemic therapy (20).

Recommendations

1. CHOP-type chemotherapy is the standard treatment of PTCLs (Grade 1B).
2. Patients with localized NK/T-cell lymphoma should be treated primarily with involved field radiation therapy (Grade 1C). The role of routine use of chemotherapy either as a radio-sensitizer or as consolidation therapy is uncertain (Grade 2C).
3. Patients with primary cutaneous PTCL can be treated with localized excision with or without radiotherapy and overly aggressive treatment should be avoided (Grade 1C).

Should patients with PTCL receive primary autologous stem cell transplantation in their primary therapy?

Given the poor outcome observed with anthracyline-based chemotherapy, attempts have been made to consolidate therapy in patients with PTCL with high dose chemotherapy (HDC) and autologous stem call transplantation (ASCT). A PubMed review was undertaken to evaluate the outcome of PTCL who have received primary ASCT. This review was restricted to studies published after 1999. Initially, 60 reports were identified using the terms "peripheral T-cell lymphoma(s)" and "transplant or transplantation"; however, only four studies were identified that reported outcome analyses exclusively on patients who were transplanted in first remission (Table 45.5), and one was excluded as it only evaluated 11 patients. Of the three included trials, two were prospective case series and one was a retrospective series (32–34) (Table 45.5). An additional nine reviews were also identified that evaluated the role of transplant in PTCL. No phase III studies comparing CHOP or CHOP-like chemotherapy to upfront transplantation specifically in PTCL were identified. Thus, a separate search of PubMed during the same treatment period limited to randomized control trials using the terms "aggressive lymphoma" and transplantation yielded 17 reports. Manual review yielded only one study (LNH-93) that included a subgroup analysis of patients with T-cell lymphoma (35). Another report was included that evaluated this study in addition to another phase III GELA prospective transplant trial (LNH-87) (36) and performed a matched control analysis of patients treated with either consolidative sequential chemotherapy or HDC and SCT (37).

The long-term results of two phase II trials evaluating primary transplant in PTCL was recently published (34) (Table 45.5). The majority of patients had either PTCLU or ALK-pos ALCL. The 12-year EFS and OS were 30% and 34%, respectively. Patients with ALK-pos ALCL had a superior EFS (54%) and OS (62%) compared to the other subtypes (19% 10-year EFS, 21% OS%), which is similar to outcome studies evaluating CHOP-type chemotherapy in the primary therapy of PTCLs as outlined above (34) (Table 45.5). Reimer and colleagues also reported a phase II study of 30 PTCL patients, excluding ALK pos ALCL, who underwent transplantation in first remission (CR or PR) following induction chemotherapy (33). The transplantation rate was 70% and with a median follow-up of 15 months, 72% were in continuous CR (CCR). However, the updated results of 65 patients with longer follow-up demonstrates a transplant rate of 62% and a CCR of only 42% (38). This highlights the difficulty of early progression in PTCL and the need for improved initial chemotherapy. The GEL-TAMO registry results of 37 PTCL patients transplanted in first CR were more favorable with a five-year OS rate of 80% (32). Patients selected for primary transplant were considered to be "high risk" although almost a third had either 0 or 1 risk factors by the age-adjusted IPI and some pediatric patients were included. These factors in addition to the selection of only CR patients for transplant and inclusion of some ALCL patients (ALK status unknown) may have inflated survival rates.

In LNH-93 a shortened chemotherapy course and HDC and SCT was compared with Adriamycin® (doxorubicin), cyclophosphamide, vincristine, bleomycin, and prednisone (ACVBP) followed by sequential chemotherapy consolidation and found no benefit overall of transplant, including in those patients with a T-cell phenotype (35) Table 45.5. The GELA group also performed a matched control analysis of patients from this trial as well as the phase III LNH-87 trial (consolidative sequential chemotherapy vs. HDC SCT) confining the analysis to those who achieved a CR/CRu patients and who were able to receive either HDC SCT (case group) or sequential chemotherapy (control group) Table 45.5. Cases and controls were matched 1:1 by treatment protocol, histology (anaplastic or nonanaplastic PTCL), age-adjusted IPI, bone marrow involvement, number of extranodal sites. Among the 29 patients with nonanaplastic (including two LBL), there was no difference in DFS or OS between the two groups (Table 45.5).

Recommendation

In the absence of randomized trials proving superiority to conventional chemotherapy, the routine use of HDC and ASCT in the primary treatment remains investigational and cannot be recommended (Grade 1C).

Is the outcome of patients with relapsed or refractory PTCL Similar to DLBCL following autologous stem cell transplantation?

The PARMA randomized controlled study established HDC and ASCT as superior to salvage chemotherapy alone in patients with relapsed, chemosensitive aggressive lymphomas (39). Tumors were classified histologically as intermediate or high grade by the Working Formulation and thus immunophenotypic information was not available and pathologic re-review was not mandatory in this study (39). Thus, this study does not address the value of HDC and ASCT specifically in relapsed PTCL and there have been no prospective randomized studies since this report comparing transplantation to conventional salvage therapy in PTCL.

Table 45.5 Studies of primary autologous stem cell transplant in PTCLs.*

Study	n	Study Type	PTCL Subtype (n)	Pretransplant CHT	EFS	OS	Comment
Corradini (2006)	62	Prospective phase II	PTCLU (28) ALK + ALCL (19) Other	2 Intensified treatment plans†	30% (12 y)	34% (12 y)	2 prospective phase II 74% transplant rate Superior EFS ALK pos ALCL (54 vs. 18% $p = 0.006$)
Reimer (2004)	30	Prospective phase II	PTCLU (12) AILT (12)	1. CHOP 4–6 cycles 2. DexaBEAM/ESHAP 3. TBI/Cy	—	76% CCR transplanted patients (median f/u 15 mo)	Prospective phase II 70% transplant rate 47% bone marrow + Update ASH 2005 n = 65 42% in CCR
Rodriguez (2003)	37	Retrospective	PTCLU (unknown) ALCL AILT Other	CHOP BEAM, BEC, Cy/TBI	–	80% (5 y)	Analysis of a subset "high-risk" patients who underwent HDC SCT in first CR ALK status unknown Included some pediatric patients
Mounier (2002) (51)	34	Phase III‡	PTCLU (23) AILT (3) ALCL(8)	1. LNH-87—ACVB or NCVB then sequential consolidation§vs. HDC SCT 2. LNH-93-3 – see below	56% (sequential consolidation) vs. 54.5% (HDC SCT)	67% (sequential consolidation) vs. 64% (HDC SCT)	Randomized phase III of high dose sequential vs HDC SCT in aggressive lymphomas first CR Matched-control analysis—HDC SCT vs. sequential consolidation in CR/Cru patients ALK status unknown
Gisselbrecht (2002) (35)	76	Phase III‖	Non-anaplastic PTCL (55) Anaplastic (29)	LNH-93-3 ACVBP and sequential consolidation vs. Escalated experimental CHT¶ and HDT SCT	30% (sequential consolidation) vs. 20% (HDC SCT) $p = 0.4$	39% (ACVBP) vs. 32% (HDC SCT) $p = 0.5$	Randomized phase III trial of ACVBP vs. shortened chemotherapy and HDC SCT in aggressive lymphomas Included 12 patients with LBL Trial stopped early due to inferior results in transplant arm ALK status unknown

*MS, Median survival; mos, months; OS, overall survival; EFS, event-free survival; IPI, International Prognostic Index; CHT chemotherapy; PTCLU, peripheral T-cell lymphoma, unspecified; AILT, angioimmunoblastic T-cell lymphoma, NK/TCL Extranodal NK/T, cell lymphoma nasal and nasal type; ALCL, anaplastic large cell lymphoma; ALK pos, ALK positive; ALK neg, ALK negative; classn, classification; LBL, lymphoblastic lymphoma; CHT, chemotherapy; HDC SCT, high-dose chemotherapy and stem cell transplantation.

†subgroup analysis of patients with T-cell Lymphomas.

1. High-dose sequential (doxorubicin, vincristine, prednisone) x 2, DHAP x 2; High-dose phase Cy, araC, Cisplatin, etoposide; conditioning mitoxantrone and melphalan.

2. MACOPB; intensification with mitoxantrone, araC; conditioning carmustine, etoposide, ara-C, melphalan.

‡. Matched-control analysis of subset of patients with T-cell lymphoma in LNH-87 and LNH-93.

§. ACVB or NCVB (closed early after inferior response).

‖Subgroup analysis of T-cell lymphoma patients.

¶Escalated doses of cyclophosphamide, epirubicin, vindesine, bleomycin, prednisone.

Table 45.6 Studies of autologous stem cell transplant for relapsed and refractory PTCL.

Study	n	PTCL subtype (n)	Disease status (24)	Salvage and conditioning	5 y EFS %	5 y OS %	Comment
Kelaramani (2006) (40)	24	PTCLU (14) ALK-neg ALCL (4) AILT (4) Other	Relapsed (16) Refractory (8)	Not stated TBI or CHT	24	33%	Included only patients with chemosensitive (PR/CR) disease Similar EFS ($p = 0.14$) and OS ($p = 0.64$) to DLBCL No difference relapsed v refractory disease
Park (2005) (53)	32	NKTCL (14) PTCLU (11)	Relapsed (10) Refractory (22)	IMVP-16/pred[†] BEAM	12 (3 y)	14 (3 y)	Largest subtype NKTCL and majority had refractory disease
Jantunen (2004) (54)	14	PTCLU[†] ALCL ETTL Other	Relapsed (14)			45	ALCL included systemic and cutaneous type ALK status unknown
Song (2003) (42)	36	PTCLU (20) ALCL (9) Other (7)	Relapsed (29) "Refractory" (7)	DHAP/ESHAP or miniBEAM	23 (3 y)	48 (3 y)	Included only patients with chemosensitive disease Refractory patients included some with residual disease ALK status unknown Similar EFS ($p = 0.31$) and OS ($p = 0.55$) to DLBCL (vs. all PTCLs) EFS inferior for PTCLU vs DLBCL ($p = 0.028$), OS no difference ($p = 0.11$)
Rodriguez (2003) (32)	78	PTCLU	Relapsed Refractory	CHOP BEAM, BEAC, Cy/TBI	39	45	Relapsed included patients in first PR

*OS, overall survival; EFS, event-free survival; CHT, chemotherapy; PTCLU, peripheral T-cell lymphoma, unspecified; AILT, angioimmunoblastic T-cell lymphoma; NK/TCL, extranodal NK/T cell lymphoma nasal and nasal type; ALCL, anaplastic large cell lymphoma; ALK pos, ALK positive; ALK neg, ALK negative; classn, classification.

† IMVP-16, ifosfamide, methotrexate, etoposide (VP-16).

In the 60 reports identified above, 7 retrospective studies addressed the outcome of patients with relapsed or refractory PTCL following HDC and ASCT. Two studies were excluded on further review due to inclusion of patients treated with primary transplant and combining autologous and allogeneic transplant in outcome analyses. Relapsed PTCL that demonstrates chemosensitivity respond favorably to HDC and ASCT, with long-term survival rates of approximately 35%–45% (2) (Table 45.6). Two studies suggest that outcome in non-ALCL patients are comparable to DLBCL, in the pre-rituximab treatment era (40,41) (Table 45.6). One study found an inferior survival if only PTCLU is considered (42), however, as the survival estimates in all of these studies are comparable the differences may reflect limitations by study size. In all analyses, patients with ALCL and in particular, ALK-pos, have superior salvage rates, often exceeding that observed in DLBCL (2) (Table 45.6). The results in patients with refractory PTCL are less consistent with some studies reporting no long-term survivors and others reporting similar results to patients with relapsed disease if chemosensitivity is demonstrated (2).

Recommendation

Patients with relapsed and selected patients with refractory PTCL with documented chemosensitive disease to a salvage regimen should be offered HDC and SCT, similar to the practice in DLBCL (Grade 1B).

References

1 Armitage JO, Weisenburger DD. New approach to classifying non-Hodgkin's lymphomas: clinical features of the major histologic subtypes. Non-Hodgkin's Lymphoma Classification Project. *J Clin Oncol.* 1998;**16**(8):2780–95.

2 Savage KJ. Aggressive peripheral T-cell lymphomas (specified and unspecified types). *Hematol Am Soc Hematol Educ Program.* 2005:267–77.

3 Jaffe ES, Railfkiaer E. Mature T-cell and NK neoplasms: introduction. In: Jaffe ES, Harris NL, Stein H, Vardiman JW, editors. *World Health Organization classification of tumours: pathology and genetics of tumours of hematopoetic and lymphoid tissues.* Lyon: IARC Press; 2001. p. 191–94.

4 Gisselbrecht C, Gaulard P, Lepage E, et al. Prognostic significance of T-cell phenotype in aggressive non-Hodgkin's lymphomas. Groupe d'Etudes des Lymphomes de l'Adulte (GELA). *Blood.* 1998;**92**(1):76–82.

5 Melnyk A, Rodriguez A, Pugh WC, et al. Evaluation of the revised European-American lymphoma classification confirms the clinical relevance of immunophenotype in 560 cases of aggressive non-Hodgkin's lymphoma. *Blood.* 1997;**89**(12):4514–20.

6 Morabito F, Gallamini A, Stelitano C, et al. Clinical relevance of immunophenotype in a retrospective comparative study of 297 peripheral T-cell lymphomas, unspecified, and 496 diffuse large B-cell lymphomas: experience of the Intergruppo Italiano Linformi. *Cancer.* 2004;**101**(7):1601–8.

7 ten Berge RL, de Bruin PC, Oudejans JJ, et al. ALK-negative anaplastic large-cell lymphoma demonstrates similar poor prognosis to peripheral T-cell lymphoma, unspecified. *Histopathology.* 2003;**43**(5):462–69.

8 Sonnen R, Schmidt WP, Muller-Hermelink HK, et al. The International Prognostic Index determines the outcome of patients with nodal mature T-cell lymphomas. *Br J Haematol.* 2005;**129**(3):366–72.

9 Savage KJ, Chhanabhai M, Gascoyne RD, et al. Characterization of peripheral T-cell lymphomas in a single North American institution by the WHO classification. *Ann Oncol.* 2004;**15**(10):1467–75.

10 Pellatt J, Sweetenham J, Pickering RM, et al. A single-centre study of treatment outcomes and survival in 120 patients with peripheral T-cell non-Hodgkin's lymphoma. *Ann Hematol.* 2002;**81**(5):267–72.

11 Arrowsmith ER, Macon WR, Kinney MC, et al. Peripheral T-cell lymphomas: clinical features and prognostic factors of 92 cases defined by the revised European American lymphoma classification. *Leuk Lymphoma.* 2003;**44**(2):241–49.

12 Lopez-Guillermo A, Cid J, Salar A, et al. Peripheral T-cell lymphomas: initial features, natural history, and prognostic factors in a series of 174 patients diagnosed according to the R.E.A.L. Classification. *Ann Oncol.* 1998;**9**(8):849–55.

13 Weisenburger DD, Anderson JR, Diebold J, et al. Systemic anaplastic large-cell lymphoma: results from the non-Hodgkin's lymphoma classification project. *Am J Hematol.* 2001;**67**(3):172–78.

14 Ascani S, Zinzani PL, Gherlinzoni F, et al. Peripheral T-cell lymphomas: clinico-pathologic study of 168 cases diagnosed according to the R.E.A.L. Classification. *Ann Oncol.* 1997;**8**(6):583–92.

15 Armitage JO, Vose JM, Weisenburger DD. Towards understanding the peripheral T-cell lymphomas. *Ann Oncol.* 2004;**15**(10):1447–49.

16 Musson R, Radstone CR, Horsman JM, et al. Peripheral T-cell lymphoma: the Sheffield Lymphoma Group experience (1977–2001). *Int J Oncol.* 2003;**22**(6):1363–68.

17 ten Berge RL, Oudejans JJ, Ossenkoppele GJ, et al. ALK expression in extranodal anaplastic large cell lymphoma favours systemic disease with (primary) nodal involvement and a good prognosis and occurs before dissemination [see comments]. *J Clin Pathol.* 2000;**53**(6):445–50.

18 Gascoyne RD, Aoun P, Wu D, et al. Prognostic significance of anaplastic lymphoma kinase (ALK) protein expression in adults with anaplastic large cell lymphoma. *Blood.* 1999;**93**(11):3913–21.

19 Falini B, Pileri S, Zinzani PL, et al. ALK+ lymphoma: clinico-pathological findings and outcome. *Blood.* 1999;**93**(8):2697–706.

20 Willemze R, Jaffe ES, Burg G, et al. WHO-EORTC classification for cutaneous lymphomas. *Blood.* 2005;**105**(10):3768–85.

21 Liu HL, Hoppe RT, Kohler S, et al. CD30+ cutaneous lymphoproliferative disorders: the Stanford experience in lymphomatoid papulosis and primary cutaneous anaplastic large cell lymphoma. *J Am Acad Dermatol.* 2003;**49**(6):1049–58.

22 Fisher RI, Gaynor ER, Dahlberg S, et al. Comparison of a standard regimen (CHOP) with three intensive chemotherapy regimens for advanced non-Hodgkin's lymphoma. *N Engl J Med.* 1993;**328**(14):1002–6.

23 Pfreundschuh M, Trumper L, Kloess M, et al. Two-weekly or 3-weekly CHOP chemotherapy with or without etoposide for the treatment of young patients with good-prognosis (normal LDH) aggressive lymphomas: results of the NHL-B1 trial of the DSHNHL. *Blood.* 2004;**104**(3):626–33.

24 Pfreundschuh M, Trumper L, Kloess M, et al. Two-weekly or 3-weekly CHOP chemotherapy with or without etoposide for the treatment of elderly patients with aggressive lymphomas: results of the NHL-B2 trial of the DSHNHL. *Blood.* 2004;**104**(3):634–41.

25 Kwong YL. Natural killer-cell malignancies: diagnosis and treatment. *Leukemia.* 2005;**19**(12):2186–94.

26 Miller TP, Dahlberg S, Cassady JR, et al. Chemotherapy alone compared with chemotherapy plus radiotherapy for localized intermediate- and high-grade non-Hodgkin's lymphoma. *N Engl J Med.* 1998;**339**(1): 21–6.

27 You JY, Chi KH, Yang MH, et al. Radiation therapy versus chemotherapy as initial treatment for localized nasal natural killer (NK)/T-cell lymphoma: a single institute survey in Taiwan. *Ann Oncol.* 2004; **15**(4):618–25.

28 Li YX, Yao B, Jin J, et al. Radiotherapy as primary treatment for stage IE and IIE nasal natural killer/T-cell lymphoma. *J Clin Oncol.* 2006;**24**(1):181–89.

29 Li CC, Tien HF, Tang JL, et al. Treatment outcome and pattern of failure in 77 patients with sinonasal natural killer/T-cell or T-cell lymphoma. *Cancer.* 2004;**100**(2):366–75.

30 Chim CS, Ma SY, Au WY, et al. Primary nasal natural killer cell lymphoma: long-term treatment outcome and relationship with the International Prognostic Index. *Blood.* 2004;**103**(1):216–21.

31 Cheung MM, Chan JK, Lau WH, et al. Early stage nasal NK/T-cell lymphoma: clinical outcome, prognostic factors, and the effect of treatment modality. *Int J Radiat Oncol Biol Phys.* 2002;**54**(1):182–90.

32 Rodriguez J, Caballero MD, Gutierrez A, et al. High-dose chemotherapy and autologous stem cell transplantation in peripheral T-cell lymphoma: the GEL-TAMO experience. *Ann Oncol.* 2003;**14**(12):1768–75.

33 Reimer P, Schertlin T, Rudiger T, et al. Myeloablative radiochemotherapy followed by autologous peripheral blood stem cell transplantation as first-line therapy in peripheral T-cell lymphomas: first results of a prospective multicenter study. *Hematol J.* 2004;**5**(4):304–11.

34 Corradini P, Tarella C, Zallio F, et al. Long-term follow-up of patients with peripheral T-cell lymphomas treated up-front with high-dose chemotherapy followed by autologous stem cell transplantation. *Leukemia.* 2006;**20**(9):1533–38.

35 Gisselbrecht C, Lepage E, Molina T, et al. Shortened first-line high-dose chemotherapy for patients with poor-prognosis aggressive lymphoma. *J Clin Oncol.* 2002;**20**(10):2472–79.

36 Haioun C, Lepage E, Gisselbrecht C, et al. Survival benefit of high-dose therapy in poor-risk aggressive non-Hodgkin's lymphoma: final analysis of the prospective LNH87-2 protocol—a groupe d'Etude des lymphomes de l'Adulte study. *J Clin Oncol.* 2000;**18**(16):3025–30.

37 Mounier N, Gisselbrecht C, Briere J, et al. All aggressive lymphoma subtypes do not share similar outcome after front-line autotransplantation: a matched-control analysis by the Groupe d'Etude des Lymphomes de l'Adulte (GELA). *Ann Oncol.* 2004;**15**(12):1790–97.

38 Reimer P, Rudiger T, Schertlin E, et al. Autologous stem cell transplantation as first-line therapy in peripheral T-cell lymphomas: a prospective multicenter study. *Blood.* 2005;**106**(11):2074a.

39 Philip T, Guglielmi C, Hagenbeek A, et al. Autologous bone marrow transplantation as compared with salvage chemotherapy in relapses of chemotherapy-sensitive non-Hodgkin's lymphoma. *N Engl J Med.* 1995;**333**(23):1540–45.

40 Kewalramani T, Zelenetz AD, Teruya-Feldstein J, et al. Autologous transplantation for relapsed or primary refractory peripheral T-cell lymphoma. *Br J Haematol.* 2006;**134**(2):202–7.

41 Jagasia M, Morgan D, Goodman S, et al. Histology impacts the outcome of peripheral T-cell lymphomas after high dose chemotherapy and stem cell transplant. *Leuk Lymphoma.* 2004;**45**(11):2261–67.

42 Song KW, Mollee P, Keating A, et al. Autologous stem cell transplant for relapsed and refractory peripheral T-cell lymphoma: variable outcome according to pathological subtype. *Br J Haematol.* 2003;**120**(6):978–85.

43 Gallamini A, Stelitano C, Calvi R, et al. Peripheral T-cell lymphoma unspecified (PTCLU): a new prognostic model from a retrospective multicentric clinical study. *Blood.* 2004;**103**(7):2474–79.

44 Rudiger T, Weisenburger DD, Anderson JR, et al. Peripheral T-cell lymphoma (excluding anaplastic large-cell lymphoma): results from the Non-Hodgkin's Lymphoma Classification Project. *Ann Oncol.* 2002;**13**(1):140–49.

45 Kim K, Kim WS, Jung CW, et al. Clinical features of peripheral T-cell lymphomas in 78 patients diagnosed according to the Revised European-American lymphoma (REAL) classification. *Eur J Cancer.* 2002;**38**(1):75–81.

46 Lee SS, Cho KJ, Kim CW, et al. Clinicopathological analysis of 501 non-Hodgkin's lymphomas in Korea according to the revised European-American classification of lymphoid neoplasms. *Histopathology.* 1999;**35**(4):345–54.

47 Isobe K, Tamaru J, Harigaya K, et al. Clinicopathological evaluation of the Revised European-American Classification of Lymphoid Neoplasms (REAL) in Japan. *Leuk Lymphoma.* 1999;**34**(1–2):143–49.

48 Kim SJ, Kim BS, Choi CW, et al. Treatment outcome of front-line systemic chemotherapy for localized extranodal NK/T cell lymphoma in nasal and upper aerodigestive tract. *Leuk Lymphoma.* 2006;**47**(7):1265–73.

49 Kim TM, Park YH, Lee SY, et al. Local tumor invasiveness is more predictive of survival than International Prognostic Index in stage I(E)/II(E) extranodal NK/T-cell lymphoma, nasal type. *Blood.* 2005;**106**(12):3785–90.

50 Kim BS, Kim TY, Kim CW, et al. Therapeutic outcome of extranodal NK/T-cell lymphoma initially treated with chemotherapy—result of chemotherapy in NK/T-cell lymphoma. *Acta Oncol.* 2003;**42**(7):779–83.

51 Mounier N, Simon D, Haioun C, et al. Impact of high-dose chemotherapy on peripheral T-cell lymphomas. *J Clin Oncol.* 2002;**20**(5):1426–27.

52 Coiffier B, Gisselbrecht C, Herbrecht R, et al. LNH-84 regimen: a multicenter study of intensive chemotherapy in 737 patients with aggressive malignant lymphoma. *J Clin Oncol.* 1989;**7**(8):1018–26.

53 Park BB, Kim WS, Lee J, et al. IMVP-16/Pd followed by high-dose chemotherapy and autologous stem cell transplantation as a salvage therapy for refractory or relapsed peripheral T-cell lymphomas. *Leuk Lymphoma.* 2005;**46**(12):1743–48.

54 Jantunen E, Wiklund T, Juvonen E, et al. Autologous stem cell transplantation in adult patients with peripheral T-cell lymphoma: a nation-wide survey. *Bone Marrow Transplant.* 2004;**33**(4):405–10.

46 Selected Management Issues of Patients with Hodgkin Lymphoma

Ralph M. Meyer

Introduction

The management of Hodgkin lymphoma has evolved to include strategies that reduce therapy for patients who are at low risk of suffering progressive disease and testing new strategies in those with higher-risk disease. Tailoring therapy according to risk is desired so that durable disease control is provided while long-term treatment-related toxicities or "late-effects" are minimized (1). Late-effects include an increased risk of second cancers and cardiovascular events, which are principally related to radiation therapy, and acute leukemia and infertility, which are associated with the use of chemotherapy regimens that include alkylating agents or epipodophyllotoxins (2). As patients with Hodgkin lymphoma are young (median age 37 years) (3), and have fewer competing risks of mortality unrelated to their disease and its treatment, it is particularly important to provide therapies that balance disease control with avoidance of late-effects. Future directions are likely to include enhanced use of functional imaging with positron emission tomographic (PET) scanning in order to adapt therapy according to baseline risk and initial treatment response.

Grading of the quality of evidence and strengths of recommendations in this chapter are based on the guidelines proposed by the international Grading of Recommendations Assessment, Development, and Evaluation Working Group (GRADE) adopting the modification used by the American College of Chest Physicians that merges the very low and low categories of quality of evidence (see chapter 1).

Questions

1. What is optimum management of patients with previously untreated limited-stage Hodgkin lymphoma?

Evidence-based Hematology. Edited by Mark A. Crowther, Jeff Ginsberg, Holger J. Schünemann, Ralph M. Meyer, and Richard Lottenberg.

2. What is optimum management of patients with previously untreated advanced-stage Hodgkin lymphoma?

Literature search and inclusion

By 2002, specific treatments were established as standard. Patients with limited-stage Hodgkin lymphoma were treated with combined-modality therapy consisting of an abbreviated course of chemotherapy and involved-field radiation therapy (1,2,4). Treatment with doxorubicin (Adriamycin®), bleomycin, vinblastine, and dacarbazine (ABVD) was more effective than the combination of nitrogen mustard, vincristine (Oncovin®), prednisone, and procarbazine (MOPP) and as effective and less toxic than MOPP-ABVD for patients with advanced-stage disease (1). Therefore, the search of MEDLINE using PubMed, conducted in February 2007, dated back only to January 1, 2002. The MeSH search terms included "Hodgkin disease" and "Hodgkin Disease/therapy" and used the limiting terms "randomized controlled trials" and "meta-analysis" and English language. Computerized searches were also performed for abstract reports from the 2002 to 2006 annual meetings of the American Society of Hematology (ASH) and American Society of Clinical Oncology (ASCO). Abstracts were obtained by using the search engines associated with these websites and through review of relevant session agenda.

The PubMed search identified 55 citations. After excluding citations that were not randomized controlled trials (RCTs) describing primary therapy of previously untreated adult patients with Hodgkin lymphoma or involved updated reporting, 24 article citations remained. The ASH and ASCO searches identified 19 citations. Five abstracts were reported in duplicate, and four others were subsequently reported in article form, leaving 10 citations. The unique 24 articles and 10 abstract citations include reports of 31 RCTs, two meta-analyses, and one population-based report. Of the 31 RCTs, 12 addressed limited-stage disease (question 1) and 19 addressed advanced-stage disease (question 2).

What is optimum management of patients with previously untreated limited-stage Hodgkin lymphoma?

Staging of Hodgkin lymphoma is based on the Ann Arbor classification (5), including modifications from the Cotswold meeting (6). In North America, cooperative group trials have defined limited-stage as clinical stage I-IIA and an absence of bulky disease. Bulky disease is defined a mass greater than 10 cm in diameter or a mediastinal mass that measures more than one-third the maximum transthoracic diameter as assessed by a standard chest radiograph. Patients with IIB or bulky stage I-IIA disease are treated with the same protocols as those with III-IV disease (1,4). In Europe, the term "favorable early-stage disease" includes patients less than 50 years old with stage I-II presentations, without B symptoms or bulky mediastinal disease, with a low erythrocyte sedimentation rate, and fewer than four sites of involvement (7). Other patients with stage I-II disease are considered to have "unfavorable early-stage disease." For the purposes of this section, limited-stage is as defined by the North American cooperative groups and favorable early-stage disease as defined in Europe.

The evolution of standard therapy for patients with limited-stage Hodgkin lymphoma has been previously described (2,4). By 2002, an individual patient-data meta-analysis had demonstrated that combined-modality therapy, as compared with radiation therapy alone, provided meaningful improvements in disease control (8), and multiple RCTs had demonstrated that the chemotherapy component of the combination could be abbreviated to two to three cycles (9–11). In addition, preliminary analysis of one RCT, the H8-F trial of the European Organization for Research and Treatment of Cancer (EORTC), clearly demonstrated that the radiation therapy component could be confined to the involved-field (11) [While finalizing the publication of this chapter, an updated analysis of this trial in article form was published (11a) and confirms the preliminary report.] A second RCT, which was previously reported in abstract form (12) and was included in article form (13) as one of the 12 citations identified in the current literature search, further supported that radiation could be confined to the involved-field as no differences in outcomes were detected between patients receiving four cycles of ABVD in combination with involved or extended-field radiation. This trial was not specifically designed as a noninferiority trial and included a small sample size. The conclusions from this trial, taken with consideration of other data, support that combined-modality therapy need only include radiation to the involved-field, together with an abbreviated course of chemotherapy. Recent directions of therapy have attempted to further reduce the extent of this treatment; of the remaining 11 RCTs identified, 5 specifically test such strategies and are reviewed (14–18).

Two abstract reports describe short-term follow-up of large RCTs that evaluate multiple principles, including the dose of involved-field radiation within the context of combined-modality therapy (14,15). Noordijk (14) reported results of the EORTC H9-F trial in which 783 patients were treated with six cycles of epirubicin, bleomycin, vinblastine, and prednisone (EBVP); 619 patients achieved a complete remission (CR) and were randomized to observation or to receive involved-field radiation therapy consisting of 36 Gy or 20 Gy. The observation arm will be described below; no differences in four-year event-free (87% vs. 84%) or overall survivals (98% in both groups) were detected between those receiving 36 Gy or 20 Gy, respectively. Similarly, Diehl (15) has reported the results of the German Hodgkin Study Group (GHSG) HD10 factorial designed RCT that included comparing involved-field radiation consisting of 30 Gy versus 20 Gy; no differences in the two-year freedom from progressive disease (FFP) or overall survival were detected. More mature follow-up and assessment of results, according to principles of noninferiority trial design, are required to confirm whether 20 Gy should be considered standard. Currently, when radiation is administered, it should be limited to the involved-field and a maximum dose of 30 Gy.

The above trials also addressed additional questions. The EORTC H9-F tested the principle of chemotherapy alone. Outcomes of patients allocated to observation (without radiation) were inferior, with four-year event-free survival of only 70%. However, another citation captured in the current search was the H7 trial of the EORTC (19), which demonstrated inferior outcomes with EBVP in comparison with MOPP-ABV (and thus ABVD). The H9-F trial does not therefore reflect an adequate test of chemotherapy alone for patients with limited-stage disease. The GHSG HD10 trial also compared two versus four cycles of ABVD and, allowing for the limitations of reporting outcomes at two years, no differences in outcomes are apparent.

To avoid late-effects associated with radiation therapy, trials testing chemotherapy alone have been performed and previously summarized (4,20). Three trials have recently reported outcomes of adult patients with limited-stage disease who have been treated with ABVD alone (16–18) (Table 46.1). Previous trials in adult patients have tested regimens known to be inferior to ABVD, and therefore do not adequately test this hypothesis (4).

Of the three RCTs testing ABVD alone, two failed to detect differences in disease control or overall survival (16,17). One report is a subset analyses from a trial evaluating patients with all stages of Hodgkin lymphoma (16). The second trial (17) was from a single institution and compared combined modality therapy with ABVD alone in patients with stages I-II A+B and IIIA disease. This trial was associated with limitations resulting from the inclusion of a more heterogeneous patient group and a sample size of only 152 patients and thus limited statistical power to detect meaningful differences. The third trial (18) was the HD.6 trial of the National Cancer Institute of Canada Clinical Trials Group (NCIC CTG) and Eastern Cooperative Oncology Group (ECOG), which included 399 evaluable patients. Patients were randomized to receive either four to six cycles of ABVD (the number of cycles was determined by the degree of antitumor response observed following the first two cycles) or to treatment that included extended-field radiation therapy (as a single modality in low-risk patients and with two cycles of ABVD in higher-risk patients). In both the overall

Table 46.1 Randomized trials comparing ABVD alone with treatment that includes radiation therapy in adult patients with limited-stage Hodgkin lymphoma.*

Author	Control therapy	Experimental therapy	Number	Disease control outcome†	Overall survival†
Laskar (16)	ABVD + IF RT	ABVD	99	8-y EFS: 97% vs. 94%; $p = 0.29$	8-y: 100% vs. 98%; $p = 0.26$
Straus (17)	ABVD + EF RT	ABVD	152	5-y FFP: 86% vs. 81%; $p = 0.61$	5-y: 97% vs. 90%; $p = 0.08$
Meyer (18)	EF RT (favorable cohort) or CMT (unfavorable cohort): ABVD + EF RT	ABVD	399	5-y FFP: 93% vs. 87%; $p = 0.006$	5-y: 94% vs. 96%; $p = 0.4$

*IF RT, involved-field radiation; EF RT, extended-field radiation; CMT, combined modality therapy; EFS, event-free survival; FFP, freedom from progression.
†Results reported for control group followed by experimental group.

analysis, and in a subset analysis comparing the higher-risk stratum where patients in the control arm received combined-modality therapy, FFP was superior in patients randomized to receive radiation, but no differences in overall survival were seen. With a median follow-up of 4.2 years, second cancers and cardiovascular events appeared to be more frequent in patients allocated to radiation treatment. Mature results will be required to thoroughly address the underlying hypothesis related to overall survival, and even then, limitations will exist related to the trial design that is based on superiority (as opposed to noninferiority) of ABVD alone and the use of extended-field radiation in the control arm. This trial also evaluated time to CR as a prognostic factor in the ABVD alone group. The five-year FFP was 95% in those achieving a CR after two cycles compared with 81% in those not meeting this endpoint. These data support the hypothesis to test response-adapted therapy, including with PET scanning.

Based on these data, current treatment options are associated with trade-offs. One option is combined-modality therapy that includes two cycles of ABVD and radiation, 30 Gy, to the involved-field. More mature data from the EORTC H9-F and the GHSG HD10 studies may permit reduction of the radiation dose to 20 Gy. This approach maximizes disease control but, based on the continued inclusion of radiation, subsequent risks of cardiovascular events and second cancers will remain. A second option is treatment with ABVD alone. The advantage of this approach is avoidance of late-effects associated with radiation therapy but is associated with reduced long-term disease control, with the magnitude of decrement estimated at 7%. Preliminary data suggest that patients with disease progression after receiving chemotherapy alone can achieve states of durable disease control with second-line therapy (21). These options and trade-offs require thorough discussions with patients and determination of personal preferences, and preclude offering a single "strong" (level 1) recommendation.

Recommendations

1. Patients with limited-stage Hodgkin lymphoma can be treated with combined modality therapy consisting of two cycles of ABVD and 30 Gy involved-field radiation therapy (Grade 2A). This recommendation is based principally on the EORTC H8-F trial (11) in conjunction with the preliminary abstract publications reporting the EORTC H9-F (14) and GHSG HD 10 (15) trials. Patients should be informed of the risks of radiation therapy-related late-effects.

2. An alternative option is treatment with four to six cycles of ABVD alone. (Grade 2A). This recommendation is based principally on the NCIC CTG/ECOG HD.6 trial (18). This therapy is not associated with radiation therapy-related late-effects, but patients should be aware that ultimate disease control may be inferior (and thus the lower strength of the recommendation). Patients achieving a remission after two treatment cycles have a particularly good prognosis.

What is optimum management of patients with previously untreated advanced-stage Hodgkin lymphoma?

In North America, cooperative group trials have defined advanced-stage as bulky stage I-II, stage IIB, and stage III-IV disease. The International Prognostic Index (22) may be used to further define eligibility for clinical trials. In Europe, advanced-stage disease is more commonly defined as stage III-IV disease, but practices in Europe have also identified a group of patients with "intermediate-stage" or "unfavorable early-stage" disease (7). These include those with stage I-II A+B disease and the presence of at least one risk factor that would separate these patients from those with "favorable early-stage" disease as defined above. Often the risk factor is the presence of bulky disease or a B symptom.

By 2002, previous RCTs had demonstrated that the regimens MOPP-ABVD, MOPP-ABV, and ABVD all provided long-term disease control in approximately 65% of patients (1,23). Of the 19 citations related to advanced-stage disease identified in the current search, one was a report of the North American Intergroup study (24) that failed to detect differences in efficacy outcomes of 856 patients randomized to ABVD or MOPP-ABV; MOPP-ABV was associated with greater toxicity. Another identified RCT also compared ABVD with "hybrid" chemotherapy; the LY09 trial of the United Kingdom Lymphoma Group (UKLG) (25) also failed

Table 46.2 Recent randomized trials for patients with advanced-stage Hodgkin lymphoma: testing of shorter courses of weekly chemotherapy.*

Author; number of patients	Regimen	Principle	Disease control outcomes	Overall survival
			5-y FFP	5-y
Radford (31); N = 282	VAPEC-B	Weekly, short course	62%	79%
	ChlVPP-EVA	Hybrid	82% $p = 0.0006$	89% $p = 0.04$
			5-y EFS	5-y
Aviles (32); N = 264	7 drug regimen	Weekly, short course	65%	59%
	EBVD	ABVD (derivative)	83% $p < 0.01$	87% $p < 0.01$
			5-y FFP	5-y
Gobbi (33); N = 355	Stanford V	Weekly, Short course	54%	82%
	ABVD	ABVD	78% $p < 0.01^{\dagger}$	90% $p = 0.04$*
	MOPPEBVCAD	Intensification	81%	89%
			CR Rate	
Johnson (34)‡; N = 150	Stanford V	Weekly, short course	86%	Not compared
	ABVD	ABVD	88% *p* not stated	

*VAPEC-B, vincristine, doxorubicin (Adriamycin®), prednisolone, etoposide, cyclophosphamide, bleomycin; ChlVPP-EVA, chlorambucil, vinblastine, prednisone, procarbazine, etoposide, vincristine, doxorubicin (Adriamycin®); EBVD, epirubicin, bleomycin, vinblastine, dacarbazine; ABVD, doxorubicin (Adriamycin®), bleomycin, vinblastine, and dacarbazine; MOPPEBVCAD, nitrogen mustard, vincristine (Oncovin®), prednisone, procarbazine, epirubicin, bleomycin, vinblastine, lomustine (CCNU), melphalan (Alkeran®), vindesine; FFP, freedom from progression; EFS, event-free survival; CR, complete remission.

† *p* values compares Stanford V and ABVD.

‡ Randomized phase II trial.

to detect differences in event-free or overall survival and demonstrated that hybrid therapy was more toxic. As ABVD is not associated with the risks of infertility and leukemogenesis observed with MOPP-ABV, treatment with ABVD has become standard.

In addition, by 2002, an individual patient-data meta-analysis of trials evaluating therapy in patients with advanced-stage disease (26) failed to detect improvement in disease control and demonstrated inferior overall survival when radiation was added to a conventional course of chemotherapy. Three RCTs identified in the current search (27–29) also tested radiation therapy in patients with stage III-IV disease and confirmed that outcomes were not improved by adding radiation therapy. Thus, other than for potential specific indications related to confirmed residual disease at an original bulky site, inclusion of radiation therapy is not considered standard.

Fourteen trials were reported that tested other chemotherapy strategies. The first of these strategies relates to the use of weekly chemotherapy that is administered over a shorter time course than ABVD. Regimens are based on principles that additional agents will be associated with "non-cross resistance" and will therefore improve disease control, and that cumulative doses of any one agent are reduced so that late-effects associated with that agent can be minimized. The Stanford V regimen is the prototype that tests these principles and is associated with promising results a phase II trial (30). As shown in Table 46.2, this strategy has been tested in three RCTs (31–33) and one randomized phase II trial (34). The RCTs all reported inferior outcomes in comparison with ABVD or equivalent regimen. A large North American Intergroup study, led by ECOG, has completed accrual to an RCT comparing Stanford V with ABVD; analyses of these results are pending. This trial differs in comparison with the studies included in Table 46.2 as radiation therapy is incorporated as an integral component of the experimental arm.

A second strategy tested is treatment intensification relative to ABVD. The prototype of such a regimen is bleomycin, etoposide, doxorubicin (Adriamycin®), cyclophosphamide, vincristine (Oncovin®), prednisone, and procarbazine (BEACOPP), which was developed by the GHSG. This regimen can be administered in "standard" (std-BEACOPP) or "escalated" (esc-BEACOPP) doses (35). Landmark testing of these regimens was a three-arm RCT comparing the two BEACOPP regimens with a MOPP-ABVD-like regimen that included cyclophosphamide (COPP-ABVD). After an interim analysis demonstrated inferior disease control with COPP-ABVD (36), the trial continued accrual to only the two BEACOPP arms. The reporting of the final analysis included a comparison of all patients randomized to each of the three arms, even though technically, patients accrued to the BEACOPP arms after closure of the COPP-ABVD arm do not represent a randomized comparison with COPP-ABVD. As shown in Table 46.3, outcomes were superior in the BEACOPP arms. The BEACOPP regimens are associated with more treatment-related toxicities and late-effects including infertility (37,38). Results of a subsequent GHSG study (28) suggest that the doses of esc-BEACOPP can be reduced to standard after completing four treatment cycles without loss of efficacy; more mature analyses of this RCT are pending.

Table 46.3 Recent randomized trials for patients with advanced-stage Hodgkin lymphoma: testing of BEACOPP chemotherapy.*

Author; Patient Number	Regimen	Population	Disease Control Outcomes	Overall Survival
			5-y FFTF‡	5 y‡
Diehl (35);†	COPP-ABVD	Ages 15–65	69%	83%
N = 1,195	std-BEACOPP	Bulky Stage IIB;	76% $p = 0.04$	87% $p = 0.16$
	esc-BEACOPP	Stage III-IV	87% $p < 0.001$	91% $p = 0.06$
			5-y FFTF	5 y
Ballova (39);†	COPP-ABVD	Ages 66–75	46% (pooled);	50% (pooled);
N = 68	std-BEACOPP	Stage IIB-IV	$p = 0.83$	$p = 0.62$
			FFTF	
Diehl (40);	ABVD	Ages 16–75	87%	97%
N = 1,293	std-BEACOPP	Stage I-IIA§	88%	96%
		Stage IIB	(Time point not stated; Median follow-up 3 y *p* not significant)	(Time point not stated; Median follow-up 3 y *p* not significant)
			4-y EFS	4-y
Ferme (41);	ABVD × 6	Stage I-II	91%	95%
N = 808	ABVD × 4	Presence of	87%	94%
	std-BEACOPP	Risk factors‖	90%	93%
			Global $p = 0.38$	Global $p = 0.98$
			4-y FFTF	4-y
Engert (28)	esc/std-BEACOPP × 4/4	Ages 15–65	86%	93%
N = 1,498	esc-BEACOPP × 8	Bulky Stage IIB;	88%	91%
		Stage III-IV		

* COPP-ABVD, cyclophosphamide, vincristine (Oncovin ®), prednisone, procarbazine, doxorubicin (Adriamycin ®), bleomycin, vinblastine and dacarbazine; BEACOPP:bleomycin, etoposide, doxorubicin (Adriamycin®), cyclophosphamide, vincristine (Oncovin®), prednisone and procarbazine; std: standard dose; esc, escalated dose; FFTF, freedom from treatment failure; EFS, event-free survival;

† These two trials included patients entered onto the BEACOPP arm(s) after closing accrual to the COPP-ABVD arm.

‡ *p* values represent the comparison of the indicated BEACOPP arms with COPP-ABVD.

§ Patients with stage I-IIA disease must have also had specific risk factors: increased erythrocyte sedimentation rate (ESR) and/or ≥3 nodal sites of disease.

‖ Risk factors present included at least one of age 50 years, ≥4 nodal sites of disease, ESR >50 if no B symptoms, ESR >30 if B symptoms, or bulky mediastinal disease.

The BEACOPP regimens were tested in three other RCTs. In one trial, older patients (ages 66–75) were randomized to COPP-ABVD or std-BEACOPP; the comparison also includes additional patients from case series testing of std-BEACOPP (39). No differences in efficacy outcomes were detected and more toxicities were observed in the std-BEACOPP group. Two RCTs compared std-BEACOPP with ABVD, both in combination with radiation therapy, for patients with unfavorable early-stage Hodgkin lymphoma (40,41). No differences in efficacy were detected in either of these trials.

Of the remaining five RCTs identified in this search, two tested the addition of ifosphamide, methotrexate, etoposide, and prednisone to the COPP-ABV regimen (COPP-ABV-IMEP) in comparison with COPP-ABVD and failed to detect differences in efficacy outcomes in patients with intermediate (42) and advanced-stage (43) disease. One trial tested the addition of prednisone and procarbazine to ABV (ABVPP) and compared this with MOPP-ABV in patients with advanced-stage disease (29). This trial also included randomization to consolidative radiation therapy and is included in the above analysis of radiation therapy. The 10-year overall survival was superior with ABVPP alone, mainly because of fewer deaths from other causes in comparison with MOPP-ABV. Finally, two RCTs have tested the role of autologous stem cell transplantation as part of initial therapy (44–45); both failed to detect or suggest advantages associated with transplantation.

Recommendations

1. Treatment with ABVD is as effective as and less toxic than hybrid chemotherapy (e.g., MOPP-ABV) and is recommended as a choice of therapy for patients with advanced-stage disease (Grade 1A).

2. The results of one RCT demonstrate that treatment with esc-BEACOPP provides superior disease control and overall survival in comparison with COPP-ABVD, and, by inference, ABVD (35). The BEACOPP regimens are associated with more acute and long-term toxicities, including important risks of infertility. In addition, the power to demonstrate that the BEACOPP regimens provided significantly superior overall survival in comparison with

COPP-ABVD appeared to require the inclusion of patients allocated to the BEACOPP regimens after closing randomization to COPP-ABVD arm; technically these patients do not contribute to a randomized comparison. Patients should be informed of the potential outstanding efficacy results associated with esc-BEACOPP but should also be aware of the trade-offs related to associated toxicities and the potential methodologic limitation related to the reporting of the superior overall survival. Provided patients are aware of these limitations, treatment with esc-BEACOPP is a reasonable option (Grade 2B). Treatment with BEACOPP is not recommended for patients older than 65 years (Grade 1C) or for those with intermediate or unfavorable early-stage disease (Grade 1B).

3. Based on results of currently available RCTs, the following treatments are not recommended:

a. Weekly short-course chemotherapy (Grade1A).

b. Autologous stem cell transplantation as a component of initial therapy (Grade 1B).

c. Routine inclusion of radiation therapy (Grade 1A).

References

1 Connors JM. State-of-the-art therapeutics: Hodgkin's lymphoma. *J Clin Oncol.* 2005;**23**:6400–408.

2 Meyer RM, Ambinder RF, Stroobants S. Hodgkin' lymphoma: evolving concepts with implications for practice. *Hematology (Am Soc Hematol Educ Program).* 2004;184–202.

3 Ries LAG, Harkins D, Krapcho M, et al., editors. *SEER Cancer Statistics Review, 1975-2003,* National Cancer Institute. Bethesda, MD, http://seer.cancer.gov/csr/1975_2003/, based on November 2005 SEER data submission, posted to the SEER Web site, 2006.

4 Gospodarowicz MK, Meyer RM. The management of patients with limited stage classical Hodgkin lymphoma. *Hematology (Am Soc Hematol Educ Program).* 2006;253–258.

5 Carbone PP, Kaplan HS, Musshoff K, et al. Report of the Committee on Hodgkin's Disease Staging Classification. *Cancer Res.* 1971;**31**:1860–61.

6 Lister TA, Crowther D, Sutcliffe SB, et al. Report of a committee convened to discuss the evaluation and staging of patients with Hodgkin's disease: Cotswolds meeting. *J Clin Oncol.* 1989;**7**:1630–36.

7 Diehl V, Thomas RK, Re D. Part II: Hodgkin's lymphoma—diagnosis and treatment. *Lancet Oncol.* 2004;**5**:19–26.

8 Specht L, Gray RG, Clarke MJ, et al. Influence of more extensive radiotherapy and adjuvant chemotherapy on long-term outcome of early-stage Hodgkin's disease: a meta-analysis of 23 randomized trials involving 3,888 patients. International Hodgkin's Disease Collaborative Group. *J Clin Oncol.* 1998;**16**:830–43.

9 Press OW, LeBlanc M, Lichter AS, et al. Phase III randomized intergroup trial of subtotal lymphoid irradiation versus doxorubicin, vinblastine, and subtotal lymphoid irradiation for stage IA to IIA Hodgkin's disease. *J Clin Oncol.* 2001;**19**:4238–44.

10 Sieber M, Franklin J, Tesch H, et al. Two cycles ABVD plus extended field radiotherapy is superior to radiotherapy alone in early stage Hodgkin's disease: results of the German Hodgkin's Lymphoma Study Group (GHSG) Trial HD7 [abstract]. *Blood.* 2002;**100**:93a.

11 Hagenbeek A, Eghbali H, Fermé C, et al. Three cycles of MOPP/ABV hybrid and involved-field irradiation is more effective than subtotal nodal irradiation in favorable supradiaphragmatic clinical stages I–II Hodgkin's disease: preliminary results of the EORTC-GELA H8-F randomized trial in 543 patients [abstract]. *Blood.* 2000;**96**:575a.

11a Ferme C, Eghbali H, Meerwaldt JH et al. Chemotherapy plus Involved-Field Radiation in Early-Stage Hodgkin's Disease. *N Engl J Med.* 2007; **357**:1916-27.

12 Santoro A, Bonfante V, Viviani S, et al. Subtotal nodal versus involved field irradiation after 4 cycles of ABVD in early stage Hodgkin's disease [abstract]. *Proc Am Soc Clin Oncol.* 1996;**15**:415.

13 Bonadonna G, Bonfante V, Viviani S, et al. ABVD plus subtotal nodal versus involved-field radiotherapy in early-stage Hodgkin's disease: long-term results. *J Clin Oncol.* 2004;**22**:2835–41.

14 Noordijk EM, Thomas J, Fermé C, et al. First results of the EORTC-GELA H9 randomized trials: the H9-F trial (comparing 3 radiation dose levels) and H9-U trial (comparing 3 chemotherapy schemes) in patients with favorable or unfavorable early stage Hodgkin's lymphoma [abstract]. *J Clin Oncol.* 2005;**23**:561s.

15 Diehl V, Engert A, Mueller RP, et al. HD10: investigating reduction of combined modality treatment intensity in early stage Hodgkin's lymphoma: interim analysis of a randomized trial of the German Hodgkin Study Group [abstract]. *J Clin Oncol.* 2005;**23**:561s.

16 Laskar S, Gupta T, Vimal S, et al. Consolidation radiation after complete remission in Hodgkin's disease following six cycles of doxorubicin, bleomycin, vinblastine, and dacarbazine chemotherapy: is there a need? *J Clin Oncol.* 2004;**22**:62–68.

17 Straus DJ, Portlock CS, Qin J, et al. Results of a prospective randomized clinical trial of doxorubicin, bleomycin, vinblastine, and dacarbazine (ABVD) followed by radiation therapy (RT) versus ABVD alone for stages I, II, and IIIA nonbulky Hodgkin disease. *Blood.* 2004;**104**: 3483–89.

18 Meyer RM, Gospodarowicz MK, Connors JM, et al. Randomized comparison of ABVD chemotherapy with a strategy that includes radiation therapy in patients with limited-stage Hodgkin's lymphoma: National Cancer Institute of Canada Clinical Trials Group and the Eastern Cooperative Oncology Group. *J Clin Oncol.* 2005;**23**:4634–42.

19 Noordijk EM, Carde P, Dupouy N, et al. Combined-modality therapy for clinical stage I or II Hodgkin's lymphoma: long-term results of the European Organisation for Research and Treatment of Cancer H7 randomized controlled trials. *J Clin Oncol.* 2006;**24**:3128–35.

20 Meyer RM. Is there convincing evidence for the use of chemotherapy alone in patients with limited-stage Hodgkin's lymphoma. *Eur J Haematol.* 2005;**75** Suppl 66:115–20.

21 Macdonald DA, Gospodarowicz MK, Wells WA, et al. Relapse patterns and subsequent outcomes of patients treated on the NCIC CTG HD.6 (ECOG JHD06) randomized trial evaluating ABVD alone in patients with limited stage Hodgkin Lymphoma (HL) [abstract]. *Blood.* 2005;**106**:241a.

22 Hasenclever D, Diehl V, Armitage JO, et al. A prognostic score for advanced Hodgkin's disease. *N Engl J Med.* 1998;**339**:1506–14.

23 Canellos GP, Anderson JR, Propert KJ, et al. Chemotherapy of advanced Hodgkin's disease with MOPP, ABVD, or MOPP alternating with ABVD. *N Engl J Med.* 1992;**327**:1478–84.

24 Duggan DB, Petroni GR, Johnson JL, et al. Randomized comparison of ABVD and MOPP/ABV hybrid for the treatment of advanced Hodgkin's disease: report of an intergroup trial. *J Clin Oncol.* 2003;**21**:607–14.

25 Johnson PW, Radford JA, Cullen MH, et al. Comparison of ABVD and alternating or hybrid multidrug regimens for the treatment of advanced Hodgkin's lymphoma: results of the United Kingdom Lymphoma Group LY09 trial. *J Clin Oncol.* 2005;**23**:9208–218.

26 Loeffler M, Brosteanu O, Hasenclever D, et al. Meta-analysis of chemotherapy versus combined modality treatment trials in Hodgkin's

disease. International Database on Hodgkin's Disease Overview Study Group. *J Clin Oncol.* 1998;**16**:818–29.

27 Aleman BM, Raemaekers JM, Tomisic R, et al. Involved-field radiotherapy for patients in partial remission after chemotherapy for advanced Hodgkin's lymphoma. *Int J Radiat Oncol Biol Phys.* 2007;**67**:19–30.

28 Engert A, Franklin J, Maueller RP, et al. HD12 randomised trial comparing 8 dose-escalated cycles of BEACOPP with 4 escalated and 4 baseline cycles in patients with advanced stage Hodgkin lymphoma: an analysis of the German Hodgkin Lymphoma Study Group (GHSG) [abstract]. 2006;**108**:33a.

29 Ferme C, Mounier N, Casasnovas O, et al. Long-term results and competing risk analysis of the H89 trial in patients with advanced-stage Hodgkin lymphoma: a study by the Groupe d'Etude des Lymphomes de l'Adulte (GELA). *Blood.* 2006;**107**:4636–42.

30 Horning SJ, Hoppe RT, Breslin S, et al. Stanford V and radiotherapy for locally extensive and advanced Hodgkin's disease: mature results of a prospective clinical trial. *J Clin Oncol.* 2002;**20**:630–37.

31 Radford JA, Rohatiner AZ, Ryder WD, et al. ChlVPP/EVA hybrid versus the weekly VAPEC-B regimen for previously untreated Hodgkin's disease. *J Clin Oncol.* 2002;**20**:2988–94.

32 Aviles A, Cleto S, Neri N, et al. Treatment of advanced Hodgkin's disease: EBVD versus intensive brief chemotherapy. *Leuk Lymphoma.* 2003;**44**:1361–65.

33 Gobbi PG, Levis A, Chisesi T, et al. ABVD versus modified Stanford V versus MOPPEBVCAD with optional and limited radiotherapy in intermediate- and advanced-stage Hodgkin's lymphoma: final results of a multicenter randomized trial by the Intergruppo Italiano Linfomi. *J Clin Oncol.* 2005;**23**:9198–207.

34 Johnson P, Hoskin P, Horwich A, et al. Stanford V regimen versus ABVD for the treatment of advanced Hodgkin lymphoma: results of a UK NCRI/LTO randomised phase II trial [abstract]. *Blood.* 2004;**104**:93a.

35 Diehl V, Franklin J, Pfreundschuh M, et al. Standard and increased-dose BEACOPP chemotherapy compared with COPP-ABVD for advanced Hodgkin's disease. *N Engl J Med.* 2003;**348**:2386–95.

36 Diehl V, Franklin J, Hasenclever D, et al. BEACOPP, a new dose-escalated and accelerated regimen, is at least as effective as COPP/ABVD in patients with advanced-stage Hodgkin's lymphoma: interim report from a trial of the German Hodgkin's Lymphoma Study Group. *J Clin Oncol.* 1998;**16**:3810–21.

37 Sieniawski M, Reineke T, Josting A, et al. Fertility in male Hodgkin lymphoma patients—a report of German Hodgkin Study Group [abstract]. *Blood.* 2006;**108**:34a.

38 Behringer K, Breuer K, Reineke T, et al. Secondary amenorrhea after Hodgkin's lymphoma is influenced by age at treatment, stage of disease, chemotherapy regimen, and the use of oral contraceptives during therapy: a report from the German Hodgkin's Lymphoma Study Group. *J Clin Oncol.* 2005;**20**:7555–64.

39 Ballova V, Ruffer JU, Haverkamp H, et al. A prospectively randomized trial carried out by the German Hodgkin Study Group (GHSG) for elderly patients with advanced Hodgkin's disease comparing BEACOPP baseline and COPP-ABVD (study HD9elderly). *Ann Oncol.* 2005;**16**:124–31.

40 Diehl V, Brillant C, Engert A, et al. Recent interim analysis of the HD11 trial of the GHSG: intensification of chemotherapy and reduction of radiation dose in early unfavorable stage Hodgkin's lymphoma [abstract]. *Blood.* 2005;**106**:240a.

41 Ferme C, Diviné M, Vranovsky A, et al. Four ABVD and involved-field radiotherapy in unfavorable supradiaphragmatic clinical stages (CS) I-II Hodgkin's lymphoma (HL): preliminary results of the EORTC-GELA H9-U trial [abstract]. *Blood.* 2005;**106**:240a.

42 Sieber M, Tesch H, Pfistner B, et al. Rapidly alternating COPP/ABV/IMEP is not superior to conventional alternating COPP/ABVD in combination with extended-field radiotherapy in intermediate-stage Hodgkin's lymphoma: final results of the German Hodgkin's Lymphoma Study Group Trial HD5. *J Clin Oncol.* 2002;**20**:476–84.

43 Sieber M, Tesch H, Pfistner B, et al. Treatment of advanced Hodgkin's disease with COPP/ABV/IMEP versus COPP/ABVD and consolidating radiotherapy: final results of the German Hodgkin's Lymphoma Study Group HD6 trial. *Ann Oncol.* 2004;**15**:276–82.

44 Saghatchian M, Djeridane M, Escoffre-Barbe M, et al. Very high risk Hodgkin's disease: ABVD (4 cycles) plus BEAM followed by autologous stem cell transplantation and radiotherapy versus intensive chemotherapy (3 cycles) (INT-CT) and RT: four-year results of the GOELAMS H97-GM multicentric randomized trial [abstract]. *J Clin Oncol.* 2002;**21**: 263a.

45 Federico M, Bellei M, Brice P, et al. High-dose therapy and autologous stem-cell transplantation versus conventional therapy for patients with advanced Hodgkin's lymphoma responding to front-line therapy. *J Clin Oncol.* 2003;**21**:2320–25.

47 Lymphocyte Predominant Hodgkin Lymphoma

Brandon McMahon, Jonathan W. Friedberg

Introduction

Lymphocyte predominant Hodgkin lymphoma (LPHL) was first described in 1937 based on its characteristic small lymphocyte-rich background with coexistent histiocytes (1). It is a rare condition, with a reported rate of 0.11 per 100,000 person-years and accounting for only approximately 4% of all cases of Hodgkin lymphoma (HL) (2). Over the past 70 years, significant data have emerged to further classify the disease both pathologically and clinically. Unfortunately, due to its rarity, most of what is known about LPHL is derived from retrospective reviews and case series, with no large randomized controlled trials (RCTs) carried out to date. This makes distillation of data on LPHL to best clinical evidence difficult, with recommendations on treatment and surveillance limited to small trials (3). What is known is that this tends to be an indolent lymphoma, often diagnosed at early stages, with extremely favorable long-term outcomes.

Questions

1. Is LPHL a distinct clinical/pathologic entity from classical HL?
2. Should de novo LPHL be treated differently from classical Hodgkin lymphoma?
3. Should detection and treatment of LPHL progression or relapse be different from classical Hodgkin lymphoma?
4. Should rituximab be included as "standard" therapeutic modality for LPHL?

Literature-search strategy and inclusions

Because of the rarity of this disease, we were not able to identify large randomized controlled trials or meta-analyses. There were no studies identified in the Cochrane database that specifically focused on LPHL. Studies for inclusion were identified using the search term "nodular lymphocyte predominant Hodgkin lymphoma" through PubMed and Ovid. This resulted in a small number of studies returned, and therefore no restrictions were placed on the returned publications, but those included for review had some focus on LPHL. Particular attention was given to those studies restricting the confirmed diagnosis to the pathognomonic immunohistochemical imprint of LPHL. Further studies were identified through cross-referencing citations on returned publications.

Where evidence is available, the quality of evidence and strengths of recommendations in this chapter are based on the guidelines proposed by the international Grading of Recommendations Assessment, Development, and Evaluation Working Group (GRADE) adopting the modification used by the American College of Chest Physicians that merges the "very low" and "low" categories of quality of evidence (see chapter 1).

Evidence-based Hematology. Edited by Mark A. Crowther, Jeff Ginsberg, Holger J. Schünemann, Ralph M. Meyer, and Richard Lottenberg.

Is LPHL a distinct clinical/pathologic entity from classical HL?

Morphologically, LPHL reveals a background of small lymphocytes and rare Reed-Sternberg cells in favor of lager lymphocyte/histiocyte "L&H," or "popcorn," cells. These cells typically have a folded, lobulated nucleus with inconspicuous nucleoli. The rarity of the disease, coupled with paucity of the L&H cells in affected lymph nodes, has made understanding disease biology difficult. Recent work demonstrating immunoglobulin gene rearrangements in the neoplastic cells indicates this is a monoclonal B lymphocyte disorder, with relation of the L&H cells to germinal center B cells at the centroblastic stage of differentiation (4,5). Histologically, these cells are typically found in nodules, with a background of reactive polyclonal B cells, dendritic cells, and macrophages (6–8). Immunophenotypically, they characteristically are negative for CD30 and CD15, while being positive for

Table 47.1 Comparison of clinicopathologic features of lymphocyte predominant Hodgkin lymphoma (LPHL) and classical Hodgkin lymphoma (HL).

	LPHL	Classical HL
Neoplastic cells	L&H, or "popcorn" cells	Reed–Sternberg cells
CD15	Negative	Positive
CD20	Positive	Rare
CD30	Negative	Positive
CD45	Positive	Negative
Gender	Men > women	Women > men
Mediastinal involvement	Rare	Variable
B symptoms	Rare	Variable
Stage IV at presentation	Rare	Variable
Survival	>90%	~80%

CD20. The REAL classification proposal separated LPHL based on the histomorphology and immunophenotypic imprint, as a distinct pathologic entity from "classical" Hodgkin lymphoma, which demonstrates CD15 and CD30 positivity, while being CD20 negative (6). An important study was carried out by the European Task Force on Lymphoma (ETFL), who evaluated 388 adult (>15 years) cases previously diagnosed as LPHL between 1970 and 1994 (9). Paraffin-embedded tissue blocks were reevaluated by an expert panel of pathologists, blinded to clinical data and previous diagnosis. Each pathologist evaluated both standard morphology on H&E stain, as well as immunostains. Results showed that without immunohistochemical confirmation, the diagnosis of LPHL is difficult and often inaccurate, as only 56.5% of the cases were confirmed. Ninety-four percent of confirmed cases had a nodular growth pattern, 98% expressed CD20, and all lacked CD30 and CD15 expression. Over 43% of the cases were reassigned, the majority (68%) were diagnosed lymphocyte-rich classical Hodgkin lymphoma (LRCHL). Although LRCHL is pathologically distinct from LPHL, the two diseases have many clinical similarities, including male predilection, early stage at diagnosis (70% Stage I or II), and favorable prognosis (10). Reported relapse rates are similar (17% vs. 21%), but those with LRCHL have a worse prognosis at relapse (Table 47.1).

LPHL presents distinctively from classical HL, and although immunophenotypically is similar to a B cell non-Hodgkin lymphoma, it is clinically very different. Clinical information gathered from the ETFL study above, in addition to smaller retrospective studies, reveals that LPHL has a male predilection (3:1) with a median age at diagnosis of 35 (9,10). Most (~80%) present at stage I or II, while few (~6%) patients are found to have stage IV disease. Extranodal involvement rarely occurs (1%–3%) in patients with advanced disease, occurring most commonly in liver, lung, and bone. Only ~13% of cases qualify as bulky disease, and B symptoms are reported in approximately 10%. Disease tends to be peripherally located, with mediastinal involvement in ~7%. Despite the immunophenotypic similarities with B-cell lymphomas, these clinical features are in contrast to the usual presentation of indolent, CD20+ B-cell lymphomas, which tend to present in later decades and many times at advanced stages and with associated B-symptoms.

The disease tends to behave indolently, and most patients have a very favorable long-term outcome. Most studies limiting LPHL to CD20+/CD15-/CD30- cases report a 10-year overall survival >90%, with overall survival (OS) rates as high as 99% in patients with stage I disease (11). Advanced stage and age predict for a less favorable outcome.

In summary, there are no large prospective studies evaluating the clinical and pathologic features of LPHL. The best evidence currently available investigating the clinicopathologic features of LPHL comes from retrospective reviews. Given the rarity of the disease (3%–5% of all Hodgkin lymphoma cases), it is unlikely that large prospective studies will be completed in the near future. Based on the best available evidence, LHPL clearly has both clinical and pathologic features, which distinguish it from both classical Hodgkin lymphoma and other indolent B-cell lymphomas.

Conclusion

LPHL is a unique clinicopathologic entity, readily diagnosed with standard immunohistochemical techniques.

Should de novo LPHL be treated differently from classical Hodgkin lymphoma?

As demonstrated by the previously mentioned studies, the majority of patients with LPHL present with early-stage disease with extremely favorable long-term overall survival rates. Historically, the majority of patients with LPHL are treated according to stage-appropriate regimens used for classical Hodgkin lymphoma. Complete remission (CR) rates with this approach are similar to those with classical Hodgkin lymphoma (12).

Early-stage LPHL is generally treated with either radiation therapy (RT) alone, or with RT combined with a brief course of systemic chemotherapy typically used to treat classical Hodgkin. This generally results in both high CR and OS rates. A retrospective study evaluating outcomes of 71 patients with LPHL found that 86% of patients were treated with RT alone (72% either mantle field alone or mantle plus para-aortic), with the remainder being treated with chemotherapy alone or combined modality chemotherapy plus RT (11). Over a median follow up of 10.8 years, the OS rate was 93%, and freedom from first relapse was 80%. Of the nine total deaths, only one was due to underlying Hodgkin lymphoma. Five deaths were from secondary malignancies, and two from cardiac disease. These results are similar to those found by the ETFL (10). The majority (88%) of stage I disease was treated with RT alone, with increasing reliance on systemic chemotherapy (MOPP, ABVD, or MOPP/ABVD hybrid) in more advanced stages. This approach led to a high CR (96%) and only a 14% death rate. Similar to the previous study, only 26% of deaths were secondary to Hodgkin lymphoma, with approximately one-third from secondary malignancies.

With high OS rates, and deaths often occurring secondary to long-term treatment toxicities, there is much interest in limiting treatment as much as possible without affecting disease-specific outcomes (8). This was addressed in a recent prospective study of 42 patients diagnosed with stage IA or IIA LPHL without mediastinal involvement (13). Patients were treated with one to three courses of anthracycline-based chemotherapy followed by extended field RT; over half received only one course of chemotherapy. This resulted in high CR (98%) and 15-year OS rates (86%). The Hodgkin-specific mortality rate at 15 years was 2.4% in patients with LPHL, with the authors noting a 6.3% incidence of secondary malignancies and 10.6% incidence of angina or myocardial infarction in that time period.

This attempt at decreasing long-term treatment-related toxicities was explored in a single-institution study of pediatric patients presenting with early-stage LPHL (14). Six patients were given no additional treatment after excisional biopsy and no evidence of remaining disease, five patients received nine weeks of CHOP, and one patient received involved-field RT. At a median of six years out, all patients were alive without evidence of active disease. There was only one local recurrence reported after initial chemotherapy with the patient sustaining a second CR after involved-field RT.

In summary, patients with LPHL have traditionally been treated with regimens used for stage-specific classical Hodgkin lymphoma. Data available demonstrate that patients with LPHL approached in this way have very favorable long-term OS. Currently, there are no prospective RCTs that exclusively address the treatment of LPHL. The best available data are mainly retrospective studies from cooperative groups. In addition, recent large, prospective interventional trials in Hodgkin lymphoma often specifically exclude patients with LPHL subtype. This will undoubtedly make optimizing treatment strategies for this rare subtype all the more difficult in the future.

Although there are no studies that convincingly show that de novo LPHL should be treated differently from classical Hodgkin lymphoma at the same stage, there are some data demonstrating that minimizing treatments especially for early-stage disease may not affect disease specific outcomes. This approach has the added benefit of limiting long-term treatment-related toxicities, and is the subject of currently accruing clinical trials. Until these studies mature, the recommendation is that de novo LPHL should be approached with curative intent, with a similar treatment paradigm to that used for classical Hodgkin lymphoma (15). In the situation of nonbulky stage IA disease, involved-field radiation without chemotherapy may be another reasonable option (16,17).

Recommendation

Upfront therapy for LPHL has not been well defined. Very early stage disease may have excellent outcomes with involved-field radiation therapy. We otherwise recommend treatment with curative intent in a manner similar to that used for classical Hodgkin lymphoma (Grade 1C).

Should detection and treatment of LPHL progression or relapse be different from classical Hodgkin lymphoma?

There have been reports of higher rates of relapse of LPHL compared with classical Hodgkin lymphoma, not uncommonly with late occurrences. In addition, up to ~25% of patients may experience multiple relapses, but this does not correlate with a decrease in OS compared with those whose disease does not multiply recur (10). Recurrences have been reported as far out as 30 years from original diagnosis (18). This has led many to reconsider strategies for detecting relapsed LPHL. Unlike classical Hodgkin lymphoma, however, patients with LPHL who recur tend to have favorable outcomes using salvage treatment regimens or even local RT, without proceeding with aggressive systemic chemotherapy or pursuit of autologous stem cell transplant.

Rates of relapse vary based on study and follow up period, with ranges of 11%–21% over a median follow up of 10–15 years (9,11,12). Those with more advanced stage at diagnosis relapse more frequently than earlier-stage disease, with one study reporting a 14.7% relapse rate in patients with stage IIA or earlier disease but 50% for those at higher stages; the median time to relapse was 53 months (11). In one of the larger series of patients, those with confirmed LPHL had an overall recurrence rate of 21%, which was comparable to the 17% rate in those with a diagnosis reassignment to lymphocyte-rich classical Hodgkin lymphoma (10). The median age at relapse was somewhat lower at 34 years for LPHL compared with 40 years in LRCHL. The eight-year freedom from treatment failure ranged from 24% for those with stage IV disease to 85% in stage I. Despite these figures, the eight-year OS was 94% and higher for those with stage III disease or earlier. Relapses tend to be treated with local RT or brief courses of systemic chemotherapy. There are no trials investigating the utility of autologous stem cell transplant for relapsed LPHL, and given the favorable prognosis of recurrent disease using less aggressive therapy, this modality cannot be uniformly endorsed at this time.

Unlike other lymphoma subtypes, LPHL can often recur after prolonged quiescent periods. The ETFL study showed no plateau for failure-free survival (Figure 47.1), with five relapses occurring 13 years or more past original diagnosis (10). Two phase II studies evaluating the efficacy of rituximab in treatment of LPHL enrolled patients with relapsed disease (18,19). The median times from original diagnosis to most recent relapse were 9 and 11.9 years, with active disease being found as far out as 33 years from original diagnosis. Although the best available data indicates that relapses can occur after prolonged periods of disease inactivity, these are selected patients with a small number of total events. There are no compelling data at present to suggest that all patients with LPHL should be monitored more intensely for disease recurrence

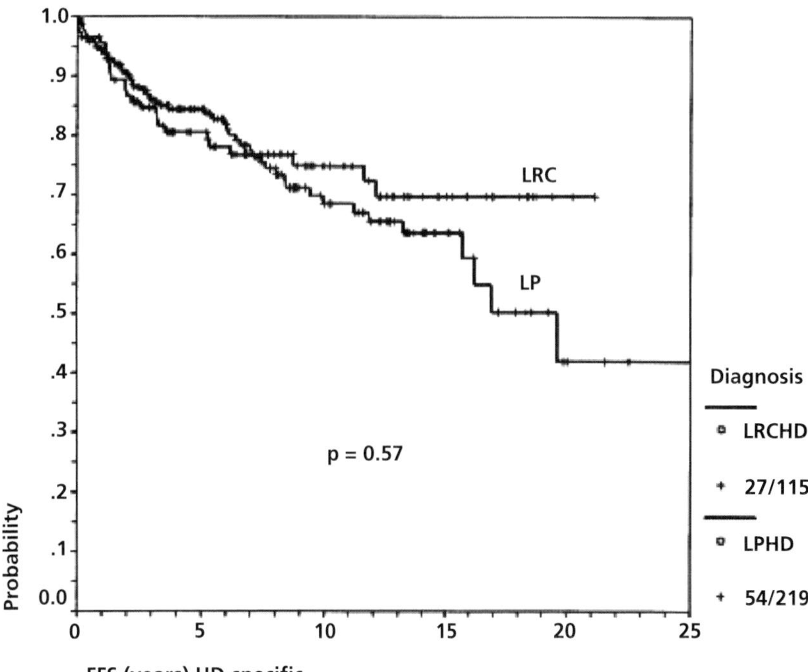

Figure 47.1 Hodgkin lymphoma-specific failure-free survival for lymphocyte predominant and lymphocyte rich disease (reproduced with permission [10]).

for longer periods when compared with other lymphoma subtypes.

Given the variability of reported relapse rates and time from original diagnosis, it is difficult to generalize currently available data to all cases of LPHL. To date, recurrence rates are largely based on retrospective studies with small numbers of overall events. However, based on the best available data, relapses may occur several years if not decades after original diagnosis of LPHL. Areas suspicious for relapse should be biopsied to ensure histologic transformation has not occurred despite no compelling data that LPHL has a higher transformation rate to aggressive B- or T-cell lymphomas compared with classical Hodgkin disease. Once relapse has been confirmed, given the indolent nature of disease and favorable outcomes even after recurrence, consideration should be given to focal RT, monoclonal antibodies, or brief courses of chemotherapy. There have been no prospective studies to date supporting the role for autologous stem cell transplant in relapsed disease, and this approach could subject patients with otherwise potentially very favorable long-term survival to high short-term treatment-related morbidity and mortality. Autologous stem cell transplant should therefore be reserved for specific clinical situations, including early recurrences or aggressive or advanced disease not responding to standard therapy.

Recommendation

Because of its unique natural history, including late recurrences, we do not routinely recommend autologous stem cell transplant for relapsed disease unless high-risk features are present (Grade 2C).

Should rituximab be included as "standard" therapeutic modality for LPHL?

Given the indolent nature of LPHL, and the expression of CD20 on the surface of the malignant cells, there has been much interest in the use of the anti-CD20 monoclonal antibody rituximab (Rituxan, Genentech/Biogen Idec, San Francisco, CA) in its treatment, both up-front and in relapsed disease.

Unfortunately, a comprehensive search of the literature of rituximab use in this setting only returned case reports, a case series, and two small phase II studies. No randomized controlled studies were identified. This is likely due to the relatively recent discovery of rituximab efficacy in other CD20+ lymphomas, as well as the rarity of LPHL, making large RCT unfeasible.

Two case reports published complete remission in two patients with relapsed, chemorefractory stage IV disease following rituximab treatment, one of whom had pulmonary involvement (20,21). A third case, however, reported failure of sustained response in a young patient also with pulmonary involvement, with evidence of disease progression within three months of completing four weekly infusions of rituximab (22). In an effort to limit treatment toxicity, Ibom et al. (22) treated four previously untreated patients and two patients with relapsed disease with upfront weekly rituximab at 375 mg/m^2 × 4 doses, followed by either radiation therapy or chlorambucil. Follow-up was relatively short; however, none of the patients exhibited disease progression or significant treatment-related toxicities at a median of 19 months following completion of rituximab and either RT or chlorambucil.

Rituximab as monotherapy in LPHL was evaluated in two phase II studies (18,19). The German Hodgkin Lymphoma Study Group (GHLSG) investigated use in *relapsed-only* disease, whereas rituximab was used as initial therapy in >50% of patients in the study by Ekstrand et al. Both had high overall response rates, 86% and 100%, respectively. Complete responses were similar in the two studies (57% vs. 41%), however relapse rates were quite disparate. Ekstrand et al. (19) reported 9/22 patients relapsing during a median follow up of 12 months, giving an overall median freedom from progression (FFP) of 10.2 months. In contrast, 9/12 responders in the GHLSG remained in remission a median duration of over 20 months, with the FFP not yet being reached by study publication. Toxicities were mainly limited to mild to moderate infusion-related reactions.

At this time, clinical evidence for use of rituximab in LPHL as either initial therapy or for relapsed disease is limited to case reports, a case series, and two phase II studies. Ideally, more convincing data on long-term efficacy and safety from larger RCT would be needed before routine endorsement of rituximab in LPHL treatment could be made. However, given the rarity of the disease, this will likely not occur in the near future. Therefore, based on efficacy in other CD20+ lymphomas, and the limited data on use in LPHL, consideration should be given to rituximab as an active treatment option for relapsed disease. At present, we do not recommend rituximab as part of upfront therapy of LPHL.

Recommendation

Rituximab is an active agent in LPHL, and clearly has a role in therapy of relapsed disease. Further studies are needed before this treatment can be routinely recommended as part of upfront therapy (Grade 1C).

Acknowledgments

Dr. Friedberg is supported in part by a career development award from the National Cancer Institute (CA-102216) and by support from the National Childhood Cancer Foundation.

References

1 Jackson H. Classification and prognosis of Hodgkin's disease and allied disorders. *Surg Gynecol Obstet.* 1937;**64**:465.

2 Morton LM, Wang SS, Devesa SS, et al. Lymphoma incidence patterns by WHO subtype in the United States, 1992–2001. *Blood.* 2006;**107**: 265–76.

3 Connors JM. Lymphocyte predominance Hodgkin's lymphoma. *Am Soc Hematol Educ Book.* 2001:744–46.

4 Marafioti T, Hummel M, Anagnostopoulos I, et al. Origin of nodular lymphocyte-predominant Hodgkin's disease from a clonal expansion of highly mutated germinal-center B cells. *N Engl J Med.* 1997;**337**: 453–58.

5 Ohno T, Stribley JA, Wu G, et al. Clonality in nodular lymphocyte-predominant Hodgkin's disease. *N Engl J Med.* 1997;**337**:459–65.

6 Harris NL, Jaffe ES, Stein H, et al. A revised European-American classification of lymphoid neoplasms: a proposal from the International Lymphoma Study Group. *Blood.* 1994;**84**:1361–92.

7 Harris NL, Jaffe ES, Diebold J, et al. World Health Organization classification of neoplastic diseases of the hematopoietic and lymphoid tissues: report of the Clinical Advisory Committee meeting-Airlie House, Virginia, November 1997. *J Clin Oncol.* 1999;**17**:3835–49.

8 Aster JC. Lymphocyte-predominant Hodgkin's disease: how little therapy is enough? *J Clin Oncol.* 1999;**17**:744–46.

9 Anagnostopoulos I, Hansmann ML, Franssila K, et al. European Task Force on Lymphoma project on lymphocyte predominance Hodgkin disease: histologic and immunohistologic analysis of submitted cases reveals 2 types of Hodgkin disease with a nodular growth pattern and abundant lymphocytes. *Blood.* 2000;**96**:1889–99.

10 Diehl V, Sextro M, Franklin J, et al. Clinical presentation, course, and prognostic factors in lymphocyte-predominant Hodgkin's disease and lymphocyte-rich classical Hodgkin's disease: report from the European Task Force on Lymphoma Project on Lymphocyte-Predominant Hodgkin's Disease. *J Clin Oncol.* 1999;**17**:776–83.

11 Bodis S, Kraus MD, Pinkus G, et al. Clinical presentation and outcome in lymphocyte-predominant Hodgkin's disease. *J Clin Oncol.* 1997;**15**:3060–66.

12 Nogova L, Reineke T, Josting A, et al. Lymphocyte-predominant and classical Hodgkin's lymphoma—comparison of outcomes. *Eur J Haemotol.* 2005;**75** Suppl. 66:106–10.

13 Feugier P, Labouyrie E, Djeridane M, et al. Comparison of initial characteristics and long-term outcome of patients with lymphocyte-predominant Hodgkin lymphoma and classical Hodgkin lymphoma at clinical stages IA and IIA prospectively treated by brief anthracycline-based chemotherapies plus extended high-dose irradiation. *Blood.* 2004;**104**:2675–81.

14 Murphy SB, Morgan ER, Katzenstein HM, et al. Results of little or no treatment for lymphocyte-predominant Hodgkin disease in children and adolescents. *J Pediatr Hematol Oncol.* 2009;**25**:684–87.

15 Friedberg JW, Ng AK, Canellos GP. Hodgkin's lymphoma: diagnosis and treatment. In: Canellos GP, Lister TA, Young B, editors. *The lymphomas.* 2nd ed. Philadelphia: Elsevier; 2006. pp. 476–99.

16 Wirth A, Yuen K, Barton M, et al. Long-term outcome after radiotherapy alone for lymphocyte-predominant Hodgkin lymphoma: a retrospective multicenter study of the Australasian Radiation Oncology Lymphoma Group. *Cancer.* 2005;**104**:1221–29.

17 Nogova L, Rudiger T, Engert A. Biology, clinical course, and management of nodular lymphocyte-predominant Hodgkin lymphoma. *Hematol Am Soc Hematol Educ Program.* 2006;266–72.

18 Rehwald U, Schulz H, Reiser M, et al. Treatment of relapsed CD20+ Hodgkin lymphoma with the monoclonal antibody rituximab is effective

and well tolerated: results of a phase 2 trial of the German Hodgkin Lymphoma Study Group. *Blood.* 2003;**101**:420–24.

19 Ekstrand BC, Lucas JB, Horwitz SM, et al. Rituximab in lymphocyte-predominant Hodgkin disease: results of a phase 2 trial. *Blood.* 2003;**101**:4285–89.

20 Lush RJ, Jones SG, Haynes AP. Advanced-stage, chemorefractory lymphocyte-predominant Hodgkin's disease: long-term follow-up of allografting and monoclonal antibody therapy. *Br J Haematol.* 2001;**114**:734–35.

21 Boulanger E, Meignin V, Leverger G, et al. Rituximab monotherapy in nodular lymphocyte-predominant Hodgkin's disease. *Ann Oncol.* 2003;**14**:171.

22 Ibom VK, Prosnitz RG, Gong JZ, et al. Rituximab in lymphocyte predominance Hodgkin's disease: a case series. *Clin Lymphoma.* 2003;**4**:115–18.

48 Management of Patients with Essential Thrombocythemia

Guido Finazzi, Giovanni Barosi, Tiziano Barbui

Introduction

Essential thrombocythemia (ET) is currently classified as a myeloproliferative disorder (MPD), which is a heterogeneous category of clonal stem cell diseases that also includes polycythemia vera (PV), primary myelofibrosis (MF), chronic myeloid leukemia, and atypical MPDs (1). A major advance in our understanding of the pathogenesis of MPDs was made with the recent identification of the V617F JAK2 mutation in a substantial proportion of patients, especially with PV (2). This discovery has had a major impact on disease classification, diagnostic approach and in addressing research strategies in these disorders. Among the classic MPDs (1), patients with ET have the most favorable outcome. In large cohort studies, ET patients showed equal or slightly shorter survival than an age- and sex-matched healthy population (3,4). Major causes of death were disease-related, thrombotic, or hemorrhagic complications or malignant progression to MF or acute leukemia, both due to natural history of the disease and possibly induced by the use of chemotherapeutic agents (5). Hence, the goal of therapy is to limit the use of cytotoxic drugs to patients stratified on the basis of their risk for developing vascular events (6).

Questions

1. When should cytoreductive agents be commenced for patients with ET?
2. What is the treatment of choice for those patients who require therapy?
3. When should antiplatelet therapy be used?
4. How should ET be managed in patients who are pregnant or of childbearing age?

Evidence-based Hematology. Edited by Mark A. Crowther, Jeff Ginsberg, Holger J. Schünemann, Ralph M. Meyer, and Richard Lottenberg.

Literature-search strategy and inclusion

For the purpose of the present review, we used the database developed for the production of the Italian guidelines for the therapy of ET, described in detail elsewhere (7). Briefly, an expert panel systematically reviewed the published literature from 1980 to October 2003, graded articles according to their quality, and formulated proper recommendations through a formal consensus process. In addition, we updated the database up to November 2006 through a computerized search of MEDLINE, PubMed, CANCERLIT, Cochrane Library, and EMBASE using the same standardized criteria previously described (7). We further reviewed reference lists and articles from the authors' libraries. Previously, we graded the quality of the evidence according to the statements of the Scottish Intercollegiate Guidelines Network (SIGN) (8). Grading of the quality of evidence and strengths of recommendations in this chapter are based on the guidelines proposed by the international Grading of Recommendations Assessment, Development, and Evaluation Working Group (GRADE) adopting the modification used by the American College of Chest Physicians that merges the "very low" and "low" categories of quality of evidence (see chapter 1).

When should cytoreductive agents be commenced for patients with ET?

The evidence used to reach recommendations about when therapy to reduce the platelet count should begin is described in Table 48.1. The recommendations described below are based on these data and take into account generalizations of management strategies for other known risk factors for venous and arterial thrombosis. The major candidates for platelet-lowering treatment are patients who are older than age 60 years or have a history of major thrombosis or major bleeding, or have a platelet count over $1{,}500 \times 10^9$/L ("high-risk" patients) because these variables were consistently associated with an increased rate of bleeding and thrombosis in cohort studies

Table 48.1 Cohort studies of risk factors for thrombosis and bleeding in essential thrombocythemia, including at least 100 patients.*

Study (Reference no.)	Patients, no.	Risk factors for thrombosis (RR or P)				Cardiovascular risk factors†
		Age >60	Previous thrombosis	Platelet count	Leukocytosis	
Cortelazzo et al. (9)	100	10.3 (2.05–51.5)	13 (4.1–41.5)	NS	—	NS
Besses et al. (31)	148	3.3 (1.5–7.4)	3.0 (1.5–6.0)	NS	—	4.7 (1.8–11.8)
Colombi et al. (32)	103	NS	$p < 0.001$	NS	—	—
Jantunen et al. (33)	132	NS	—	NS	—	$p = 0.01$
Bazzan et al. (34)	187	NS (age >55)	—	NS	—	NS
Wolanskyi et al. (4)	322	1.51 (1.05–2.18)	2.3 (1.25–4.24) (arterial only)	—	1.74 (1.15–2.66) (WBC $\geq 15 \times 10^9$/L)	NS
Carobbio et al. (17)	439	2.3 (1.3–3.9) (age >60 and previous thrombosis evaluated together)		NS	2.3 (1.4–3.9) (WBC $\leq 8.7 \times 10^9$/L)	—

Study (Ref)	Patients, no.	Risk factor for bleeding: Platelet count
van Genderen et al. (35)	200 (review of published cases)	$p < 0.001$ (platelets >1.000 × 10^9/L)
Fenaux et al. (36)	147	"higher risk" (platelets >2.000 × 10^9/L)
Wolanskyi et al. (4)	322	NS

*NS, not significant; WBC, white blood count.

†At least one of the following: smoking, hypertension, hypercholesterolemia, diabetes.

and were used for risk stratification in controlled clinical trials (9–11). Other potential determinants of vascular risk, including age in the range of 40–60 years, platelet count in the range of 1,000–1,500 × 10^9/L, cardiovascular risk factors (i.e., smoking, hypertension, hypercholesterolemia, diabetes mellitus) or the presence of thrombophilic conditions, are more contentious (5).

The presence of the V617F JAK2 mutation in about 50% of patients with ET raised the question whether mutated and non-mutated patients differ in terms of thrombotic risk. The largest prospective study on 806 patients suggested that JAK2 mutation in ET was associated with venous but not arterial events (12). An increased risk of thrombosis in JAK2 mutated patients was also retrospectively observed by other investigators (13,14). However, the rate of vascular complications was not affected by the presence of the mutation in two other relatively large retrospective studies, including 150 and 130 ET patients, respectively (15,16). It is possible that the higher age distribution and hematocrit and leukocyte levels consistently found in mutation-positive patients (12–16) contributed to the apparent association between JAK2 V617F and thrombosis reported in some studies.

Recently, a prognostic role for leukocytosis in MPDs has been advocated. Three large cohort studies have demonstrated that an increased leukocyte count is a novel independent risk factor for both thrombosis and inferior survival in ET (4,17) and for thrombosis in PV (18). In one study, a correlation between leukocytosis and the V617F JAK2 mutation was reported (17). In ET and PV, in vivo leukocyte activation has been shown to occur and to be associated with signs of activation of both platelets and endothelial cells (19). Platelet activation is increased in ET patients carrying the V617F JAK2 mutation (20). Thus, leukocyte and platelet activation may play a role in the generation of the prethrombotic state that characterizes ET, although further studies are required to translate these findings into clinical recommendations.

Recommendations

1. Patients who are older than age 60 years or have a history of major thrombosis or major bleeding or have a platelet count over 1,500 × 10^9/L (high-risk patients) should receive therapy to lower their platelet count (Grade 1B).

2. The Italian expert panel reached a consensus in considering candidates for cytoreductive therapy those patients who are between the ages of 40 to 60 years if their platelet count is over 1,000 × 10^9/L and they have a cardiovascular risk factor or familial thrombophilia, are younger than 40 years of age if they carry a comorbid condition that greatly increases their thrombotic risk (homocystinuria, familial dominant hypercholesterolemia) or suffer from severe microcirculatory symptoms, such as erythromelalgia, despite antiplatelet therapy (7) (Grade 1C).

3. Once the decision to start cytoreduction is made the target platelet count to reach and maintain ranges between 400 and 600 × 10^9/L. The lower threshold was recommended for patients with a history of a major thrombotic event. A platelet count of

Table 48.2 Retrospective studies of aspirin in essential thrombocythemia.*

Study (Reference no.)	Patients and follow-up	Dosage of ASA (mg/d)	Outcomes ASA treatment		
			Yes	No	p
Jensen et al. (37)	96 pts; 70 months (median)	100–150	Thrombosis or microvascular disturbances		
			21%	45%	0.017
van Genderen et al. (38)	68 pts; 1974–1993	100–500	Thrombosis or microvascular disturbances		
			3.6% pt-y	32.3 %pt-y	<0.001
			Bleeding		
			7.2% pt-y	1.6 % pt-y	0.032
Randi et al. (39)	195 pts; 6.3 years (median)	100	Thrombosis (primary prevention)		
			6.3%	2.5%	n.r.
			Thrombosis (secondary prevention)		
			13.6%	6.2%	n.r.
			Bleeding		
			12.9%	5.4%	n.r.

*n.r., not reported; pt-y, patient-year.

600×10^9/L may be more appropriate target for those patients with a high risk of toxicity, that is, patients who require higher than standard drug doses (7) (Grade 1C).

What is the treatment of choice for those patients who require therapy?

The main cytoreductive drugs currently in use for the treatment of "high-risk" ET patients are hydroxyurea (HU), anagrelide, and interferon-alpha. Only HU and anagrelide have been studied in randomized clinical trials (RCTs). The first RCT was performed about 10 years ago in Italy and evaluated 114 ET patients who were randomized to HU or no cytoreductive treatment (10). With a median follow-up of 27 months, two thromboses were recorded in the HU-treated group (1.6%/patient-year[pt-y]) compared with 14 in the control group (10.7%/pt-y; $p = 0.003$). This study provided the basis for considering HU as the standard therapy for high-risk ET patients and the reference arm for other randomized trials.

The second trial was carried out in the United Kingdom and compared HU and aspirin with anagrelide plus aspirin in 809 high risk ET patients analyzed with a median follow up of 39 months (21). Patients randomized to anagrelide and aspirin were more likely to reach the composite primary endpoint of major thrombosis (arterial or venous), major hemorrhage or death from a vascular cause ($p = 0.03$). When individual endpoints were assessed, arterial thrombosis, major hemorrhage and myelofibrosis were all significantly more frequent for patients treated with anagrelide ($p = 0.004$, 0.008, and 0.01, respectively). Intriguingly, venous thrombosis was however less frequent in patients treated with anagrelide ($p = 0.006$).

Based on the results of these two RCTs, HU is considered the drug of first choice in most high-risk ET patients who are candidates for platelet-lowering therapy. Importantly, the leukemogenicity of this agent is still debated. Some retrospective studies found that a proportion of ET patients treated with HU developed acute leukemia (22,23). In other prospective analysis, however, this drug was rarely associated with secondary malignancies when used alone, both in ET (24–26) and PV (27). To date, there are no randomized studies powered to assess the relative risk of malignant transformation in HU-treated patients. Nevertheless, most investigators agreed on using a cautionary principle against the use of hydroxyurea in very young subjects (below 40 years of age), even in the absence of strong evidence about the risk of malignant transformation due to the drug (5,7). Data evaluating the leukemogenicity of HU is discussed in Chapter 49 with respect to the use of this agent in treating patients with PV.

Interferon-alpha (IFN-α) has been evaluated in 27 clinical studies including 292 ET patients (reviewed in 7). No RCTs, systematic review, or meta-analysis has been found. Using the original response criteria of each study, the overall response rate in reducing platelet count was 85%, while 15% of the patients were resistant to the treatment and achieved no response. A reduction of splenomegaly, when present, was found in 66% of patients. A positive effect on clinical symptoms was reported, with their complete disappearance when platelet count was normalized. No controlled data on hard clinical endpoints, such as thrombosis, major bleeding, or death were available. At the beginning of IFN-α treatment, side effects (mainly flu-like syndrome) occurred in virtually all patients but thereafter they generally subsided, requiring drug discontinuation in 16% of patients. No deaths or leukemic transformations related to IFN-α are reported. This agent is not known to be teratogenic and does not cross the placenta.

Table 48.3 Case series of pregnancies in essential thrombocythemia, including at least 5 patients.

Study (Reference no.)	Patients no.	Pregnancies no.	Treatment during pregnancy (no. of pts.)	Outcomes	
				Maternal thrombohemorrhagic complications	Live births no. (%)
Beard et al. (40)	6	9	None (3) Aspirin alone (4) Aspirin + heparin (2) + ante-partum platelet apheresis (1)	1 hemorrhage post-partum 1 hemorrhage after abortion 1 superficial thrombophlebitis	8 (89%)
Beressi et al. (41)*	18	34	None (10) Aspirin alone (18) Other antiplatelet drugs (2) Cytoreductive drugs (4) + ante-partum platelet apheresis (3)	5 vaginal bleeding (mild to moderate)	17 (50%) (2 elective abortions; 1 ectopic pregnancy)
Pagliaro et al. (42)	9	15	None (5) Aspirin alone (3) Aspirin + heparin (7)	1 abdominal vein thrombosis	9 (60%) (1 elective abortion)
Randi et al. (43)	13	16	None (9) Aspirin alone (7)	1 cerebral thrombosis 2 abdominal vein thrombosis	13 (81%)
Bangerter et al. (44)	9	17	None (11) Aspirin alone (1) Aspirin + heparin (5)	3 major vaginal bleeding 2 minor bleeding (epistaxis) 1 transient visual loss	11 (65%)
Wright et al. (45)*	20	43	None (16) Aspirin alone (24) Heparin (1) Cytoreductive drugs (2) + ante-partum platelet apheresis (3)	3 vaginal bleeding (mild to moderate)	22 (51%) (2 elective abortions; 1 ectopic pregnancy)
Niittyvuopio et al. (46)	16	40	None (27) Aspirin alone (5) Aspirin + Interferon-alpha (5) Cytoreductive drugs (3)	2 cerebral and visual disturbances	25 (62%)

*Case series coming from the same Institution.

Recommendations

1. For patients who require therapy to lower their platelet count, HU is the agent of choice (Grade 1A).
2. For patients younger than age 40 who are candidates for platelet-lowering therapy, interferon or anagrelide can be considered an alternative first-line therapy. In case of side effects that impair patients' quality of life or, if there is a high toxicity risk (i.e., requirement of higher than standard doses) with the use of interferon and anagrelide, hydroxyurea is recommended (Grade 1C).
3. Interferon and anagrelide should also be considered as second-line therapy in high-risk ET patients refractory or intolerant of HU. The criteria for defining resistance or intolerance to hydroxyurea have been recently established by an International Working Group (28) and include: platelet count greater than 600 × 10^9/L after three months of at least 2 g/d of HU (2.5 g/d in patients with a body weight over 80 kg); platelet count greater than 400 × 10^9/L and WBC less than 2.5 × 10^9/L or Hb less than 10 g/dL at any dose of HU; presence of leg ulcers or other unacceptable mucocutaneous manifestations at any dose of HU; HU-related fever (Grade 1C).

When should antiplatelet therapy be used?

Only retrospective studies aimed at evaluating the antithrombotic efficacy of antiplatelet agents in ET are available (reviewed in 7 and summarized in Table 48.2). A randomized clinical trial showing a clear benefit/risk ratio of low-dose aspirin (100 mg/d) has been carried out in patients with PV (29), but translating this evidence to ET is questionable.

Recommendations

1. Low-dose aspirin is recommended for patients with microcirculatory symptoms or with a recent major arterial vascular event (ischemic stroke, transient ischemic attack, peripheral arterial occlusion, myocardial infarction, unstable angina) or clinical or laboratory evidence of coronary artery disease (Grade 1C).
2. Clopidogrel, 75 mg per day, should be reserved to patients who have major contraindications to aspirin therapy (aspirin intolerance or allergy, documented gastritis or peptic ulcer) (Grade 2C).
3. Antiplatelet therapy should be interrupted promptly in case of clinically significant bleeding while on treatment and withheld at least one week before elective surgery in interventions at high-risk of bleeding or in which even minor bleeding could result in life-threatening complications, like neurosurgery, or requiring heparin prophylaxis. Prescription or self-administration of nonsteroidal anti-inflammatory drugs in association with antiplatelet therapy should be strictly avoided (Grade 1C).

How should ET be managed in patients who are pregnant or of childbearing age?

No controlled studies addressing the management of pregnancy in ET have been published and current recommendation are based on pooled data from small-sized case series summarized in Table 48.3 (7,30).

Recommendations

1. Pregnant women are candidates for platelet-lowering therapy (high-risk pregnancy) when there is a history of major thrombosis, or major bleeding, or severe pregnancy complications or when the platelet count is greater than 1,500 × 10^9/L (Grade 1C).
2. In "low-risk" patients, antiplatelet therapy is recommended, particularly in the presence of a history of microvascular symptoms or with previous pregnancy failures (at least one event) (Grade 1C).
3. All pregnant women should also receive low- molecular-weight heparin at prophylactic doses (4,000 U daily) for six weeks in the puerperium (Grade 2C).
4. "High-risk" patients should receive prophylactic low-molecular-weight heparin throughout pregnancy and for at least six weeks in the puerperium (Grade 2C).
5. Women with a thrombotic episode (peripheral, placental) during pregnancy should receive low molecular weight heparin at therapeutic doses (100 U/kg twice daily) until at least six weeks in the puerperium (Grade 1C).
6. Pregnant women who are candidates for platelet-lowering therapy should receive interferon (Grade 2C).
7. Females with childbearing potential who are candidates to platelet-lowering therapy should receive first-line interferon therapy. In the presence of therapy side effects that impair patients' quality of life, these patients should receive anagrelide or hydroxyurea. Patients on anagrelide or hydroxyurea should be advised to stop taking the drug in the presence of menstrual delay, until the result of a pregnancy test is available (Grade 1C).

References

1 Tefferi A, Barbui T. *bcr/abl* negative, classic myeloproliferative disorders: diagnosis and treatment. *Mayo Clin Proc.* 2005;**80**:1220–32.
2 Schafer AI. Molecular basis of the diagnosis and treatment of polycythemia vera and essential thrombocythemia. *Blood.* 2006;**107**:4214–22.
3 Rozman C, Giralt M, Feliu E, et al. Life expectancy of patients with chronic nonleukemic myeloproliferative disorders. *Cancer.* 1991;**67**:2658–63.
4 Wolanskyj AP, Schwager SM, McClure RF, et al. Essential thrombocythemia beyond the first decade: life expectancy, long-term complication rates, and prognostic factors. *Mayo Clin Proc.* 2006;**81**:159–166.

5 Finazzi G, Harrison C. Essential thrombocythemia. *Semin Hematol.* 2005;**42**:230–8.

6 Barbui T, Finazzi G. When and how to treat essential thrombocythemia. *N Engl J Med.* 2005;**353**:85–86.

7 Barbui T, Barosi G, Grossi A, et al. Evidence- and consensus-based practice guidelines for the therapy of essential thrombocythemia:. a statement from the Italian Society of Hematology. *Haematologica.* 2004;**89**: 215–32.

8 Harbour R, Miller J for the Scottish Intercollegiate Guidelines Network Grading Review Group. A new system for grading recommendations in evidence based guidelines. *Br Med J.* 2001;**323**:334–36.

9 Cortelazzo S, Viero P, Finazzi G, et al. Incidence and risk factors for thrombotic complications in a historical cohort of 100 patients with essential thrombocythemia. *J Clin Oncol.* 1990;**8**:556–62.

10 Cortelazzo S, Finazzi G, Ruggeri M, et al. Hydroxyurea in the treatment of patients with essential thrombocythemia at high risk of thrombosis: a prospective randomized trial. *N Engl J Med.* 1995;**332**:1132–36.

11 Ruggeri M, Finazzi G, Tosetto A, et al. No treatment for low-risk essential thrombocythemia: results from a prospective study. *Br J Haematol.* 1998;**103**:772–77.

12 Campbell PJ, Scott LM, Buck G, et al. Definition of subtypes of essential thrombocythaemia and relation to polycythaemia vera based on JAK2 V617F mutation status: a prospective study. *Lancet.* 2005;**366**: 1945–53.

13 Cheung B, Radia D, Pantedelis P, et al. The presence of the JAK2 V617F mutation is associated with higher haemoglobin and increased risk of thrombosis in essential thrombocythaemia. *Br J Haematol.* 2005;**132**:244–50.

14 Finazzi G, Rambaldi A, Guerini V, et al. Risk of thrombosis in patients with essential thrombocythemia and polycythemia vera according to JAK2 V617F status. *Haematologica.* 2007; **92**:135–136.

15 Wolanskyj AP, Lasho TL, Schwager SM, et al. JAK2 V617F mutation in essential thrombocythaemia: clinical associations and long-term prognostic relevance. *Br J Haematol.* 2005;**131**:208–13.

16 Antonioli E, Guglielmelli P, Pancrazzi A, et al. Clinical implications of the JAK2 V617F mutation in essential thrombocythemia. *Leukemia.* 2005;**19**:1847–49.

17 Carobbio A, Finazzi G, Guerini V, et al. Leukocytosis is a risk factor for thrombosis in essential thrombocythemia: interaction with treatment, standard risk factors and JAK2 mutation status. *Blood.* 2007; **109**:2390–93.

18 Landolfi R, Di Nisio M, Finazzi G, et al. Leukocytosis as a major thrombotic risk factor in patients with polycythemia vera. *Blood.* 2007; **109**:2446–52.

19 Falanga A, Marchetti M, Barbui T, et al. Pathogenesis of thrombosis in essential thrombocythemia and polycythemia vera: the role of neutrophils. *Semin Hematol.* 2005;**42**:239–47.

20 Arellano-Rodrigo E, Alvarez-Larran A, Reverter JC, et al. Increased platelet and leukocyte activation as contributing mechanisms for thrombosis in essential thrombocythemia and correlation with the JAK2 mutation status. *Haematologica.* 2006;**91**:169–75.

21 Harrison CN, Campbell P, Buck G, et al. Hydroxyurea compared with anagrelide in high-risk essential thrombocythemia. *N Engl J Med.* 2005;**353**:33–45.

22 Lofvenberg E, Nordenson I, Walhlin A. Cytogenetic abnormalities and leukemic transformation in hydroxyurea-treated patients with Philadelphia chromosome negative chronic myeloproliferative disease. *Cancer Genet Cytogenet.* 1990;**49**:57–67.

23 Sterkers Y, Preudhomme C, Lai J-L, et al. Acute myeloid leukemia and myelodyslastic syndromes following essential thrombocythemia treated with hydroxyurea: high proportion of cases with 17p deletion. *Blood.* 1998;**91**:616–22.

24 Murphy S, Peterson P, Iland H, et al. Experience of the Polycythemia Vera Study Group with essential thrombocythemia: a final report on diagnostic criteria, survival and leukemic transition by treatment. *Semin Hematol.* 1997;**34**:29–39.

25 Finazzi G, Ruggeri M, Rodeghiero F, et al. Second malignancies in patients with essential thrombocythemia treated with busulphan and hydroxyurea: long-term follow-up of a randomized clinical trial. *Br J Haematol.* 2000;**110**:577–83.

26 Finazzi G, Ruggeri M, Rodeghiero F, et al. Efficacy and safety of long-term use of hydroxyurea in young patients with essential thrombocythemia and a high risk of thrombosis. *Blood.* 2003;**101**:3749.

27 Finazzi G, Caruso V, Marchioli R, et al. Acute leukemia in polycythemia vera: an analysis of 1638 patients enrolled in a prospective observational study. *Blood.* 2005;**105**:2664–70.

28 Barosi G, Besses C, Birgegard G, et al. A unified definition of clinical resistance/intolerance to hydroxyurea in essential thrombocythemia: results of a consensus process by an international working group. *Leukemia.* 2007;**21**:277–80.

29 Landolfi R, Marchioli R, Kutti J, et al. Efficacy and safety of low-dose aspirin in polycythemia vera. *N Engl J Med.* 2004;**350**:114–24.

30 Harrison C. Pregnancy and its management in the Philadelphia negative myeloproliferative diseases. *Br J Haematol.* 2005;**129**:293–306.

31 Besses C, Cervantes F, Pereira A, et al. Major vascular complications in essential thrombocythemia: a study of the predictive factors in a series of 148 patients. *Leukemia.* 1999;**13**:150–54.

32 Colombi M, Radaelli F, Zocchi L, et al. Thrombotic and hemorrhagic complications in essential thrombocythemia: a retrospective study of 103 patients. *Cancer.* 1991;**67**:2926–30.

33 Jantunen R, Juvonen E, Ikkala E, et al. The predictive value of vascular risk factors and gender for the development of thrombotic complications in essential thrombocythemia. *Ann Hematol.* 2001;**80**:74–78.

34 Bazzan M, Tamponi G, Schinco P, et al. Thrombosis-free survival and life expectancy in 187 consecutive patients with essential thrombocythemia. *Ann Hematol.* 1999;**78**:539–43.

35 Van Genderen PJJ, Michiels JJ. Erythromelalgic, thrombotic and haemorrhagic manifestations of thrombocythaemia. *Presse Med.* 1994;**23**: 73–77.

36 Fenaux P, Simon M, Caulier MT, et al. Clinical course of essential thrombocythemia in 147 cases. *Cancer.* 1990;**66**:549–56.

37 Jensen MK, de Nully Brown P, Nielsen OJ, et al. Incidence, clinical features and outcome of essential thrombocythaemia in a well defined geographical area. *Eur J Haematol.* 2000;**65**:132–39.

38 Van Genderen PJJ, Mulder PGH, Waleboer M, et al. Prevention and treatment of thrombotic complications in essential thrombocythemia: efficacy and safety of low-dose aspirin. *Br J Haematol.* 1997;**97**: 179–84.

39 Randi ML, Rossi C, Fabris F, et al. Aspirin seems as effective as myelosuppressive agents in the prevention of rethrombosis in essential thrombocythemia. *Clin Appl Thromb Hemost.* 1999;**5**:131–35.

40 Beard J, Hillmen P, Anderson CC, et al. Primary thrombocythemia in pregnancy. *Br J Haematol.* 1991;**77**:371–74.

41 Beressi AH, Tefferi A, Silverstein MN, et al. Outcome analysis of 34 pregnancies in women with essential thrombocythemia. *Arch Intern Med.* 1995;**155**:1217–22.

42 Pagliaro P, Arrigoni L, Muggiasca ML, et al. Primary thrombocythemia in pregnancy: treatment and outcome in fifteen cases. *Am J Hematol.* 1996;**53**:6–10.

43 Randi ML, Rossi C, Fabris F, et al. Essential thrombocythemia in young adults: treatment and outcome of 16 pregnancies. *J Intern Med.* 1999;**246**:517–18.

44 Bangerter M, Guthner C, Beneke H, et al. Pregnancy in essential thrombocythemia: treatment and outcome of 17 patients. *Eur J Haematol.* 2000;**65**:165–69.

45 Wright CA, Tefferi A. A single institutional experience with 43 pregnancies in essential thrombocythemia. *Eur J Haematol.* 2001;**66**:152–59.

46 Niittyvuopio R, Juvonen E, Kaaja R, et al. Pregnancy in essential thrombocythemia: experience with 40 pregnancies. *Eur J Haematol.* 2004;**73**:431–36.

49 Management of Patients with Polycythemia Vera

Guido Finazzi, Roberto Marchioli, Tiziano Barbui

Introduction

Polycythemia vera (PV) is a chronic myeloproliferative disorder (MPD) characterized by trilineage expansion of red cells, white cells and platelets without significant bone marrow fibrosis (1,2). Our understanding of pathophysiology of PV has advanced considerably with the recent discovery of an acquired mutation of JAK2 in the vast majority of patients. JAK2 is a member of the Janus kinase family of cytoplasmic tyrosine kinases that are associated with the intracellular domains of cytokine and growth factors receptors. The mutation replaces valine with phenylalanine in position 617 (V617F) of the JAK2 protein and causes cytokine-independent activation of several biochemical pathways implicated in erythropoietin receptor signaling (3–7). Besides molecular pathogenesis, the discovery of JAK2 V617F has had a major impact on the diagnostic approach to PV. Traditionally, PV was diagnosed on the basis of a set of internationally recognized criteria established by the Polycythemia Vera Study Group (PVSG) and then the World Health Organization (8,9). However, the observation that more than 90% of patients with PV carry JAK2 V617F supports the recommendation that peripheral blood mutation screening for the mutation be incorporated into the initial evaluation of all patients with suspected PV (1,2).

Early studies in untreated PV patients found a high incidence of thrombotic events and a life expectancy of about 18 months after diagnosis (10). Cytoreductive treatments of blood hyperviscosity by phlebotomy or chemotherapy have dramatically reduced the number of thrombotic events, even though haematological transformations towards myelofibrosis and acute leukemia (AL) still represent a major cause of death (11). Since there is a concern that myelosuppressive drugs given to control the proliferative phase of the disease might be implicated in the long-term complications, current treatment recommendations should be adapted on the expected risk for thrombosis of the patient (12).

Evidence-based Hematology. Edited by Mark A. Crowther, Jeff Ginsberg, Holger J. Schünemann, Ralph M. Meyer, and Richard Lottenberg.
 ISBN: 978-1-4051-5747-6.

Questions

1. How should patients be stratified into risk categories?
2. Which therapy should low-risk patients receive?
3. Which therapy should high-risk patients receive?
4. When myelosupressive therapy is required, how can the risk of leukemogenesis be reduced?

Literature-search strategy and inclusion

MEDLINE, PubMed, CANCERLIT, Cochrane Library, and EMBASE were systematically searched for publication in English from 1980 to November 2006. Reference lists and articles from the authors' libraries and older references generated from initial papers were also examined. Randomized clinical trials (RCTs), longitudinal studies and case series were considered if appropriate. A summary of RCTs published in PV is reported in Table 49.1.

Grading of the quality of evidence and strengths of recommendations in this chapter are based on the guidelines proposed by the international Grading of Recommendations Assessment, Development, and Evaluation Working Group (GRADE) adopting the modification used by the American College of Chest Physicians that merges the "very low" and "low" categories of quality of evidence (see chapter 1).

How should patients be stratified into risk categories?

The largest and most recent prospective study evaluating risk factors for survival and thrombosis is the European Collaboration on Low-dose Aspirin in Polycythemia (ECLAP) (11). In this cohort of 1,638 patients, the incidence of cardiovascular complications

Table 49.1 Randomized clinical trials in polycythemia vera.*

Study (Reference)	Patients and follow-up	Treatments and main results			p
PVSG-01 (8)	**431 pts; 18 y (max)**	**32P**	**Phlebotomy**	**Chlorambucil**	
			Median survival		
		11.8 y	13.9 y	8.9 y	0.02
			Thrombosis		
		30%	34%	25%	0.08
			Acute Leukemia		
		10%	1.5%	13%	<0.0012
EORTC (35)	**293 pts; 8 y (median)**	**32P**		**Busulphan**	
			10-y survival		
		55%		70%	0.02
			Vascular deaths		
		18%		5%	n.r.
Najean et al. (36)	**461 pts** (age >65 y); **16 y (max)**	**32P**		**32P+Hydroxyurea**	
			Median survival		
		10.9 y		9.3 y	n.s.
Najean et al. (21)	**292 pts** (age <65 y); **16 y (max)**	**Hydroxyurea**		**Pipobroman**	
			14-y survival		
		70%		70%	n.s.
			Myelofibrosis		
		17%		2.1%	0.03
PVSG-05 (37)	**166 pts; 1.2 y (median)**	**ASA (900 mg/d)***		**32P**	
			Thrombosis		
		8%		2%	n.r.
			Bleeding		
		7%		0%	0.02
GISP (38)	**112 pts; 1.4 y (median)**	**ASA (40 mg/d)**		**Placebo**	
			Thrombosis		
		5%		7.7%	n.s.
			Bleeding		
		1.7%		1.9%	n.s.
ECLAP (19)	**518 pts; 2.8 y (median)**	**ASA (100 mg/d)**		**Placebo**	
			Death from any cause		
		3.6%		6.8%	n.s.
			Thrombosis		
		6.7%		15.5%	0.003
			Major bleeding		
		1.2%		0.8%	n.s.

*n.r., not reported; n.s., not significant.

†plus phlebotomy and dypiridamole.

was higher in those ages more than 65 years (5.0% patient-year, hazard ratio [HR] 2.0, 95% confidence interval [CI] 1.22–3.29, $p < 0.006$) or with a history of thrombosis (4.93% patient-year, HR 1.96, 95% CI 1.29–2.97, $p = 0.0017$) than in younger subjects with no history of thrombosis (2.5% patient-year, reference category). These data confirm previous findings that increasing age and a history of thrombosis are the two most important prognostic factors for development of vascular complications (8). Actually, age is a continuous variable and the cut-off dividing low from high risk patients is in part arbitrary. Since most authorities establish this threshold at 60 years (1,12), we used this value in the recommendation given in Table 49.2.

The ECLAP and other prospective studies failed to show any association between platelet count and thrombotic events (8,11). Thus, current treatment does not primarily aim at lowering the platelet count. Interestingly, leukocytosis was recently found to be an independent risk factor for thrombosis both in PV and in essential thrombocythemia (ET) (13–15). Leukocytes may play

Table 49.2 Risk stratification in polycythemia vera based on thrombotic risk.

Risk category	Age > 60 years or history of thrombosis	Cardiovascular risk factors*
Low	NO	No
Intermediate	NO	Yes
High	YES	

* Hypertension, hypercholesterolemia, diabetes, smoking, congestive heart failure.

an important and hitherto underestimated role in the generation of the prethrombotic state of MPDs that is worth to be further explored (16).

Other significant risk factors for cardiovascular morbidity in PV are hypertension, hypercholesterolemia, smoking, diabetes mellitus, and congestive heart failure. These disorders should be managed aggressively (17) and, when present in a young patient without prior thrombosis ("low-risk" patient), define an "intermediate risk" category (1).

Recommendations

1. Patients with PV can be stratified into three risk categories on the basis of their probability of developing thrombotic complications (Table 49.2). This classification forms the rationale for the indication of therapy (Grade 1C).
2. Patients in an intermediate-risk category (Table 49.2) should be managed as per patients in the low-risk category and in addition, should have aggressive management of their cardiovascular risk factors (Grade 1C).

Which therapy should low-risk patients receive?

The treatment options that have been considered for these patients have included phlebotomy, myelosuppressive therapy, and aspirin. A single randomized study comparing phlebotomy with myelosuppressive therapy was done by the PVSG more than 20 years ago (8). Between 1967 and 1974, 431 patients were randomized to one of the following treatments: (a) phlebotomy alone; (b) radiophosphorus (32P) plus phlebotomy, and (c) chlorambucil plus phlebotomy. Patients randomized to the phlebotomy arm showed a higher incidence of thrombosis in the first three years of treatment. According to the authors, a major determinant of this high risk was the fact that over the first few years of the study the target hematocrit marking adequate treatment was below 0.52. When subsequently hematocrit was lowered to less than 0.45, the rate of thrombosis in the phlebotomy arm was reduced. However, the recent ECLAP study failed to show a clear effect of hematocrit values in the range of 0.45–0.50 on the thrombotic rate (18). Future prospective studies are going to be planned to answer the question of the target hematocrit to be pursued in low-risk PV patients. After 3 to 5 years of study, the rate of thrombosis in all three arms of the PVSG trial became similar but patients treated with 32P or chlorambucil began to develop an excess incidence of acute leukemia, lymphoma, and carcinomas of the gastrointestinal tract and skin. Patients treated in the phlebotomy arm of the PVSG trial therefore had a better overall median survival at 13.9 years than the other two arms (chlorambucil 8.9 years, radiophosphorus 11.8 years) (8). The efficacy and safety of low-dose aspirin (100 mg daily) in PV has been formally assessed in a double-blind, placebo-controlled, randomized clinical trial carried out in the setting of the ECLAP project (19). Aspirin lowered significantly the risk of a primary combined endpoint including cardiovascular death, nonfatal myocardial infarction, nonfatal stroke and major venous thromboembolism (relative risk 0.4 [95% CI 0.18–0.91], $p = 0.0277$). Total and cardiovascular mortality were also reduced by 46% and 59%, respectively. Major bleeding was slightly increased by aspirin (relative risk 1.6, 95% CI 0.27–9.71).

Recommendations

1. Low-risk patients should not receive myelosuppressive therapy (Grade 1A).
2. Phlebotomy should be considered the cornerstone of therapy of PV and is recommended to all patients (Grade 1A).
3. Antithrombotic preventive strategy with low-dose aspirin is recommended to all PV patients who do not have a contraindication to this therapy (Grade 1A).

Which therapy should high-risk patients receive?

In PV, the evidence for selecting cytotoxic therapy comes from very few randomized clinical trials (Table 49.1), and the most relevant treatment options for consideration have included hydroxyurea and interferon-alpha (IFN-alpha). In the seminal PVSG 01 trial (8), patients given myelosuppressive drugs had an excess of AL documented in 13% of patients in chlorambucil arm; in contrast only 1.5% of AL was reported in the phlebotomy arm. To reduce the AL incidence related to chlorambucil and 32P, the PVSG investigated hydroxyurea (HU), an antimetabolite that prevents DNA synthesis. At that time, HU was assumed not to be leukemogenic. After a median follow-up treatment of 8.6 years, 51 patients had an incidence of leukemia of 9.8% (vs. 3.7% in the historical phlebotomized controls) but less myelofibrosis (7.8% vs, 12.7%) and fewer total deaths (39.2% vs. 55.2%) (20).

The efficacy and safety of HU in PV have also been analyzed in a randomized clinical trial carried out in France (21); 292 patients age less than 65 years were randomized to treatment with HU or pipobroman and followed from 1980 until 1997. Pipobroman is a bromide derivative of piperazine with a chemical formula similar to the alkylating agents but a mechanism of action also involving metabolic competition of pyrimidine bases. No significant differences between the two groups were observed in overall survival, rate of thrombotic complications and incidence of secondary leukemia (about 5% at the 10th and 10% at the 13th year).

A significant increase in risk of progression to myelofibrosis was seen in the patients treated with HU (26 cases) compared to those treated with pipobroman (3 cases).

These studies, and translated evidence from randomized clinical trials carried out in ET (22,23) (reviewed in chapter 48), indicate that HU is the drug of choice in PV patients at high risk of thrombosis, despite concerns regarding its leukemogenic potential (24,25). New drugs known to be not leukemogenic have been proposed in PV. Silver, the first to report on the efficacy and safety of IFN-alpha in PV (26), found a complete response in 90% of 55 patients (median age 49 years) (27), while Lengfelder in a retrospective analysis of 16 prospective nonrandomized studies calculated a rate of complete remission, defined as a stable hematocrit of 45% without concomitant phlebotomies, in 50% of patients (28). Noteworthy, no case of leukemia was registered. Recently, semisynthetic pegylated forms of IFN-alpha (peg-IFN alpha) have been used to treat MPDs, which in a limited number of studies have been shown to be superior to unmodified IFN-alpha as related to its adverse event profile and efficacy (29). In one study, the use of peg-IFN alpha-2a was able to decrease the percentage of mutated JAK2 allele in 24 of 27 treated PV patients from a mean of 49% to a mean of 27% (30). Overall, the role of IFN- alpha in PV therapy requires controlled clinical trials evaluating long-term clinical endpoints.

Recommendations

1. In high-risk patients who will require myelosuppressive therapy, HU is the treatment of choice (Grade 1B).
2. Due to its high cost and toxicity, IFN-alpha should be reserved to selected categories of patients such as pregnant women, very young subjects or those with intolerance to HU or intractable pruritus (Grade 2C).

When myelosuppressive therapy is required, how can the risk of leukemogenesis be reduced?

Because HU still remains the most used cytotoxic drug in PV patients requiring myelosuppression the issue of its leukemogenic potential is of crucial clinical importance. Two studies from France (24) and Italy (31) revealed a high frequency of 17p chromosomal deletions in patients with acutely transformed disease who were treated with HU, suggesting that these cytogenetic abnormalities might represent a possible leukemogenic mechanism of the drug. However, the 17p deletion also occurs in other hematological disorders, including both de novo and treatment-related cases of AL and myelodysplastic syndromes. Moreover, further analysis of the French data revealed a stronger association of 17p- with advanced age than with HU treatment (32). In another study, in vivo exposure to HU was not associated with any increase of acquired DNA mutations (33).

To date there are no randomized studies powered to assess the relative risk of malignant transformation in HU-treated MPD patients. These disorders have an inherent tendency to evolve into AL, even in the absence of specific therapy. Thus, studies that enrolled patients in need of therapy automatically selected patients with more active disease and thus with a higher propensity to malignant transformation. Furthermore, leukemic transformation occurs after a lead time of several years. Consequently, only long-term studies with a large number of patients are suitable to assess this issue. The 1,638 patients prospectively enrolled in the ECLAP study, with a median disease duration of 6.3 years, represent a particularly appropriate population to reach this goal. In a recent analysis of the leukemogenic risk in these patients, HU alone did not enhance the risk of leukemia in comparison with patients treated with phlebotomy only (HR 0.86, 95% CI 0.26–2.88; $p = 0.8$) whereas this risk was significantly increased by exposure to radiophosphorus, busulphan, or pipobroman (HR 5.46, 95% CI 1.84–16.25; $p = 0.002$) (1). The use of HU in patients already treated with alkylating agents or radiophosphorus also enhanced the leukemic risk (HR 7.58, 95% CI 1.85–31; $p = 0.0048$) (34).

Recommendations

1. The bulk of evidence briefly discussed here does not support a clear leukemogenic role for HU and therefore this drug remains the best option in most PV patients at high-risk for thrombosis (1,2,12,17) (Grade 2C).
2. Because of remaining uncertainty about the true risk of leukemogenesis, HU should be used with caution in very young subjects and in those carrying cytogenetic abnormalities and should be avoided in pregnant women and in patients previously exposed to radiophosphorus or alkylating drugs (Grade 1C).

References

1 Tefferi A, Barbui T. *bcr/abl* negative, classic myeloproliferative disorders: diagnosis and treatment. *Mayo Clin Proc.* 2005;**80**:1220–32.
2 Campbell PJ, Green AR. The myeloproliferative disorders. *N Engl J Med.* 2006;**355**:2452–66.
3 James C, Ugo V, Le Couedic JP, et al. A unique clonal JAK2 mutation leading to constitutive signaling causes polycythemia vera. *Nature.* 2005;**434**:1144–48.
4 Levine RL, Wadleigh M, Cools J, et al. Activating mutation of the tyrosine kinase JAK2 in polycythemia vera, essential thrombocythemia, and myeloid metaplasia with myelofibrosis. *Cancer Cell.* 2005;**7**: 387–97.
5 Baxter EJ, Scott LM, Campbell PJ, et al. Acquired mutation of the tyrosine kinase JAK2 in human myeloproliferative diseases. *Lancet.* 2005;**365**:1054–61.
6 Kralovics R, Passamonti F, Buser AS, et al. A gain-of-function mutation of JAK2 in myeloproliferative disorders. *N Engl J Med.* 2005;**352**:1779–90.
7 Jones AV, Kreil S, Zoi K, et al. Widespread occurrence of the JAK2 V617 mutation in chronic myeloproliferative disorders. *Blood.* 2005;**106**:2162–68.
8 Berk PD, Goldberg JD, Donovan PB, et al. Therapeutic recommendations in polycythemia vera based on Polycythemia Vera Study Group protocols. *Semin Hematol.* 1986;**23**:132–43.

9 Pierre R, Vardiman JW, Imbert M, et al., editors. *WHO pathology and genetics of tumours of haematopoietic and lymphoid tissues.* Lyon: IARC Press; 2001. p. 32–34.
10 Chievitz E, Thiede T. Complications and causes of death in poliycythemia vera. *Acta Med Scand.* 1962;**172**:513–23.
11 Marchioli R, Finazzi G, Landolfi R, et al. Vascular and neoplastic risk in a large cohort of patients with polycythemia vera. *J Clin Oncol.* 2005;**23**:2224–32.
12 Barbui T, Finazzi G. Evidence-based management of polycythemia vera. *Best Pract Res Clin Haematol.* 2006; **19**:483–93.
13 Landolfi R, Di Gennaro L, Barbui T, et al. Leukocytosis as a major thrombotic risk factor in patients with Polycythemia Vera. *Blood.* 2007;2446–52.
14 Wolanskyj AP, Schwager SM, McClure RF, et al. Essential thrombocythemia beyond the first decade: life expectancy, long-term complication rates, and prognostic factors. *Mayo Clin Proc.* 2006;**81**: 159–66.
15 Carobbio A, Finazzi G, Guerini V, et al. Leukocytosis is a risk factor for thrombosis in essential thrombocythemia: interaction with treatment, standard risk factors and JAK2 mutation status. *Blood.* 2007;**109**:2310–36.
16 Falanga A, Marchetti M, Vignoli A, et al. Leukocyte-platelet interaction in patients with essential thrombocythemia and polycythemia vera. *Exp Hematol.* 2005;**33**:523–30.
17 McMullin MF, Bareford D, Campbell P, et al. Guidelines for the diagnosis, investigation and management of polycythaemia/erythrocytosis. *Br J Haematol.* 2005;**130**:174–95.
18 Di Nisio M, Barbui T, Di Gennaro L, et al. The hematocrit and platelet target in polycythemia vera. *Br J Haematol.* 2007;**136**:249–59.
19 Landolfi R, Marchioli R, Kutti J, et al. Efficacy and safety of low-dose aspirin in polycythemia vera. *N Engl J Med.* 2004;**350**:114–24.
20 Fruchtman SM, Mack K, Kaplan ME, et al. From efficacy to safety: a polycythemia vera study group report on hydroxyurea in patients with polycythemia vera. *Semin Hematol.* 1997;**34**:17–23.
21 Najean Y, Rain JD for the French Polycythemia Study Group. Treatment of polycythemia vera: the use of hydroxyurea and pipobroman in 292 patients under the age of 65 years. *Blood.* 1997;**90**:3370–77.
22 Cortelazzo S, Finazzi G, Ruggeri M, et al. Hydroxyurea in the treatment of patients with essential thrombocythemia at high risk of thrombosis: a prospective randomized trial. *N Engl J Med.* 1995;**332**:1132–36.
23 Harrison CN, Campbell PJ, Buck G, et al. Hydroxyurea compared with anagrelide in high-risk essential thrombocythemia. *N Engl J Med.* 2005;**353**:33–45.
24 Sterkers Y, Preudhomme C, Lai J-L, et al. Acute myeloid leukemia and myelodyslastic syndromes following essential thrombocythemia treated with hydroxyurea: high proportion of cases with 17p deletion. *Blood.* 1998;**91**:616–22.
25 Nand S, Stock W, Godwin J, et al. Leukemogenic risk of hydroxyurea therapy in polycythemia vera, essential thrombocythemia and myeloid metaplasia with myelofibrosis. *Am J Hematol.* 1996;**52**:42–46.
26 Silver RT. Interferon alpha2b: a new treatment for polycythemia vera. *Ann Intern Med.* 1993;**119**:1091–92.
27 Silver RT. Long-term effects of the treatment of polycythemia vera with recombinant interferon-alpha. *Cancer.* 2006;**107**:451–58.
28 Lengfelder E, Berger U, Hehlmann R. Interferon alpha in the treatment of polycythemia vera. *Ann Hematol.* 2000;**79**:103–9.
29 Quintas-Cardama A, Kantarjian HM, Giles F, et al. Pegylated interferon therapy for patients with Philadelphia chromosome-negative myeloproliferative disorders. *Semin Thromb Hemost.* 2006;**32**:409–16.
30 Kiladjian JJ, Cassinat B, Turlure P, et al. High molecular response rate of polycythemia vera patients treated with pegylated interferon alpha-2a. *Blood.* 2006;**108**:2037–40.
31 Bernasconi P, Boni M, Cavigliano PM, et al. Acute myeloid leukemia (AML) having evolved from essential thrombocythemia (ET): distinctive chromosomal abnormalities in patients treated with pipobroman or hydroxyurea. *Leukemia.* 2002;**16**:2078–83.
32 Liu TC, Suri R. Multiple factors in the transformation of essential thrombocythemia to acute leukemia or myelodysplastic syndromes. *Blood.* 1998;**92**:1465–66.
33 Hanft VN, Fruchtman SR, Pickens CV, et al. Acquired DNA mutations associated with in vivo hydroxyurea exposure. *Blood.* 2000;**95**:3589–93.
34 Finazzi G, Caruso V, Marchioli R, et al. Acute leukemia in polycythemia vera. An analysis of 1,638 patients enrolled in a prospective observational study. *Blood.* 2005;**105**:2664–70.
35 Haanen C, Mathe G, Hayat M. Treatment of polycythemia vera by radiophosphorus or busulphan: a randomised clinical trial. *Br J Cancer.* 1981;**44**:75–78.
36 Najean Y, Rain JD for the French Polycythemia Study Group. Treatment of polycythemia vera: use of 32P alone or in combination with maintenance therapy using hydroxyurea in 461 patients greater than 65 years of age. *Blood.* 1997;**89**:2319–27.
37 Tartaglia AP, Goldberg JD, Berk PD, et al. Adverse effects of antiaggregating platelet therapy in the treatment of polycythemia vera. *Semin Hematol.* 1986;**23**:172–76.
38 Gruppo Italiano Studio Policitemia. Low-dose aspirin in polycythemia vera: a pilot study. *Br J Haematol.* 1997;**97**:453–56.

50 Evidence-based Review of Therapies in Multiple Myeloma

Michael Sebag, A. Keith Stewart

Multiple myeloma (MM) is the second most common hematological malignancy in adults with an annual incidence of 4.3 cases per 100,000 people (1). For many decades, the therapeutic standard of care has been oral melphalan with prednisone (2). However, the last decade has seen tremendous advances in our understanding of this disease and has rewarded us with a range of therapeutic options that were previously unavailable. These options range from high-dose chemotherapy with autologous stem cell transplant to newer agents with novel mechanisms of action such as bortezomib, thalidomide, and lenalidomide. In this chapter, we systematically review the literature regarding specific aspects of myeloma therapy.

Grading of the quality of evidence and strengths of recommendations in this chapter are based on the guidelines proposed by the international Grading of Recommendations Assessment, Development, and Evaluation Working Group (GRADE) adopting the modification used by the American College of Chest Physicians that merges the very low and low categories of quality of evidence (see chapter 1).

Questions

1. In patients who are to undergo autologous transplantation as initial therapy, is dexamethasone with thalidomide superior to dexamethasone alone as initial therapy for untreated MM?
2. Does the addition of thalidomide to melphalan and prednisone improve outcomes in untreated patients?
3. Does high dose therapy followed by stem cell transplant improve outcomes compared with conventional therapy?
4. Is bortezomib superior to dexamethasone in relapsed/ refractory myeloma?
5. What is the role of lenalidomide in patients with relapsed or refractory myeloma?

Evidence-based Hematology. Edited by Mark A. Crowther, Jeff Ginsberg, Holger J. Schünemann, Ralph M. Meyer, and Richard Lottenberg.
 ISBN: 978-1-4051-5747-6.

Literature-search strategy and inclusions

For all questions, MEDLINE(OVID), CANCERLIT, and the Cochrane Library were searched and review articles were screened and discarded while all clinical trials were evaluated for inclusion. The specific literature searches are included within the sections dealing with each question.

In patients who are to undergo autologous transplantation as initial therapy is dexamethasone with thalidomide superior to dexamethasone alone as initial therapy for untreated multiple myeloma?

The use of multiagent cytotoxic chemotherapy pre-transplantation in newly diagnosed multiple myeloma patients confers unique disadvantages, including myelosuppression and the use of central indwelling catheters, which predispose to infection and sepsis. Less toxic approaches to induction therapy would therefore be advantageous and welcome. Dexamethasone remains one of the most powerful antimyeloma agents, said to account for 85% of response rates seen in newly diagnosed patients treated with the well known induction regimen VAD (vincristine, adriamycin, dexamethasone) (3). Thalidomide has shown considerable activity as a single agent in relapsed or refractory myeloma (4). In this section, we will examine the clinical efficacy of dexamethasone alone versus dexamethasone in combination with thalidomide in newly diagnosed multiple myeloma patients. The search strategy included the combination of the following terms (myeloma OR plasmacytoma) AND (thalidomide AND dexamethasone). Trials were included if they evaluated thalidomide alone or in combination with dexamethasone in patients that have not had any prior therapy for a diagnosis of multiple myeloma. Trials evaluating dexamethasone and/or thalidomide in combination with any other agent(s) were excluded. This search yielded several phase II studies and only one randomized phase III trial.

The first phase II study was published in 2002 and included a series of 50 previously untreated symptomatic (stage II/III) MM patients from the Mayo Clinic who received either dexamethasone alone or dexamethasone in combination with thalidomide (5). Following four cycles of therapy patients proceeded to autologous stem cell transplant if eligible. Thalidomide was given at doses ranging from 100 mg/d to the very high dose of 800 mg/d. A response was observed in 68%, while another 28% demonstrated stable disease. The largest phase II trial showed similar results (66% response rate) in 71 preautologous stem cell transplantation patients who received a more reasonable 200mg/d dose (6).

Only one randomized controlled trial has been published to date (7). Two hundred and seven untreated symptomatic patients were randomly assigned to 200 mg/d of thalidomide for four weeks in addition to 40 mg/d of dexamethasone for four days on days 1–4, 9–12, and 17–20 or to dexamethasone on the same schedule as the single agent. Response in the thalidomide-dexamethasone arm was significantly higher than with dexamethasone alone (63% vs. 41%). Four percent of patients in the combination arm had complete responses by ECOG criteria versus none in the dexamethasone alone arm. The study was not powered to look at survival or relapse rate postautologous stem cell transplantation.

Toxicities reported in the single randomized trial included a 4%–5% treatment-related mortality rate in both arms of the study (7). The overall rates of grade 3 nonhematologic toxicities were 67% of patients treated with thalidomide plus dexamethasone and 43% of patients with dexamethasone alone. The most impressive toxicity was that of thrombosis/embolism, seen 19.6% of patients treated with thalidomide plus dexamethasone and in only 3% in dexamethasone treated patients and no thromboprophylaxis was used.

Although data supporting the use of thalidomide and dexamethasone as initial myeloma therapy is still evolving, in one randomized controlled trial the combination of thalidomide and dexamethasone has demonstrated superior response rates in comparison with dexamethasone alone for untreated myeloma patients that are candidates for autologous stem cell transplantation. This combination has possible advantages over combination chemotherapy for initial myeloma therapy such as VAD, although these are only now being directly and prospectively compared (8). As serious toxicities exist, including a very high incidence of thrombosis, the benefits of this combination must be weighed against the inherent risks. Although not adequately addressed in these studies, and beyond the scope of this review, the use of thromboprophylaxis is advisable prior to starting therapy. Readers should also be aware that results of randomized controlled trials testing bortezomib and lenalidomide in newly diagnosed patients are now emerging.

Recommendations

1. Based on a superior response rate, the combination of thalidomide plus dexamethasone is recommended over dexamethasone alone as induction therapy for patients who are to undergo autologous stem cell transplantation. As there is a high incidence of thrombosis and no evidence of a survival benefit, the strength of the recommendation is downgraded (Grade 2A).

2. The issues of thromboprophylaxis and the relative comparison of thalidomide plus dexamethasone in comparison with VAD require further study.

Does the addition of thalidomide to melphalan and prednisone improve outcomes in untreated patients?

The combination of melphalan and prednisone (MP) has been the mainstay of myeloma therapy for over 40 years (2). As the alkylator, melphalan can interfere with successful peripheral stem cell collection and MP is now reserved for primary therapy in patients who are not eligible for transplantation because of advanced age, poor performance status, or significant comorbidities. To improve this outcome, thalidomide has been advanced as a nonchemotherapeutic modality to be added to this standard therapy. This section will examine the evidence for the addition of thalidomide to standard MP therapy. The search strategy included the combination of the following terms (myeloma OR plasmacytoma) AND (thalidomide AND melphalan). All trials were included if they evaluated the combination of melphalan, prednisone, and thalidomide in patients that have not had any prior therapy for a diagnosis of multiple myeloma and are ineligible for autologous stem cell transplantation. This search strategy yielded seven clinical trials. Of these, only two were in untreated patients and only two are randomized clinical trials (9,10); Palumbo 2006). A third randomized trial was presented at the 2006 American Society of Clinical Oncology is also included (11).

The sole published phase III clinical trial randomized 331 stage II-III patients that were at least 65 years old or older and ineligible for stem cell transplantation (10). These patients received either standard therapy (melphalan 4 mg/m^2 on day 1–7 and prednisone at 40 mg/m^2 on days 1–7 every 4 weeks for six cycles) or standard therapy with the addition of thalidomide at 100 mg/d (MPT) continuously and continued as maintenance therapy until confirmed evidence of relapse or progression. The trial was stopped prematurely at the second interim analysis when it became evident that the MPT group demonstrated a significantly improved response rate and event-free survival rate compared with the MP group. Overall response rate in the MPT group was 76% as compared with 45% in the MP group. Of significance, there were 15.5% complete responders in the MPT group versus only 2.4% in the MP group. The 2-year event-free survival (a composite endpoint of time to relapse or death from any cause) was 54% in the MPT group and significantly higher than in the MP group (hazard ratio [HR] 0.51, 95% confidence interval [CI] 0.35–0.75, $p = 0.0006$). Although the overall survival (OS) was not statistically different, the trial design did not include the statistical power to address this question. Powered to look at overall survival, a large French cooperative study, presented in abstract form, confirmed the latter study and showed an improved median OS of 32.2% with MP alone compared with 53.6% in the MPT arm (HR 1.8, 95% CI 1.3–2.6, $p = 0.001$) (11). In these trials, significant toxicities were

Table 50.1 Results of Phase III Trials Comparing Stem Cell Transplantation with Conventional Chemotherapy.*

		% CR		Median EFS		Median OS	
Trial	**No. of patients**	**SD**	**HDT**	**SD**	**HDT**	**SD**	**HDT**
IFM90	200	5	22†	18	28†	44	57†
MRC VII	401	8	44†	20	32†	42	54†
MAG91	190	NR	NR	19	24†	50	55
Pethema	164	11	30†	33	42	61	66
HOVON	379	13	29†	21	22	50	47
NACG	427	15	17	7y EFS 14%	7y EFS 17%	7y OS 38%	7y OS 39%

*SD, standard dose; HDT, high-dose therapy; CR, complete remission; EFS, event-free survival; OS, overall survival.
†Significantly different from SD group.

observed more frequently in patients receiving thalidomide, including neuropathy, infection, and venous thromboembolism.

Recommendation

Based on the results of two randomized trials that provide consistent results, induction treatment with melphalan, prednisone plus thalidomide is recommended for patients who will not be considered for autologous stem cell transplantation (Grade 1A).

Does high dose therapy followed by stem cell transplant improve outcomes compared with conventional therapy?

The rationale of treating MM with high dose therapy followed by autologous stem cell rescue is borne from the observation that there is a dose responsive effect of melphalan chemotherapy in myeloma (12). Early reports showed that high-dose therapy and stem cell transplantation could be performed safely and may have a beneficial effect on survival. However, subsequent publications have somewhat muddied these promises showing modest, if any long-term survival benefit. In this section, we will address these conflicting results. The search strategy included the combination of the following terms (myeloma OR plasmacytoma) AND (bone marrow transplantation OR peripheral blood stem cell transplantation OR autologous stem cell transplant OR high dose therapy). While 42 articles were selected for review, only 15 specifically addressed the question of high dose therapy versus conventional therapy by clinical trial. Of these, six are randomized phase III clinical trials. One meta-analysis was also included in this review.

Results of the six trials reviewed for this evaluation are summarized in Table 50.1. The first randomized controlled trial comparing high-dose to conventional therapy was the French IFM90 trial, which randomized 200 patients (13). The conventional chemotherapy arm consisted of VMCP/VBAP for 12 months while the high dose arm received four to six cycles followed by an intermediate dose of melphalan (140 mg/m^2) with TBI and bone marrow rescue. The complete response rate, event-free survival and overall survival were all significantly higher in the high dose therapy arm (Table 50.1). Long-term follow-up of these patients also confirmed the survival benefits of high-dose therapy (OS 43% vs. 25%, $p = 0.03$) (14). Echoing these results, an MRC trial demonstrated an increased median survival with high dose therapy in a study including 401 patients, 54% versus 42% in patients receiving conventional chemotherapy alone (15).

In contrast, three other randomized trials did not show a survival benefit to high-dose therapy and transplantation. The second French study MAG91 and its long-term follow-up report showed a benefit in EFS but no significant improvement in overall survival (16,17). A Belgian-Dutch (HOVON) study as well as a North American cooperative (NACG) study also reported improved EFS but no improvement in OS (18,19). These last three trials, however, all allowed patients to undergo autologous transplantation once they had failed conventional therapy. Delayed transplantation may shed light as to why these trials all showed improved EFS but equivalent OS. A smaller Spanish trial (PETHEMA), which also allowed delayed transplantation for relapse, showed superior EFS and OS with high-dose therapy compared with conventional therapy, but these were not statistically significant (20). However, a smaller percentage of relapsed patients received transplantation than in other similarly designed studies. A recently published meta-analysis that combined only the three French studies, including the MAG91, concluded that high-dose therapy improved EFS but not overall survival. However, the result of the meta-analysis may have been weighed against transplantation because of its inclusion of the MAG91 trial, which allowed delayed transplantation (21).

Prognostic factors related to transplantation were assessed prospectively only in the above randomized trials. None of these reports included specific evaluations, including statistical testing for an interaction to evaluate predictive properties of the prognostic variable. Most important variables appear to include an elevated beta 2 microglubulin (>3.5 mg/dL) and age (>60 years), Variables of uncertain importance are an elevated plasma cell labeling index, elevated lactate dehydrogenase (LDH) and anemia (<10 g/dL). Cytogenetics also appear important; loss of chromosome 13 was reported to have a strong correlation with adverse outcome, specifically shortened event free survival (19). Independent retrospective studies have suggested that patients with 13q deletions, t(4;14), t(14;16) or p53 (chromosome 17) deletions do not benefit from transplantation and should be considered for alternate or investigational approaches (22,23).

Recommendations

1. As patients 65 years of age or younger without significant comorbidities are likely to benefit from a prolonged event-free survival and possibly longer overall survival following initial therapy with high-dose therapy and autologous stem cell transplantation, this treatment is recommended over conventional dose therapy (Grade 2B).
2. Patients with high-risk disease as defined by a high serum ß 2 microglobulin (>3.5 mg/dL) or deletion of chromosome 13 by cytogenetics may not be as likely to benefit from high-dose therapy. Additionally, patients with deletion 13, t(4;14), t(14;16), or deletion 17 by fluorescence in situ hybridization analysis are also unlikely to benefit from transplantation. These patients should be considered for investigational strategies (Grade 1C)

Is bortezomib superior to dexamethasone in relapsed/refractory myeloma?

Most, if not all, patients with MM will relapse following either conventional or high-dose therapy. Second-line treatment for these patients is often dexamethasone to attempt a further remission despite low remission rates and poor survival outcomes (24). A new and promising therapeutic option, bortezomib (Velcade, formerly PS-341), is a peptide boronate inhibitor of the 26S proteosome, responsible for the timely degradation of various regulators of cell cycle progression or apoptosis. This section will address the use of bortezomib in patients that have relapsed after primary antimyeloma therapy. The search strategy included the combination of the following terms (myeloma OR plasmacytoma) AND (Bortezomib OR Velcade OR PS-341). Of all the articles that specifically addressed the question of bortezomib in relapsed/refractory disease, two are phase II trials; only one is a randomized phase III clinical trial.

Two multi-institutional, open-label nonrandomized phase II trials (SUMMIT, CREST) have been published, suggesting the efficacy of bortezomib in relapsed/refractory myeloma (25,26). These data led to the completion of the lone phase III trial (APEX), in which 669 patients with relapsed myeloma that had received at least one previous treatment, were randomized to receive bortezomib at 1.3 mg/m^2 or dexamethasone 40 mg (27). In this intention-to-treat but open-label study, the overall response rates were 38% in the bortezomib group versus 18% in the dexamethasone group. Median time to progression was six months in the bortezomib group versus 3.5 months in the dexamethasone group. Overall survival at one year was significantly higher in the bortezomib group, 80% versus 66%, and included those who crossed over from the dexamethasone to receive bortezomib after disease progression.

In all trials, adverse events were frequent in patients receiving bortezomib as compared with those that have received dexamethasone. In the APEX trial, 37% of patients in the bortezomib group had to discontinue therapy because of adverse events. The most common reasons for discontinuation was peripheral neuropathy followed by thrombocytopenia, GI disorder and then fatigue. The neuropathy associated with bortezomib was specifically addressed in a follow-up study to the CREST and SUMMIT phase II trials (28). More than 80% of patients in these two trials had preexisting neuropathies by either questionnaire or examination, and 35% of patients developed treatment-related (bortezomib) neuropathy. The incidence of severe neuropathy (grade 3 or higher) was higher in patients with preexistent neural damage, but this was not predictive of bortezomib induced neuropathy.

The APEX trial and the phase II trials all give an important overview of the therapeutic potential of bortezomib. Response rates with bortezomib alone were impressive in all trials. However, response duration was extended by only three months in patients given bortezomib over those on dexamethasone. Hinting at improved clinical efficacy, patients in the SUMMIT and CREST trials that had a suboptimal response to bortezomib alone, had an improvement of response with the addition of dexamethasone (29). It is possible that this combination for relapsed/refractory myeloma may extend the modest duration of response seen with bortezomib alone, but this has not been studied prospectively. Although bortezomib has impressive clinical activity in relapsed/refractory patients, this is at the expense of toxicity, especially neurotoxicity.

Recommendations

1. These data support a role for bortezomib, for patients that have relapsed or are refractory to at least one modality of antimyeloma therapy (Grade 2A).
2. It is probable that bortezomib in combination with dexamethasone may yield better outcomes (Grade 2C).

What is the role of lenalidomide in patients with relapsed or refractory myeloma?

Lenalidomide (CC4013, Revlimid) was developed as a second-generation, more potent oral analogue of thalidomide and shares most of its chemical structure. Unlike thalidomide, it is not teratogenic in rabbit preclinical models (30). Its clinical activity became apparent in the initial phase I dose escalation study where 71% of heavily pretreated patients responded to the drug and showed none of the somnolence, constipation, or neuropathy commonly associated with thalidomide (31). As is usually the case for a novel agent, the bulk of the available early literature is in the relapsed/refractory setting. Therefore, in this section, we will review the literature on the use of lenalidomide in the relapsed/refractory setting. The search strategy included the combination of the following terms (myeloma OR plasmacytoma) AND (lenalidomide OR revlimid OR CC-5013). All trials were included if they evaluated lenalidomide in multiple myeloma patients that have failed prior therapy. We have chosen to report on published phase I and II trials as well as two published phase III trials.

A phase I trial assessed escalating doses of lenalidomide (31) and a follow-up phase II trial (32) assessed a total of 129 patients. All patients had received and failed at least one line of chemotherapy, most had received three or more. In the phase II trial, the total response rate (CR+ PR+ MR) was 25% with higher rates of response in a group receiving 30 mg once daily. Progression-free survival was reported to be up to 8.3 months for the once daily arm with overall survival of 28 months.

Two phase III trials, one North American and one European (MM-009 and MM-010), randomly assigned patients to receive either lenalidomide 25 mg/d PO for 21 of a 28-day cycle, with dexamethasone 40 mg/d PO on days 1–4, 9–12, and 17–20 or dexamethasone with placebo at the same dosing schedule. Both trials had to be stopped because of superior response rates and progression-free survival rates in the lenalidomide plus dexamethasone group (33, 34). Response rates for lenalidomide and dexamethasone were 59.4% and 21.1% with dexamethasone alone. Time-to-disease progression with lenalidomide plus dexamethasone was 11 months and only 4.7 months with dexamethasone alone. Finally, overall survival was significantly better with lenalidomide and dexamethasone than with dexamethasone alone (29.6 months vs. 20.2 months). The European trial showed similar results (overall relative risk 59% vs. 24%; time to progression 11.3 vs. 4.7 months) (34).

In the phase II study, significant adverse events were cytopenias (neutropenia and thrombocytopenia). Thromboses were seen only when dexamethasone was added to either dosage of lenalidomide (35). Importantly, somnolence, neuropathy, and constipation were not observed with lenalidomide. Interim analysis of the European Phase III trial reported that grade 3 or 4 neutropenic events were more common with lenalidomide than with dexamethasone alone (16.5% vs. 1.2%), but the number of infectious episodes were no different between groups.

Recommendation

Lenalidomide is a recommended treatment option for patients with relapsed or refractory myeloma. While this recommendation is based on the results of two randomized trials, the publication of these results in abstract from limits the strength of the possible recommendation at the time of this writing (Grade 1B).

References

1 Jemal A, et al. Cancer statistics, 2006. *CA Cancer J Clin.* 2006;**56**:106.

2 Myeloma Trialists Collaborative Group. Combination chemotherapy versus melphalan plus prednisone as treatment for multiple myeloma: an overview of 6,633 patients from 27 randomized trials. *J Clin Oncol.* 1998;**16**(12):3832–42.

3 Alexanian R, Dimopoulos MA, Delasalle K, et al. Primary dexamethasone treatment of multiple myeloma. *Blood.* 1992;**80**(4):887–90.

4 Singhal S, Mehta J, Desikan R, et al. Antitumor activity of thalidomide in refractory multiple myeloma. *N Engl J Med.* 1999;**341**(21):1565–71.

5 Rajkumar SV, Hayman S, Gertz MA, et al. Combination therapy with thalidomide plus dexamethasone for newly diagnosed myeloma. *J Clin Oncol.* 2002;**20**(21):4319–23.

6 Cavo M, Zamagni E, Tosi P, et al. First-line therapy with thalidomide and dexamethasone in preparation for autologous stem cell transplantation for multiple myeloma. *Haematologica.* 2004;**89**(7):826–31.

7 Rajkumar SV, Blood E, Vesole D, et al. Phase III clinical trial of thalidomide plus dexamethasone compared with dexamethasone alone in newly diagnosed multiple myeloma: a clinical trial coordinated by the Eastern Cooperative Oncology Group. *J Clin Oncol.* 2006;**24**(3):431–36.

8 Macro M, Divine M, Uzunhan Y, et al. Dexamethasone+thalidomide (dex/thal) compared to VAD as a pre-transplant treatment in newly diagnosed multiple myeloma. *Blood.* 2006 (ASH Annual Meeting Abstracts):57.

9 Dimopoulos MA, Anagnostopoulos A, Terpos E, et al. Primary treatment with pulsed melphalan, dexamethasone and thalidomide for elderly symptomatic patients with multiple myeloma. *Haematologica.* 2006;**91**(2):252–54.

10 Palumbo A, Bringhen S, Caravita T, et al. Oral melphalan and prednisone chemotherapy plus thalidomide compared with melphalan and prednisone alone in elderly patients with multiple myeloma: randomised controlled trial. *Lancet.* 2006;**367**(9513):825–31.

11 Facon T, Mary J, Harousseau J, et al. Superiority of melphalan-prednisone (MP) + thalidomide (THAL) over MP and autologous stem cell transplantation in the treatment of newly diagnosed elderly patients with multiple myeloma. *J Clin Oncol.* 2006;1(24 Suppl 18):1 [data updated on webcast]. Available at http://www.asco.org/portal/site/ASCO.

12 McElwain TJ, Powles RL. High-dose intravenous melphalan for plasma-cell leukaemia and myeloma. *Lancet.* 1983;**2**(8354):822–24.

13 Attal M, Harousseau JL, Stoppa AM, et al. A prospective, randomized trial of autologous bone marrow transplantation and chemotherapy in multiple myeloma. Intergroupe Français du Myelome. *N Engl J Med.* 1996;**335**(2):91–97.

14 Attal M, Harousseau JL. Randomized trial experience of the Intergroupe Francophone du Myelome. *Semin Hematol.* 2001;**38**:226.

15 Child JA, Morgan GJ, Davies FE, et al. High-dose chemotherapy with hematopoietic stem-cell rescue for multiple myeloma. *N Engl J Med.* 2003;**348**(19):1875–83.

16 Fermand JP, Ravaud P, Chevret S, et al. High-dose therapy and autologous peripheral blood stem cell transplantation in multiple myeloma: up-front or rescue treatment? Results of a multicenter sequential randomized clinical trial. *Blood.* 1998;**92**(9):3131–36.

17 Fermand JP, Katsahian S, Divine M, et al. High-dose therapy and autologous blood stem-cell transplantation compared with conventional treatment in myeloma patients aged 55 to 65 years: long-term results of a randomized control trial from the Group Myelome-Autogreffe. *J Clin Oncol.* 2005;**23**(36):9227–33.

18 Segeren CM, Sonneveld P, van der Holt B, et al. Overall and event-free survival are not improved by the use of myeloablative therapy following intensified chemotherapy in previously untreated patients with multiple myeloma: a prospective randomized phase 3 study. *Blood.* 2003;**101**(6):2144–45.

19 Barlogie B, Kyle RA, Anderson KC, et al. Standard chemotherapy compared with high-dose chemoradiotherapy for multiple myeloma: final results of phase III US Intergroup Trial S9321. *J Clin Oncol.* 2006;**24**(6):929–36.

20 Blade J, Rosinol L, Sureda A, et al. High-dose therapy intensification compared with continued standard chemotherapy in multiple myeloma patients responding to the initial chemotherapy: long-term results from a prospective randomized trial from the Spanish cooperative group PETHEMA. *Blood.* 2005;**106**(12):3755–59.

21 Glasmacher A, Hahn C, Hoffmann F, et al. A systematic review of phase-II trials of thalidomide monotherapy in patients with relapsed or refractory multiple myeloma. *Br J Haematol.* 2006;**132**(5):584–93.

22 Moreau P, Facon T, Leleu X, et al. Recurrent 14q32 translocations determine the prognosis of multiple myeloma, especially in patients receiving intensive chemotherapy. *Blood.* 2002;**100**(5):1579–83.

23 Chang H, Qi XY, Samiee S, et al. Genetic risk identifies multiple myeloma patients who do not benefit from autologous stem cell transplantation. *Bone Marrow Transplant.* 2005;**36**(9):793–96.

24 Gertz MA, Garton JP, Greipp PR, et al. A phase II study of high-dose methylprednisolone in refractory or relapsed multiple myeloma. *Leukemia.* 1995;**9**(12):2115–18.

25 Richardson PG, Barlogie B, Berenson J, et al. A phase 2 study of bortezomib in relapsed, refractory myeloma. *N Engl J Med.* 2003;**348**(26):2609–17.

26 Jagannath S, Barlogie B, Berenson J, et al. A phase 2 study of two doses of bortezomib in relapsed or refractory myeloma. *Br J Haematol.* 2004;**127**(2):165–72.

27 Richardson PG, Sonneveld P, Schuster MW, et al. Bortezomib or high-dose dexamethasone for relapsed multiple myeloma. *N Engl J Med.* 2005;**352**(24):2487–98.

28 Richardson PG, Briemberg H, Jagannath S, et al. Frequency, characteristics, and reversibility of peripheral neuropathy during treatment of advanced multiple myeloma with bortezomib. *J Clin Oncol.* 2006;**24**(19):3113–20.

29 Jagannath S, Richardson PG, Barlogie B, et al. Bortezomib in combination with dexamethasone for the treatment of patients with relapsed and/or refractory multiple myeloma with less than optimal response to bortezomib alone. *Haematologica.* 2006;**91**(7):929–34.

30 Bartlett JB, Dredge K, Dalgleish AG. The evolution of thalidomide and its IMiD derivatives as anticancer agents. *Nat Rev Cancer.* 2004;**4**(4):314–22.

31 Richardson PG, Schlossman RL, Weller E, et al. Immunomodulatory drug CC-5013 overcomes drug resistance and is well tolerated in patients with relapsed multiple myeloma. *Blood.* 2002;**100**(9):3063–67.

32 Richardson PG, Blood E, Mitsiades CS, et al. A randomized phase 2 study of lenalidomide therapy for patients with relapsed or relapsed and refractory multiple myeloma. *Blood.* 2006;**108**(10):3458–64.

33 Weber DM, Chen C, Niesvizky R, et al. Lenalidomide plus high-dose dexamethasone provides improved overall survival compared to high-dose dexamethasone alone for relapsed or refractory multiple myeloma (MM): results of a North American phase III study (MM-009). *J Clin Oncol.* 2006;**24**(Pt 1, Suppl 18):7521.

34 Dimopoulos MA, Spencer, A, Attal M, et al. Study of lenalidomide plus dexamethasone versus dexamethasone alone in relapsed or refractory multiple myeloma (mm): results of a phase 3 study (MM-010). *Blood.* 2006(ASH Annual Meeting Abstracts)**106**:6.

35 Richardson PG, Barlogie B, Berenson J, et al Extended follow-up of a phase II trial in relapsed, refractory multiple myeloma: final time-to-event results from the SUMMIT trial. *Cancer.* 2006;**106**(6):1316–19.

51 Management of Waldenstrom's Macroglobulinemia

Christine I. Chen

Introduction

Waldenstrom's macroglobulinemia (WM) is a rare B-cell lymphoproliferative disorder categorized by the World Health Organization as an indolent lymphoplasmacytic lymphoma. It is characterized by a serum monoclonal IgM paraprotein and bone marrow infiltration of plasma cells, mature lymphocytes, and lymphoplasmacytoid cells. Although some patients are asymptomatic, heterogeneous clinical features are observed, including IgM-related complications (e.g., hyperviscosity, bleeding, peripheral neuropathy) or features of tumor infiltration (e.g., adenopathy, organomegaly, cytopenias). Treatment options can range from watchful waiting to aggressive combination chemotherapy regimens. The heterogeneity and rarity of this disease (incidence 1 per million) make it difficult to perform large randomized trials and require that results be generalized from smaller studies. Although treatment options have traditionally resembled those used for indolent lymphoma or myeloma, WM has unique treatment-related responses and toxicity that may warrant distinct therapeutic approaches. However, present determinations of best practices require generalizing principles gleaned from these other diseases.

Questions

1. When should therapy be initiated?
2. What is the best initial treatment for symptomatic patients?
3. What treatment options exist for a patient who has relapsed after initial therapy with fludarabine?
4. What are the indications for plasmapheresis?

Evidence-based Hematology. Edited by Mark A. Crowther, Jeff Ginsberg, Holger J. Schünemann, Ralph M. Meyer, and Richard Lottenberg.

Literature-search strategy and inclusions

A PubMed search was performed using the terms "Waldenstrom macroglobulinemia therapy," "lymphoplasmacytic lymphoma therapy," and "immunocytoma therapy." A total of 927, 948, and 115 articles, respectively, were identified, of which 62 in total were therapeutic studies. Of these, only two were randomized controlled trials (RCT). As well, both American Society of Hematology and American Society of Clinical Oncology abstracts from 1996 to 2006 were searched for relevant studies. Only those studies with at least 10 patients were reviewed for this article. Much of the data to be reviewed will deal with an evaluation of clinical response to therapy. Standardized response criteria in WM were developed by a consensus panel at the Second International Workshop on WM (1,2). These criteria include evaluation of both monoclonal IgM levels and bidimensional disease (nodal or tumor masses) and are more stringent than older studies assessing monoclonal protein levels alone. Most studies reviewed for this chapter fall into this latter category. Until the new criteria are uniformly adopted, comparison of response rates between studies must account for these differences. The role of response as a surrogate outcome measure for the more important outcomes of durable disease control, quality of life, and overall survival has not been widely evaluated and poses a major limitation in reaching treatment recommendations.

Grading of the quality of evidence and strengths of recommendations in this chapter are based on the guidelines proposed by the international Grading of Recommendations Assessment, Development, and Evaluation Working Group (GRADE)adopting the modification used by the American College of Chest Physicians that merges the "very low" and "low" categories of quality of evidence (see chapter 1).

When should therapy be initiated?

Treatment for WM is generally reserved until there are disease-related symptoms or complications. Although there are no prospective RCTs evaluating WM, three RCTs in various indolent lymphomas support this watch-and-wait approach (3–5). With initial observation only, the median survival of WM patients is 5–10 years (6) and a subset of patients may enjoy survival well beyond 10 years. Indications for initiating therapy include cytopenias (hemoglobin <100 g/L or platelets $<100 \times 10^9$/L), bulky lymphadenopathy or hepatosplenomegaly, lymphoproliferative-related symptoms (e.g., fever, night sweats, weight loss) manifestations related to the paraprotein production (e.g., hyperviscosity) or evidence of disease transformation (7). The clinical status of the patient, not the level of the IgM paraprotein, determines the need to treat.

Recommendation

Based on generalization of data from other lymphoproliferative disorders, "watch and wait" with follow-up every three to six months is recommended for asymptomatic patients (Grade 1B).

What is the best initial treatment for symptomatic patients?

There are no RCTs demonstrating a specific therapeutic agent or regimen as the treatment of choice as initial therapy. Decisions must therefore be based on individual patient considerations such as presence of cytopenias, need for rapid disease control and age (8). Options should be weighed with consideration of toxicity, mode of administration, and cost to the individual patient. Use of single agent alkylator agents or nucleoside analogues has been traditional choices of initial therapy. Rituximab has recently been evaluated as an initial alternative.

Alkylating agents. Chlorambucil is the most common single-agent alkylator agent used in WM and other indolent lymphomas. It is well tolerated orally when given either continuously (0.1 mg/kg/d) or intermittently (0.3 mg/kg $\times$ 7 days or 8 mg/m^2 $\times$ 10 days every six weeks) (9,10). No significant differences in responses or survival have been demonstrated between these dosing options (9). Chlorambucil is associated with responses in up to 75% of symptomatic WM patients, but complete responses (CR) are rare (9,10) and maximum responses may require a median of 18–21 months to occur. Thus, treatment durations may be prolonged as symptoms are slow to resolve (9). Therefore, this option is not recommended for urgent therapy, but given its favorable toxicity profile is reasonable for elderly or debilitated patients. There is no evidence of enhanced efficacy associated with using multiple alkylator agents in comparison with a single agent (11,12).

When treating patients with indolent lymphoma, cyclophosphamide, vincristine, and prednisone (CVP) is considered to have similar efficacy as single-agent alkylator therapy but with a faster onset of response; the addition of rituximab (CVP-R) prolongs the time to progression when compared with CVP alone and is generally well tolerated (13). Though there are no data specific for WM, CVP-R has been widely adopted for use in WM and may be appropriate initial therapy for selected patients requiring rapid control of disease who are not candidates for nucleoside analogue therapy. Although other combination chemotherapy regimens (e.g., DRC (dexamethasone, rituximab, and cyclophosphamide), CHOP or CHOP with rituximab) have also been used in WM (14,15,16), there are no prospective comparative data available that permit a thorough evaluation of these options.

Nucleoside analogues. Fludarabine and cladribine (2-chlorodeoxyadenosine) are nucleoside analogues with activity in indolent lymphomas and chronic lymphocytic leukemia (CLL). No RCTs comparing either of these agents to alternative strategies in previously untreated patients were identified. In seven phase II studies testing fludarabine or cladribine as initial therapy, reported responses ranged from 38% to 85% (CR 3%–10%) (17–23). In the largest published study, 118 symptomatic patients were treated with at least four cycles of fludarabine (30 mg/m^2/d $\times$ 5 days) (17). In contrast to most other studies, this U.S. Intergroup study reported a modest 38% response rate (CR 3%). Updated results from this study reported a median PFS of 59 months and overall survival of 84 months (24). When used as initial therapy, fludarabine and cladribine lead to prompt responses, usually within the first two to three cycles. With CR rates no greater than 10%, however, they are clearly not curative. Toxicities, such as myelosuppression and immunosuppression can be limiting. Even in previously untreated patients, fludarabine is associated with severe or life-threatening neutropenia in half of patients and thrombocytopenia can be prolonged (25). Secondary myelodysplasia can follow cladribine or fludarabine therapy and is not only restricted to those with heavy exposure to alkylator agents (26). Treatment-related deaths, usually due to infections, occurred in 3% of patients entered into the Intergroup study) (27). In contrast, death due to toxicity from single agent alkylators is extremely rare.

Treatment of WM with fludarabine or cladribine is administered as in other lymphoproliferative disorders. Intravenous fludarabine is given at doses of 25–30 mg/m^2/d intravenously for five days per cycle. Although oral fludarabine is in common usage in Europe and Canada, there are no studies evaluating this formulation in WM. The target number of treatment cycles is debatable but convention and experience dictate a minimum of four to six cycles. Cladribine is generally given at doses 0.6–0.7 mg/kg/cycle in either a continuous infusion or daily two-hour bolus for five days. Cladribine can be repeated every four to six weeks to maximal response but cumulative myelosuppression may preclude repeated dosing. Hence, a course of two to three cycles is common. Considering the toxicity, cost, and inconvenience of nucleoside analogues, it is debatable whether initial use should be recommended over alkylating agents. The WM1 study, an open-label randomized trial comparing chlorambucil with single-agent fludarabine (oral or intravenous), is anticipated to clarify this first-line treatment dilemma (28). Combinations of purine analogues with alkylating agents are hypothesized to be synergistic, but there is limited experience testing this concept in WM and use outside of a clinical trial cannot be recommended (29,30).

Rituximab. In evaluating previously untreated patients, no RCTs and only three prospective phase II studies reporting results of at least 10 WM patients were identified (31–34). In an ECOG study, 69 patients, 34 of whom were previously untreated, received 375 mg/m^2 as four consecutive weekly infusions (2,31). Response rates of 35.3% in previously untreated and 20% in previously treated patients were observed. The median response duration for previously untreated patients was 27 months. In an attempt to enhance clinical efficacy, Dimopoulos et al. (32) and Treon et al. (34) both studied an extended rituximab schedule using a total of eight rituximab infusions (the standard four weekly infusions plus an additional four weekly infusions at week 12). Dimopoulos et al. reported a 35% response rate (no CR) in 15 untreated patients with a median time to progression (TTP) of 13 months (32). Treon et al. reported similar results with responses in 48.3% in 29 patients, 12 of whom were previously untreated (34); the TTP was 17 months in the previously untreated group. Hence, it is reasonable to conclude that single-agent rituximab has moderate activity in previously untreated patients, but response durations are relatively short, even with extended schedules. The role of rituximab maintenance therapy is under investigation. When using single-agent rituximab, treating physicians should beware of an IgM "flare" that may occur in up to half of patients (35,36). This flare, particularly occurring in patients with baseline total IgM levels >60g/L or monoclonal protein >40g/L, typically develops after one month of therapy (but as early as 1 week) and resolves in most patients by four months. If unsuspected, this flare can be misinterpreted as disease progression. Rituximab is otherwise well tolerated in WM and with its nonmyelosuppressive profile, it may be useful in first-line therapy where severe cytopenias preclude the use of cytotoxic agents. Because of the risk of IgM flare, single-agent rituximab is not recommended for use in hyperviscosity syndrome.

Recommendations

1. In previously untreated, symptomatic patients, treatment with a single-agent alkylator agent or a nucleoside analogue (either fludarabine or cladribine alone) or rituximab are reasonable choices for initial treatment (Grade 1C).

2. Based on the slow rate of response, treatment with a single agent alkylating agent is not recommended for urgent therapy. This option may be the treatment of choice for elderly or debilitated patients (Grade 1C).

3. For patients requiring a more rapid response to treatment, it is reasonable to generalize the use of CVP-R, which is well tolerated and effective in other indolent lymphomas, as an option for initial therapy when avoidance of nucleoside analogue toxicities is desired (Grade 1C).

4. Based principally on data demonstrating a high response rate, initial therapy with a nucleoside analogue is a reasonable option for patients requiring more rapid control of their disease and who do not have important comorbidities (Grade 1C).

What treatment options exist for a patient who has relapsed after initial therapy with fludarabine?

In patients with relapsed WM, there is a single RCT demonstrating superior event-free survival in patients treated with fludarabine in comparison with cyclophosphamide, doxorubicin, and prednisone (37). However, this trial excluded patients who had previously received fludarabine. Thus, while fludarabine is a reasonable option for patients who have not initially received this agent, data evaluating options in patients who received initial therapy with fludarabine are limited. No RCTs were identified and most other options have been evaluated either retrospectively or in small phase II studies. Again, generalizing principles from other lymphoproliferative disorders does influence treatment prioritization.

Retreatment with single-agent nucleoside analogues. For those patients who experience a period of prolonged disease control after prior therapy with fludarabine or cladribine, retreatment with the same agent may be reasonable. Weber et al. (2a) retreated 10 patients with prior responses to cladribine and achieved a second remission in 8 patients (80%). Second response duration was similar to first response duration (23 vs. 24 months, respectively) (29). In the same series, similar retreatment sensitivities were noted with cladribine combinations.

Combination Therapies. Nucleoside analogues and alkylator agent combinations have been evaluated retrospectively. Given the limitations of these data, the highest level of justification for these options comes from generalizing the data from other lymphoproliferative disorders, including chronic lymphocytic leukemia. For instance, combination regimens used in CLL such as fludarabine, cyclophosphamide, and rituximab (FCR) and pentostatin, cyclophosphamide, with or without rituximab are being investigated (38,39). Anthracycline-containing chemotherapy regimens used for aggressive histology lymphoma (CHOP, CAP) have been used as subsequent-line therapy for patients with indolent lymphomas and although used with some frequency in WM, there is little evidence to support this approach (37,40). The addition of rituximab to CHOP (CHOP-R) significantly improves efficacy in treatment of aggressive histology lymphoma and may have rationale for use in WM patients failing fludarabine. Treon et al. reported responses in 11/13 patients (85%; CR in three patients) using six cycles of CHOP-R (16). These data are promising but do not permit confident recommendations.

Rituximab. Rituximab appears to have activity in patients relapsed or refractory to fludarabine. In three prospective studies evaluating rituximab, important differences in response rates and toxicities were not observed when comparing previously treated and untreated patients (31,32,34).

Thalidomide and other immunomodulating agents. Thalidomide is an immunomodulatory agent with significant activity in myeloma. It is currently under investigation for treatment of various malignancies including WM. Dimopoulos et al reported a 25% response rate with thalidomide in 20 WM patients (41). Although toxicities were common, they were not unexpected and reversed with drug withdrawal. Use of thalidomide as part of combination therapy and development of thalidomide analogues, such as lenalidomide, are under evaluation.

Bortezomib. Bortezomib is a reversible proteasome inhibitor which is effective in myeloma and appears to be active in other hematologic malignancies including lymphoma. Two phase II trials have demonstrated activity of this agent in WM (42,43). Treon et al., using eight cycles of bortezomib, reported a paraprotein reduction of at least 50% in 40% of 27 patients, 26 of whom were previously treated (42). Chen et al. reported similar paraprotein response in 44% of 27 previously untreated and treated patients, but using serial CT scanning, noted a lag in nodal disease with a composite (paraprotein and bidimensional disease) response rate of only 26% (43). Testing of bortezomib in combination with other agents is ongoing.

Transplantation. Currently, there are only 49 reports of autologous and 37 allogeneic stem cell transplants in WM. These data are insufficient for recommendations outside of clinical trial testing.

Recommendations

1. There is insufficient evidence to recommend one therapy over another in the treatment of patients with disease progression after initial therapy with fludarabine. For patients who have had a period of durable disease control with fludarabine, retreatment with this agent is reasonable (Grade 2C).
2. Use of rituximab is reasonable for patients who are refractory to fludarabine, particularly if there are cytopenias or poor performance status that limit the tolerance of more intensive cytotoxic regimens (Grade 1C).
3. Patients who are refractory to fludarabine should be considered for treatment with a new agent, potentially as part of combination therapy, within the context of a clinical trial (Grade 2C).

What are the indications for plasmapheresis?

Currently, plasmapheresis is used as an adjunct to more definitive therapy for WM. There is extensive, though mostly anecdotal, experience with the acute use of plasmapheresis in patients with high levels of IgM paraprotein causing hyperviscosity symptoms (headache, visual blurring, bleeding, and CNS impairment). Patients typically manifest symptoms when the serum viscosity level is 4 centipoise (Cp) or greater (normal 1.6–2.4 Cp). Although the relationship between serum viscosity and M-protein level is not linear, hyperviscosity symptoms are usually seen with IgM levels greater than 40 g/L. As IgM is a large molecule of which 70%–80% remains intravascular, 50% of circulating IgM can be cleared with one exchange (44). Daily or every other day exchanges can be performed until symptoms resolve but often dramatic improvements are observed with just one exchange. Since plasmapheresis does not alter production of IgM, concurrent systemic therapy is required for long-term management. In those patients who are refractory to systemic therapy, long-term plasmaphereses at regular intervals may be considered (45) Cascade filtration, a more selective approach to removal of macromolecules without causing loss of other plasma components, has not been shown to be more effective than standard plasmapheresis (46,47). The American Society for Apheresis and the American Association of Blood Banks both categorize hyperviscosity as a Category II indication for plasmapheresis (i.e., disease for which apheresis is generally accepted but considered to be supportive or adjunctive) (48). Plasmapheresis has also been used anecdotally for complications of WM such as symptomatic neuropathy, cryoglobulinemia, or cold agglutinins, coagulation inhibitors with bleeding, and for preoperative preparation to minimize bleeding/thrombosis. There are limited data to support efficacy of routine apheresis in these complications.

Recommendations

1. Plasmapheresis is recommended as an urgent adjunct therapy for patients with symptomatic hyperviscosity (Grade 1C).
2. Plasmapheresis is recommended as a palliative measure for patients with disease that is refractory to systemic treatment and who are vulnerable to chronic features of increased viscosity (Grade 2C).
3. Plasmapheresis may be considered as an adjunct therapy for patients with the uncommon antibody-mediated complications of WM such as neuropathy, cryoglobulinemia or cold agglutinins, coagulation inhibitors with bleeding, and for preoperative preparation to minimize bleeding/thrombosis (Grade 2C).

References

1 Kimby E, Treon S, Anagnostopoulos A, et al: Update on recommendations for assessing response from the Third International Workshop on Waldenstrom's macroglobulinemia. *Clin Lymph & Myeloma.* 2006; **6**:380–383.

2 Weber D, Treon S, Emmanouilides C, et al: Uniform response criteria in Waldenstrom's macroglobulinemia consensus panel recommendations from the Second International Workshop on Waldenstrom's Macroglobulinemia. *Semin Oncol.* 2003;**30**:127–131.

3 Brice P, Bastion Y, Lepage E, et al: Comparison in low-tumor-burden follicular lymphomas between an initial no-treatment policy, prednimustine, or interferon alfa: a randomized study from the Groupe D'Etude des Lymphomes Folliculaires. *J Clin Oncol.* 1997;**15**:1110–1117.

4 Young R, Longo D, Glatstein E, et al: The treatment of indolent lymphomas: watchful waiting versus aggressive combined modality treatment. *Semin Hematol.* 1988;**25**:11–16.

5 Ardeshna K, Smith P, Norton A, et al: Long-term effect of a watch and wait policy versus immediate systemic treatment for asymptomatic

advanced-stage non-Hodkgin lymphoma: a randomised controlled trial. *Lancet.* 2003;**362**:516–522.

6 Garcia-Sanz R, Montoto S, Torrequebrada A, et al: Waldenstrom's macroglobulinemia: presenting features and outcome in a series with 217 patients. *Br J Haematol.* 2001;**115**:575–582.

7 Kyle R, Treon S, Alexanian R, et al: Prognostic markers and criteria to initiate therapy in Waldenstrom's macroglobulinemia: Consensus Panel Recommendations from the Second International Workshop on Waldenstrom's macroglobulinemia. *Semin Oncol.* 2003;**30**:116–120.

8 Gertz M, Anagnostopoulos A, Anderson K, et al: Treatment recommendations in Waldenstrom's macroglobulinemia: consensus panel recommendations from the Second International Workshop on Waldenstrom's Macroglobulinemia. *Semin Oncol.* 2003;**30**:121–126.

9 Kyle R, Greipp P, Gertz M, et al: Waldenstrom's macroglobulinemia: a prospective study comparing daily with intermittent oral chlorambucil. *Br J Haematol.* 2000;**108**:737–742.

10 Dimopoulos M, Alexanian R: Waldenstrom's macroglobulinemia. *Blood.* 1994;**83**:1452–1459.

11 Case D, Ervin T, Boyd J, et al: Waldenstrom's macroglobulinemia: Long-term results with the M-2 protocol. *Cancer Invest.* 1991;**9**:1–7.

12 Petrucci M, Avvisati G, Tribalto M, et al: Waldenstrom's macroglobulinaemia: results of a combined oral treatment in 34 newly diagnosed patients. *J Intern Med.* 1989;**226**:443–447.

13 Marcus R, Imrie K, Belch A, et al: CVP chemotherapy plus rituximab compared with CVP as first-line treatment for advanced follicular lymphoma. *Blood.* 2005;**105**:1417–1423.

14 Dimopoulos M, Anagnostopoulos A, Kyrtsonis M, et al: Primary treatment of Waldenstrom Macroglobulinemia with dexamethasone, rituximab, and cyclophosphamide. *J Clin Oncol.* 2007;**25**:3344–3349.

15 Weber D, Dimopoulos M, Gavino M, et al: Nucleoside analogues: new combinations for the treatment of Waldenstrom's macroglobulinemia, 1st International Symposium on Waldenstrom's Macroglobulinemia. Banff, Canada, 2001, pp 10–11a.

16 Treon S, Hunter Z, Branagan A: CHOP plus rituximab therapy in Waldenstrom's Macroglobulinemia (WM). *Clinical Lymphoma.* 2005;**5**:273–277.

17 Dhodapkar M, Jacobson J, Gertz M, et al: Prognostic factors and response to fludarabine therapy in patients with Waldenstrom's macroglobulinemia: results of United States intergroup trial (Southwest Oncology Group S9003). *Blood.* 2001;**98**:41–48.

18 Foran J, Rohatiner A, Coiffier B, et al: Multicenter phase II study of fludarabine phosphate for patients with newly diagnosed lymphoplasmacytoid lymphoma, Waldenstrom's macroglobulinemia, and mantle-cell lymphoma. *J Clin Oncol.* 1999;**17**:546–553.

19 Lewandowski K, Zaucha J, Bieniaxzewska M, et al: 2-Chlorodeoxyadenosine treatment of Waldenstrom's Macroglobulinemia – the analysis of own experience and the review of literature. *Med Sci Monit.* 2000;**6**:740–745.

20 Fridrik M, Jager G, Baldinger C, et al: First-line treatment of Waldenstrom's disease with cladribine. *Ann Hematol.* 1997;**74**:7–10.

21 Delannoy A, Ferrant A, Martiat P, et al: 2-Chlorodeoxyadenosine therapy in Waldenstrom's macroglobulinemia. *Nouv Rev Fr Hematol.* 1994;**36**:317–320.

22 Delannoy A, Neste VD, Michaux J, et al: Cladribine for Waldenstrom's macroglobulinemia. *Br J Haematol.* 1999;**104**:933.

23 Dimopoulos M, Kantarjian J, Weber D, et al: Primary therapy of Waldenstrom's macroglobulinemia with 2-chlorodeoxyadenosine. *J Clin Oncol.* 1994;**12**:2694–2698.

24 Fassas A, Dhodapkar M, Barlogie B, et al: Fludarabine for Waldenstrom's Macroglobulinemia: Update of Southwest Oncology Intergroup S9003. *Trial. Blood.* 2002;**100**:396a.

25 Dimopoulos M, Weber D, Delasalle K, et al: Treatment of Waldenstrom's macroglobulinemia resistant to standard therapy with 2-chlorodeoxyadenosine: Identification of prognostic factors. *Ann Oncol.* 1995;**6**:49–52.

26 Van Den Nest E, Louviaux I, Michaux J, et al: Myelodysplastic syndrome with monosomy 5 and/or 7 following therapy with 2-chloro-2-deoxyadenosine. *Br J Haematol.* 1999;**105**:268–270.

27 Dhodapkar M, Jacobson J, Gertz M, et al: Phase II intergroup trial of fludarabine in Waldenstrom's macroglobulinemia: results of Southwest Oncology Group trial (SWOG 9003) in 220 patients. *Blood.* 1997;**90**: 577a.

28 Johnson S, Owen R, Oscier D, et al: Phase III study of chlorambucil versus fludarabine as initial therapy for Waldenstrom's macroglobulinemia and related disorders. *Clin Lymphoma.* 2005;**5**:294–297.

29 Weber D, Dimopoulos M, Delasalle K, et al: 2-Chlorodeoxyadenosine alone and in combination for previously untreated Waldenstrom's Macroglobulinemia. *Semin Oncol.* 2003;**30**:243–247.

30 Tamburini J, Levy V, Chaleteix C, et al: Fludarabine plus cyclophosphamide in Waldenstrom's macroglobulinemia: results in 49 patients. *Leukemia.* 2005;**19**:1831–1834.

31 Gertz M, Rue M, Blood E, et al: Multicenter phase 2 trial of rituximab for Waldenstroms Macroglobulinemia (WM): An Eastern Cooperative Oncology Group Study (E3A98). *Leuk Lymph.* 2004;**45**:2047–2055.

32 Dimopoulos M, Zervas C, Zomas A, et al: Extended rituximab therapy for previously untreated patients with Waldesntrom's Macroglobulinemia. *Clinical Lymphoma.* 2002;**3**:163–166.

33 Dimopoulos M, Zervas C, Zomas A, et al: Treatment of Waldenstrom's macroglobulinemia with rituximab. *J Clin Oncol.* 2002;**20**:2327–2333.

34 Treon S, Emmanouilides C, Kimby E, et al: Extended rituximab therapy in Waldenstrom's macroglobulinemia. *Ann Oncol.* 2005;**16**:132–138.

35 Treon S, Branagan A, Hunter Z, et al: Paradoxical increases in serum IgM and viscosity levels following rituximab in Waldenstrom's macroglobulinemia. *Ann Oncol.* 2004;**15**:1481–1483.

36 Ghobrial I, Fonseca R, Greipp P, et al: Initial immunoglobulin M 'flare' after rituximab therapy in patients diagnosed with Waldenstrom Macroglobulinemia. An Eastern Cooperative Oncology Group Study. *Cancer.* 2004;**101**:2593–2598.

37 Leblond V, Levy V, Maloisel F, et al: Multicenter, randomized comparative trial of fludarabine and the combination of cyclophosphamide-doxorubicin-prednisone in 92 patients with Waldenstrom macroglobulinemia in first relapse or with primary refractory disease. *Blood.* 2001;**98**:2640–2644.

38 Tam C, Wolf M, Prince H, et al: Fludarabine, cyclophosphamide, and rituximab for the treatment of patients with chronic lymphocytic leukemia or indolent non-Hodgkin's lymphoma. *Cancer.* 2005;**106**:2412–2420.

39 Hensel M, Villalobos M, Kornacker M, et al: Pentostatin, cyclophosphamide and rituximab: an effective regimen for patients with Waldenstrom's macroglobulinemia. *Clin Lymphoma.* 2005;**2**:131–135.

40 Clamon G, Corder M, Patrick Burns C: Successful doxorubicin therapy of primary macroglobulinemia resistant to alkylating agents. *Am J Hematol.* 1980;**9**:221–223.

41 Dimopoulos M, Tsatalas C, Zomas A, et al: Treatment of Waldenstrom's macroglobulinemia with single-agent thalidomide or with the combination of clarithromycin, thalidomide and dexamethasone. *Semin Oncol.* 2003;**30**:265–269.

42 Treon S, Hunter Z, Matous J, et al: Phase II study of bortezomib in Waldenstrom's macroglobulinemia: Results of WMCTG Trial 03–248. *Blood.* 2005;**106**:147a.

43 Chen C, Kouroukis C, White D, et al: Bortezomib is active in patients with untreated or relapsed Waldenstrom's Macroglobulinemia:A phase II study of the National Cancer Institute of Canada Clinical Trials Group. *J Clin Oncol.* 2007, p 25.

44 Brecher M: Plasma exchange: Why we do what we do. *J Clin Apheresis.* 2002;**17**:207–211.

45 Buskard N, Galton D, Goldman J, et al: Plasma exchange in the long-term management of Waldenstrom's macroglobulinemia. *Can Med Assoc J.* 1977;**117**:135–137.

46 Valbonesi M, Montani F, Guzzini F, et al: Efficacy of discontinuous flow centrifugation compared with cascade filtration in Waldenstrom's macroglobulinemia. *Int J Artif Organs.* 1985;**8**:165–168.

47 Hoffkes H-G, Heemann U, Teschendorf C, et al: Hyperviscosity syndrome: efficacy and comparison of plasma exchange by plasma separation and cascade filtration in patients with immunocytoma of Waldenstrom 's type. *Clin Nephrol.* 1995;**43**:335–338.

48 McLeod B: Introduction to the Third Special Issue: Clinical applications of therapeutic apheresis. *J Clin Apheresis.* 2000;**15**:1–5.

52 The Role of Hematopoietic Growth Factors in Managing Patients with Hematologic Malignancies

Heloisa P. Soares, Ambuj Kumar, Charles Bennett, Benjamin Djulbegovic

Introduction

The hematopoietic growth factors are potent regulators of blood-cell proliferation and development (1). These factors, including erythropoietin (EPO), granulocyte colony-stimulating factor (G-CSF), and granulocyte-macrophage stimulating factor (GM-CSF) are currently used in the management of myelosuppression and anemia following chemotherapy in cancer patients (2). They play an important role as supportive tools to decrease morbidity and mortality related to chemotherapy regimens (2).

Questions

1. Do patients with hematologic malignancies benefit from the addition of EPO in the treatment of chemotherapy-induced anemia?
2. What are the benefits and harms associated with the use of CSFs as primary and secondary prophylaxis for chemotherapy-induced febrile neutropenia?

Literature-search strategy and inclusions

We performed a search from 2000 to 2006 on MEDLINE/PubMed database and *Cochrane Database for Systematic Reviews* to identify all systematic reviews (SR) that were relevant to address the questions listed below. We adopted the search strategies described by Montori et al. (3). If no SR was identified, we performed a complementary search to identify potentially relevant randomized controlled trials (RCTs) using the search strategy techniques described by Haynes et al. (4).

Evidence-based Hematology. Edited by Mark A. Crowther, Jeff Ginsberg, Holger J. Schünemann, Ralph M. Meyer, and Richard Lottenberg.
 ISBN: 978-1-4051-5747-6.

Grading of the quality of evidence and strengths of recommendations in this chapter are based on the guidelines proposed by the international Grading of Recommendations Assessment, Development, and Evaluation Working Group (GRADE) adopting the modification used by the American College of Chest Physicians that merges the "very low" and "low" categories of quality of evidence (see chapter 1).

Do patients with hematologic malignancies benefit from the addition of EPO in the treatment of chemotherapy-induced anemia?

Within this section, we will address whether EPO increases hematological response and decreases transfusion requirements, affects tumor response, produces symptomatic and quality of life (QoL) improvement, improves survival, and which important side effects are associated with use of EPO in cancer patients. In the United States, two erythropoietic products are licensed for commercial use: epoetin alfa (commercially distributed as Procrit® by Johnson & Johnson for clinical indications other than chronic kidney disease and distributed by AMGEN as Epogen® for treatment anemia of chronic kidney disease) and darbepoetin alfa (commercially available as Aransep® and distributed as an agent for management of chronic kidney disease as well as anemia related to cancer chemotherapy). Human EPO and epoetin are a 30,400 dalton heavily glycosylated protein hormone; 40% of their mass of the molecule is composed by carbohydrate (5). Darbepoetin alfa differs from epoetin as it contains 5 *N*-linked oligosaccharide chains, two more than EPO. It has a molecular weight of 37,100 daltons and a carbohydrate composition of 51%. The additional carbohydrates result in longer half-life, increased biologic activity, and decreased receptor affinity (5). The half-life of epoetin is 8.5 ± 2.4 hours and the darbopoetin half-life is 25.3 ± 2.2 hours.

Out of 72 titles related to EPO, 20 SRs were initially selected for our analysis, including 14 published in the last three years. The most comprehensive meta-analysis published so far is that by Bohlius et al (6). The authors reported a priori defined subgroup analysis of patients with hematological malignancies that mainly included patients with non-Hodgkin's lymphoma, multiple myeloma, and myelodysplastic syndrome (MDS).

EPO or darbepoetin treatment compared with control (observation or transfusion when needed) was associated with improvement in hematological response, which was defined as the proportion of participants with an increase in hemoglobin level of 2 g/dL or more, or increase in hematocrit of six percentage points or more, unrelated to transfusion or a decrease in requirement for RBC transfusions. This meta-analysis reported separately data for MDS and all other hematological disorders. Table 52.1 summarizes data on benefits and harms. Most of the studies included patients receiving chemotherapy. As shown in Table 52.1, the use of EPO or darbopoetin was associated with more frequent hematologic responses, including a reduction in transfusions. Improvements in tumor response rates and overall survival were not detected and in fact very recent evidence suggests that the use of ESA may actually compromise survival. Treatment was associated with an increased risk of thrombotic events.

In a separate study, we evaluated the impact of EPO on hematological response in myeloma patients only (7). The results are similar to those shown in Table 52.1 [hematological response was improved in myeloma patients receiving EPO, relative risk = 7.75 (95% confidence interval [CI] 4.19 to 14.35, four trials, n = 272)].

No trial evaluated the role of darbepoetin exclusively in myeloma patients. However, the results of the recent large, multicenter, randomized, placebo-controlled study showed that darbepoetin was ineffective in reducing red blood cell transfusions or fatigue in patients with cancer who have anemia that is not due to concurrent chemotherapy. The study also showed higher mortality in patients receiving darbepoetin including a subgroup of patients with myeloma.(http://www.fda.gov/medwatch/safety/2007/Aranesp_DHCP_012707.htm).

Published guidelines

Several organizations developed guidelines for the use of EPO in cancer patients (not exclusively hematological malignancies). Most popular ones are from the American Society of Clinical Oncology/American Society of Hematology (8) and from the 2008 National Comprehensive Cancer Network (9). These recommendations are both evidence and consensus-based. They are freely available on the Web.

Recommendation

We conclude that overall there are trade-offs regarding the use of EPO for treatment of anemia because EPO increases hemoglobin levels, decrease the need for transfusions and have potential favorable impact on patients' quality of life. In quantitative terms, for every seven patients treated with EPO, one will have avoid red-blood cell transfusion.

However, patients should be aware of the risk of the development of potential life-threatening adverse reaction, such as thrombotic events. In fact, 1 in 45 patients treated with EPO/Darbepo will have such a complication.

One should also be aware that the accumulated evidence (as of January 2008) raises possibility that administration of EPO may be associated with increased mortality and that effort to improve survival or tumor response rate is potentially dangerous (i.e., when EPO is administered in an effort to treat beyond the correction of anemia) (10,11). We classify the recommendation for the use of EPO as Grade 2A.

The recommendation did not take into account costs. We, therefore, conclude this brief presentation with cost considerations in the United States, EPO and darbepoetin accounted for the first and second largest clinic expenditures in 2004 ($3.9 billion; 17.7% of all clinic related pharmaceutical expenditures) and $1.2 billion (5.5%), respectively, and the first and third greatest hospital expenditure $1.2 billion (4.8% of hospital pharmaceutical expenditures) and $380 million (1.5%), respectively (12). In contrast, the United Kingdom's National Institute for Clinical Excellence in July 2006, which looks at the cost-effectiveness of drugs prescribed under the United Kingdom's National Health Service, concluded that EPO and darbepoetin should not be used for cancer chemotherapy-related anemia, except in the context of research studies. At the time, the institute's technology appraisal committee said that EPO drugs cost approximately $10,000 per course of treatment.

What are the benefits and harms associated with the use of CSFs as primary prophylaxis of chemotherapy-induced febrile neutropenia?

Colony-stimulating factors (CSF) have been proposed for the prevention and treatment of chemotherapy-induced neutropenia and the associated problem of febrile neutropenia (FN) (13). Febrile neutropenia may lead to life-threatening infections, result in costly hospitalization, affect the quality of life, and cause delays or reductions in dose of chemotherapy agents, which may ultimately affect survival (14). Most studies that evaluated the role of CSF in febrile neutropenia enrolled patients with an absolute neutrophil count (ANC) $<1{,}000/\mu L$ or $< 500/\mu L$. The risk of infections is a function not only of ANC count but also duration of neutropenia. Earlier studies show that patients with ANC $<500/\mu L$ have about 50% of chance of getting infected while those with ANC $<100/\mu L$ have more than 90% chance of developing infections (15). Likewise, the patients with low ANC that lasted ≤ 1 week have 10% and lasting ≥ 6 weeks have 65% chance of getting infected, respectively (16). Granulocyte colony stimulating factors (G-CSF) and granulocyte-macrophage colony stimulating factors (GM-CSF) have been most widely studied in cancer patients with febrile neutropenia (17).

Primary prophylaxis

Primary prophylaxis refers to use of the growth factor before there has been any occurrence of neutropenia. We found four SRs addressing the use of CSF for prevention of myelosupressive therapy-induced febrile neutropenia (18–21). These are summarized in Table 52.2. The SR by Bohlius et al. (18) that exclusively evaluated

Table 52.1 Summary of evidence of the use of EPO the treatment of hematological malignancy-related anemia.*

Quality assessment						Summary of findings				
						No. of patients		Effect		
No. of studies	Design	Limitations	Consistency	Directness	Other considerations	EPO/ Darbepo	Control (observation and transfusion when required)	Relative (95% CI)	Absolute risk (AR) (95% CI) NNT or NNH (number need to treat or harm)	Quality
Benefits: Hematological response for hematological malignancies (a proportion of patients with an increase in hemoglobin level of 2 g/dL or more, or increase in hematocrit of 6% points or more)										
7	Randomized trials	No limitations	No important inconsistency	Some uncertainty*	High probability of reporting bias†	518/872 (59.4%)	116/631 (18.4%)	Relative risk = 3.31 (2.77 to 3.94)	AR = 41% (36 to 46) NNT = 2 (2 to 3)	⊕⊕○○ Low
Hematological response for myelodysplastic syndrome (a proportion of patients with an increase in hemoglobin level of 2 g/dl or more, or increase in hematocrit of 6% points or more)										
2	Randomized trials	No limitations	No important inconsistency	No uncertainty	Imprecise or sparse data‡ High probability of reporting bias†	9/88 (10.2%)	1/63 (1.6%)	Relative risk = 4.27 (0.86 to 21.19)	AR = 9% (0.6 to 16) NNT = 11 (NNH 167 to ∞ to NNT 6)	⊕⊕○○ Low
Change in HB levels (change in hemoglobin level from baseline until end of study)										
2	Randomized trials	No limitations	No important inconsistency	No uncertainty	Imprecise or sparse data‡	243	264	—	Weighted mean difference = 1.73 (1.41 to 2.05)	⊕⊕⊕○ Moderate
Patients receiving red cell transfusions										
8	Randomized trials	No limitations	No important inconsistency	No uncertainty	High probability of reporting bias†	324/869 (37.3%)	329/640 (51.4%)	Relative risk = 0.72 (0.64 to 0.80)	AR = 14% (9 to 19) NNT = 7 (5 to 11)	⊕⊕⊕○ Moderate
Number of red cell transfusions required per patient										
5	Randomized trials	No limitations	No important inconsistency	No uncertainty	None	529	396	—	Weighted Mean Difference = −0.71 (−1.37 to −0.06)	⊕⊕⊕⊕ High
Tumor response rate (complete responses only)										
3	Randomized trials	No limitations	No important inconsistency	No uncertainty	High probability of reporting bias‡	28/267 (10.5%)	16/250 (6.4%)	Relative risk = 1.61 (0.91 to 2.84)	AR = 4% (−0.7 to 9) NNT = 25 (NNH 143 to ∞ to NNT 11)	⊕⊕⊕○ Moderate
Overall Survival (longest follow-up or the highest number of death events)										
7	Randomized trials	No limitations	No important inconsistency	No uncertainty	None	229/856 (26.8%)	197/598 (32.9%)	Hazard ratio = 1.12 (0.93 to 1.36)	ARR = 4% (−2 to 12) NNT = 25 (NNH 50 to ∞ to NNT 8)	⊕⊕⊕⊕ High

Harms: Thrombotic events (all type of cancers, not exclusively hematological malignancies)										
35	Randomized trials	No limitations	No important inconsistency	No uncertainty	None	229/3728 (6.1%)	118/3041 (3.9%)	Relative risk = 1.67 (1.35 to 2.06)	AR = 2% (1 to 3) NNH[§] = 50 (33–100)	⊕⊕⊕⊕ High
Hypertension events (all type of cancers, not exclusively hematological malignancies)										
16	Randomized trials	No limitations	No important inconsistency	No uncertainty	None	150/1311 (11.4%)	70/952 (7.4%)	Relative risk = 1.24 (1.00 to 1.54)	AR = 4% (1 to 6) NNH = 25 (17 to 100)	⊕⊕⊕⊕ High
Thrombocytopenia events (all type of cancers, not exclusively hematological malignancies)										
10	Randomized trials	No limitations	No important inconsistency	No uncertainty	None	84/875 (9.6%)	45/613 (7.3%)	Relative risk = 1.13 (0.80 to 1.60)	AR = 2% (−0.6 to 5) NNH = 50 (NNH 20 to ∞ to NNT 167)	⊕⊕⊕⊕ High
Quality of life outcomes (measure according to the following scales: Cancer Linear Analog Scale [CLAS]; the Functional Assessment of Cancer Therapy [FACT], Eastern Cooperative Oncology Group scale [ECOG])										
13	Randomized trials out of 28 trials	Serious limitations[‖]	Important inconsistency[¶]	No uncertainty	Dose response[¶]	—	—	CLAS Activity: 9.9 (6.4–13.5) Energy levels: 8.7 (4.8–12.6) Overall QOL: 1.0 (6.0–14.0) FACT total: 6.2 (0.6–11.7) ECOG: −0.1 (−0.3 – [−0.1])	NA	⊕⊕○○ Low

Intervention: The use of EPO/Darbepo (Erythropoietin or darpoboetin) for the treatment of hematological malignancy-related anemia
Patient or population: patients with hematologic malignancies (mainly non-Hodgkin lymphoma, myeloma multiple and myelodysplastic syndrome)
Systematic reviews:
a) For all outcomes, except quality of life (6): Bohlius J, Wilson J, Seidenfeld J, et al. Erythropoietin or darbepoetin for patients with cancer. *Cochrane Database Syst Rev.* 2006;(3):CD003407. Review.
b) For quality of life outcome: Jones M, Schenkel B, Just J, et al. Epoetin alfa improves quality of life in patients with cancer: results of meta-analysis. *Cancer* 2004;**101**(8):1720–32.
* Different doses and schedules of EPO/ Darbo were used among studies.
† The funnel plot analysis was asymmetric ($p < 0.005$), suggesting that "negative" results were underreported.
‡ Few studies with small sample sizes.
§ The authors calculated numbers needed to harm for several hypothetical baseline risks. These results described below show that the potential harmfulness of Epo/Darbepo depends on the underlying risk for thromboembolic complications.

a) In a population with an underlying risk of 2%: NNH = 75 patients (95% CI 47 to 143),
b) In a population with an underlying risk of 5%: NNH = 30 patients (95% CI 19 to 57),
c) In a population with a hypothetical baseline risk of 10%: NNH = 15 (95% CI 9 to 29).

NB. The annual average risk of thromboembolic complications in general population is 0.1%, while in cancer patients that received at least one cycle of chemotherapy, the risk is 0.8%/month, representing an annual risk of 9.6% (Khorana, Cancer 2005). In the hospitalized cancer patients with neutropenia the risk of the development of thromboembolic complications is 8% (Khorana, JCO 2006).
‖ The analysis included trials that were a mix of single arm trials and randomized controlled trials.
¶ There was some variation of in the magnitude of the QOL response according to duration of EPO treatment and type of studies analyzed (single arm versus randomized trials)
See http://www.fda.gov/medwatch/safety/2007/Aranesp_DHCP_012707.htm for the results of the trial in which Epo (Aranesp) was not found effective and may have been harmful. As of January 2008, both NCCN and ASH/ASCO guidelines recommend against using ESA for anemia of cancer and exercising caution in using these agents in chemo-related anemia.

Table 52.2 Summary of evidence of prophylactic use of granulopoiesis-stimulating factors (G-CSF or GM-CSF) for chemotherapy-induced febrile neutropenia.

Quality assessment						Summary of findings				
						No. of patients		Effect		
No. of studies	Design	Limitations	Consistency	Directness	Other considerations	Prophylactic Granulopoiesis-stimulating factor (G-CSF or GM-CSF)	No treatment (observation and transfusion when required)	Relative (95% CI)	Absolute (95% CI)	Quality[†,‡]
BENEFITS:										
Overall Survival (presented as overall mortality. Follow up: average 4.4 years)										
9	Randomized trials	No limitations	No important inconsistency	No uncertainty	None	357/728 (49%)	358/709 (50.5%)	HR 1.00 (0.86 to 1.16)	0% (−7%, 8%) NNT = ∞ (NNH = 14 to ∞ to NNT = 12)	⊕⊕⊕⊕ High
Freedom from treatment failure (defined as freedom from progression, relapse of disease, or death of any cause)										
5	Randomized trials	No limitations	No important inconsistency	No uncertainty	None	216/366 (59%)	191/352 (54.3%)	HR 1.11 (0.91 to 1.35)	6% (5%, 19%) NNT = 17 (NNH 5 to ∞ to NNT 20)	⊕⊕⊕⊕ High
Neutropenia (defined as absolute neutrophil count (ANC) below 0.5×10^9/L)										
7	Randomized trials	No limitations	No important inconsistency	No uncertainty	Please refer to footnote §and ‖	255/512 (49.8%)	377/501 (75.2%)	RR‖ 0.67 (0.60 to 0.73)	25% (20%, 30%) NNT = 4 (3, 5)	⊕⊕⊕⊕ High
Febrile neutropenia (Defined as absolute neutrophil count (ANC) $<1.0 \times 10^9$/L and fever ≥38°C)										
4	Randomized trials	No limitations	No important inconsistency	No uncertainty	None	84/184 (45.7%)	109/176 (61.9%)	RR 0.74 (0.62 to 0.89)	16% (6%, 26%) NNT = 6 (4, 17)	⊕⊕⊕⊕ High
Febrile neutropenia (defined as ANC below 0.5×10^9/L and fever ≥ 38°C)										
2	Randomized trials	No limitations	No important inconsistency	No uncertainty	None	92/303 (30.4%)	155/301 (51.5%)	RR 0.59 (0.48 to 0.72)	21% (13%, 29%) NNT = 5 (3, 7)	⊕⊕⊕⊕ High
Infection (infections were documented by both microbiological and clinical methods; however, only the microbiologically documented infections were included)										
9	Randomized trials	No limitations	No important inconsistency	No uncertainty	None	201/657 (30.6%)	265/635 (41.7%)	RR 0.74 (0.64 to 0.85)	11% (6%, 16%) NNT = 9 (6, 17)	⊕⊕⊕⊕ High
Risk of requiring parenteral antibiotic treatment										
4	Randomized trials	No limitations	No important inconsistency	No uncertainty	Please refer to footnote¶	34/186 (18.3%)	39/173 (22.5%)	RR 0.82 (0.57 to 1.18)	4% (−4%, 12%) NNT = 25 (NNH 25 to ∞ to NNT 8)	⊕⊕⊕○ Moderate¶
Infection-related mortality										
9	Randomized trials	No limitations	No important inconsistency	No uncertainty	None	16/533 (3%)	11/518 (2.1%)	RR 1.37 (0.66 to 2.82)	1% (−1%, 3%) NNT = 100 (NNH 100 to ∞ to NNT 33)	⊕⊕⊕⊕ High

(*Continued.*)

Complete response									
10	Randomized trials	No limitations	No important inconsistency	No uncertainty	Would have increased the effect for RR close or equal to 1 (+1)[#]	455/798 (57%)	438/786 (55.7%)	RR 1.02 (0.94 to 1.11)	1% (−4%, 6%) NNT = 100 (NNH 25 to ∞ to NNT 17)	⊕⊕⊕○ Moderate[#]
HARMS:									
Bone pain									
8	Randomized trials	No limitations	No important inconsistency	No uncertainty	None	56/606 (9.2%)	14/598 (2.3%)	RR 3.57 (2.09 to 6.12)	7% (4%, 10%) NNH = 15 (11, 23)	⊕⊕⊕⊕ High
Thromboembolic complications									
5	Randomized trials	No limitations	No important inconsistency	No uncertainty	None	10/216 (4.6%)	7/209 (3.3%)	RR 1.29 (0.56 to 3.01)	1% (−2%, 5%) NNH = 100 (NNT 50 to ∞ to NNH 20)	⊕⊕⊕⊕ High
Skin rash									
2	Randomized trials	No limitations	No important inconsistency	No uncertainty	None	33/119 (27.7%)	4/113 (3.5%)	RR 7.69 (2.84 to 20.82)	24% (15%, 33%) NNH = 4 (3, 7)	⊕⊕⊕⊕ High
Injection site reaction									
2	Randomized trials	No limitations	No important inconsistency	No uncertainty	None	43/170 (25.3%)	6/167 (3.6%)	RR 6.55 (3.01 to 14.25)	22% (15%, 29%) NNH = 5 (4, 7)	⊕⊕⊕⊕ High

Intervention: Prophylactic use of granulopoiesis-stimulating factors (G-CSF or GM-CSF) for chemotherapy-induced febrile neutropenia.

Patient or population: Adult patients with malignant lymphoma undergoing chemotherapy.

Systematic review (18): Bohlius J, Reiser M, Schwarzer G, et al.. Granulopoiesis-stimulating factors to prevent adverse effects in the treatment of malignant lymphoma. *Cochrane Database Syst Rev* 2004;(3): CD003189. DOI: 10.1002/14651858.CD003189.pub3.

*HR, hazard ratio; RR, relative risk, a value of <1 indicates a benefit for the treatment (CSF in this case) and >1 indicates a benefit for the control arm (no treatment arm in this case). NNT, number needed to treat; NNH, number needed to harm.

† Three studies with 616 patients have either never been published (Cunningham*) or not have been published as full-text articles (Bastion 1993; Björkholm 1999). However, the abstract by Björkholm 1999 is now available as a full-text article and was included in the analysis (Ösby 2003). The reviewers also obtained unreported data from several study authors. However, none of the outcomes showed a significant difference between published and unpublished or unreported data.

‡ Selection bias: Except two studies (information on allocation concealment not available) all had adequate allocation concealment. However, inclusion or exclusion of these two studies did not significantly affect any of the outcomes analyzed. Performance bias: Five studies had placebo as control. Sensitivity analysis for placebo-controlled and open label studies did not show significant differences for objective or subjective outcome measures. Attrition bias: Seven studies and one sub study undertook intention to treat analysis. The other studies were based on full set analysis and excluded patients who did not meet the eligibility criteria, had major protocol violation or did not receive any study medication. None of the results analyzed differed markedly from the pooled data reported. Publication bias: The funnel plot analysis of the data for complete response and parenteral antibiotic treatment showed an imbalance of positive and negative results, indicating that studies with negative findings might be under-represented. Taking this into consideration, the estimated benefit of G-CSF and GM-CSF in improving complete response and reducing the need for antibiotic treatment may be overestimated.

§ There was significant statistical heterogeneity among the trials (chi squared = 14.98, df = 7, $p = 0.04$), indicating that the variation in the effect of G-CSF and GM-CSF was larger than would be expected to result from chance alone. Sensitivity analyses revealed significant between group heterogeneity for prophylactic administration of antibiotic treatment during chemotherapy ($p = 0.0042$). A stronger treatment effect was observed in trials with antibiotic prophylaxis (RR 0.43; 95% CI 0.31 to 0.60, 2 trials with n = 229) compared to trials without antibiotic prophylaxis (RR 0.72; 95% CI 0.65 to 0.79, 5 trials with n = 784).

‖ Sensitivity analysis showed no significant differences with respect to G-CSF versus GM-CSF, HD versus NHL, age, hematological toxicity, blinded versus open label, concealment of allocation, quality and size of study and publication type. There was no indication of bias in the meta-analysis.

A funnel plot to test for publication bias ($p = 0.026$) indicated that both the RR and its 95% CI may be overestimated.

‖ A subgroup analysis of study size showed a bigger treatment effect in small studies (RR 1.31; 95% CI 1.08 to 1.60, 5 trials of n = 258) compared to large studies (RR 0.97; 95% CI 0.88 to 1.07, 5 studies of n = 1.326). However, a sensitivity analysis (type of drug, tumor entity, patient age, antibiotic prophylaxis, quality of study and publication type) did not show any significant differences.

patients with hematological malignancies, concluded that G-CSF and GM-CSF, when used as a prophylaxis in patients with malignant lymphoma undergoing conventional chemotherapy, reduce the risk of neutropenia, febrile neutropenia, and infection. However, there was no evidence showing significant advantage in terms of complete tumor response, and overall survival (see Table 52.2). The SR by Sasse et al. (20) evaluating children with ALL concluded that prophylactic use of CSF resulted in shorter hospitalization and fewer infections. However, there was no evidence for a shortened duration of neutropenia nor fewer treatment delays, or increase in survival.

The SR by Lyman and colleagues (19) with mixed group of patients (hematologic malignancies and solid tumors) concluded that there is a benefit for the prophylactic use of G-CSF in terms of reducing the risk of febrile neutropenia, and infections. However, the use of G-CSF was not effective in reducing the infection- related mortality. Similarly SR by Wittman et al. (21) reported that prophylactic CSFs significantly decrease the incidence of FN and the duration of severe neutropenia, hospitalization, and antibiotic use in pediatric cancer patients, but had no significant effect on documented infections.

An alternative management option in these patients has included use of prophylactic antibiotics. A meta-analysis that included 95 randomized controlled trials (RCT) enrolling 2,910 patients (22) evaluated the role of antibiotic prophylaxis in neutropenic patients in terms of reducing mortality and incidence of infection. It concluded that antibiotic prophylaxis significantly decreased the risk for death when compared with placebo or no treatment (relative risk, 0.67 [95% CI 0.55 to 0.81]). However, it also reported an increased risk for adverse events (relative risk, 1.69 [95% CI 1.14 to 2.50]) and increased risk of developing antibacterial resistance with the use of prophylactic antibiotics. Two subsequent RCTs (23,24) were consistent with the findings of this meta-analysis.

Consensus guidelines of National Comprehensive Cancer Network (25) and American Society for Clinical Oncology (13) recommend using CSF as primary prophylaxis for the prevention of FN in patients who have a high risk (>20%) of FN. The models to determine the risk of FN based on age, medical history, disease characteristics, and myelotoxicity of the chemotherapy regimen have been published (25).

Secondary prophylaxis

Secondary prophylaxis refers to the use of G-CSF in subsequent chemotherapy cycles after the occurrence of neutropenia in at least of one previous cycles. We found only one RCT that studied the role of G-CSF versus placebo as secondary prophylaxis to prevent FN in patients with small-cell lung cancer (26). Only 40% of the patients in the G-CSF arm compared with 77% in the placebo arm had at least one episode of febrile neutropenia ($p < 0.001$). The median duration of grade IV neutropenia over the course of chemotherapy was one day in the G-CSF versus six days in the placebo arm. Use of intravenous antibiotics, length of hospitalization, and the incidence of confirmed infections were reduced by 50% with G-CSF use when compared with placebo. However, 20% of patients receiving G-CSF suffered from medullary bone pain.

Patients in both the arms received the same doses of chemotherapy. The result from this RCT provides some evidence that use of G-CSF as secondary prophylaxis reduces the incidence of FN in patients with a prior episode of FN.

Established fever and neutropenia

We found one SR meta-analysis (27) addressing the role of CSF for chemotherapy-induced febrile neutropenia which included data from 13 RCTs enrolling patients with hematological malignancies as well as mixed tumors. In all of these RCTs, the treatment arm included the use of G-CSF or GM-CSF with antibiotics, which was compared against antibiotics alone. In this SR, the outcome measures were overall mortality, infection-related mortality, length of hospitalization, time to neutrophil recovery, and assessment of side effects, including deep vein thrombosis, bone pain, joint pain, and flu-like symptoms associated with CSF use. These data are summarized in Table 52.3.

The findings from this SR concluded that use of CSF in patients with febrile neutropenia associated with cancer chemotherapy reduces the duration of time spent in hospital and the duration of neutrophil recovery. There was a slight trend for benefit in terms of overall mortality and infection-related mortality in the CSF arm. However, the trend for benefit disappeared when one trial (28) was excluded from the analysis (odds ratio $= 0.87$; 95% CI 0.51 to 1.49; $p = 0.6$). This trial included only patients with hematologic malignancies and accounted for 33% of the total deaths (15 of 45 deaths) in the control group among all trials (see Table 52.3).

Published Guidelines

Consensus guidelines of National Comprehensive Cancer Network (25) and American Society for Clinical Oncology (13) are freely available on the Web.

Recommendations

1. Based on the evidence from the SRs (Table 52.2), administration of G-CSF or GM-CSF as *primary prophylaxis* is associated with significant reductions in the relative risk of febrile neutropenia. However, neither GCSF nor GM-CSF reduce the requirement for intravenous antibiotics, lower infection-related mortality, improve complete tumor response, or result in improved overall survival. Therefore, use as primary prophylaxis is recommended for the purposes of reducing febrile neutropenia only when this risk is greater than 20% (Grade 1A).

2. Use of G-CSF as *secondary prophylaxis* helps in preventing the incidence of FN, reducing the number of days of treatment with intravenous antibiotics, the number of days of hospitalization, and the incidence of confirmed infections. Secondary prophylaxis is recommended for patients experiencing a neutropenic complication from a prior cycle of chemotherapy (for which no previous primary prophylaxis was received), and dose reduction

Table 52.3 Summary of evidence of treatment use of granulopoiesis-stimulating factors (G-CSF or GM-CSF) for chemotherapy-induced febrile neutropenia.*

Quality assessment						Summary of findings				
						No. of patients		Effect		
No. of studies	Design	Limitations	Consistency	Directness	Other considerations	Colony-stimulating factors plus antibiotics (CSF + ATB)	Antibiotics (ATB) alone	Relative (95% CI)	Absolute (95% CI)	Quality
BENEFITS:										
Overall mortality (presented as overall mortality)										
12	Randomized trials	No limitations	No important inconsistency	No uncertainty	Please refer to footnote[†].	34/670 (5.1%)	45/670 (6.7%)	HR 0.68[†] (0.43 to 1.08)	21% (5%, 38%) NNT = 5 (NNH 3 to ∞ to NNT 19)	⊕⊕⊕○ Moderate[‡]
Infection-related mortality										
9	Randomized trials	No limitations	No important inconsistency	No uncertainty	Please refer to footnote ‡ .	14/453 (3.1%)	24/419 (5.7%)	HR 0.51[‡] (0.26 to 1.00)	28% (0%, 48%) NNT = 4 (2, ∞)	⊕⊕⊕○ Moderate[‡]
Length of hospitalization										
8	Randomized trials	No limitations	No important inconsistency	No uncertainty	None	144/630 (22.9%)	189/591 (32%)	HR 0.63 (0.49 to 0.82)	9% (4%, 14%) NNT = 11 (7, 24)	⊕⊕⊕⊕ High
Time to neutrophil recovery										
5	Randomized trials	No limitations	No important inconsistency	No uncertainty	Please refer to footnote §.	105/419 (25.1%)	170/375 (45.3%)	HR 0.32 (0.23 to 0.46)	20% (14%, 26%) NNT = 5 (4, 7)	⊕⊕⊕○ Moderate
HARMS:										
Deep vein thrombosis										
4	Randomized trials	No limitations	No important inconsistency	No uncertainty	None	9/194 (4.6%)	5/195 (2.6%)	HR 2.49 (0.72 to 8.66)	39% (7%, 199%) NNH = 3 (NNT 0.5 to ∞ to NNH 14)	⊕⊕⊕⊕ High
Bone pain, joint pain and flu like symptoms										
6	Randomized trials	No limitations	No important inconsistency	No uncertainty	None	47/328 (14.3%)	25/294 (8.5%)	HR 2.05 (1.22 to 3.46)	6% (1%, 11%) NNH = 17 (9, 118)	⊕⊕⊕⊕ High

Intervention: Colony-stimulating factors plus antibiotics (CSF+ATB) vs. Antibiotics (ATB) alone for treatment of chemotherapy-induced febrile neutropenia Patient or population: Cancer patients undergoing chemotherapy who experienced neutropenia. Systematic review (27): Clark OA, Lyman GH, Castro AA, et al. Colony-stimulating factors for chemotherapy-induced febrile neutropenia: a meta-analysis of randomized controlled trials. *J Clin Oncol.* 2005;**23**(18):4198–214.

* HR, hazard ratio; RR, relative risk, a value of <1 indicates a benefit for the treatment (CSF+antibiotics in this case) and >1 indicates a benefit for the control arm (antibiotics in this case). NNT = Number needed to treat, NNH = Number needed to harm.

† The trend to benefit patients receiving CSF disappeared when one trial by Aviles et al. was excluded from the analysis (OR = 0.87; 95% CI, 0.51 to 1.49; $p = 0.6$). This trial included only patients with hematologic malignancies and accounted for 33% of the total deaths (15 of 45 deaths) in the control group among all trials.

‡ The benefit for patients receiving CSF disappeared when one trial by Aviles et al. was excluded from the analysis (OR = 0.85; 95% CI, 0.33 to 2.20; $p = 0.7$). 63% of the events in the control group occurred in this trial (15/24). Significant heterogeneity was observed by the X^2 test ($X^2 = 26.39$; df = 7; P = 0.0004). Because of significant heterogeneity, the magnitude of this effect cannot be precisely estimated with currently available data. Exploring the possible causes of heterogeneity, it was found that all trials but one by Mayordomo et al indicated a much stronger effect than detected in all other trials. Repeating the analysis excluding the trial by Mayordomo et al resulted in substantial reduction in heterogeneity ($X^2 = 11.67$; df= 6; P = 0.07). However the significance of the treatment effect remained (HR= 0.72; 95% CI, 0.55 to 0.95; $p = 0.02$[QU5]).

§Small statistical heterogeneity ($X^2 = 8.97$; df = 4; $p = 0.062$) was observed as a result of the magnitude of the CSF effect detected in the Mayordomo et al trial. Excluding this trial from the analysis, did not result in the decrease of the effect (HR = 0.37; 95% CI, 0.26 to 0.53; $p = 0.00001$), and the heterogeneity disappeared ($X^2 = 1.61$; df = 3; $p = 0.66$).

in chemotherapy may compromise disease-free or overall survival or treatment outcome (Grade 1B).

3. a) For patients with established febrile neutropenia, *routine treatment* with CSF in patients who are not at high risk for infection-related life threatening complications is not recommended. However, administration of CSF significantly reduces the length of hospitalization and time to neutrophil recovery, which may be cost-effective in some settings (Grade 1B).

b) In addition, in patients with fever and neutropenia who are at high-risk for infection associated complications, or who have prognostic factors that are predictive of poor clinical outcomes *therapeutic CSF use* is recommended. Patients are considered high risk if they had expected prolonged (>10 days) and profound ($<0.1 \times 10^9/L$) neutropenia, age greater than 65 years, uncontrolled primary disease, pneumonia, hypotension and multiorgan dysfunction (sepsis syndrome), invasive fungal infection, or being hospitalized at the time of the development of fever (Grade 2A).

As in case of EPO, these recommendations did not take into account costs. In the United States, pegfilgastrim and filgastim account for $1.2 billion (5.3% of all expenditures) and $230 million (1%), in-clinic pharmaceutical expenditures respectively. In the hospital setting, pegfilgastrim and filgastrim account for $430 million and $340 million in pharmaceutical expenditures (4.8% and 1%, respectively) (12). Few studies have reported on the cost-effectiveness of these agents, although these studies suggest that the agents are cost-effective when used following treatment of chemotherapy regimens with a 20% or greater rate of febrile neutropenia (for primary prophylaxis) (13,25).

References

1 Groopman JE, Molina JM, Scadden DT. Hematopoietic growth factors: biology and clinical applications. *N Engl J Med.* 1989;**321**(21):1449–59.

2 Goodnough LT, Anderson KC, Kurtz S, et al. Indications and guidelines for the use of hematopoietic growth factors. *Transfusion.* 1993;**33**(11):944–59.

3 Montori VM, Wilczynski NL, Morgan D, et al. Optimal search strategies for retrieving systematic reviews from Medline: analytical survey. *BMJ.* 2005;**330**(7482):68.

4 Haynes RB, McKibbon KA, Wilczynski NL, et al. Optimal search strategies for retrieving scientifically strong studies of treatment from Medline: analytical survey. *BMJ.* 2005;**330**(7501):1179–1182.

5 Egrie JC, Browne JK. Development and characterization of novel erythropoiesis stimulating protein (NESP). *Br J Cancer.* 2001;**84** Suppl 1:3–10.

6 Bohlius J, Wilson J, Seidenfeld J, et al. Erythropoietin or darbepoetin for patients with cancer. *Cochrane Database Syst Rev.* 2006;(3): CD003407.

7 Soares HP KA, Silvestris F, Djulbegovic B. Systematic review and meta-analysis of randomized trials which tested erythropoietin in the treatment of anemia in multiple myeloma [abstract 232]. *Blood.* 2004;**104**(11): 70a.

8 Rizzo JD, Somerfield MR, Seidenfield KR, et al. Use of epoetin and dubopoietin in patients with cancer: 2007 American Society of Clinical Oncology / American Society of Hematology Clinical Practice Guideline update. *J Clin Oncol.* 2008;**26**:139–49.

9 Rodgers GM, Becker PS, Bennett CL et al. NCCN Practice guidelines in oncology: cancer and treatment-related anemia, version V.I 2008. Available at: www.nccn.org/professionals/physician_gls/PDF/anemia.pdf, NCCN National Comprehensive Cancer Network (Accessed January 2008).

10 Henke M, Laszig R, Rube C, et al. Erythropoietin to treat head and neck cancer patients with anaemia undergoing radiotherapy: randomised, double-blind, placebo-controlled trial. *Lancet.* 2003;**362**(9392): 1255–60.

11 Leyland-Jones B, Semiglazov V, Pawlicki M, et al. Maintaining normal hemoglobin levels with epoetin alfa in mainly nonanemic patients with metastatic breast cancer receiving first-line chemotherapy: a survival study. *J Clin Oncol.* 2005;**23**(25):5960–72.

12 Meropol NJ, Schulman KA. Cost of cancer care: issues and implications. *J Clin Oncol.* 2007;**25**(2):180–86.

13 Smith TJ, Khatcheressian J, Lyman GH, et al. 2006 update of recommendations for the use of white blood cell growth factors: an evidence-based clinical practice guideline. *J Clin Oncol.* 2006;**24**(19):3187–205.

14 Caggiano V, Weiss RV, Rickert TS, et al. Incidence, cost, and mortality of neutropenia hospitalization associated with chemotherapy. *Cancer.* 2005;**103**(9):1916–24.

15 Djulbegovic B. *Reasoning and decision making in hematology.* New York: Churchill Livingstone; 1992.

16 Crawford J, Dale DC, Lyman GH. Chemotherapy-induced neutropenia: risks, consequences, and new directions for its management. *Cancer.* 2004;**100**(2):228–37.

17 Griffin JD: Hematopoietic growth factors, in DeVita VT, Hellman S, Rosenberg SA (eds): *Principles and Practice of Oncology*, 6th ed, Philadelphia, Lippincott Williams & Wilkins; 2001.

18 Bohlius J, Reiser M, Schwarzer G, et al. Granulopoiesis-stimulating factors to prevent adverse effects in the treatment of malignant lymphoma. *Cochrane Database Syst Rev.* 2006;(4):CD003189. DOI: 10.1002/14651858.CD003189.pub3.

19 Lyman GH, Kuderer NM, Djulbegovic B. Prophylactic granulocyte colony-stimulating factor in patients receiving dose-intensive cancer chemotherapy: a meta-analysis. *Am J Med.* 2002;**112**(5): 406–11.

20 Sasse EC, Sasse AD, Brandalise S, et al. Colony stimulating factors for prevention of myelosupressive therapy induced febrile neutropenia in children with acute lymphoblastic leukaemia. *Cochrane Database Syst Rev.* 2005(3):CD004139.

21 Wittman B, Horan J, Lyman GH. Prophylactic colony-stimulating factors in children receiving myelosuppressive chemotherapy: a meta-analysis of randomized controlled trials. *Cancer Treat Rev.* 2006;**32**(4):289–303.

22 Gafter-Gvili A, Fraser A, Paul M, Leibovici L. Meta-analysis: antibiotic prophylaxis reduces mortality in neutropenic patients. *Ann Intern Med.* 2005;**142**(12 Pt 1):979–95.

23 Bucaneve G, Micozzi A, Menichetti F, et al. Levofloxacin to prevent bacterial infection in patients with cancer and neutropenia. *N Engl J Med.* 2005;**353**(10):977–87.

24 Cullen M, Steven N, Billingham L, et al. Antibacterial prophylaxis after chemotherapy for solid tumors and lymphomas. *N Engl J Med.* 2005;**353**(10):988–98.

25 Lyman GH. Guidelines of the National Comprehensive Cancer Network on the use of myeloid growth factors with cancer chemotherapy: a review of the evidence. *J Natl Compr Canc Netw.* 2005;**3**(4):557–71.

26 Crawford J, Ozer H, Stoller R, et al. Reduction by granulocyte colony-stimulating factor of fever and neutropenia induced by chemotherapy in patients with small-cell lung cancer. *N Engl J Med.* 1991;**325**(3):164–70.

27 Clark OA, Lyman GH, Castro AA, et al. Colony-stimulating factors for chemotherapy-induced febrile neutropenia: a meta-analysis of randomized controlled trials. *J Clin Oncol.* 2005;**23**(18):4198–214.

28 Aviles A, Guzman R, Garcia EL, et al. Results of a randomized trial of granulocyte colony-stimulating factor in patients with infection and severe granulocytopenia. *Anticancer Drugs.* 1996;**7**(4):392–97.

Index

Page numbers in *italic* refer to figures; page numbers in **bold** refer to tables.